Cutaneous Hematopathology

Hernani D. Cualing • Marshall E. Kadin
Mai P. Hoang • Michael B. Morgan
Editors

Cutaneous Hematopathology

Approach to the Diagnosis of
Atypical Lymphoid-Hematopoietic
Infiltrates in Skin

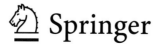 Springer

Editors
Hernani D. Cualing, MD
Department of Hematopathology
IHCFLOW Diagnostic Laboratory
Lutz, FL
USA

Marshall E. Kadin, MD
Department of Dermatology
Roger Williams Medical Center
Boston University School of Medicine
Providence, RI
USA

Mai P. Hoang, MD
Department of Pathology
Harvard Medical School
Massachusetts General Hospital
Boston, MA
USA

Michael B. Morgan, MD
Pensacola and Atlanta
Dermpath Diagnostics
University of South Florida
College of Medicine
Tampa, FL
USA

ISBN 978-1-4939-0949-0   ISBN 978-1-4939-0950-6   (eBook)
DOI 10.1007/978-1-4939-0950-6
Springer New York Heidelberg Dordrecht London

Library of Congress Control Number: 2014945353

Printed on acid-free paper

Springer is part of Springer Science+Business Media (www.springer.com)

Foreword

This effort fills a much needed niche for the fields of both dermatopathology and hematopathology. The interpretation of lymphoid infiltrates in the skin is one of the most challenging problems for practitioners from both disciplines. Dermatopathologists, while comfortable examining lymphocytic reaction patterns, are often confused by the subtleties of immunohistochemical profiles, cytometric studies, and molecular data that further delineate the nature of the infiltrating cells. In general, their experience with various, relatively uncommon, subtypes of lymphoma is limited and the data seems overwhelming. In contrast, hematopathologists have a great deal of experience interpreting these ancillary tests, but do not frequently encounter the subtle histologic patterns that characterize cutaneous lymphoid infiltrates, benign or malignant.

The authors have attempted to and have succeeded in conquering a difficult task. The divergent approaches to the study of cutaneous lymphoid infiltrates are no better exemplified than in the long history of lymphoma classification schemes that have populated the literature (and confused practitioners) for many decades. In this work, the authors, a group of well-known and experienced hematopathologists and dermatopathologists, have worked together to create a rational, logical, and thoughtful approach to these difficult cutaneous lesions. Virtually all of the malignant lymphocytic infiltrates that are encountered in the skin are described within the volume alongside benign lymphocytic reaction patterns that might provide the observer with a diagnostic dilemma. Routine histologic changes are presented as a starting point to which the authors have added a comprehensive discussion of immunohistochemistry, molecular and flow cytometry data that characterize each of the entries. The authors have included lucid photomicrographs that capture the salient diagnostic features. The organizational structure of the book enables the reader to refer to the section of the book that addresses a particular histologic pattern. Within this section, both benign and malignant infiltrates are described, with the text and accompanying photographic images highlighting the most useful discriminating data. This logical approach more realistically addresses the concerns of the pathologist attempting to arrive at a correct diagnosis than does the frequent approach in which benign entities are described sequentially, followed by a description of the cutaneous lymphomas.

Several features differentiate this work from previous volumes that address similar topics. Other works that describe cutaneous lymphomas have concentrated almost entirely upon this body of diseases with only passing comments dedicated to histologic mimics of these malignancies. In this volume, the authors confront the real-world situation of presenting to the reader differential diagnoses that go beyond subtyping lymphoma but also provide side-by-side discussions of benign lesions that might give rise to diagnostic confusion. This volume provides up-to-date information regarding the ancillary tests that are crucial for arriving at a precise diagnosis in this rapidly evolving field. Such information was not readily available to practitioners when the classic books in the field were written. Perhaps most importantly, this work demonstrates a collaborative effort by hematopathologists and dermatopathologists. By putting together a text that accurately portrays the observations and conclusions from each of the disciplines, the authors have created a unifying approach and have succeeded in giving the reader a comprehensive and logical approach to this very complicated set of diagnoses.

Rochester, NY, USA   Bruce Smoller, MD

Cutaneous Atypical Lymphoid Infiltrate: A Morphologic Approach to Diagnosis

The difficulty in diagnosis of cutaneous atypical lymphoid infiltrate is well known to both hematopathologists and dermatologists. Hence, it is not uncommon to have multiple biopsies to arrive at a diagnosis of cutaneous lymphoma. Part of the difficulty is the wide clinical and pathological overlap between reactive and malignant lymphoid infiltrate in the skin. The other reason may be the lack of a framework to classify these lesions, which may also be related to the fact that a select few hematopathologists and dermatopathologists specialize in these relatively rare, difficult to diagnose and confusing disease. Often the lack of clinical history exacerbates the limited microscopic view that a pathologist initially sees. In addition, many autochthonous and exotic tropical infectious diseases present with features that mimic lymphomas in skin.

This book was written to address a need for a systematic pattern-based framework to diagnose lymphomas and pseudolymphomas in the skin. In this handbook, we use an approach used by many hematopathologists and dermatopathologists, in their approach to diagnose lymphomas and atypical lymphoid infiltrates: begin with the histologic and phenotypic pattern that point to a classification subset, and use clinical, morphological, immunohistochemical, and molecular criteria to differentiate pseudolymphomatous and lymphomatous entities under consideration. This book is written to address these issues for the benefit of hematopathologists and dermatopathologists who will entertain a diagnosis of an atypical infiltrate in skin that looks like a lymphoma. Hence, the selection of contributors was based on active practitioners who diagnose pseudolymphomas, lymphomas, and infections of the skin. Trainees and residents of both disciplines may also find these references basic in their understanding of these diseases. Finally, clinicians may refer to these categories and find covered terms useful in reading reports.

This handbook addresses this topic using a unique approach proffered from the perspective of hematopathologists together with dermatopathologists. In evaluating a complex set of nearly 120 unique diseases, there is close interaction among hematopathologists, surgical pathologists, dermatopathologists, dermatologists, and infectious disease specialists. We emphasized an architectural approach using morphologic and immunologic patterns as a starting point and providing an algorithmic path leading to the correct diagnosis. Along with ancillary tests like flow cytometry, cytochemistry, immunohistochemistry, and clonal and molecular cytogenetic studies, the hematopathologist approaches these findings systematically. These approaches are crucial in distinguishing neoplasms that present in the skin from cutaneous manifestations of immune dysregulation, infections, and other inflammatory processes of either autochthonous or exotic forms. The widely disparate entities within this domain are simplified using an approach tested in daily practice of cutaneous hematopathology. It is back to basics. Using this approach, starting with what we see under the microscope, we present an intuitive, easy to follow, and practical algorithm for the daily practice of cutaneous hematopathology.

Organization of the Text

The text is divided into three parts comprising a total of 18 chapters. Part I covers an introduction to the hematopathology of cutaneous lymphoid infiltrate. In this part, the common patterns of lymphoid reaction in the skin and its relation to skin-associated lymphoid tissue are presented followed by an overview of the skin compartments and useful markers delineating them. In this regard, practical ancillary tests needed for a successful diagnosis (immunohistology, in situ hybridization, flow cytometry, image cytometry, and molecular pathology) are included. Part II covers patterns based on histology and immunoarchitecture that are key to diagnosis. When applicable, nonneoplastic pseudolymphoma entities are presented followed by analogous neoplastic conditions in that compartment. The epidermotrophic, dermotrophic/nodular, subcutaneous, and mixed patterns are separately discussed. Subsets based on B or T predominant immunoreaction are covered and a special group of CD30-positive entities are separately discussed. Part III includes specific patterns that are seen in skin biopsies other than a lymphoid infiltrate. These include granulomas, histiocytosis, emergent and tropical infections, the new group of skin lesions associated with biological modifiers, as well as leukemias and myelomonocytic and histiocytic/dendritic infiltrates. Finally, intravascular skin lesions and non-hematologic malignancy masquerading as lymphomas or cancers obscured by pseudolymphomas are included as well.

Acknowledgments

Dr. Cualing would like to thank the cutaneous lymphoma multidisciplinary clinic, staffed by Dr. Sokol and Dr. Glass, of the University of South Florida (USF)/Moffitt Cancer Center for their support and for the clinical materials. We are indebted to Dr. George Gibbons and all DermPath Diagnostics dermatopathologists of Tampa along with their dermatologist clients, who contributed both biopsy and clinical photographs and sent many interesting cutaneous lymphoma cases for consults. He is also thankful to Drs. Debbie and John Breneman, principals of CTCL clinic at the Cutaneous Lymphoma Cooperative Group at University of Cincinnati Medical Center, for furthering his hematopathology interest in these lesions back in the 1990s. Special thanks to USF Dermatology department chair Neil Feinske and senior dermatopathologist Frank Glass who both contributed slide materials and pictures from the Cutaneous Lymphoma Clinic.

Dr. Kadin would like to acknowledge his continuous collaboration with Eric C. Vonderheid, MD, Professor of Oncology at Johns Hopkins Medical Institute, who provided patient material and many helpful suggestions for his contribution. He acknowledges the many opportunities provided to him by Vincent Falanga, MD, former Chair of Dermatology and Skin Surgery at Roger Williams Medical Center in Providence, RI. He is grateful to Guenter Burg, former Dean and Chair of Dermatology, for providing clinical photographs and warmly hosting his sabbatical at the University of Zurich, Switzerland. He thanks Katie Breen, MD, at Roger Williams Medical Center in Providence, RI, and Steve Tahan, MD, of Beth Israel Deaconess Medical Center in Boston, for sharing dermatopathology cases. He thanks Deborah Christian, the publications manager of the American Society of Hematology, for permission to reuse pathology images he submitted to the ASH Image Bank while he was the associate editor. We also thank Dr. Bruce Smoller, a prominent dermatopathologist, for writing the foreword.

Finally, this book would not be in production without the help from the Springer medical team. On behalf of the editors and contributors, we thank the senior editor Richard Hruska, the assistant editor Joanna Perey, and the invaluable guidance and communication provided by Jennifer Schneider, this book's developmental editor. This book would not have been possible also without the tireless work by all authors and their contributors and the continuing dedication of the editors. We send special thanks to Dr. Shieh of Centers for Disease Control for providing clinical pictures and contributing a unique chapter of emergent and tropical infections in skin. Needless to say, we are all indebted to the workers and scientists of the US and International Society of Cutaneous Lymphoma and the WHO-EORTC contributors for their continuing advancement of knowledge in cutaneous lymphomas: our basis for this book.

We also thank Springer's Andy Kwan and the art division for their help as well as the services of Suganya Selvaraj- the project manager of Springer-SPi Content Solutions- for getting the proofs and book through the last hurdle of printing.

Contents

Contributors

Phyu P. Aung, MD, PhD Dermatopathology Section, Department of Dermatology, Boston Medical Center, Boston University School of Medicine, Boston, MA, USA

May P. Chan, MD Departments of Pathology and Dermatology, University of Michigan Health System, Ann Arbor, MI, USA

Hernani D. Cualing, MD Department of Hematopathology and Cutaneous Lymphoma, IHCFLOW Diagnostic Laboratory, Lutz, FL, USA

Samir Dalia, MD Department of Malignant Hematology, H. Lee Moffitt Cancer Center and Research Institute, Tampa, FL, USA

Mai P. Hoang, MD Department of Pathology, Harvard Medical School, Massachusetts General Hospital, Boston, MA, USA

Marshall E. Kadin, MD Department of Dermatology, Roger Williams Medical Center, Boston University School of Medicine, Providence, RI, USA

Jennifer R. Kaley, MD Department of Pathology, University of Arkansas for Medical Sciences, Little Rock, AR, USA

Jonathan J. Lee, BA Department of Pathology, Harvard Medical School, Boston, MA, USA

Vincent Liu, MD Department of Dermatology and Pathology, University of Iowa Hospitals and Clinics, Iowa City, IA, USA

Meera Mahalingam, MD, PhD, FRCPath Dermatopathology Section, Department of Dermatology, Boston University School of Medicine, Boston, MA, USA

Mark C. Mochel, MD Department of Pathology, Massachusetts General Hospital, Boston, MA, USA

Summer D. Moon, DO Department of Dermatology, Largo Medical Center, Nova Southeastern University, Largo, FL, USA

Michael B. Morgan, MD Department of Pathology, University of South Florida College of Medicine, Tampa, FL, USA

Department of Dermatology, Michigan State University College
of Medicine, East Lansing, MI, USA

Primary Care Diagnostics Institute, Quest Diagnostics,
Palm Beach Gardens, FL, USA

Tampa, Pensacola and Atlanta Dermpath Diagnostics, Tampa, FL, USA

Manojkumar T. Patel, MD, FCAP Department of Dermatopathology,
Dermpath Diagnostics, Bay Area, Tampa, FL, USA

Alicia Schnebelen, MD Department of Pathology, University of Arkansas
for Medical Sciences, Little Rock, AR, USA

M. Angelica Selim, MD Dermatopathology Unit, Department of
Pathology, Duke University Medical Center, Durham, NC, USA

Sara C. Shalin, MD, PhD Department of Pathology, University of
Arkansas for Medical Sciences, Little Rock, AR, USA

Wun-Ju Shieh, MD, MPH, PhD Infectious Disease Pathology Branch,
Centers for Disease Control and Prevention, Atlanta, GA, USA

Bruce Smoller, MD Department of Pathology, University of Rochester
School of Medicine and Dentistry, Rochester, NY, USA

Lubomir Sokol, MD, PhD Department of Malignant Hematology,
Moffitt Cancer Center, Tampa, FL, USA

Uma N. Sundram, MD, PhD Department of Pathology,
Stanford Hospital and Clinics, Stanford, CA, USA

Kara M. Trapp, BA Department of College of Medicine,
Georgetown University School of Medicine, Washington, DC, USA

Part I

Introduction to Hematopathology of Skin Infiltrates

Patterns of Lymphohistiocytic Reaction in Skin: An Approach to Cutaneous Lymphohematopoietic Infiltrate Using Histologic Patterns and Immunostains

Hernani D. Cualing and Marshall E. Kadin

Introduction

It is helpful to think of cutaneous lymphomas in the context of their relationship to normal skin structures. Here, we proffer an approach using guidelines based on the usual patterns seen in reactive histology of skin with lymphocytic and histiocytic reactions. There is increasing evidence that neoplastic histomorphologic patterns are superimposed on normal physiologic patterns. See Chap. 2 on this evidence. Morphologic and immunophenotypic reactions show a relatively consistent pattern.

Many advances have been made through the cooperation of international medical groups, such as the European Organization for Research and Treatment of Cancer (EORTC) and the World Health Organization (WHO), and their joint classification of primary cutaneous lymphomas (Willemze et al. 2005) (partly shown in Table 1.1). Thanks to this excellent effort by these dedicated groups, a common language is now spoken by dermatopathologists, hematopathologists, and clinicians in diagnosing and treating cutaneous

lymphomas. Continuous progress especially in the application of molecular pathology brought forth new information and facilitated better understanding, not only of neoplastic but also of nonneoplastic cutaneous lymphoid infiltrates. Foremost is the recognition that cutaneous lymphomas are different from the similarly named nodal or systemic lymphomas and have to be approached and treated differently.

Extranodal lymphomas, especially those arising from the most visible organ, i.e., the skin, present, for the most part a different biology, pathogenesis, and, for the common types, a better response to therapy. In addition, access to skin lesions is relatively easy compared to nodal and other systemic lesions. Hence, workup of a suspected lump or growth almost always involves a biopsy. The histology may be nonlymphoid or a lymphohematopoietic process. Rarely, the monomorphic infiltrate can resemble lymphoma though upon further comprehensive analysis it is discovered to be a poorly differentiated sarcoma, leukemia, carcinoma, or melanoma.

Hence, this book addresses the issue of approaching a biopsy with an open viewpoint that the lesion confronted could be lymphoid or nonlymphoid, neoplastic, dysplastic (but not frankly neoplastic), or reactive in nature. The first step in analyzing the biopsy begins with the microscope. Because most books in this subject organize the topics into known diseases or lymphoproliferations, we chose to differ in

H.D. Cualing, MD (✉)
Department of Hematopathology and Cutaneous Lymphoma, IHCFLOW Diagnostic Laboratory, 18804 Chaville Rd, Lutz, FL 33558, USA
e-mail: ihcflow@verizon.net

M.E. Kadin, MD
Department of Dermatology, Roger Williams Medical Center, Boston University School of Medicine, Providence, RI, USA

H.D. Cualing et al. (eds.), *Cutaneous Hematopathology*,
DOI 10.1007/978-1-4939-0950-6_1, © Springer Science+Business Media New York 2014

Table 1.1 Overview of nonneoplastic and neoplastic cutaneous lymphohematopoietic infiltrates

Nonneoplastic	Neoplastic
Reactive epidermotropic and lichenoid dermatitis	*Cutaneous T-cell and NK-cell lymphomas*
Langerhans cell hyperplastic vesicles, SD	Mycosis fungoides (MF)
Epidermotropic T-cell pseudolymphomas	MF variants and subtypes
Pseudolymphomatous folliculitis/idiopathic FM	Folliculotropic MF
"Spongiotic dermatitides (SD)"/lymphomatoid keratosis	Pagetoid reticulosis
Benign granulomatous dermatitis/dyscrasia	Granulomatous slack skin
Inflammatory vitiligo/hypopigmented T-cell dyscrasia	Hypopigmented MF
Syringolymphoid T-cell hyperplasia/dyscrasia	Syringolymphoid MF
Benign erythroderma/T-cell lymphocytosis of uncertain significance	Sézary syndrome
Benign lymphocytosis/ T-cell pseudolymphomas	Adult T-cell leukemia/lymphoma
CD30 pseudolymphomas	Cutaneous CD30+ lymphoproliferative disorders
Nonclonal "regressing histiocytosis"	Anaplastic large cell lymphoma
Scabies, other CD30(+) infections, PLEVA	Lymphomatoid papulosis
Lupus profundus and other reactive panniculitis	Subcutaneous panniculitis-like T-cell lymphoma (SPCTL)
Reactive drug-induced/idiopathic vasculitis	Extranodal NK/T-cell lymphoma, nasal type
Nodular T-cell pseudolymphomas	Cutaneous peripheral T-cell lymphoma (large cell), unspecified
Pityriasis lichenoides et varioliformis acuta (PLEVA) and chronica (PLC)	Cutaneous aggressive epidermotropic CD8+ T-cell lymphoma
Spongiosis and reactive panniculitis	Cutaneous γ/δ T-cell lymphoma
Solitary T-cell nodules uncertain significance	Cutaneous small-/medium-sized lymphomas (CD8, CD4)
Germinal center hyperplasia	*Cutaneous B-cell lymphomas*
Cutaneous B-cell lymphoid hyperplasia	Primary cutaneous marginal zone B-cell lymphoma
(B-cell pseudolymphomas)	Primary cutaneous follicle center lymphoma
Drug-induced hyperplasia (i.e., phenytoin)	Primary cutaneous diffuse large B-cell lymphoma, leg type
Solitary B-cell pseudolymphomas	Primary cutaneous diffuse large B-cell lymphoma, others
Granulomatous dermatitis	Lymphomatoid granulomatosis
Cutaneous IgG4 plasmacytosis	Plasmacytoma
Intravascular (intralymphatic) histiocytosis	Intravascular lymphoma
Sinus histiocytosis with massive lymphadenopathy	Hodgkin lymphoma
Langerhans cell hyperplasia	Langerhans cell histiocytosis
Immature extramedullary hematopoiesis	*Cutaneous plasmacytoid dendritic leukemia*
	Cutaneous granulocytic sarcoma
	Mastocytosis/Mast cell sarcoma
	Lymphoblastic T- or B-cell lymphoma

FM follicular mucinosis

proffering an approach based on morphologic *patterns*. In this way, the microscopic findings provide the point of departure to seek the most precise diagnosis based first on tissue patterns, then on cytomorphology, immunophenotypic results, and when necessary molecular genetic analysis. Furthermore, we subscribe to the state-of-the-art cutaneous lymphoma consensus classifications and atypical lymphoproliferations (Cerroni et al. 2009; Magro et al. 1997, 2003; Magro and Crowson 1996; Swerdlow

et al. 2008; Isaacson and Norton 1994). See Table 1.1 for the overview of benign and malignant cutaneous lymphohematopoietic infiltrates listing topics covered in this book.

Synonyms

Cutaneous lymphoid hyperplasia (Lymphadenosis benigna cutis, Lymphocytoma cutis, Pseudolymphoma)

Granulocytic sarcoma (leukemia cutis, myeloid sarcoma, myelomonocytic sarcoma, extramedullary leukemic skin infiltrate)

Definitions

Cutaneous lymphoid hyperplasia (CLH) with band-like and perivascular pattern is a reactive pattern of the skin that histologically resemble mycosis fungoides.

Cutaneous lymphoid hyperplasia with nodular pattern ("nodular pattern of cutaneous lymphoid hyperplasia") is a reactive histologic pattern in skin characterized by solitary or localized nodules predominantly in the dermis that clinically appear as a reddish to violaceous lump. The presence of germinal centers forming most nodules indicates a B-cell type. It is our experience that dermal compact nodules often mark as a T-cell type of nodular cutaneous lymphoid hyperplasia instead of a B-cell type.

Pseudolymphomas of skin are reactive proliferations that clinically or histologically resemble cutaneous lymphomas (Cerroni et al. 2009; Cerroni 2006). Pseudolymphoma is not a specific diagnosis and encompasses cutaneous lymphoid hyperplasia and drug-induced or infection-induced skin lymphoid lesions of varied pathogenesis, appearance, and clinical behaviors. Although progression from a reactive process to a lymphoma is not a usual course of pseudolymphomas, lymphomas in preexisting hyperplasia do sometimes occur (Bergman 2010). Hence, recurrent or persistent lesions with an appearance suggestive of lymphoma require careful follow-up to rule out progression to malignancy. See Chaps. 5, 7, and 8 on expanded discussion of pseudolymphomas.

Atypical cutaneous lymphoid hyperplasias may include abnormal, disorganized, or transformed germinal centers (Kojima et al. 2010a, b) associated with atypical cells or as dense dermal or subcutaneous lymphoid diffuse infiltrates with atypical cells. Lesions are usually persistent or recurrent over several years.

Cutaneous lymphomas are a diverse group of heterogeneous entities arising from malignant lymphoproliferation of either T-cell, B-cell, or natural killer-cell lineage, which primarily originate, present, or remain confined to the skin without detectable extracutaneous manifestations at diagnosis.

Epidemiology

Primary cutaneous lymphomas have an estimated annual incidence of 1.0–1.5/100,000 and are the second most common group of extranodal lymphomas. Despite their relative low frequency, there has been an increasing incidence of cutaneous lymphomas in the United States from 5 to 13 per million person-years over 25 years reported in 2005 (SEER data) (Bradford et al. 2009). The incidence of cutaneous T-cell lymphomas (CTCL) is 3–9 per million, and like all cutaneous lymphomas, this incidence appears to be increasing both in North America and in Europe (Criscione and Weinstock 2007; Jenni et al. 2011). Mycosis fungoides (MF) and Sézary syndrome (SS) represent the most common cutaneous lymphomas and account for 4.1 per million person-years (Bradford et al. 2009). Although MF is an indolent lymphoma, histologic and clinical progression often occurs over time. Large cell transformation of MF occurs in up to 7 % of early clinical stages but up to 23 % in advanced clinical stages of MF (Lai et al. 2012). Diagnosis of these rare cutaneous T-cell lymphomas which vary from focally epidermotropic early MF to non-epidermotropic dense dermal infiltrates is challenging.

Cutaneous Lymphoid Hyperplasia

Although there is no exact data on the actual incidence of CLH or cutaneous pseudolymphoma, the frequency of diagnosis of cutaneous lymphoid hyperplasia in premodern pathology practice is higher than the frequency of diagnosis of cutaneous lymphoma. In an early seminal study comparing 225 skin biopsies for benign and malignant lymphoid infiltrates, benign diagnoses accounted for 61 % and malignant lymphoid infiltrates comprised 39 % (Caro 1978; Caro and Helwig 1969).

In our current referral consultation practice, however, pseudolymphomas comprise about 30 % and lymphomas 60 %, with myelomonocytic/non-hematopoietic diagnosis comprising about 10 %. B-cell pseudolymphomas account for about 5 % (defined as having 70 % or more of B-cell nodules), T-cell pseudolymphoma account for about 10 % (defined as a band or nodular infiltrate with 90 % or more T cells), and mixed T- and B-cell pseudolymphomas account for about 15 % (with mixed T cells and B cells, usually of approximately equal proportion plus a range that does not fit the defined brackets for either previous types).

Borrelia-associated lymphoid hyperplasia is uncommon, occurring in about 1 % of cases reported in Europe (Colli et al. 2004) and in North America; a variety of skin infiltrative patterns is also observed (Lipsker 2007). Drug-induced pseudolymphoma is an equally rare condition with more than 100 individual cases reported in the literature worldwide, and may easily be mistaken for lymphoma if a drug etiology is not uncovered. When associated with systemic symptoms and hypersensitivity such as those typical for a drug reaction with systemic symptoms (DRESS), mortality is reported in up to 10 % of patients (Bocquet et al. 1996).

Cutaneous lymphoid hyperplasia (CLH) is generally classified according to clinicopathologic entities or placed into broad spectrums of B-cell or T-cell predominance or co-dominance (Bergman et al. 2011). The predominant immunologic type usually can be inferred from the histopathologic pattern supplemented by immunohistochemistry, and in correlation with molecular genetic analysis using appropriate T-cell antigen receptor or immunoglobulin, gene primers and PCR can usually distinguish cutaneous lymphoid hyperplasia from cutaneous lymphoma. A recent study suggests that using a panel of cytotoxic markers, the expression of granulysin, may be differentially expressed more in CLH more than in cutaneous large B-cell lymphoma (Furudate et al. 2013). Granulysin or granzyme B is a cytolytic substance released by cytotoxic T cells (CD8+) during 3–5 days after their activation.

In cases with mild to moderately atypical cells, a clonal population that correlates clinically with a recurrent or persistent mass after repeated biopsies and clinical follow-up usually indicates a malignancy. On the other hand, the presence of clusters of plasma cells or eosinophils along with reactive histiocytes in association with "top-heavy" nodules, or spongiotic epidermis, is often indicative of a reactive proliferation with defined and specific exceptions. Care must be taken with cases that present with benign-looking germinal centers because this is a common pattern associated with lymphomas arising from the marginal zone (Arai et al. 2005; Baldassano et al. 1999).

Clinical evidence of progression is probably the ultimate determinant of whether heavy, multinodular cutaneous lymphoid infiltrates, with or without the presence of a clonal B- or T-cell population, have become a cutaneous lymphoma (Ceballos et al. 2002).

Processing of the Skin Biopsy

It is essential to obtain as much information as possible from the skin biopsy. Because of the usual small size, often a punch biopsy, we recommend immediate splitting of the biopsy into separate parts for conventional histology and possible future studies requiring unfixed cryopreserved tissue. This is especially important for cutaneous lymphomas for which immunohistochemistry, immunofluorescence, gene rearrangement, and other molecular genetic studies require optimal preservation of RNA, DNA, and cell surface proteins. In academic centers, there may be opportunities for cytogenetics, tissue culture, flow cytometry, and transplantation to immunodeficient mice. Thus, the protocol for processing skin biopsies will vary according to your practice. For dermatologists, it is obviously of great importance to establish a well-rehearsed routine with your pathologists and research associates according to your goals. For punch biopsies, we find it practical to place the skin surface down on a cutting surface and bisect the specimen with a sterile

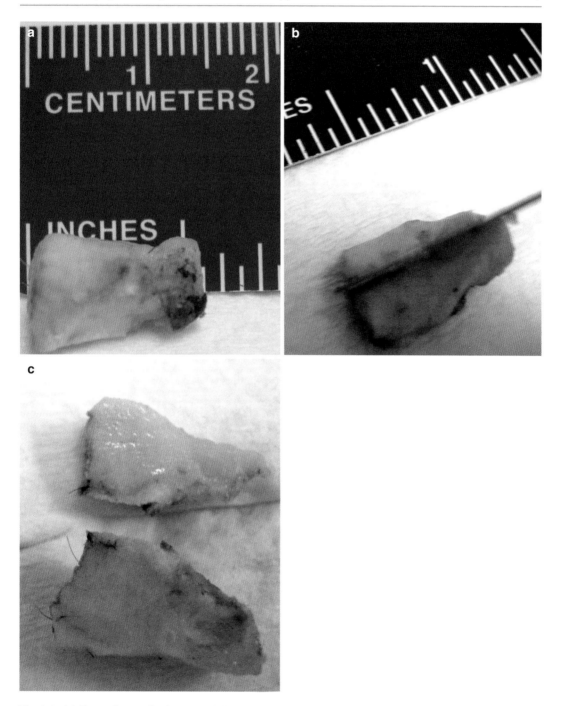

Fig. 1.1 (**a**) Gross picture of a 6 mm punch biopsy and (**b**) its bisection. (**c**) Cut section with yellow fat and whitish dermis (Courtesy of George Gibbons, Dermatopathologist, Dermpath Diagnostics, Tampa FL)

sharp scalpel or razor blade along the longitudinal axis (Fig. 1.1). One-half of the specimen can then be placed immediately into fixative, and the other one-half placed into sterile saline or on a sterile saline-soaked gauze and sent to the laboratory. With improved immunohistochemical methods including antigen retrieval and virtual flow immunohistochemistry (see Chap. 4 for this technology), much information can be available from fixed tissue. Ten percent buffered formalin is adequate for most studies. Optimal morphology and immunohistochemistry is gleaned from 4 % paraformaldehyde fixation (Muramoto and Kadin 1987).

Optimal Specimen for Work-Up of Cutaneous Lymphoid Infiltrates

Since a skin biopsy is often submitted without prior knowledge of the type of infiltrate and since epithelial and melanocytic proliferations are the usual considerations, specimens are obtained in the most common and convenient manner, either by shave, punch, or excision biopsy. Shave biopsies, if scalloped or deep to obtain deeper dermal or subcutaneous tissues, can offer a suitable specimen. However, the common thin shave biopsies we receive with associated lymphoid lesions generally do not provide adequate information on deeper dermal or subcutaneous areas, so that eccrino-syringo-tropic or subcutaneous panniculitic lesions are not recognizable.

If a lymphoid lesion is strongly suspected, superficial shave biopsies should be avoided. Many of our cases submitted for molecular assays from shave biopsies fail to provide adequate DNA for clonality analysis (see Chap. 4 on increased false-negative or oligoclonal results that are seen from thin shave biopsies). As a rule, a lymphoid infiltrate section is subjected to a battery of ancillary tests including multiple step sections for a number of immunoperoxidase stains plus DNA analysis for T- or B-cell clonality. If a molecular genetic assay is performed on the tissue section or block after sectioning for immunohistochemistry, test failures due to inadequate DNA may result. To avoid this, a routine stain and immediate submission of the tissue for molecular IgH or T-cell receptor gene rearrangement assays are recommended. This has worked in our practice with the caveat that any additional

immunohistochemistry that may be needed to classify the lesion will be delayed.

In centers equipped with the ability to process fresh tissue using tissue culture media, additional information can be obtained via flow cytometry analysis, especially useful in clonal light chain analysis or T-cell aberrancy analysis for B- and T-cell lymphoproliferations, respectively. Caution is advised in interpreting the results of flow cytometry without histologic correlation, since flow cytometry analysis requires tissue disaggregation and the neoplastic large cell population may be "lost" or obscured by the more numerous reactive small cell population. Interpreting the results of flow cytometry as negative for lymphoma must be correlated with the morphology or immunohistochemistry. This approach is similar to the work-up for nodal lymphomas or leukemias, using a multiparameter approach, as the best way to arrive at the most accurate diagnosis.

Morphologic Approach

As in evaluations of other dermatologic disorders, the first step in the pathologic assessment is to obtain an overview of the specimen using a low-power (2× or 4×) objective lens. Note whether the lymphoid infiltrate is compact or dispersed and involves the epidermis, dermis, and/or subcutaneous tissues. It is important to note the presence of reactive germinal centers of altered follicles in B-cell disorders, e.g., marginal zone lymphoma. Note if there are foreign bodies or pathogens, such as mites in scabies.

In biopsies with germinal centers, it is important to note if the germinal centers have a normal polarized appearance with a paler germinal center composed of mixed centrocytes and centroblasts and a rim of smaller perifollicular lymphocytes representing the mantle zone. If the germinal centers are transformed, simulating progressive transformation of germinal centers, or else lysed, disorganized, or admixed with other atypical cells or otherwise with expanded mantle or marginal zone lymphocytes, then these atypical findings call for a higher index of suspicion for lymphoma, prompting further ancillary work-up to distinguish B-cell lymphoma or transformation of a B-cell cutaneous lymphoid hyperplasia.

Mantle cell lymphoma is exceedingly rare as primary skin lymphoma but cutaneous involvement by nodal follicle center or marginal zone lymphoma is relatively frequent, if there are corresponding known nodal follicular or marginal zone lymphomas. If primary cutaneous lymphoma is suspected, the following histologic features would be indicative of a primary cutaneous marginal zone lymphoma: normal or colonized germinal centers, along with expanded marginal zones, composed of small- and medium-sized lymphocytes with a moderate amount of cytoplasm, centrocyte-like round to irregular nuclei, and admixed plasma cells. Indeed, many cutaneous lymphoid hyperplasias diagnosed in the past before the era of more sensitive immunohistochemistry or molecular gene rearrangement assays turned out to be cutaneous marginal zone lymphomas. (Please see Chap. 3 for differential diagnosis of primary cutaneous B-cell lymphomas.)

Using medium-power 10× and 20× objectives, one can appreciate if adnexa and blood vessels are affected and whether or not there is an interface pattern at the dermal-epidermal junction. Pautrier's microabscesses diagnostic of MF can be suspected at medium-power magnification. A general impression can also be gained of the presence or absence of inflammatory cells, e.g., neutrophils, eosinophils, plasma cells, and macrophages. Necrosis of keratinocytes and blood vessels can be determined.

High magnification with 40–60× objectives is required to note nuclear conformation, irregularities or convolutions, presence or absence of nucleoli and their prominence, presence of mitotic figures, and apoptotic bodies or karyorrhexis. Oil immersion lens of 60–100× magnification, if available, provide the clearest view to assess hyperconvoluted or cerebriform nuclei. Nuclear convolutions are especially noteworthy in assessing cutaneous T-cell lymphomas, e.g., mycosis fungoides and Sézary syndrome. It is often necessary to confirm the presence of three or more tumor cells with nuclear irregularities comprising a Pautrier's microabscess and distinguish them from Langerhans cells which also have nuclear convolutions but more elongated nuclei and pale staining cytoplasm (for illustrations and further details, see Chap. 6). Prominent nucleoli and mitotic figures are characteristic of CD30+ cutaneous lymphoproliferative disorders, as well as the presence of more than 90 % immunoblasts or centroblasts typical for the leg type of diffuse large B-cell lymphoma. Karyorrhexis is a feature of subcutaneous and gamma-delta T-cell lymphoma that may distinguish them from autoimmune disorders involving the skin, e.g., lupus profundus.

As in melanoma evaluation, immunohistochemistry can help to identify tumor cells that may otherwise escape your attention. For example, stains for CD3 and TCR beta f1 often outline the nuclear convolutions of tumor cells in mycosis fungoides/Sézary syndrome, helping to distinguish them from reactive lymphocytes. Immunohistochemical enumeration of reactive cells can also be of importance for prognosis of CTCL. We recently reported that tumor progression from early-stage (I–IIA) CD4+ MF is significantly correlated with <20 % CD8+ cells in the dermal infiltrate (Vonderheid et al. 2014).

Normal Skin Histology

This low-power view shows a typical histology of skin showing epidermis, hair follicles, and sweat and sebaceous glands (Fig. 1.2).

Epidermis

The epidermis consists of four layers (five in the soles and palms) starting from the most superficial or outward layer: a cornified layer (stratum corneum), a granular layer (stratum granulosum) in which keratinocytes lose their nuclei and their cytoplasm appears granular, a spinous layer (stratum spinosum), and a basal/germinal

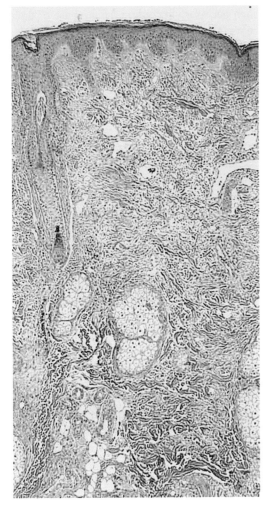

Fig. 1.2 Low power of normal skin showing epidermis with rete ridges and hair follicle on left with sebaceous and eccrine glands below, some endothelial vessels with minimal lymphoid elements

layer (stratum basale/germinativum) composed mainly of proliferating and nonproliferating keratinocytes. In CTCL, lymphocytes initially line up in the basal layer of the epidermis (lymphocyte tagging) and are often surrounded by a clear space (halo) (Fig. 1.3). Clusters of three or more lymphocytes within the epidermis comprise a Pautrier's microabscess which is a diagnostic feature of MF/SS (Fig. 1.4). In CTCL, tumor cells are CD4+ in >90 % of cases. It should be appreciated that CD8+ cells are also commonly found in the epidermis in CTCL. See Chap. 6 for discussion of neoplastic epidermotropic patterns.

Keratinocytes comprise the predominant cell type in the epidermis, the outermost layer of the skin, constituting 90 % of the cells found there.

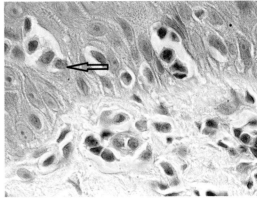

Fig. 1.4 Early Pautrier's or Darier's nest with six atypical lymphocytes (*arrow*) surrounding a Langerhans cell

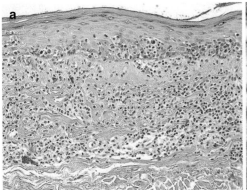

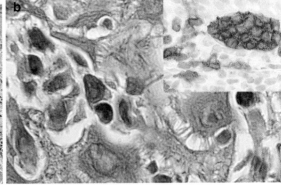

Fig. 1.3 (**a**) Typical mycosis fungoides basal layer localization of haloed atypical lymphocytes with Pautrier's microabscesses. (**b**) Oil power view of cerebriform cells and of *inset* CD3 stain, highlighting the nuclear hyperconvolutions

The primary function of keratinocytes is the formation of a barrier against environmental damage such as pathogens (bacteria, fungi, parasites, viruses), heat, UV radiation, and water loss. Once pathogens start to invade the upper layers of the epidermis, keratinocytes can react with the production of proinflammatory mediators and in particular chemokines such as CXCL10 and CCL2 which attract leukocytes to the site of pathogen invasion. Keratinocytes also produce stem cell factor (SCF) which stimulate the SCF receptor (also called cKIT or CD117) on the surface of melanoblasts and melanocytes. The cytolytic effect of junctional CD8 T cells against these receptors or against keratinocytes, leading to cell death, is implicated in the pathogenesis of hypopigmented MF (Singh et al. 2006) (Fig. 1.5). In turn, keratinocyte growth and differentiation can be affected by lymphocyte-derived cytokines, in particular IL-22 which we have found to promote pseudoepitheliomatous keratinocyte hyperplasia, a condition mimicking squamous cell carcinoma (Guitart et al. 2013).

Antigen presenting cells within the epidermis are known as Langerhans cells (LC). LC have abundant pale staining cytoplasm and an elongated convoluted nucleus with clear nucleoplasm and inconspicuous nucleoli and stain readily with S100 antibody. When hyperplastic and forming vesicles, they must be distinguished from tumor cells in MF/SS which have only a

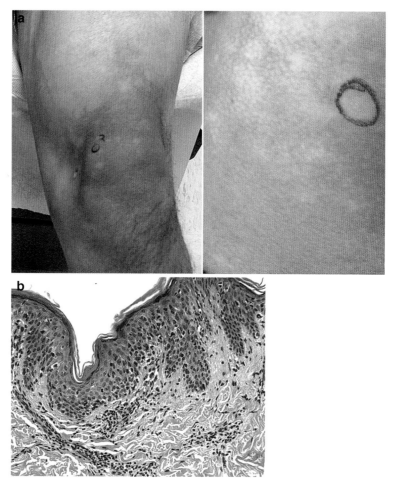

Fig. 1.5 (**a**) Hypopigmented MF in a young Asian, knee and elbow. (**b**) Histopathology (Courtesy of Neil Fenske, Chair Dermatology and Frank Glass, University of South Florida)

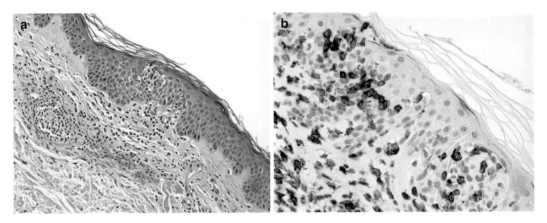

Fig. 1.6 (**a**) Langerhans cell hyperplastic vesicle in contact dermatitis. (**b**) CD3 staining of epidermotropic lymphocytes is largely absent in vesicle with Langerhans cell hyperplasia

narrow rim of cytoplasm, dark and sometimes mottled nucleoplasm, and occasional nucleoli (Fig. 1.6). See Chap. 5 for discussion of reactive lichenoid and epidermotropic disorders.

Intercellular edema or spongiosis is more common in reactive processes but can occur in CTCL and does not discount a diagnosis of CTCL. Necrotic keratinocytes can be found exceptionally in lichenoid CTCL (Guitart et al. 1997) but are more common in interface dermatitides, e.g., PLEVA and lichen planus.

Dermis

The dermis is the main compartment involved in most nodular patterns seen in subtypes of cutaneous B-cell lymphomas (Fig. 1.7). See Chap. 9 for discussion of neoplastic nodular B-cell patterns. The dermis is the site of the major tumor T-cell infiltrate in plaque and tumor stages of mycosis fungoides and in anaplastic large cell lymphoma. The dermis is also the location of most T-cell lymphomas with a nodular dermal pattern such as primary cutaneous small-medium T-cell lymphoma and angioimmunoblastic and extranodal NK/T-cell lymphomas. See Chap. 10 for discussion of T-cell lymphomas with nodular pattern, including transformed MF. Dermal infiltration is uncharacteristic of SPTCL but is common in gamma-delta T-cell lymphoma and other cytotoxic lymphomas such as extranodal NK/T-cell lymphomas.

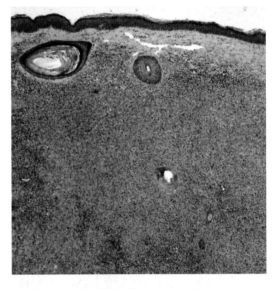

Fig. 1.7 Cutaneous B-cell lymphoma with dermal nodular and sparing of grenz zone pattern

Subcutaneous Tissue

Fat necrosis and rimming of fat cells by atypical neoplastic cells is characteristic of SPTCL and some cases of gamma-delta T-cell lymphoma. Subcutaneous fat is also infiltrated by lymphocytes in lupus, but fat necrosis and rimming of fat cells by atypical pleomorphic lymphocytes is unusual. The involvement of fat is seen in anaplastic large cell lymphoma, large cell transformation of MF, and precursor blastic tumors of either B- or T-cell type as well (Fig. 1.8).

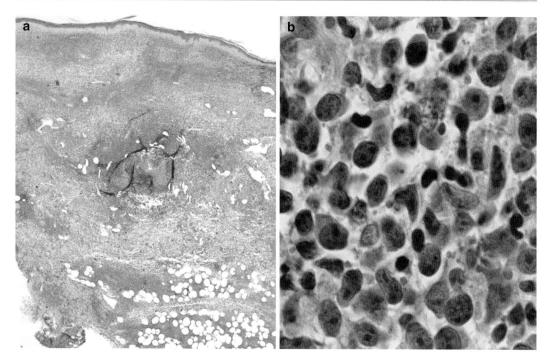

Fig. 1.8 (**a**) Precursor B-cell lymphoblastic lymphoma with deep fat involvement. (**b**) Oil magnification, with lymphoblasts with fine blastic chromatin and abnormal mitosis

Septal panniculitis is more common in reactive or infectious process (erythema nodosum or induratum), and nodular or mixed nodular patterns with minimal septal fat involvement are more common in SPTCL and fat involvement of gamma-delta T-cell lymphoma. See Chap. 11 for further discussion of subcutaneous neoplastic and reactive patterns.

Patterns of Lymphoid Reactions in Skin

Epidermotropic

Lichenoid Pattern

Lichenoid pattern is a band-like pattern with lymphocytes closely apposed to the epidermis with minimal epidermal vacuolar changes. It is a common pattern seen in both reactive and malignant processes. It is often associated with varying upper dermal perivascular lymphoid pattern and may be associated or delineated from an interface pattern which shows prominent vacuolar changes (Guitart et al. 1997; Magro and Crowson 2000; Oliver et al. 1989). Discussion of epidermotropic as well as dermotropic changes in association with reactive lichenoid patterns is in Chaps. 5 and 8, respectively.

Minimal vacuolar change is seen in MF, which is often grouped with vacuolar interface dermatitis (Ramos-Ceballos and Horn 2010). A subset of MF patients with lichenoid reaction pattern is often associated with pruritus (Guitart et al. 1997). Extensive vacuolar change and spongiosis are unusual in MF and are more often seen in reactive vacuolar interface dermatitides such as drug eruptions, viral exanthems, graft versus host disease, connective tissue disorders, and pityriasis lichenoides. Vacuolar change and tagging of basal epidermis by atypical lymphocytes are seen in an example of hypopigmented MF; see Fig. 1.5.

In association with variable hypo- or hyperpigmented atrophic epidermis, with melanophages and/or band-like or perivascular

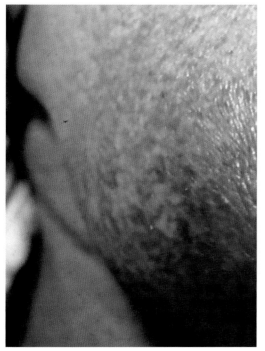

Fig. 1.9 Poikilodermatous MF on skin of breast

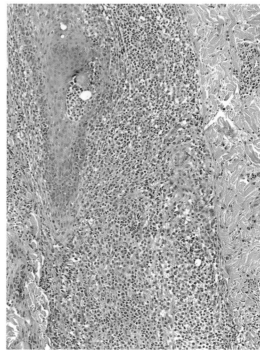

Fig. 1.10 Pseudolymphomatous folliculitis

lymphoid infiltrate, poikilodermatous lichenoid changes could be seen in a variety of sun-damaged dermatitis, rare childhood poikilodermatitis, and dermatomyositis as well as in regressive phases of classic MF or a subtype called poikilodermatous MF. This subtype, which has predilection to certain locations such as on the breasts, is indolent and has reduced risk for disease progression by multivariate analysis (Agar et al. 2010) (Fig. 1.9).

Histiocytes and inflammatory elements are also seen in lichenoid inflammatory infiltrates (Magro and Crowson 2000), but when extensive and appear as a lymphoid-rich sarcoid-like pattern, granulomatous MF should be considered. Clusters of histiocytes and foreign body giant cells are common features of cutaneous lymphoid hyperplasia or pseudolymphomas (Rijlaarsdam and Willemze 1993, 1994). Infections show histiocytic or acute inflammatory reactions. See Chap. 14 for cutaneous infections and tropical diseases.

Folliculotropic Pseudolymphomatous Folliculitis (PLF)

Pseudolymphomatous folliculitis is a common pattern with exclusive involvement of the hair follicles by a dense lymphoid infiltrate (Fig. 1.10). In those cases, PLF is a subset of lymphoid hyperplasia with characteristic clinical and pathologic features showing perifollicular clustering of T-cell-associated dendritic cells with activation of pilosebaceous units. PLF is a reactive group of patterns of varied etiologies, including lupus, rosacea, acne, and nonspecific bacterial infections, that have to be differentiated from malignant lymphomas and other cutaneous pseudolymphomas (Arai et al. 1999).

Hair follicles can be infiltrated by tumor cells in CTCL in a variant known as pilotropic or folliculotropic mycosis fungoides or follicular mucinosis-associated CTCL. Syringotropic and basaloid lymphomatous folliculitis is one of the five patterns seen in follicular MF (Gerami et al. 2008). Infiltration of hair follicles and sebaceous

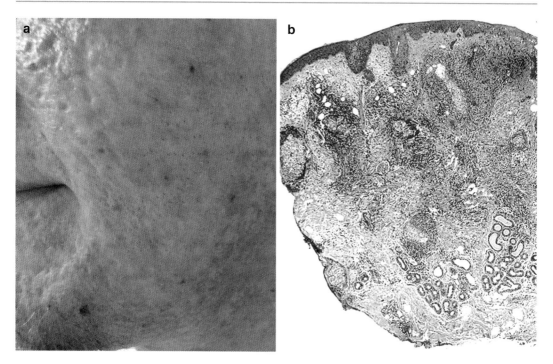

Fig. 1.11 (**a**) Head and neck folliculotropic MF in a young male. (**b**) Histopathology (Courtesy of Neil Fenske, Chair Dermatology and Frank Glass, Dermatopathologist, University of South Florida)

units can be accompanied by mucinous change in a phenomenon known as follicular mucinosis (Cerroni et al. 2002; Cerroni 2010; Cerroni and Kerl 2004). This event appears to forecast a poorer prognosis in MF; folliculotropic MF appears to be an aggressive variant of MF (Gerami et al. 2008; van Doorn et al. 2002). Folliculotropic MF without mucinosis is seen in about 50 %, epidermotropism along with folliculotropic MF in 25 %, and syringotropic involvement with folliculotropic MF in less than 10 % (Gerami et al. 2008) (Fig. 1.11).

Dermotropic

Nodules with Germinal Centers: Pseudolymphomatous B-Cell Pattern

This pattern is conventionally applied to a dense lymphoid infiltrate in the dermis or subcutaneous tissue showing discrete germinal centers (Burg et al. 2006) (Fig. 1.12). In studies that reviewed cutaneous lymphoid hyperplasia or cutaneous pseudolymphomas, Arai et al. detected up to 7 %

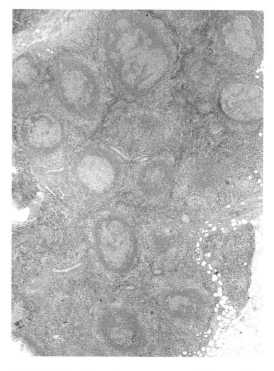

Fig. 1.12 Pseudolymphomatous pattern with several discrete follicles with germinal centers

with cutaneous lymphomas, typically of the cuta-neous marginal zone type (Arai et al. 2005).

Nodules with Granulomas: Granulomatous Pattern

Granulomas are frequently seen in T- and B-cell pseudolymphomas. Granulomas consisting of aggregates of histiocyte/macrophages, without the necrosis, are also seen in infectious disease, e.g., tuberculosis, fungal infections, and others. Granulomas may be the prominent histopathology of a peculiar variant of mycosis fungoides known as granulomatous slack skin, or granulomatous

Fig. 1.13 Histiocytosis pattern seen in cutaneous Rosai-Dorfman. Also typical of Lennert's lymphohistiocytic pattern

MF, a mycosis fungoides variant without slack skin. According to a recent multicenter study of the Cutaneous Lymphoma Histopathology Task Force Group of the European Organization for Research and Treatment of Cancer (EORTC), granulomatous CTCLs show a therapy-resistant, slowly progressive course. The prognosis of GMF appears worse than that of classic non-granuloma-tous mycosis fungoides (Kempf et al. 2008). See Chap. 6 for discussion of granulomatous MF.

A reactive granulomatous dermatitis is com-mon in both T- and B-cell lymphomas. See Fig. 1.13 sarcoidosis involves the skin with spher-oids of epithelioid granulomas with minimal lymphocytic component; see Chap. 13.

Histiocytosis Pattern. Reactive necrotizing his-tiocytic granulomatous dermatitis is the hallmark of Kikuchi-Fujimoto's disease involving the skin (Fig. 1.14). The presence of loose array of plump giant epithelioid histiocytes with cytophagocytosis or emperipolesis is seen in cutaneous Rosai-Dorfman disease (Fig. 1.15). See Chap. 13 for dis-cussion of cutaneous histiocytic disorders.

Nodular T-Cell Cell Pattern: Nodules without germinal centers

Although this pattern is often associated with a B-cell pseudolymphomatous pattern, in our experience, the nodules of T cells is a common presentation of idiopathic nonclonal T-cell

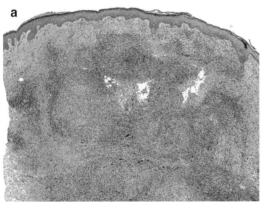

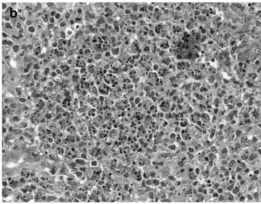

Fig. 1.14 Kikuchi's granulomatous dermatitis. (**a**) Low-power view with skin and underlying granulomatous nec-rotizing pattern. (**b**) Typical numerous apoptotic histiocytes with densely pyknotic nuclear debris and lack of neutrophils

pseudolymphoma and in many non-MF T-cell neoplasms (Fig. 1.16). See Chaps. 8 and 10.

Nodules with Increased Vessels

Capillary hemangiomas or granulation wound healing shows increased vessels with thin-walled endothelial lining cells. When "high," cuboidal or

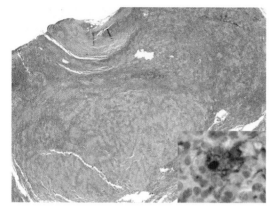

Fig. 1.15 Rosai-Dorfman in skin with *inset* of S100-positive histiocyte with emperipolesis of lymphocytes bounded by the irregular pinkish dendritic borders

plump endothelial cells are seen, in concert with atypical small and medium pleomorphic T cells, cutaneous involvement of angioimmunoblastic T-cell lymphoma should be suspected, if the clinical presentation shows typical systemic wide features (Fig. 1.17). Prominent endothelial venules with plump pink cytoplasm, sometimes arborizing, surrounded by perivascular atypical small- and medium-sized pleomorphic lymphocytes that coexpress T cell and follicle center cell-associated markers, such as CD10, Bcl-6, and PD-1, suggest a cutaneous involvement by angioimmunoblastic T-cell lymphoma, a systemic disease with frequent skin involvement (Martel et al. 2000; Patsouris et al. 1989).

Medium-sized vessels are prominently involved in (angiocentric) NK/T-cell lymphomas, nasal type of extranodal or extranasal lymphomas. Vessel walls are often necrotic and occluded with resulting infarct and eschar formation in the skin. Angionecrotic, occluded vessels with cutaneous eschars have been described in a variant of lymphomatoid papulosis, type E (Kempf et al. 2013)

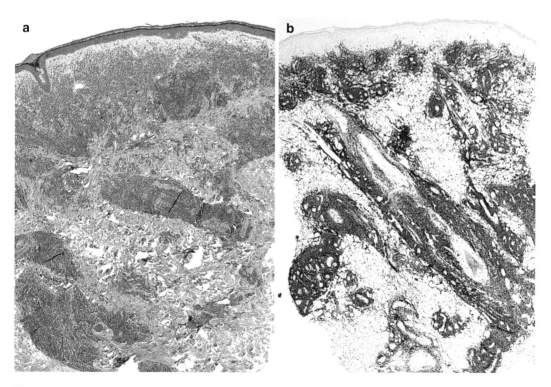

Fig. 1.16 (**a**) Nodular T-cell pseudolymphoma secondary to persistent reaction after a spider bite. (**b**) Low-power view of CD4-positive lymphocytes; T-cell receptor gene is germline

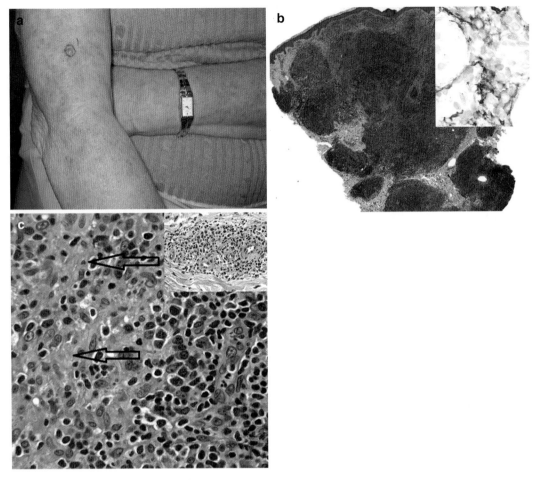

Fig. 1.17 (**a**) Clinic photo of erythematous rash with a nodule that was biopsied. (**b**) Nodular form of AITL with *inset* of CD10+ T cells. (**c**) High-power view with plasma cells and pink vessel deposits (*arrows*), *inset*. Subtle

AITL histopathology with plump endothelial venules surrounded by atypical pleomorphic lymphocytes (Courtesy of Neil Fenske, Chair Dermatology and Frank Glass, University of South Florida)

(Fig. 1.18). Scant perivascular lymphoid infiltrates are a common manifestation of early MF or many reactive lymphoid infiltrates in a nonspecific reaction to autoimmune or drug-induced dermatitis.

Nodules with Increased Vessels and Eosinophils

Angiolymphoid hyperplasia with eosinophilia presents with concentrated eosinophils, some form of vascular malformation, and reactive lymphocytes (Fig. 1.19). Kimura's disease is a differential diagnosis, when no arteriovenous malformation is seen. Drug hypersensitivity reactions may show increased vessels and eosino-

phils. History is critical and previous therapy may disclose findings seen in cutaneous reactions to biological modifiers. See Chap. 15 for discussion of skin reactions secondary to biological modifiers and chemokine treatment.

Nodules with Increased Plasma Cells

Plasma cells at the edges of nodules of T cells are commonly seen in T-cell pseudolymphomas. When sheets of plasma cells are associated with expanded marginal zones and reactive germinal centers, cutaneous marginal zone lymphoma has to be considered (Fig. 1.20). Nodules of plasma cells that express high IgG4 subset are pathognomonic of

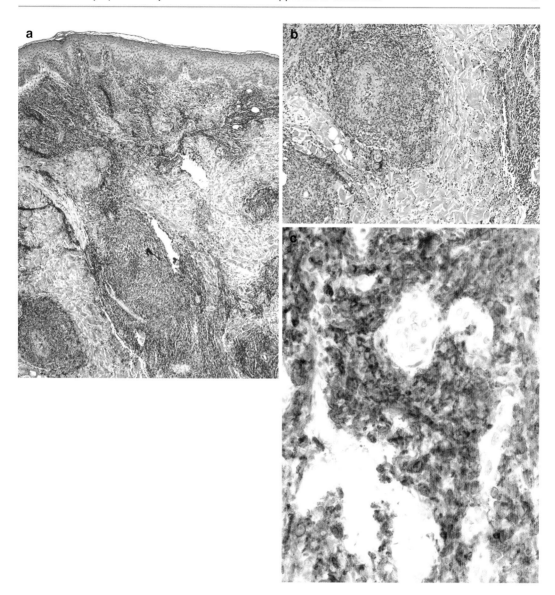

Fig. 1.18 (**a**) Lymphomatoid papulosis type E, low-power view. (**b**) Medium-power view of angiocentric pattern with occluded vessel. (**c**) CD30-positive infiltrate in cutaneous manifestation of IgG4 disease (Cheuk and Chan 2010; Divatia et al. 2012).

LyP E subtype (Courtesy of Frank Glass, Aurora and USF Dermatopathology, Tampa, FL)

Dermal Wedge-Shaped and Perivascular Pattern

This pattern is almost always described with lymphomatoid papulosis type A (Burg et al. 2006) but may not be present or clearly wedge shaped but nodular or perivascular in superficial biopsies or where the biopsy only shows part or half of the wedge or in other types of LyP. See Chap. 12 for discussion of these diseases.

Diffuse Pattern

Diffuse pattern is commonly associated with a nodular pattern, at least focally, and is seen in the dermis, subcutaneous tissue, or both. It can be seen in cases of T-cell pseudolymphomas

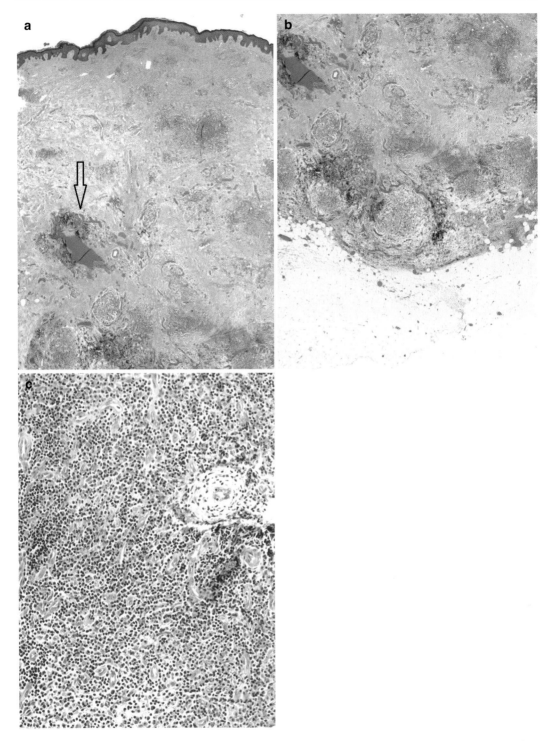

Fig. 1.19 (**a**) Angiolymphoid hyperplasia with eosinophilia showing vascular malformation (*arrow*), sclerosis, and lymphoid hyperplasia. (**b**) Medium-power view of arteriovenous malformation. (**c**) Vascular congestion, eosinophilia, and lymphoid infiltrate

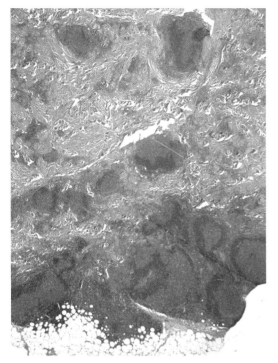

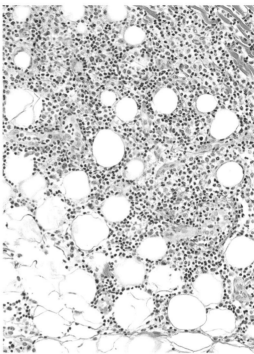

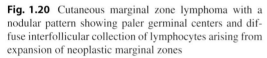

Fig. 1.20 Cutaneous marginal zone lymphoma with a nodular pattern showing paler germinal centers and diffuse interfollicular collection of lymphocytes arising from expansion of neoplastic marginal zones

Fig. 1.21 Subcutaneous panniculitis in a patient with lupus profundus

secondary to drugs or to antigen-induced hypersensitivity reactions, and these cases are often associated with tissue eosinophils and plasma cells. When eosinophils or plasma cells are associated with a diffuse pattern with atypical small to medium or medium to large cells, with increased mitosis, lymphoma should be suspected.

Cytologic examination on high-power view will reveal whether the cells are predominantly of one or two types. In the diffuse large B-cell lymphoma, leg type, immunoblasts, or centroblasts predominate. In transformed MF, at least 25 % are large cells with small cerebriform cells in the background. If the large cells are less than 25 % and the lump is solitary or few, with lymphocytes composed of atypical small- and medium-sized population that are monoclonal by T-cell gene rearrangement, then a primary cutaneous small- and medium-sized T-cell lymphoma is a prime consideration (see Chap. 10 for discussion of these entities).

Subcutaneous Pattern

Subcutaneous pattern is seen in both reactive and neoplastic processes. A predominantly septal panniculitis is typical of erythema nodosum, often bilateral on extensor surfaces of the lower extremities, and secondary to varied etiology; foremost are infections, i.e., mycobacteria or leprosy.

Predominantly nodular panniculitis is typical of lupus profundus, cytophagic histiocytic panniculitis, atypical lobular lymphocytic panniculitis, and subcutaneous panniculitic T-cell lymphoma (see Chap. 11 for discussion of subcutaneous pattern) (Fig. 1.21).

Miscellaneous Patterns

Intravascular Pattern

This is a rare pattern which occasionally baffles the pathologist because of the peculiar localization of the atypical cells within dermal blood vessels.

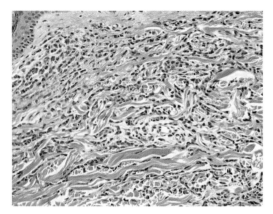

Fig. 1.22 Single-file pattern in hematodermic or blastic plasmacytoid dendritic cell neoplasm. Note the plasmacytoid violaceous appearance of the blasts

This pattern upon further immunohistologic stains would be seen in a variety of lymphomas including intravascular large B- and T-cell lymphomas, intravascular histiocytosis, and/or even the rare recently described cases simulating intravascular CD30+ lymphomas. Intravascular involvement of lymphomas is readily detected in skin biopsies. Please see Chap. 17 for discussion of intravascular lymphomas.

Single-File Pattern

Single-file pattern could be seen in myelomonocytic and lymphoid leukemias involving the skin. Please see Chap. 16 for discussion of leukemic, histiocytic, and myelomonocytic skin pattern. Caution has to be exercised in interpreting a low-grade lymphoma insinuating small non-blastic lymphoid cells between collagen fibers as a single-file pattern. Often the single-file pattern in leukemia is seen next to the epidermis in a horizontal array, without sclerosis, and admixed with a targetoid or diffuse pattern deeper in the dermal and subcutaneous tissue (Fig. 1.22).

References

Agar NS, Wedgeworth E, Crichton S, Mitchell TJ, Cox M, Ferreira S, Robson A, Calonje E, Stefanato CM, Wain EM, Wilkins B, Fields PA, Dean A, Webb K, Scarisbrick J, Morris S, Whittaker SJ. Survival outcomes and prognostic factors in mycosis fungoides/ Sezary syndrome: validation of the revised International Society for Cutaneous Lymphomas/ European Organisation for Research and Treatment of Cancer staging proposal. J Clin Oncol. 2010;28(31): 4730–9.

Arai E, Okubo H, Tsuchida T, Kitamura K, Katayama I. Pseudolymphomatous folliculitis: a clinicopathologic study of 15 cases of cutaneous pseudolymphoma with follicular invasion. Am J Surg Pathol. 1999;23(11): 1313–9.

Arai E, Shimizu M, Hirose T. A review of 55 cases of cutaneous lymphoid hyperplasia: reassessment of the histopathologic findings leading to reclassification of 4 lesions as cutaneous marginal zone lymphoma and 19 as pseudolymphomatous folliculitis. Hum Pathol. 2005;36(5):505–11.

Baldassano MF, Bailey EM, Ferry JA, Harris NL, Duncan LM. Cutaneous lymphoid hyperplasia and cutaneous marginal zone lymphoma: comparison of morphologic and immunophenotypic features. Am J Surg Pathol. 1999;23(1):88–96.

Bergman R. Pseudolymphoma and cutaneous lymphoma: facts and controversies. Clin Dermatol. 2010;28(5): 568–74.

Bergman R, Khamaysi K, Khamaysi Z, Ben AY. A study of histologic and immunophenotypical staining patterns in cutaneous lymphoid hyperplasia. J Am Acad Dermatol. 2011;65(1):112–24.

Bocquet H, Bagot M, Roujeau JC. Drug-induced pseudolymphoma and drug hypersensitivity syndrome (Drug Rash with Eosinophilia and Systemic Symptoms: DRESS). Semin Cutan Med Surg. 1996;15(4):250–7.

Bradford PT, Devesa SS, Anderson WF, Toro JR. Cutaneous lymphoma incidence patterns in the United States: a population-based study of 3884 cases. Blood. 2009;113(21):5064–73.

Burg G, Kempf W, Cozzio A, Dobbeling U, Feit J, Golling P, Michaelis S, Scharer L, Nestle F, Dummer R. Cutaneous malignant lymphomas: update 2006. J Dtsch Dermatol Ges. 2006;4(11):914–33.

Caro WA. Biopsy in suspected malignant lymphoma of the skin. Cutis. 1978;21(2):197–201.

Caro WA, Helwig HB. Cutaneous lymphoid hyperplasia. Cancer. 1969;24(3):487–502.

Ceballos KM, Gascoyne RD, Martinka M, Trotter MJ. Heavy multinodular cutaneous lymphoid infiltrates: clinicopathologic features and B-cell clonality. J Cutan Pathol. 2002;29(3):159–67.

Cerroni L. Lymphoproliferative lesions of the skin. J Clin Pathol. 2006;59(8):813–26.

Cerroni L. Pilotropic mycosis fungoides: a clinicopathologic variant of mycosis fungoides yet to be completely understood. Arch Dermatol. 2010;146(6):662–4.

Cerroni L, Kerl H. Primary follicular mucinosis and association with mycosis fungoides and other cutaneous T-cell lymphomas. J Am Acad Dermatol. 2004;51(1):146–7.

Cerroni L, Fink-Puches R, Back B, Kerl H. Follicular mucinosis: a critical reappraisal of clinicopathologic features and association with mycosis fungoides and Sezary syndrome. Arch Dermatol. 2002;138(2):182–9.

Cerroni L, Gatter K, Kerl H. Skin lymphoma: the illustrated guide, Wiley-Blackwell, Hoboken, NJ, USA; 3rd. 2009.

Cheuk W, Chan JK. IgG4-related sclerosing disease: a critical appraisal of an evolving clinicopathologic entity. Adv Anat Pathol. 2010;17(5):303–32.

Colli C, Leinweber B, Mullegger R, Chott A, Kerl H, Cerroni L. Borrelia burgdorferi-associated lymphocytoma cutis: clinicopathologic, immunophenotypic, and molecular study of 106 cases. J Cutan Pathol. 2004;31(3):232–40.

Criscione VD, Weinstock MA. Incidence of cutaneous T-cell lymphoma in the United States, 1973–2002. Arch Dermatol. 2007;143(7):854–9.

Divatia M, Kim SA, Ro JY. IgG4-related sclerosing disease, an emerging entity: a review of a multi-system disease. Yonsei Med J. 2012;53(1):15–34.

Furudate S, Fujimura T, Kambayashi Y, Aiba S. Profiles of cytotoxic T lymphocytes in cutaneous lymphoid hyperplasia of the face. Case Rep Dermatol. 2013;5(1):88–92.

Gerami P, Rosen S, Kuzel T, Boone SL, Guitart J. Folliculotropic mycosis fungoides: an aggressive variant of cutaneous T-cell lymphoma. Arch Dermatol. 2008;144(6):738–46.

Guitart J, Deonision J, Kadin M. CD30 lymphoproliferative disorders with pseudoepitheliomatous hyperplasia: a possible role for Th17 cytokines, neutrophils and eosinophils. 2nd world congress on cutaneous lymphomas, Berlin; 2013. Abstract 48.

Guitart J, Peduto M, Caro WA, Roenigk HH. Lichenoid changes in mycosis fungoides. J Am Acad Dermatol. 1997;36(3 Pt 1):417–22.

Isaacson PG, Norton AJ. Cutaneous lymphomas. In: Extranodal lymphomas. Edinburgh: Churchill Livingstone; 1994. p. 131–91.

Jenni D, Karpova MB, Seifert B, Golling P, Cozzio A, Kempf W, French LE, Dummer R. Primary cutaneous lymphoma: two-decade comparison in a population of 263 cases from a Swiss tertiary referral centre. Br J Dermatol. 2011;164(5):1071–7.

Kempf W, Kazakov D, Scharer L, et al. Angioinvasive lymphomatoid papulosis: a new variant simulating aggressive lymphomas. Am J Surg Pathol. 2013; 37:1–3.

Kempf W, Ostheeren-Michaelis S, Paulli M, Lucioni M, Wechsler J, Audring H, Assaf C, Rudiger T, Willemze R, Meijer CJ, Berti E, Cerroni L, Santucci M, Hallermann C, Berneburg M, Chimenti S, Robson A, Marschalko M, Kazakov DV, Petrella T, Fraitag S, Carlotti A, Courville P, Laeng H, Knobler R, Golling P, Dummer R, Burg G. Granulomatous mycosis fungoides and granulomatous slack skin: a multicenter study of the Cutaneous Lymphoma Histopathology Task Force Group of the European Organization For Research and Treatment of Cancer (EORTC). Arch Dermatol. 2008;144(12):1609–17.

Kojima M, Nakamura N, Sakamoto K, Sakurai S, Tsukamoto N, Itoh H, Ikota H, Enomoto Y, Shimizu K, Motoori T, Hoshi K, Igarashi T, Masawa N, Nakamine H. Progressive transformation of the germinal center of extranodal organs: a clinicopathological, immunohistochemical, and genotypic study of 14 cases. Pathol Res Pract. 2010a;206(4):235–40.

Kojima M, Sakurai S, Shimizu K, Itoh H. B-cell cutaneous lymphoid hyperplasia representing progressive transformation of germinal center: a report of 2 cases. Int J Surg Pathol. 2010b;18(5):429–32.

Lai P, Hsiao Y, Hsu J, Wey SJ. Early stage mycosis fungoides with focal CD30-positive large cell transformation. Dermatol Sin. 2012;31(2):1–5. doi:http://dx.doi.org/10.1016/j.dsi.2012.06.006.

Lipsker D. Dermatological aspects of Lyme borreliosis. Med Mal Infect. 2007;37(7–8):540–7.

Magro CM, Crowson AN. Drug-induced immune dysregulation as a cause of atypical cutaneous lymphoid infiltrates: a hypothesis. Hum Pathol. 1996;27(2):125–32.

Magro CM, Crowson AN. Lichenoid and granulomatous dermatitis. Int J Dermatol. 2000;39(2):126–33.

Magro CM, Crowson AN, Harrist TJ. Atypical lymphoid infiltrates arising in cutaneous lesions of connective tissue disease. Am J Dermatopathol. 1997;19(5):446–55.

Magro CM, Crowson AN, Kovatich AJ, Burns F. Drug-induced reversible lymphoid dyscrasia: a clonal lymphomatoid dermatitis of memory and activated T cells. Hum Pathol. 2003;34(2):119–29.

Martel P, Laroche L, Courville P, Larroche C, Wechsler J, Lenormand B, Delfau MH, Bodemer C, Bagot M, Joly P. Cutaneous involvement in patients with angioimmunoblastic lymphadenopathy with dysproteinemia: a clinical, immunohistological, and molecular analysis. Arch Dermatol. 2000;136(7):881–6.

Muramoto L, Kadin M. Improved detection of lymphoid cell surface antigens in tissues fixed in periodate-lysine-paraformaldehyde. Am J Clin Pathol. 1987;88:589–95.

Oliver GF, Winkelmann RK, Muller SA. Lichenoid dermatitis: a clinicopathologic and immunopathologic review of sixty-two cases. J Am Acad Dermatol. 1989;21(2 Pt 1):284–92.

Patsouris E, Noel H, Lennert K. Angioimmunoblastic lymphadenopathy–type of T-cell lymphoma with a high content of epithelioid cells. Histopathology and comparison with lymphoepithelioid cell lymphoma. Am J Surg Pathol. 1989;13(4):262–75.

Ramos-Ceballos F, Horn TD. Interface dermatitis. In: Barnhill RL, Crowson AN, Magro CM, et al., editors. Dermatopathology. 3rd ed. China: McGraw Hill Medical; 2010. pp. 342–344.

Rijlaarsdam JU, Willemze R. Diagnosis and classification of cutaneous pseudolymphoma. Historical review and perspectives. Ann Dermatol Venereol. 1993;120(1):100–6.

Rijlaarsdam JU, Willemze R. Cutaneous pseudolymphomas: classification and differential diagnosis. Semin Dermatol. 1994;13(3):187–96.

Singh ZN, Tretiakova MS, Shea CR, Petronic-Rosic VM. Decreased CD117 expression in hypopigmented mycosis fungoides correlates with hypomelanosis: lessons learned from vitiligo. Mod Pathol. 2006;19(9):1255–60.

Swerdlow SJ, Campo E, Harris NL, Jaffe ES, Pileri S, Stein H, Thiele J, Vardiman JW, editors. WHO classification of tumors of haematopoieitic and lymphoid tissues, WHO press, Geneva, Switzerland; 4th ed. 2008.

van Doorn R, Scheffer E, Willemze R. Follicular mycosis fungoides, a distinct disease entity with or without associated follicular mucinosis: a clinicopathologic and follow-up study of 51 patients. Arch Dermatol. 2002;138(2):191–8.

Vonderheid EC, Pavlov I, Delgado JC, Martins TB, Telang GH, Hess AD, Kadin M, et al. Prognostic factors and risk stratification in early mycosis fungoides. Leuk Lymphoma. 2014;55(1):44–50. doi: 10.3109/10428194.2013.790541. Epub 2013 May 7.

Willemze R, Jaffe ES, Burg G, Cerroni L, Berti E, Swerdlow SH, Ralfkiaer E, Chimenti S, az-Perez JL, Duncan LM, Grange F, Harris NL, Kempf W, Kerl H, Kurrer M, Knobler R, Pimpinelli N, Sander C, Santucci M, Sterry W, Vermeer MH, Wechsler J, Whittaker S, Meijer CJ. WHO-EORTC classification for cutaneous lymphomas. Blood. 2005;105(10):3768–85.

Functional Organization of the Skin as an Immune Response Organ: Skin, Immune Response, and Useful Immunohistochemistry

Marshall E. Kadin and Hernani D. Cualing

Introduction to Cutaneous Lymphoid Tissue

Skin Meets Environment

The skin is the body's major interface with the environment where it is exposed to a diverse repertoire of foreign antigens. It is also a highly susceptible portal of entry for infectious organisms. For its protective role, the skin has therefore developed highly effective immediate and long-term immune responses. The patterns of inflammatory responses may set the stage for the development of subsequent malignant lymphomas. Accordingly, malignant lymphocytes that traffic to and through the skin share many immunologic and genotypic features of their benign counterparts involved in cutaneous immune surveillance.

M.E. Kadin, MD (✉)
Department of Dermatology, Roger Williams
Medical Center, Boston University School of Medicine,
50 Maude Street, Elmhurst Bldg.,
Providence, RI 02908, USA
e-mail: mkadin@chartercare.org

H.D. Cualing, MD
Department of Hematopathology and Cutaneous
Lymphoma, IHCFLOW Diagnostic Laboratory,
Lutz, FL, USA

Innate Immune Response

The innate immune system, also known as nonspecific immune system and first line of defense, comprises the cells and mechanisms that defend the host from infection by other organisms in a nonspecific manner. This "innate" response is focused on early (minutes to hours) response to pathogens. Triggers of the innate immune response include microbial and foreign glycolipids, glycoproteins, and DNA complexes (Beetz et al. 2008; Holtmeier and Kabelitz 2005; Kabelitz 2011; Kabelitz et al. 2000). Cellular components of the innate immune system include neutrophils, mast cells, macrophages, dendritic cells, and effector lymphocytes. The immediate effector lymphocytes include natural killer (NK) cells and gamma-delta T cells (γ/δ T cells) (Kabelitz 1992; Kabelitz et al. 2005; Kim et al. 2005). The γ/δ T cells, which comprise 10 % of skin T lymphocytes, along with B cells and NK cells, are largely localized in the dermis and subcutaneous tissue and, for their role as immune effector cells, are also predisposed to the basal layer of the epidermis and outer root sheaths of hair follicles (Kabelitz 2011; Kabelitz et al. 2000).

Secondary Immune Response

The secondary immune responses require the regulation of circulating and peripheral memory T cells, and the skin is postulated to be an active peripheral lymphoid organ, hosting 20 billion T cells, twice that in circulation (Egawa and Kabashima 2011). The adaptive or long-term component of the immune response is composed mainly of T cells bearing α/β T-cell antigen receptors (alpha-beta T cells). These so-called α/β T cells, which comprise 90 % of the cutaneous T cells, acquire homing capacity to the epidermis through the activation of surface addressins enabling them to interact with epidermal Langerhans cells for microbial recognition. Differential expression of surface receptors appears to determine T-cell localization. More than 90 % of these cells express cutaneous lymphocyte antigen (CLA), CD45RO and CCR4 receptors, which are characteristic surface antigens of effector memory T cells (Fig. 2.1). Unlike memory T cells common in the blood circulation and in lymph nodes (which additionally express CCR7 chemokine receptor), memory T cells resident in the skin lack the central memory T-cell marker CCR7 (Egawa and Kabashima 2011). The circulating central memory T-cell pool transiently expresses lymph node homing CCR7 and CD62L (L-selectin). Upon encountering its cognate antigens within the lymph nodes, these central memory T cells downregulate these markers and upregulate CLA + and other skin-specific homing addressins necessary for homing to the skin.

Cutaneous Trafficking of Lymphocytes

A subset of T lymphocytes migrate to the skin via dermal postcapillary venules and recirculate to regional lymph nodes that drain the skin, creating a local network of immune surveillance. For a detailed pictorial review, see (Clark 2010), (Fig. 2.1). This decades-old hypothesis by Streilein (Streilein 1978, 1983, 1985, 1989; Streilein and Bergstresser 1984) is supported by in vivo and in vitro observations and is validated in live mammalian studies by two-photon microscopy which visualize this regional network and

its dynamic stepwise development (Egawa et al. 2011). In addition, live animal skin color changes and microscopy of skin-associated lymphocytes trafficking from the lymph nodes is visualized using a technique relying on new fluorescent-tagged cells (Tomura 2012) which changes from fluorescent green to red upon exposure to skin-directed UV (ultraviolet) light (Kaplan et al. 2005, 2008). Accumulating evidence indicates that skin is a crucial modulator of the global immune response and is considered to be a crucial peripheral lymphoid organ akin to the lymph nodes (Egawa and Kabashima 2011).

An orchestrated set of ligand-receptor and chemokine exchanges between immune effector cells, epithelia, and dermal high endothelial venules lead to cutaneous lymphoid infiltrates. These lymphoid infiltrates generate a pattern of reaction that may appear more or less concentrated within the epidermis, dermis, and/or subcutaneous tissue depending on the main participating cells and the signals they receive. Remarkable inroads into the origin and function of the normal components of the immune response provide insights into the histologic architecture, phenotype, and behavior of malignant lymphoma/leukemia counterparts.

Cytokines Define Functional T Helper Subsets

Cytokines are the soluble hormonelike messengers active in mediating the immune response. Deregulation or overproduction of select cytokines is known to play a major role in the pathogenesis of common cutaneous inflammatory diseases, e.g., psoriasis (Schaerli et al. 2004; Wolk et al. 2009) and atopic dermatitis (Asarch et al. 2008; Koga et al. 2008). Ongoing research indicates that cytokines also are involved in the pathogenesis of cutaneous lymphomas (Saed et al. 1994; Vowels et al. 1994a, b). Clinical trials targeting cytokines and their receptors have shown promise for the treatment of cutaneous inflammatory and autoimmune diseases (Asarch et al. 2008; Miossec et al. 2009).

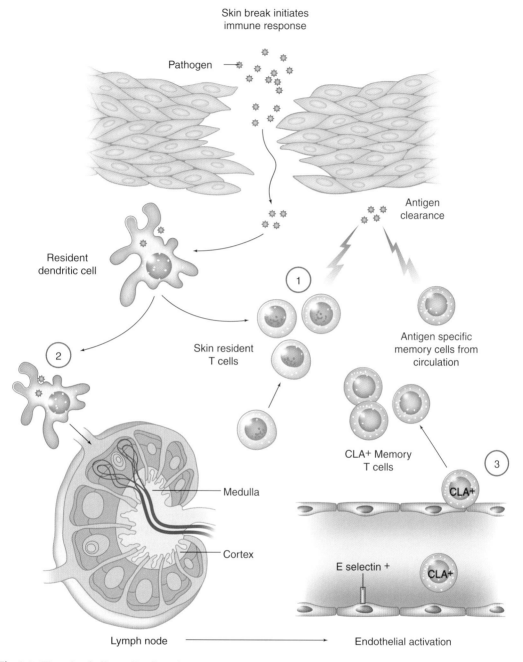

Fig. 2.1 The role of effector T cells and memory T cells in recall immune responses (Modified from Clark 2010). Memory immune responses can be divided into three stages. First, dendritic cells (DC) take up antigen following pathogen reexposure and present it to effector T resident locally within the skin. These cells proliferate and effect clearance of the pathogen. Second, DC carry endo- cytosed antigen to the skin-draining lymph nodes where it is presented to central memory T cells. These cells then give rise to new populations of skin homing T effector cells that migrate to the skin and clear the infection; third, inflammation leads to endothelial activation and nonspe- cific recruitment of T cells from the blood

The interaction between proinflammatory T cells and regulatory T cells also determines cutaneous manifestations of graft-versus-host disease (Beres and Drobyski 2013). Serum cytokine/receptor levels are useful markers of disease activity and quantification of tumor burden (Wasik et al. 1996; Kadin et al. 2012). Therefore, we feel it is essential for our readers to have a basic understanding of cytokines and the cells that produce them.

Of the two main subsets of T lymphocytes, CD4 and CD8, the CD4 T helper subset (Th) is the main cytokine producer. Initially two main Th subset groups were defined by the cytokines they secrete. Th1 cells, regulated by transcription factors Tbet and STAT4, secrete IFN-gamma and induce inflammatory responses to intracellular pathogens. Th2 cells, regulated by GATA3 and STAT5, are represented by interleukins 4, 5, and 13, respond to extracellular parasites, and are associated with the promotion of IgE and eosinophilia. Th9 cells are closely related to Th2 cells but have the capacity to produce IL-9 and IL-10. IL-9 is produced by tumor cells in some anaplastic large cell lymphomas and Hodgkin lymphomas (Merz et al. 1991). More recently described Th17 cells, which recruit neutrophils and macrophages to sites of inflammation, are regulated by ROR and STAT3, convey autoimmune responses, and promote antimicrobial immunity at the body's borders, e.g., linings of the respiratory and gastrointestinal tracts and the skin. Th17 cells also can produce interleukin 22 which induces epithelial and mucosal cells to secrete antimicrobial peptides active against fungi and bacteria. The proinflammatory and autoimmune effects of Th17 cells are counterbalanced by natural and induced regulatory T cells (Tregs), regulated by the transcription factor FoxP3 and the secretion of immunosuppressive cytokines TGF-beta and IL-10. T cells associated with follicular center differentiation employ transcription factor Bcl-6 and appear to be the source of neoplastic cells in some primary cutaneous CD4+ small-/medium-sized pleomorphic T-cell lymphomas (Rodriguez Pinilla et al. 2009) and mycosis fungoides/Sezary syndrome cases (Meyerson et al. 2013).

CD4+ T cells demonstrate remarkable plasticity (Zhou et al. 2009). It appears that expression of Foxp3 by induced Treg cells (iTregs) or IL-17 by Th17 cells may not be stable. TGF-beta promotes Th17 cell differentiation in a concentration-dependent manner. At low concentrations, TGF-beta synergizes with interleukin IL-6 and IL-21 to promote IL-23 receptor (IL23R) expression, favoring Th17 cell differentiation. High concentrations of TGF-beta repress IL23R expression and favor the development of Foxp3+ Treg cells (Zhou et al. 2008). See Fig. 2.2 on the Th subset cytokines and transcription factors.

Duhen characterized a population of human skin-homing memory CD4+ T cells that express the chemokine receptors CCR10, CCR6, and CCR4 and produce IL-22 but neither IL-17 nor IFN-gamma. The differentiation of T cells producing only IL-22 is efficiently induced in naive T cells by plasmacytoid dendritic cells in an IL-6- and tumor necrosis factor-dependent manner (Duhen et al. 2009). Notch signaling drives IL-22 secretion in CD4+ T cells by stimulating the aryl hydrocarbon receptor (Alam et al. 2010).

An overview of Th subsets and the cytokines they produce is presented in Fig. 2.2 (and Table 2.1). For more detailed descriptions, readers are referred to several review articles (Maddur et al. 2012; Miossec et al. 2009; Zhou et al. 2009).

Functional Compartments

Epidermis: Generation of Lichenoid Infiltrate

Following antigen stimulation or injury to the skin, there is epidermal keratinocyte activation with lymphokine release. In addition, Toll-like receptors of dendritic antigen-presenting cells (APC) located in the epidermis and dermis are activated with antigenic epitopes from microbes or foreign bodies. Following antigen activation, Langerhans cells and plasmacytoid dendritic cells migrate to the lymph nodes draining the skin to recruit more lymphocytes.

Fig. 2.2 Overview of Th cell differentiation from naive CD4+ T cells. This diagram depicts the cytokines and transcription factors which determine naive CD4 T cell fates, the cytokines they produce, and their main effects

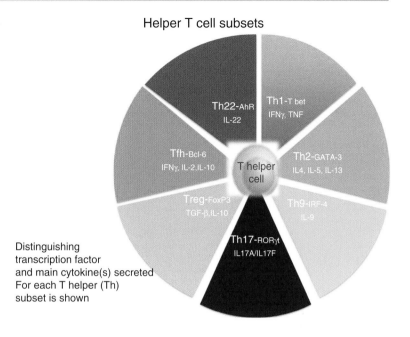

Helper T cell subsets

Distinguishing transcription factor and main cytokine(s) secreted For each T helper (Th) subset is shown

Table 2.1 T helper cell subsets

Th subset	Th1	Th2	Th17	Th9	Th22	Treg	Tfh
Transcription factors	Tbet, Stat4	GATA-3	RORγτ/ RORC	IRF-4	AhR	FoxP3	Bcl-6
		Stat-5	Stat3	PU.1	Stat3	Stat5	Stat3
Secreted cytokines	IFNγ, IL2 IL-10	IL-4, IL-5, IL-10, IL-13	IL-17A, IL-17F, IL21, IL-22	IL-9, IL-10	IL-22, IL-21, IL10, IL-13	TGF-β, IL-10	IFNγ, IL2, IL-4, IL-10, IL-17A, IL-17F
Main functions	Delayed hypersensitivity, macrophage activation, cytotoxic T-cell proliferation, nitric oxide production. Promote skin inflammatory disorders and autoimmunity	Humoral immunity, eosinophil activation Response to large extracellular pathogens	Response to fungi, extracellular bacteria Recruitment of neutrophils and macrophages, promote acute inflammation and autoimmunity	Defense against helminth infections, chronic allergic reaction	Synergize with Th17 cells to promote innate immunity in the skin and GI and respiratory tracts, promote tissue regeneration, involved in skin inflammatory disorders	Suppress immune responses including inflammation, autoimmunity, and graft-versus-host disease	Regulate antigen-specific B-cell immunity
Cell surface receptors	CCR1, CCR5, CCR3, IFNγ-R1, IFNγ-R2	CCR3, CCR4, CCR8, CXCR4 IFNγ-R1, IFNγ-R2	IL-1RI L-21R. IL23R, TGFβRII	TGFβRII, IL17RB	CCR4, CCR10, CCR6, TGFβRII	CD62L/L-selectin, CD25, OX40/ CD134	PD-1 CXCR4, CXCR5, ICOS CD40L, IL-6Rα

Fig. 2.3 Perivascular lymphoid infiltrate as a beginning of trafficking of lymphocytes (SALT early pattern)

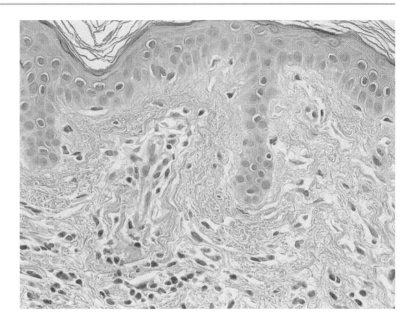

Antigen-Presenting Cells

A skin-associated lymphoid tissue (SALT) develops (Fig. 2.3). This pattern resembles the distribution of neoplastic skin lymphoid infiltrates. SALT initially are composed of T cells that are attracted to Langerhans cells, the epidermal sentinel immune cells, which are also epidermal antigen-presenting cells. It is postulated that Langerhans cells contribute or perhaps initiate the pathogenesis and recruitment of the malignant T cells in the skin, particularly in mycosis fungoides (Edelson 2001; Berger et al. 2002).

Cytology

A small population of reactive T cells, upon stimulation with certain antigens, demonstrate small cell cerebriform nuclear morphology. Anti-CD3 stimulation is one such trigger (Reinhold et al. 1994). Ultrastructural and monoclonal antibody analysis shows that a normal subset of peripheral blood cells have a cerebriform appearance (Matutes et al. 1983). In practice, less than 3 % of epidermal or dermal T cells have cerebriform nuclei. Although genetic lesions are known to be correlated with blastic transformation of these small cells, certain mitogens/antigen triggers in vitro also appear to cause blastic cytologic

transformation of neoplastic cerebriform cells (Kadin et al. 1984).

Dermis: Generation of Nodular Infiltrate

Subsequently, lymphocytes primed within the epidermis accumulate in the dermis around dermal postcapillary venules and dendritic cells, likely leading to nodular and sometimes diffuse dermal lymphoid infiltrates. Recruitment and help from circulating B cells and Thf cells also come into play. B cells are seen early around capillaries and venules, then later form follicles containing germinal centers composed of B cells, with scattered follicular T helper (Tfh) cells. These cells accumulate in the T-cell ridge between the mantle and light zone. These cells, unlike the interfollicular T cells, coexpress several follicle center associated markers including CD10, Bcl-6, PD1, and CXCL13. Lymphomas arising from this subset tend to form nodules in the dermis with the expression of CD3 plus the aforementioned Tfh subset markers. Angioimmunoblastic T-cell lymphomas, primary cutaneous small- and medium-sized T-cell lymphomas, and some PTCL not otherwise specified (NOS) have been reported to express these markers. See Chap. 10 for further discussion.

NK T Cells and Gamma-Delta T Cells

Gamma-delta T and NK cells respond to stress-associated factors and are present in the normal epithelial tissues as well as in normal human dermis. They are well-known effectors of the immediate immune response but also have other unique surveillance abilities. These cells express receptors for homing to non-inflamed skin as well as surface receptors for the recognition of allogeneic tumor cells and are reported to be part of the immune surveillance for the elimination of cutaneous tumors and distressed cells (Ebert et al. 2006).

T-Cell Reaction Followed by Accumulation of B Cells

Memory T cells expressing alpha-beta appear to be a major component of skin tropic cells with immune surveillance against previously encountered antigens (Schaerli et al. 2004). Hence, repeated stimulation of skin may induce accumulation of alpha-beta T cells along with NK and gamma-delta T cells.

In vivo findings support this accumulative cellular migration sequence with a dominant CD4+ effector T-cell subset reaction (Fuhlbrigge et al. 1997; Kupper and Edelson 1987; Hoeller et al. 2009) in the epidermis and into the dermis. These CD4+ T cells migrate from dermal venules and infiltrate between bundles of dermal collagen fibers to form nodules within the dermis (Matheu et al. 2008). Two-photon microscopy studies, which allow imaging of movement of live cells, indicate a defined sequence of cell populations trafficking to the skin from draining lymph nodes. This trafficking is more conspicuous among CD4+ T cells than CD8 T cells (Gebhardt et al. 2011). B-cell transition is slower than T-cell migration (Gebhardt et al. 2009; Mackay et al. 1988; Wakim et al. 2008; Tomura et al. 2008).

Pathogens and Dendritic Cells

The expansion of T helper subsets into defined Th1, Th2, or Th17 profiles appears to be induced by specific types of pathogens. Th1 cells function in autoimmunity and immune response to intracellular pathogens. They secrete IFN-gamma. Th2 cells, which deal with extracellular parasites and are also active in allergy and asthma. Th17 cells provide immunity against a variety of extracellular pathogens, including bacteria such as *Klebsiella pneumoniae* and fungi such as *Cryptococcus neoformans* and *Candida* (Pelletier et al. 2010). The Th17 axis is active in the pathogenesis of a range of dermatological diseases including allergic contact dermatitis, atopic dermatitis, psoriasis, and scleroderma (Asarch et al. 2008).

Th17 and MF

There is limited evidence of Th17 differentiation of tumor cells in mycosis fungoides, particularly in cases with accumulating neutrophils (Ciree et al. 2004) or with a higher rate of progression to advanced stages (Litvinov et al. 2010).

Epithelioid Histiocytes and Granulomas

Epithelioid histiocytes and tissue macrophages aggregate as discrete clusters within the dermis or subcutaneous tissue as granulomas. These arise as an immune system response to an antigen, in which epithelioid macrophages and inflammatory and immune effector cells accumulate. Chronic granulomas are often surrounded by fibrosis or a lymphocyte cuff, but early formation appears as microgranulomas or lymphohistiocytic clusters. Presence of granulomas is often equated with infections, but a variety of noninfectious triggers should also be kept in mind such as autoimmune disorders including rheumatoid skin nodules, Churg-Strauss syndrome, or iatrogenic injections, vaccinations, and lymphoproliferative disorders. Among the latter is a granulomatous form of mycosis fungoides, which can be associated with slack skin.

Histiocytosis arising from tumors of antigen-presenting cells as well as those common in children should also be considered in the proper setting. See discussion in Chap. 14 of histiocytic lesions of the skin.

Subcutaneous Tissue

The subcutaneous tissue or hypodermis is composed of fat and blood vessels. Commonly involved by transformed and diffuse lymphomas, it is seldom inflamed except in certain types of panniculitis. See Chap. 11 for discussion.

The deep vascular plexus is located just above this layer and seldom is involved by perivascular lymphoid infiltrates. In contrast, the superficial vascular plexus just beneath the epidermis is often the site of inflammatory T-cell reactions in dermatitis and psoriasis (Kunstfeld et al. 1997; Lechleitner et al. 1999). Changes in endothelial structure and acquisition of addressins facilitate skin homing above the subcutis (Lechleitner et al. 1999). Gamma-delta T cells and their malignant counterparts can be partially localized to the panniculus (Magro and Wang 2012). The less frequent skin epithelial localization of these cells and their rela-tive lower density compared to alpha-beta T cells are well recognized (Hocker et al. 2012).

Immunohistochemistry Panel for Evaluation of Lymphohemotoporetic Cutareous Diseases

An immunohistochemical panel is often used in the evaluation of lymphohematopoietic cutaneous diseases. Here we list the commonly used antibodies and show their normal tissue cross-reactions in addition to the usual targets. See list of commonly used antibodies in Table 2.2 and illustrations demonstrating their usefulness in cutaneous hematopathology (Figs. 2.3, 2.4, 2.5, 2.6, 2.7, 2.8, 2.9, 2.10, 2.11, 2.12, 2.13, 2.14, 2.15, 2.16, 2.17, 2.18, 2.19, 2.20, 2.21, 2.22, 2.23, 2.24, 2.25, 2.26, 2.27, 2.28, 2.29, 2.30, 2.31, 2.32, 2.33, and 2.34).

Table 2.2 Antibodies routinely used in paraffin-embedded tissue in the investigation of cutaneous lymphoma/leukemia

Antibody/reactivity	Main specificity	Uses	Normal skin and other reactivities
CD1a membrane	Langerhans cells and cortical thymic T cells (positive in some cases of precursor T-ALL)	Useful in investigating Rosai-Dorfman disease and other histiocytosis or T lymphoblasts but not routinely used for mature T-cell neoplasms. Reacts with dermal dendritic antigen-presenting cells and epidermal Langerhans cells	Langerhans cells
CD2 membrane	Pan T-cell marker, cortical and late thymocytes, and NK cells, antigen-presenting cells	For both NK and T cells, immature and mature	Langerhans cells. Mast cells, some AML and some B-lineage neoplasms
CD3 cytoplasmic/membrane	Pan T-cell marker, late thymocytes, and mature T cells. Expressed on many neoplasms of mature T cells	Mature T-cell marker that may be lost is T-cell lymphomas. Highlights nuclear cerebriform cell morphology Precursor T cell positive	Epsilon chain of the CD3 molecule and shows cytoplasmic positivity in NK cells
CD4 membrane	T-cell helper subset, expressed as weaker staining on monocytes and macrophages	Useful in MF and T-cell lymphomas and for CD4/CD8 ratio	Monocytes, macrophages, histiocytes
CD5 membrane	Pan T-cell marker, expressed by B cells in B-CLL, mantle cell lymphoma	Most of reactive T cells but may be lost in T-cell lymphomas. Absent in most cutaneous marginal zone and cutaneous large B-cell lymphomas	Secondary DLBCL may express CD5 in 1/5, also in secondary splenic marginal zone lymphoma, CLL, and mantle zone lymphoma
CD7 membrane	Pan T-cell marker also in NK cells	Useful in T-cell lymphoma, commonly lost on Sezary cells but not specific	Positive on blast cells in a minority of cases of myelomonocytic leukemia

Table 2.2   (continued)

Antibody/reactivity	Main specificity	Uses	Normal skin and other reactivities
CD8 membrane	T-cell cytotoxic subset. Expressed in some T-cell precursor leukemia/lymphoma	Useful in CD4/CD8 ratio, some CD8-positive cutaneous lymphomas and pagetoid variant of lymphomatoid papulosis	Large granular lymphocytic leukemia, T-CLL/T-PLL, and some gamma-delta T-cell lymphomas may express CD8
CD10 membrane	Common ALL antigen. Expressed by mature and precursors cells. Also in normal germinal center B cells and some normal B-cell precursors such as hematogones	Useful in cutaneous follicle center cell lymphoma but often weaker than Bcl6; also in angioimmunoblastic T-cell lymphoma and precursor B-lymphoblastic lymphoma/leukemia; some peripheral T-cell lymphoma, unspecified	Reacts with normal germinal centers in marginal zone lymphoma. Secondary diffuse large B-cell lymphoma or Burkitt lymphoma. Cutaneous stromal cells and nonspecifically to ischemic and infarcted lymphoid cells
CD11c membrane	Monocytes, NK cells, and neutrophils	Less commonly used in the skin but may be useful in suspected secondary lymphomas	Seen in hairy cell leukemia, some variant hairy cell leukemia, splenic marginal zone lymphoma, and some cases of CLL and B NHL
CD15 membrane	Neutrophils and myeloid precursor cells, macrophages	Useful in granulocytic sarcoma workup to determine myeloid maturation	Expressed on Reed-Sternberg cells, some large T-cell lymphomas, and rare DLBCL. Some cases of AML and B-cell precursor leukemia
CD20 membrane, cytoplasmic aberrantly in transformed	B-cell antigen	B cells; useful in getting a CD20:CD3 ratio; may be lost in rituximab-treated cases	B cells as well as nodular lymphocyte predominant Hodgkin lymphoma, some precursor B-cell tumors, some plasma cell myeloma
CD23 membrane, dendrites	Activated B cells; follicular dendritic cells	Useful in getting the pattern of germinal centers; disorganized in atypical/transformed germinal centers and lymphoma in skin	Follicular dendritic cell sarcoma; secondary CLL, some follicular lymphomas and diffuse large B-cell lymphoma
CD25 membrane	IL-2 receptor (alpha chain) on T cells and B cells	Detects an activation antigen that may be present on CTCL, LyP and transformed T- or B-cell lymphomas	Adult T-cell leukemia and anaplastic large cell lymphoma and others like hairy cell leukemia, a target antigen of Ontak
CD30 membrane cytoplasmic	Activated T and B lymphoid cell marker	Useful in CD30-positive lymphomas including lymphomatoid papulosis, cutaneous and systemic anaplastic large cell lymphoma and reactive CD30 + skin lesions like scabies, etc.	Expressed in Reed-Sternberg cells and Hodgkin cells in classical Hodgkin lymphoma, embryonal carcinoma, malignant melanoma cells, diffuse large B-cell lymphomas of mediastinal B-cell lymphoma, plasmablastic lymphomas or some myeloid leukemias
CD34 membrane cytoplasmic	Stem cells such as myelolymphoid blasts or normal vessels	Some blastic myeloid leukemia presenting as cutaneous myeloid sarcoma	Cutaneous endothelial cells and may be seen in some vascular skin tumors
CD35 cytoplasmic	Follicular dendritic cell marker	Cutaneous involvement of follicular dendritic cell sarcoma	Some AML, especially with monocytic differentiation
CD43 membrane	Normal T cells, myeloid cells	Useful in a panel of CD3, CD20, and CD43. Positive on myeloid sarcoma (chloroma) in a CD3-negative CD4-positive manner	Also in T-cell lymphomas, ALCL, and some low-grade lymphomas and proportion of diffuse large B-cell lymphoma

(continued)

Table 2.2 (continued)

Antibody/reactivity	Main specificity	Uses	Normal skin and other reactivities
CD45 membrane	Leukocyte common antigen (LCA)—pan hematopoietic marker	Useful in determining if lesion is either lymphoid or leukemic or is a sarcoma, melanoma, or carcinoma	Reacts with mature and immature B, T, myeloid cells and weakly with monocytes
CD45R0 membrane	Activated or memory T cells	Most mature T-cell lymphomas and CTCL derived from memory T cells	Many T-cell lymphomas
CD45RA membrane	Naive B or T cells	Lymphocytes before antigen activation	
CD56 membrane	NK cell marker; also stains a subset of T cells, myeloid cells	Some cutaneous NK or T-cell lymphomas and gamma-delta T cells Subtyping of myeloid sarcoma if CD4 + CD56+ blastic dendritic neoplasm	Also carcinomas such as neuroendocrine derived, some plasma cell myeloma. Some AML, mainly AML-M5. NK LGL leukemias and some T-cell LGL leukemias and extranodal NK/T-cell lymphomas
CD57 membrane	NK cell and T cells	Useful in follicle T helper cell, some NK cell large granular leukemia	Large granular lymphocytic leukemia, NK cells
CD68 cytoplasmic	Histiocytes, monocytes, and macrophages	Useful in myelomonocytic sarcoma, cutaneous Rosai-Dorfman disease, Langerhans cells and tissue macrophages	Some cells of granulocytic lineage, positive in granulomas
CD79a membrane	B cells, plasma cells	Useful in cases with lost CD20	May be expressed by some AML with aberrant B-cell antigens, staining both B and plasma cells
CD117 cytoplasmic	Stem cells, melanoblasts Melanocytes	Useful in the skin for determining loss of melanocytes	Epidermal melanocytic cells, adnexa, and in leukemia for the presence of blasts
CD123 membrane	Detects the alpha chain of the IL3 receptor	Expressed in plasmacytoid dendritic cell neoplasm and normal plasmacytoid dendritic cells	Also in NK cells, eosinophils, basophils, and monocytes; hairy cell leukemia, about half of AML and precursor B-lymphoblastic lymphoma
CD138 cytoplasmic membrane	Expressed in plasma cells and epithelia	Myeloma, plasmablastic lymphoma, plasma cells, primary effusion lymphoma, and some lymphoplasmacytic lymphoma	Normal and neoplastic epithelia
CD163 membrane	Hemoglobin scavenger receptor glycoprotein	Expressed on monocytes and macrophages and in cutaneous Rosai-Dorfman	Positive in myelomonocytic leukemia and histiocytic malignancies
CD279 (PD1) membrane	Programmed death 1 T cells, T follicle T helper cell	Expressed in both CTCL and PTCL, NOS, and in lymphomas such as AITL with helper T-cell origin	Positive in normal germinal center T cells
BCL2 cytoplasmic membrane	Apoptosis regulator	Not expressed in reactive follicle centers; seen in follicular lymphomas and DLBCL, leg type	Also stains a wide range of normal and neoplastic T cells, both inside and outside follicles
BCL6 nuclear	Transcription factor	Positive in follicular lymphoma and in a subset of diffuse large B-cell lymphoma	Also positive in nuclei of normal germinal center cells and epithelia, pattern useful in determining the organization of germinal centers
BOB-1 nuclear	Lymphocyte transcription cofactor	Marks L and H cells in nodular lymphocyte predominant	Germinal center cells Negative in RS-cells of classic Hodgkin lymphoma

Table 2.2 (continued)

Antibody/reactivity	Main specificity	Uses	Normal skin and other reactivities
Cyclin D1 nuclear	Transcription factor	Mantle cell lymphoma versus other lymphomas	Some cases of plasma cell myeloma and hairy cell leukemia Epithelia reactivity in normal tissue
EBV-LMP1/EBER ISH Cytoplasmic/nuclear	Epstein-Barr virus	Useful in extranodal NK T cell and posttransplant lymphomas	
Factor XIIIa nuclear	Histiocytes and dermal dendrocytes	Useful in distinguishing dermal dendritic cells from lymphomas	Normal dermal dendrocytes
Granzyme B cytoplasmic	Granulysin or cytotoxic granules of cytotoxic effector cells	Cytotoxic T-cell marker in CD8 or cytotoxic lymphomas; one half of LyP, advanced stage mycosis fungoides, increased in lymphoid hyperplasia	Some T-cell lymphomas especially of LGL or cytotoxic NK T-cell origin
IRF4 (MUM1) nuclear	Multiple myeloma 1 MUM1/IRF4 expressed in post-germinal center B cells including leg type of DLBCL. Often coexpressed with CD30 in ALCL and LyP	Regulator factor protein, B-cell proliferation/differentiation marker	Prognostic marker in nodal DLBCL
Kappa Lambda ISH or IHC cytoplasmic	Light chains	Useful in determining clonal restriction in plasma cells; may be useful in cutaneous B-cell lymphomas, especially marginal zone lymphoma	May not react to neoplastic B cells despite expression in nonneoplastic plasma cells in the background
Ki67/MIB1 nuclear	Proliferative marker surrogate for DNA synthesis	Useful in determining the proliferative activity and grading of cutaneous lymphomas	High in aggressive versus low in low-grade lymphoma, cross-reacts with proliferating epithelia
Herpes simplex virus 2	Immunostains HSV2	Useful in workup of herpes-induced pseudolymphoma	e.g., basal layer keratinocytes
Myeloperoxidase cytoplasmic	Granulocytes and some monocytes	Granulocytes cell marker (mature myeloid cells) useful in granulocytic sarcoma positive in most AML	Monocytes with weaker staining than those of granulocytic lineage
CD246 (p80; ALK1) nuclear cytoplasmic	Anaplastic lymphoma kinase-1	Anaplastic large cell lymphoma; ALK+; also ALK cytoplasmic + nuclear usually positive in secondary ALCL and only rarely positive (cytoplasmic) in primary cutaneous ALCL	Large cell lymphoma workup
S100 cytoplasmic	Neuroectodermal marker	Interdigitating reticulum cells and Langerhans cells and Rosai-Dorfman disease	Melanomas, most sarcomas, gamma-delta T cells and Schwann and other stromal cells
TCRβ TCR gamma-delta membrane	T-cell receptor subsets	Useful in determining the origin of a subcutaneous or other T-cell lymphomas	Normal T cells in a 9:1 ratio between beta and gamma
TdT nuclear	Terminal deoxyribonucleotidyl transferase	Immature B and T cells as well as myeloid cells	Precursor lymphoblastic leukemia, T or B and some rare AML subtypes

(continued)

Table 2.2 (continued)

Antibody/reactivity	Main specificity	Uses	Normal skin and other reactivities
TIA-1 cytoplasmic	T-cell intracellular antigen 1	Cytotoxic T-cell marker	Positive in some T-cell lymphomas, such as CD8 or gamma-delta T-cell lymphoma and T-cell LGL leukemia
Pankeratin cytoplasmic	Cocktail of AE1, AE3, Cam 5.2	Useful in carcinoma undifferentiated tumor versus lymphoma	Epithelia/keratinocytes
Pax-5	Transcription factor active in early stages of B-cell differentiation	Most B-cell neoplasms, Reed-Sternberg cells, rare ALCL	Useful in the differential diagnosis of undifferentiated neoplasms
EMA	Epithelial membrane antigen	Application in systemic ALCL versus cutaneous ALCL	EMA seen in systemic and not in cutaneous CD30 lymphomas, epithelia, plasma cells

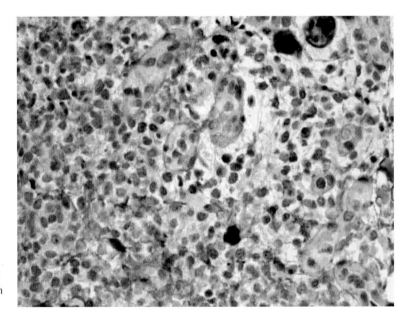

Fig. 2.4 CD1a. High-power view of CD1a brown-stained dermal Langerhans cells with dendritic processes

Fig. 2.5 CD2. Pan T-cell staining on a contact dermatitis as well as with partial staining of CD2 with receptors in Langerhans cell vesicles and with other dermal T lymphocytes

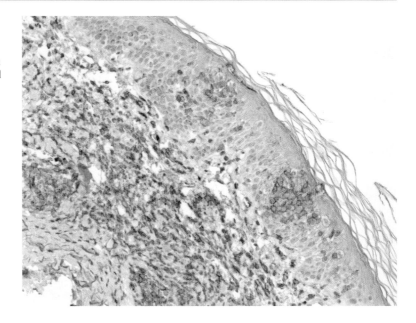

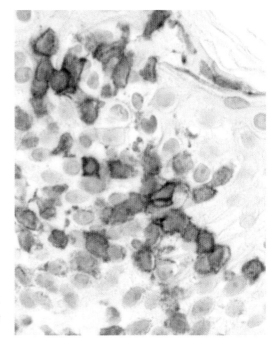

Fig. 2.6 CD3. Oil magnification view of nuclear contour highlighted by CD3 stain

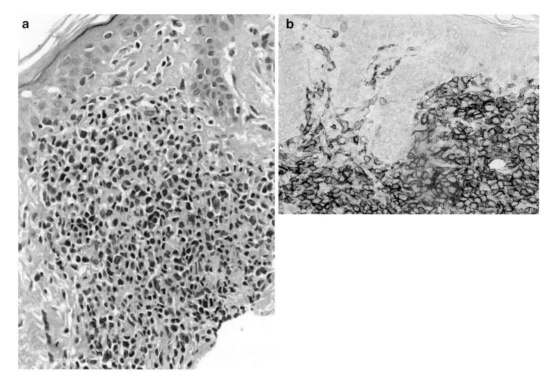

Fig. 2.7 CD4. Histology of solitary cutaneous small and medium T-cell lymphoma with corresponding CD4 immunostaining below

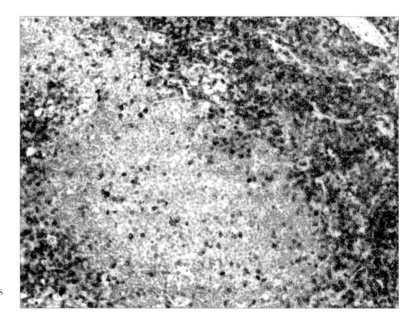

Fig. 2.8 CD5. Staining mostly of interfollicular T cells with partial weaker staining of mantle zone cells and germinal center T cells

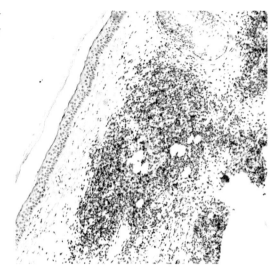

Fig. 2.9   CD7. T cells partly stained with CD7 in a solitary cutaneous small and medium T cell-lymphoma

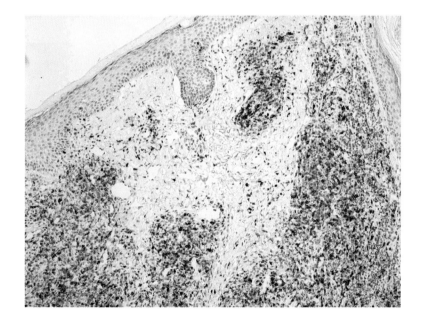

Fig. 2.10   CD8. Dermal CD8-positive T cells in lymphomatous folliculitis secondary to acneiform follicular hair plugging reaction

Fig. 2.11 CD10. Stromal fibrous interfollicular pattern of staining of CD10 in cutaneous lymphoid hyperplasia. Note the weaker staining of benign germinal center

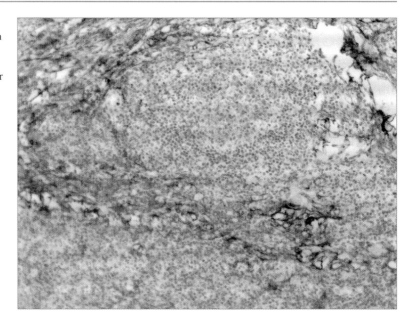

Fig. 2.12 Reed-Sternberg cell stained for CD15; adjacent granulocytes stain diffusely. Reed-Sternberg cells typically are found in the lymph nodes involved by Hodgkin lymphoma, rarely in the skin

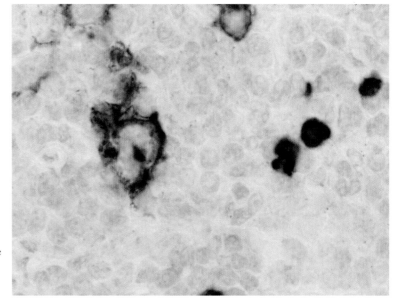

Fig. 2.13 CD20. Normal staining pattern in cutaneous lymphoid hyperplasia with paler staining centers and darker mantle zone lymphocytes separated by nonstaining interfollicular T cells

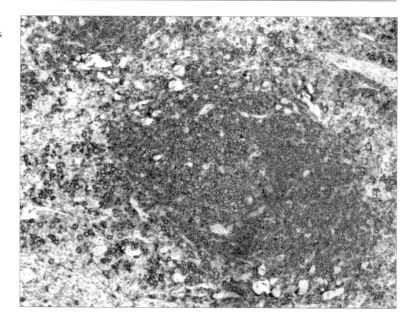

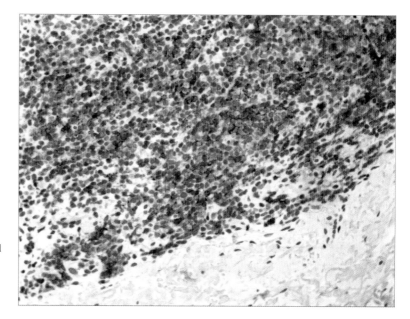

Fig. 2.14 CD23. Dense staining of CD23-positive infiltrate in the skin involved by systemic chronic lymphocytic leukemia that was also CD5 positive and CD20 positive

Fig. 2.15 CD30. Typical
high-power view of clusters
of lymphomatoid papulosis
neoplastic CD30 large cells

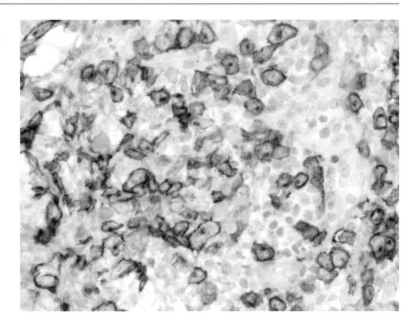

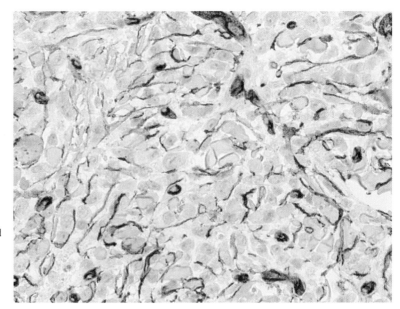

Fig. 2.16 CD34. Vessels and
endothelia show as immunoreactive internal control for
the evaluation of stem cell
blasts in the skin with blastic
infiltrate

Fig. 2.17 CD43. Sheets of myeloid sarcoma immature cells stained with CD43

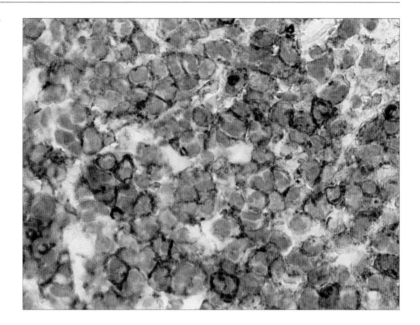

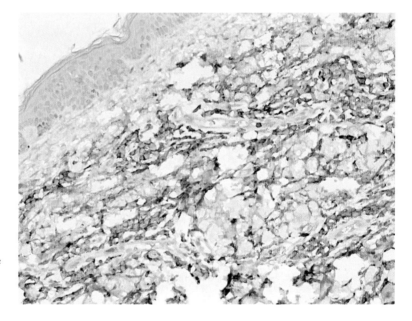

Fig. 2.18 CD45. Leukocyte common antigen (LCA) in myelomonocytic skin infiltrate

Fig. 2.19 CD56. Single-file blastic infiltrate of a leukemia cutis rare type of blastic plasmacytoid dendritic cell leukemia

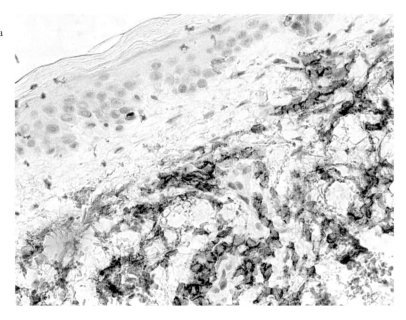

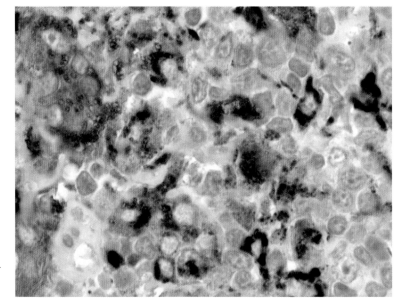

Fig. 2.20 CD68. Large epithelioid CD68 + histiocytes with lymphophagocytosis in cutaneous Rosai-Dorfman disease

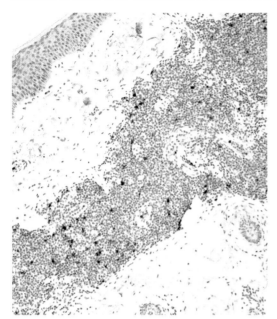

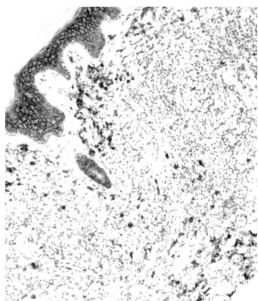

Fig. 2.21 CD79a. Scattered CD79a + B cells and plasma cells in predominantly T-cell nodular infiltrate

Fig. 2.23 CD138. Dermal plasma cells and epithelia in the skin and dermis stain with CD138

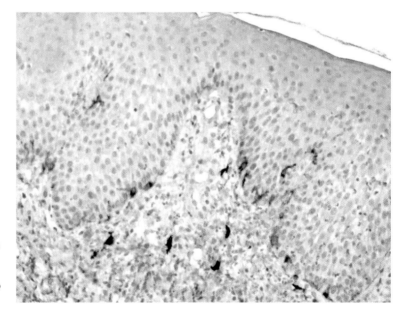

Fig. 2.22 CD117. Melanocytes, melanophages with melanin, and adnexa are CD117 (stem cell factor receptor) typical skin reactivity that may be used to determine pigmentation

Fig. 2.24 CD279 (pro-
grammed death 1, PD1).
Staining of follicle T helper
cell seen in normal germinal
centers and useful for
determining if a lymphoma in
the skin has follicle T helper
origin

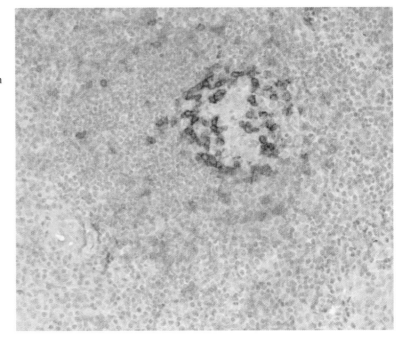

Fig. 2.25 Bcl2. Reactive T
cells in and around an
atypical cutaneous lymphoid
hyperplasia with disorganized
germinal centers, same cases
as the following Bcl6

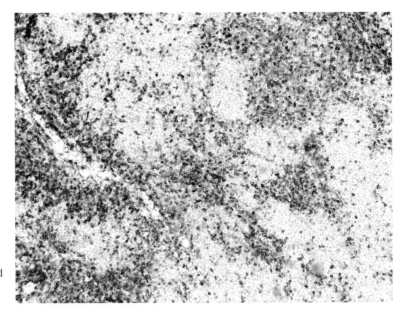

Fig. 2.26 Bcl6. Disorganized germinal centers highlighted by bcl6 nuclear stain

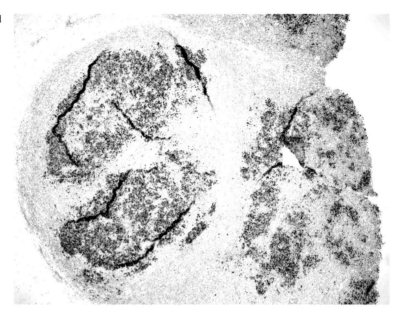

Fig. 2.27 Cyclin D1. Normal tissue reactivity of cyclin D1 (bcl-1) for mantle cell lymphoma showing reactivity to normal endothelial lining tissue and larger darker staining scattered histiocytes. Epidermis weakly stained (not shown)

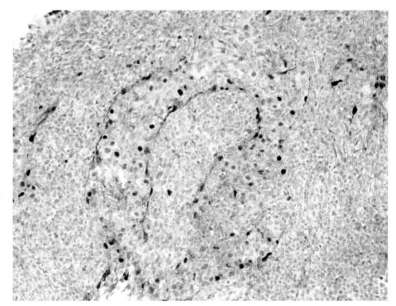

Fig. 2.28 Factor XIIIa.
Dermal dendrocytes showing
granular cytoplasmic staining
of marrow-derived histio-
cytes, putative origin of
fibrohistiocytomas in the skin

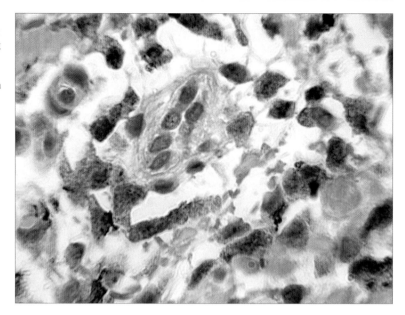

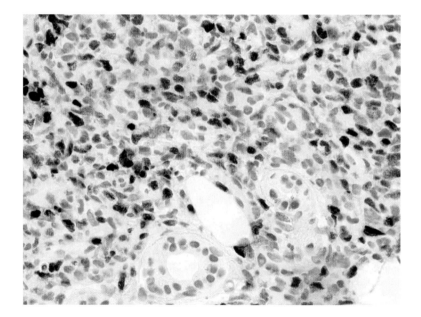

Fig. 2.29 MUM1. Diffuse
large B-cell lymphoma, leg
type with MUM1 (IRF4)
nuclear positivity

Fig. 2.30 Ki67. Proliferating lymphocytes in the dermis along with few nuclear reactive keratinocytes stained with Ki67

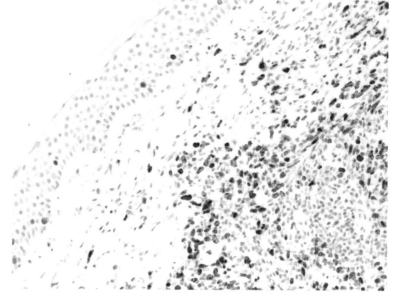

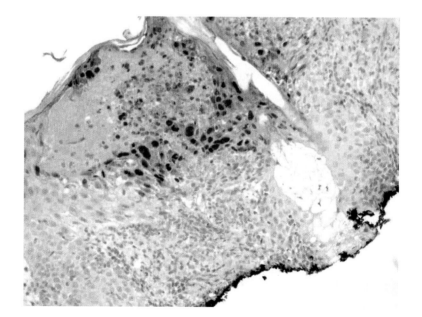

Fig. 2.31 HSV2. Herpes simplex immunostain showing nuclear reactive infected keratinocytes and intense lymphohistiocytic dermal response. Herpes infection is a rare cause of pseudolymphoma

Fig. 2.32 S100. Sentinel cells or epidermal Langerhans cells highlighted by S100b stain

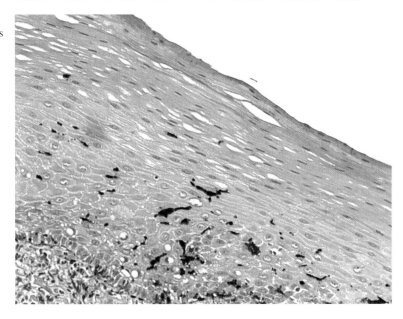

Fig. 2.33 TdT. Lymphoblasts in oil power with TdT nuclear positivity consistent with precursor lymphoblastic leukemia skin involvement

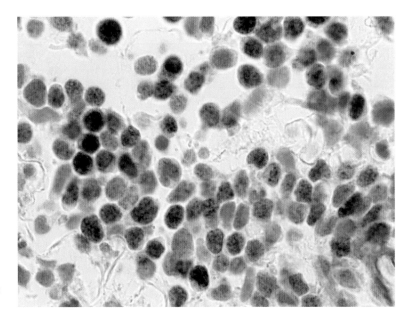

Fig. 2.34 Pankeratin. Highlighted keratinocytes with epidermotropic lymphocytes

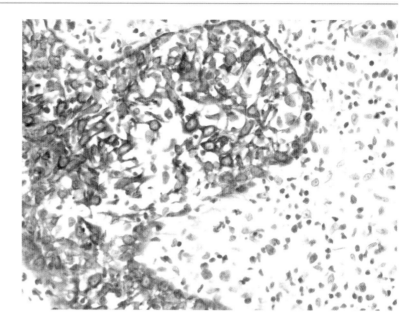

References

Alam MS, Maekawa Y, Kitamura A, Tanigaki K, Yoshimoto T, Kishihara K, et al. Notch signaling drives IL-22 secretion in CD4+ T cells by stimulating the aryl hydrocarbon receptor. Proc Natl Acad Sci U S A. 2010;107:5943–8.

Asarch A, Barak O, Loo DS, Gottlieb AB. Th17 cells: a new therapeutic target in inflammatory dermatoses. J Dermatolog Treat. 2008;19(6):318–26.

Beetz S, Wesch D, Marischen L, Welte S, Oberg HH, Kabelitz D. Innate immune functions of human gamma delta T cells. Immunobiology. 2008;213(3–4): 173–82.

Beres AJ, Drobyski WR. The role of regulatory T cells in the biology of graft versus host disease. Front Immunol. 2013;4:163.

Berger CL, Hanlon D, Kanada D, Dhodapkar M, Lombillo V, Wang N, Christensen I, Howe G, Crouch J, El-Fishawy P, Edelson R. The growth of cutaneous T-cell lymphoma is stimulated by immature dendritic cells. Blood. 2002;99(8):2929–39.

Ciree A, Michel L, Camilleri-Broet S, Jean LF, Oster M, Flageul B, Senet P, Fossiez F, Fridman WH, Bachelez H, Tartour E. Expression and activity of IL-17 in cutaneous T-cell lymphomas (mycosis fungoides and Sezary syndrome). Int J Cancer. 2004;112(1):113–20.

Clark RA. Skin-resident T, cells: the ups and downs of on site immunity. J Invest Dermatol. 2010;130(2): 362–70.

Duhen T, Geiger R, Jarrossay D, Lanzavecchia A, Sallusto F. Production of interleukin 22 but not interleukin 17 by a subset of human skin-homing memory T cells. Nat Immunol. 2009;10:857–63.

Ebert LM, Meuter S, Moser B. Homing and function of human skin gamma delta T cells and NK cells: relevance for tumor surveillance. J Immunol. 2006;176(7): 4331–6.

Edelson RL. Cutaneous T, cell lymphoma: the helping hand of dendritic cells. Ann N Y Acad Sci. 2001; 941:1–11.

Egawa G, Honda T, Tanizaki H, Doi H, Miyachi Y, Kabashima K. In vivo imaging of T-cell motility in the elicitation phase of contact hypersensitivity using two-photon microscopy. J Invest Dermatol. 2011;131(4): 977–9.

Egawa G, Kabashima K. Skin as a peripheral lymphoid organ: revisiting the concept of skin-associated lymphoid tissues. J Invest Dermatol. 2011;131(11): 2178–85.

Fuhlbrigge RC, Kieffer JD, Armerding D, Kupper TS. Cutaneous lymphocyte antigen is a specialized form of PSGL-1 expressed on skin-homing T cells. Nature. 1997;389(6654):978–81.

Gebhardt T, Wakim LM, Eidsmo L, Reading PC, Heath WR, Carbone FR. Memory T cells in nonlymphoid tissue that provide enhanced local immunity during infection with herpes simplex virus. Nat Immunol. 2009;10(5):524–30.

Gebhardt T, Whitney PG, Zaid A, Mackay LK, Brooks AG, Heath WR, Carbone FR, Mueller SN. Different patterns of peripheral migration by memory CD4+ and CD8+ T cells. Nature. 2011;477(7363):216–9.

Hocker TL, Wada DA, El-Azhary R, Gibson LE. Expression of T-cell receptor-gamma delta in normal human skin, inflammatory dermatoses and mycosis fungoides. J Cutan Pathol. 2012;39(4):419–24.

Hoeller C, Richardson SK, Ng LG, Valero T, Wysocka M, Rook AH, Weninger W. In vivo imaging of cutaneous

T-cell lymphoma migration to the skin. Cancer Res. 2009;69(7):2704–8.

Holtmeier W, Kabelitz D. gamma delta T cells link innate and adaptive immune responses. Chem Immunol Allergy. 2005;86:151–83.

Kabelitz D. Function and specificity of human gamma/delta-positive T cells. Crit Rev Immunol. 1992;11(5): 281–303.

Kabelitz D. gamma delta T-cells: cross-talk between innate and adaptive immunity. Cell Mol Life Sci. 2011;68(14):2331–3.

Kabelitz D, Glatzel A, Wesch D. Antigen recognition by human gamma delta T lymphocytes. Int Arch Allergy Immunol. 2000;122(1):1–7.

Kabelitz D, Marischen L, Oberg HH, Holtmeier W, Wesch D. Epithelial defence by gamma delta T cells. Int Arch Allergy Immunol. 2005;137(1):73–81.

Kadin ME, Nasu K, Sako D, Su IJ. Distinctive phorbol ester-induced morphological and surface antigen changes in mycosis fungoides, the Sezary syndrome, and adult T-cell leukemia. Cancer Res. 1984;44(8): 3383–7.

Kadin ME, Pavlov IY, Delgado JC, Vonderheid EC. High soluble CD30, CD25, and IL-6 may identify patients with worse survival in CD30+ cutaneous lymphomas and early mycosis fungoides. J Invest Dermatol. 2012;132(3 Pt 1):703–10.

Kaplan DH, Jenison MC, Saeland S, Shlomchik WD, Shlomchik MJ. Epidermal langerhans cell-deficient mice develop enhanced contact hypersensitivity. Immunity. 2005;23(6):611–20.

Kaplan DH, Kissenpfennig A, Clausen BE. Insights into Langerhans cell function from Langerhans cell ablation models. Eur J Immunol. 2008;38(9):2369–76.

Kim EJ, Hess S, Richardson SK, Newton S, Showe LC, Benoit BM, Ubriani R, Vittorio CC, Junkins-Hopkins JM, Wysocka M, Rook AH. Immunopathogenesis and therapy of cutaneous T cell lymphoma. J Clin Invest. 2005;115(4):798–812.

Koga C, Kabashima K, Shiraishi N, Kobayashi M, Tokura Y. Possible pathogenic role of Th17 cells for atopic dermatitis. J Invest Dermatol. 2008;128(11):2625–30.

Kunstfeld R, Lechleitner S, Groger M, Wolff K, Petzelbauer P. HECA-452+ T cells migrate through superficial vascular plexus but not through deep vascular plexus endothelium. J Invest Dermatol. 1997; 108(3):343–8.

Kupper TS, Edelson RL. The role of cytokines in the pathophysiology of T cell mediated skin disease. J Dermatol. 1987;14(6):517–23.

Lechleitner S, Kunstfeld R, Messeritsch-Fanta C, Wolff K, Petzelbauer P. Peripheral lymph node addressins are expressed on skin endothelial cells. J Invest Dermatol. 1999;113(3):410–4.

Litvinov IV, Jones DA, Sasseville D, Kupper TS. Transcriptional profiles predict disease outcome in patients with cutaneous T-cell lymphoma. Clin Cancer Res. 2010;16(7):2106–14.

Mackay CR, Kimpton WG, Brandon MR, Cahill RN. Lymphocyte subsets show marked differences in their distribution between blood and the afferent and efferent lymph of peripheral lymph nodes. J Exp Med. 1988;167(6):1755–65.

Maddur MS, Miossec P, Kaveri SV, Bayry J. Th17 cells: biology, pathogenesis of autoimmune and inflammatory diseases, and therapeutic strategies. Am J Pathol. 2012;181(1):8–18.

Magro CM, Wang X. Indolent primary cutaneous gamma/delta T-cell lymphoma localized to the subcutaneous panniculus and its association with atypical lymphocytic lobular panniculitis. Am J Clin Pathol. 2012;138(1):50–6.

Matheu MP, Beeton C, Garcia A, Chi V, Rangaraju S, Safrina O, Monaghan K, Uemura MI, Li D, Pal S, De la Maza LM, Monuki E, Flugel A, Pennington MW, Parker I, Chandy KG, Cahalan MD. Imaging of effector memory T cells during a delayed-type hypersensitivity reaction and suppression by Kv1.3 channel block. Immunity. 2008;29(4):602–14.

Matutes E, Robinson D, O'Brien M, Haynes BF, Zola H, Catovsky D. Candidate counterparts of Sezary cells and adult T-cell lymphoma-leukaemia cells in normal peripheral blood: an ultrastructural study with the immunogold method and monoclonal antibodies. Leuk Res. 1983;7(6):787–801.

Merz H, Fliedner A, Orscheschek K, Binder T, Sebald W, Muller-Hermelink HK, et al. Cytokine expression in T-cell lymphomas and Hodgkin's disease. Its possible implication in autocrine or paracrine production as a potential basis for neoplastic growth. Am J Pathol. 1991;139:1173–80.

Meyerson HJ, Awadallah A, Pavlidakey P, Cooper K, Honda K, Miedler J. Follicular center helper T-cell (TFH) marker positive mycosis fungoides/Sezary syndrome. Mod Pathol. 2013;26:32–43.

Miossec P, Korn T, Kuchroo VK. Interleukin-17 and type 17 helper T cells. N Engl J Med. 2009;361(9): 888–98.

Pelletier M, Maggi L, Micheletti A, Lazzeri E, Tamassia N, Costantini C, et al. Evidence for a cross-talk between human neutrophils and Th17 cells. Blood. 2010;115:335–43.

Reinhold U, Herpertz M, Kukel S, Oltermann I, Uerlich M, Kreysel HW. Induction of nuclear contour irregularity during T-cell activation via the T-cell receptor/CD3 complex and CD2 antigens in the presence of phorbol esters. Blood. 1994;83(3):703–6.

Rodriguez Pinilla SM, Roncador G, Rodriguez-Peralto JL, Mollejo M, Garcia JF, Montes-Moreno S, et al. Primary cutaneous CD4+ small/medium-sized pleomorphic T-cell lymphoma expresses follicular T-cell markers. Am J Surg Pathol. 2009;33:81–90.

Saed G, Fivenson DP, Naidu Y, Nickoloff BJ. Mycosis fungoides exhibits a Th1-type cell-mediated cytokine profile whereas Sezary syndrome expresses a Th2-type profile. J Invest Dermatol. 1994;103(1):29–33.

Schaerli P, Ebert L, Willimann K, Blaser A, Roos RS, Loetscher P, Moser B. A skin-selective homing mechanism for human immune surveillance T cells. J Exp Med. 2004;199(9):1265–75.

Streilein JW. Lymphocyte traffic, T-cell malignancies and the skin. J Invest Dermatol. 1978;71(3):167–71.

Streilein JW. Skin-associated lymphoid tissues (SALT): origins and functions. J Invest Dermatol. 1983; 80(Suppl):12s–616.

Streilein JW. Circuits and signals of the skin-associated lymphoid tissues (SALT). J Invest Dermatol. 1985;85(1 Suppl):10s–313.

Streilein JW. Skin-associated lymphoid tissue. Immunol Ser. 1989;46:73–96.

Streilein JW, Bergstresser PR. Langerhans cells: antigen presenting cells of the epidermis. Immunobiology. 1984;168(3–5):285–300.

Tomura M. Visualization of cellular dynamics in the entire body using the photoconvertible protein "Kaede" of transgenic mice. Seikagaku. 2012;84(3):195–202.

Tomura M, Yoshida N, Tanaka J, Karasawa S, Miwa Y, Miyawaki A, Kanagawa O. Monitoring cellular movement in vivo with photoconvertible fluorescence protein "Kaede" transgenic mice. Proc Natl Acad Sci U S A. 2008;105(31):10871–6.

Vowels BR, Lessin SR, Cassin M, Jaworsky C, Benoit B, Wolfe JT, Rook AH. Th2 cytokine mRNA expression in skin in cutaneous T-cell lymphoma. J Invest Dermatol. 1994a;103(5):669–73.

Vowels MR, Tiedemann K, Lam-Po-Tang R, Tucker DP. Use of granulocyte-macrophage colony-stimulating factor in two children treated with cord blood transplantation. Blood Cells. 1994b;20(2–3):249–54.

Wakim LM, Gebhardt T, Heath WR, Carbone FR. Cutting edge: local recall responses by memory T cells newly recruited to peripheral nonlymphoid tissues. J Immunol. 2008;181(9):5837–41.

Wasik MA, Vonderheid EC, Bigler RD, Marti R, Lessin SR, Polansky M, Kadin ME. Increased serum concentration of the soluble interleukin-2 receptor in cutaneous T-cell lymphoma. Clinical and prognostic implications. Arch Dermatol. 1996;132(1): 42–7.

Wolk K, Haugen HS, Xu W, Witte E, Waggie K, Anderson M, Vom BE, Witte K, Warszawska K, Philipp S, Johnson-Leger C, Volk HD, Sterry W, Sabat R. IL-22 and IL-20 are key mediators of the epidermal alterations in psoriasis while IL-17 and IFN-gamma are not. J Mol Med (Berl). 2009;87(5):523–36.

Zhou L, Lopes JE, Chong MM, Ivanov II, Min R, Victora GD, et al. TGF-beta-induced Foxp3 inhibits T(H)17 cell differentiation by antagonizing RORgammat function. Nature. 2008;453:236–40.

Zhou L, Chong MM, Littman DR. Plasticity of CD4+ T cell lineage differentiation. Immunity. 2009;30: 646–55.

Role of Immunohistochemistry and Chromogenic In Situ Hybridization in Diagnosis

3

Mark C. Mochel and Mai P. Hoang

Introduction

Immunohistochemistry utilizes antigen-antibody recognition in detecting specific antigens within tissues. Due to technical advances, there has been a significant increase in the number of diagnostic immunohistochemical stains and chromogenic in situ hybridization available to pathologists in recent years. The sensitivity and specificity of each antibody, its pattern of staining (nuclear, cytoplasmic, or membranous), and background artifact must be considered in its interpretation. In addition, evaluation must be done in relation to internal controls. In the diagnosis of lymphoid infiltrates, a panel of immunohistochemical markers is helpful in narrowing the differential diagnoses. In this chapter, an update of recently available immunohistochemical stains as well as selected diagnostic panels are outlined. These panels are used to distinguish reactive lymphoid hyperplasia from low-grade B-cell lymphoma, diffuse cutaneous follicle center cell lymphoma from diffuse large B-cell lymphoma, subcutaneous panniculitic T-cell lymphoma from cutaneous gamma-delta T-cell lymphoma, CD30-positive lymphoproliferative disorders from reactive processes, follicular mucinosis from folliculotropic mycosis fungoides, and lymphomatoid drug eruption from plaque-stage mycosis fungoides.

Recently Available Immunohistochemical Markers

PD1

Programmed cell death protein 1 (PD1) is a protein encoded by the *PDCD1* gene (Shinohara et al. 1995) and is a member of T-cell regulators (Ishida et al. 1992). PD-1, a marker of germinal center-associated T cells (Fig. 3.1a), is expressed by neoplastic cells in primary cutaneous CD4+ small-/medium-sized pleomorphic T-cell lymphoma (Rodriguez Pinilla et al. 2009) and angio-immunoblastic T-cell lymphoma (Dorfman et al. 2006). Its expression can be seen in cutaneous pseudo-T-cell lymphoma; thus, PD-1 is *not* a helpful diagnostic marker in the distinction of a reactive T-cell process from cutaneous CD4+ small-/medium-sized pleomorphic T-cell lymphoma (Cetinozman et al. 2012).

CD123

CD123, interleukin-3 receptor alpha (Munoz et al. 2001), is a marker of plasmacytoid dendritic cells and the blastic plasmacytoid dendritic cell neoplasm. A tumor characterized by dense

M.C. Mochel, MD
Department of Pathology, Massachusetts
General Hospital, Boston, MA, USA

M.P. Hoang, MD (✉)
Department of Pathology, Harvard Medical School,
Massachusetts General Hospital, 55 Fruit Street,
Warren 820, Boston, MA 02114, USA
e-mail: mhoang@mgh.harvard.edu

H.D. Cualing et al. (eds.), *Cutaneous Hematopathology*,
DOI 10.1007/978-1-4939-0950-6_3, © Springer Science+Business Media New York 2014

55

monomorphous infiltrates of medium-sized blastoid cells positive for CD4, CD56, and CD123 (Cota et al. 2010; Facchetti et al. 2008).

CD14

CD14 has been reported to be a specific marker for monocytic differentiation, but with low sensitivity in comparison to CD68 (Klco et al. 2011).

B-Cell Transcription Factors Including MUM1/IRF-4, PAX5, OCT2, and BOB.1

The multiple myeloma oncogene 1 (*MUM1*)/interferon regulator factor 4 (*IRF4*) gene encodes the MUM1 protein which is normally expressed in plasma cells, a small fraction of B cells, and activated T cells (Gualco et al. 2010). MUM1 expression is seen in several malignancies including plasma cell myeloma (Iida et al. 1997),

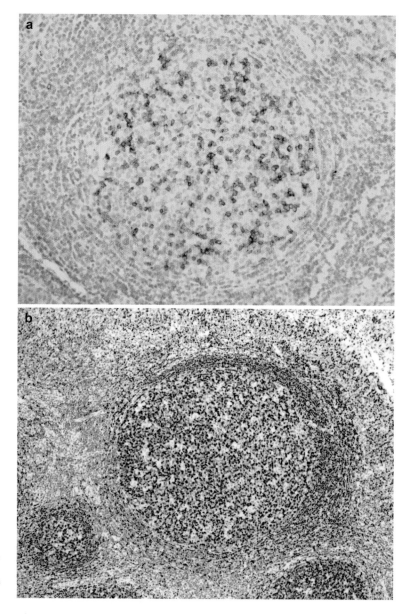

Fig. 3.1 PD1 (**a**), PAX5 (**b**), OCT2 (**c**), and BOB.1 (**d**) immunostaining of a reactive germinal center

Fig. 3.1 (continued)

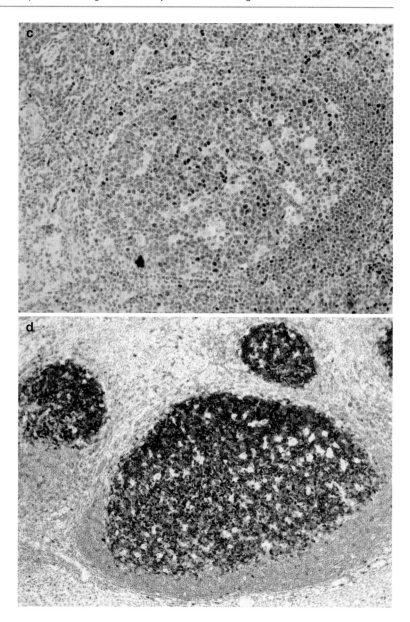

diffuse large B-cell lymphomas (especially cutaneous diffuse large B-cell lymphomas, leg type), and systemic anaplastic large cell lymphomas (Tsuboi et al. 2000; Natkunam et al. 2001; Hoefnagel et al. 2003).

PAX5 (paired box gene 5) is a pan B- and pan pre-B-cell marker present in most B-cell neoplasms (both mature and immature) (Fig. 3.1b). Approximately one-third of plasma cell neo-

plasms express PAX5. Reed-Sternberg cells of classical Hodgkin lymphoma and the L&H (lymphocyte and histiocytic) cells of nodular lymphocyte predominant Hodgkin lymphoma are PAX5 positive (Torlakovic et al. 2002). PAX5 is also expressed in some anaplastic large cell lymphomas (Feldman et al. 2010).

OCT2 is a transcription factor restricted to B lymphocytes and is associated with BOB.1, a

B-cell transcriptional coactivator (Krenacs et al. 1998) (Fig. 3.1c). BOB.1 is less lineage specific than OCT2, being expressed in T-cell as well as B-cell lymphomas (Fig. 3.1d). BOB.1 is strongly positive in a range of non-Hodgkin lymphomas. It is generally not expressed in classical Hodgkin lymphoma; however, weak expression has been reported, making interpretation challenging.

TCR Gamma

The T-cell receptor (TCR) is comprised of two ligand-binding glycoproteins containing variable regions (alpha-beta and gamma-delta) (Rojo et al. 2008). The gamma-delta T cells can comprise up to 16 % of T cells in mucosal sites, particularly the intestine and skin (Groh et al. 1989). Rodriguez-Pinilla et al. (2013) found the expression of TCR gamma to be a characteristic feature of primary cutaneous gamma-delta T-cell lymphoma (PCGD-TCL) (5/5), although its expression was also noted in other primary cutaneous lymphomas including isolated cases of mycosis fungoides (MF) and lymphomatoid papulosis (LyP) type D, representing approximately 8 % of the 146 primary cutaneous T-cell lymphoma (CTCL) cases analyzed. While TCR beta F1 antibody has been available for decades, TCR-gamma-delta antibody has become available only recently (Krajewski et al. 1989; Rodriguez-Pinilla et al. 2013).

Reactive Lymphoid Hyperplasia Versus Low-Grade B-Cell Lymphoma

The differential diagnosis of cytologically low-grade lymphoid proliferations in the skin includes reactive lymphoid hyperplasia, primary cutaneous marginal zone B-cell lymphoma (PCMZL), and primary cutaneous follicle center lymphoma (PCFCL). Nonneoplastic or reactive lymphoid proliferations mimicking lymphoma ("pseudolymphoma") typically consist of a mixed population of B and T lymphocytes (Cerroni et al. 2000). Variable quantities of scattered CD3 and CD20 staining can help to establish the reactive nature of the lymphoid infiltrate. The germinal center cells of reactive lymphoid follicles are CD20+, CD79a+, Bcl2−, and Bcl6+, while cells of the mantle zone are Bcl2+ (Hoefnagel et al. 2003). Reactive germinal center cells as well as scattered interfollicular cells may stain for CD10 (Hoefnagel et al. 2003; Cerroni et al. 2000). For reactive populations, evaluation of B lymphocytes by light chain in situ hybridization should demonstrate a mixed kappa and lambda population (Levy et al. 1977). Reactive follicles also tend to show Ki-67 staining in the vast majority of germinal center cells, whereas the cells in the neoplastic follicles of PCFCL frequently show less than 50 % positive Ki-67 staining (Cerroni et al. 2000).

PCMZL is characterized by peri- and interfollicular proliferation of marginal zone cells (small- to medium-sized cells with indented nuclei and pale cytoplasm) which are CD20+, CD79a+, Bcl2+, Bcl6−, CD5−, and CD10− (Servitje et al. 2002; de Leval et al. 2001; Cerroni et al. 2000) (Fig. 3.2). In contrast to cells of PCFCLs, cells of PCMZL are CD5−, CD10−, and Bcl6− (Hoefnagel et al. 2003). Commonly, aggregates of plasma cells are seen at the periphery of the tumor which exhibit kappa or lambda light chain restriction (de Leval et al. 2001; Servitje et al. 2002) (Fig. 3.2). The presence of Bcl2+, Bcl6−, and CD10− infiltrating lymphocytes strongly supports the diagnosis of PCMZL over PCFCL or reactive lymphoid hyperplasia (Hoefnagel et al. 2003); however, reactive interfollicular T cells may also show this staining pattern. PCMZL is often associated with reactive follicles with the CD10+, Bcl2−, and Bcl6+ immunophenotype which may represent a diagnostic pitfall if not recognized (de Leval et al. 2001; Hoefnagel et al. 2003). CD21, a marker of follicular dendritic cells (FDC), often highlights an expanded follicular dendritic meshwork due to colonized neoplastic marginal zone or plasmacytoid cells admixed with reactive follicular cells (de Leval et al. 2001). This pattern of CD21 staining, highlighting the colonized germinal centers with distorted architecture, can be helpful in establishing the diagnosis of PCMZL (Fig. 3.2).

PCFCL characteristically appears as a nodular to diffuse lymphoid proliferation with neoplastic follicle center B cells (centrocytes and centroblasts) which are CD20+, CD79a+, Bcl2−, and Bcl6+ (Cerroni et al. 2000; Hoefnagel et al. 2003). Different authors describe the neoplastic cells as CD10+ (Cerroni et al. 2000), CD10− (Hoefnagel et al. 2003), or CD10 variable (de Leval et al. 2001). CD10-negative PCFCL is often seen in diffuse form or areas of PCFCL. Besides Bcl6 and CD10 as germinal center signature differentiation markers, PAX5 and interferon regulatory factor (IRF) 8 are also useful. While the neoplastic cells of PCFCL are typically Bcl2− (Hoefnagel et al. 2003; Hoefnagel et al. 2005; Cerroni et al. 2000; Child et al. 2001) in contrast to the Bcl2 positivity demonstrated by nodal follicular lymphoma, some authors

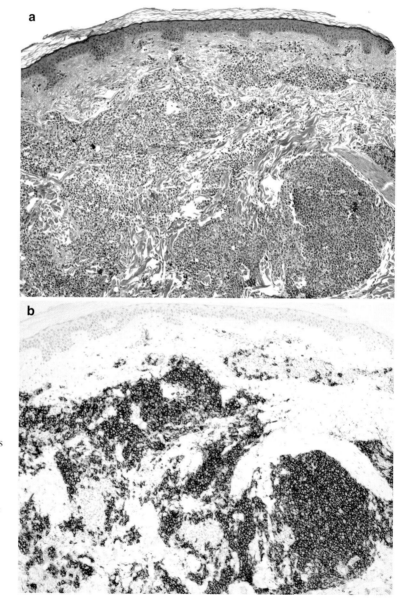

Fig. 3.2 The neoplastic cells of a marginal zone lymphoma (**a**) are positive for CD20 (**b**) and Bcl-2 (**c**). CD21 highlights the expanded follicular dendritic meshwork due to colonized neoplastic cells (**d**). Lambda (**e**) and kappa (**f**) in situ hybridization demonstrate lambda light chain restriction

Fig. 3.2 (continued)

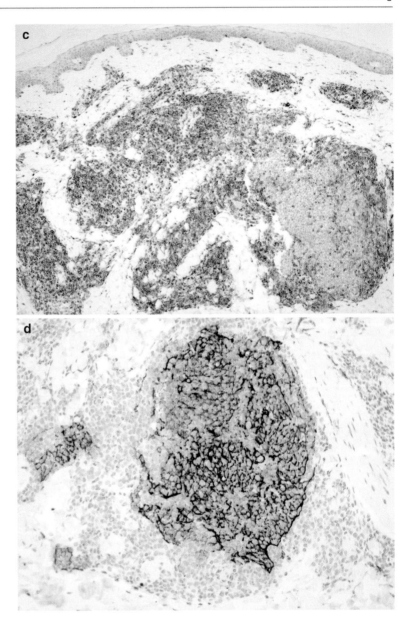

have demonstrated cases of PCFCL to be Bcl2+ (de Leval et al. 2001; Goodlad et al. 2002). Moreover, secondary cutaneous involvement of nodal follicular lymphoma is usually Bcl2+, and clinical investigations of BCL2+ cutane- ous follicular lymphomas often disclose extra- cutaneous primary disease. As mentioned above, neoplastic follicles of PCFCL often show less than 50 % positivity for Ki-67 versus reactive follicle cells which are predominately

Fig. 3.2   (continued)

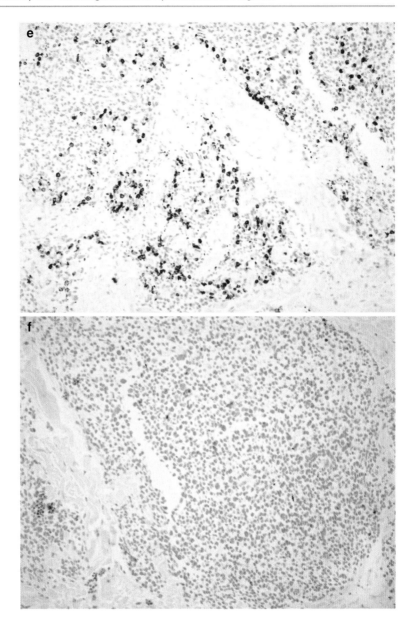

Ki-67 positive (Cerroni et al. 2000). In PCFCL with a prominent nodular arrangement, CD21+ FDCs are present as a sharply defined, thick rim surrounding neoplastic follicles (de Leval et al. 2001; Cerroni et al. 2000).

Recommended panel (Table 3.1): CD3, CD20, Bcl2, Bcl6, CD21, and kappa and lambda in situ hybridization (CD5, CD10, cyclin D1, Ki67, kappa/lambda IHC as additional informative second-line markers)

Table 3.1 Immunoprofile of reactive lymphoid hyperplasia versus low-grade B-cell lymphoma (de Leval et al. 2001; Goodlad et al. 2002)

	Reactive lymphoid hyperplasia	Marginal zone B-cell lymphoma	Follicle center cell lymphoma
CD20	Germinal center +	+	+
Bcl2	Mantle zone + Germinal center –	+	Usually – (+10–25 %)
Bcl6	Germinal center +	–	+
CD21	Intact germinal center	Expanded germinal center	Follicles – Perifollicular rim +
Kappa and lambda in situ hybridization	Mixed light chain expression	Light chain restriction	Light chain restriction

Diffuse Follicle Center Lymphoma Versus Cutaneous Diffuse Large B-Cell Lymphoma, Leg Type

The differential diagnosis for a cutaneous large cell lymphoma with a diffuse growth pattern and numerous blasts includes primary cutaneous diffuse large B-cell lymphoma (PCLBCL), leg type, and the diffuse histologic phenotype of primary cutaneous follicle center lymphoma (PCFCL). The distinction between these entities provides critical prognostic information as the 5-year disease-specific survival for PCFCL is 95 %, while that of PCLBCL is only 55 % (Willemze 2006).

As described previously in this chapter, the neoplastic cells of PCFCL are typically positive for CD20 and Bcl6, variably positive for CD10, and usually negative for Bcl2, in contrast to nodal follicular lymphoma (Cerroni et al. 2000; Hoefnagel et al. 2003; de Leval et al. 2001) (Fig. 3.3). In contrast, PCLBCL consists of diffuse proliferation of 90 % or more of medium to large centroblasts and immunoblasts which are typically positive for CD20 and Bcl2 (Fig. 3.3), variably positive for Bcl6, and usually negative for CD10 (Willemze 2006). As these basic lymphocytic markers overlap considerably, additional markers may be required to support a specific diagnosis.

IHC for MUM1, IgM, HGAL (human germinal center-associated lymphoma), and FoxP1 have also been studied for the purpose of distinguishing PCFCL and PCLBCL (Table 3.2). In one study, all cases of PCLBCL demonstrated at least 30 % of cells positive for MUM1, while all cases of PCFCL were negative for MUM1, showing 10 % or less positivity (Hoefnagel et al. 2005; Pham-Ledard et al. 2010; Xie et al. 2008). While other studies have also demonstrated the specificity of MUM1 for PCLBCL (Kodama et al. 2005; Senff et al. 2007), one study classified 50 % of PCFCL cases as MUM1+ (Xie et al. 2008). In two separate studies, IgM staining has been shown to be positive in 100 % of PCLBCL cases and negative in all or nearly all cases of PCFCL (Koens et al. 2010; Demirkesen et al. 2011). The germinal center marker HGAL is positive in 88 % of PCFCL and only 33 % of PCLBCL (Xie et al. 2008). In one series, IHC for FoxP1 was shown to stain ≥50 % of cells in all cases of PCLBCL, while the neoplastic cells of PCFCL are either entirely negative or only 5-10 % positive for FoxP1 in nearly all cases (Hoefnagel et al. 2006).

Recommended panel (Table 3.2): CD20, Bcl2, Bcl6, MUM1, and IgM (also FoxP1 and HGAL, if available)

Subcutaneous Panniculitic T-Cell Lymphoma Versus Cutaneous γ/δ T-Cell Lymphoma

The WHO-EORTC classifications of subcutaneous panniculitic T-cell lymphoma (SPTCL) and cutaneous γ/δ T-cell lymphoma (CGD-TCL) often demonstrate overlapping histopathologic features (Willemze et al. 2005, 2008; Salhany

Fig. 3.3 For both diffuse follicle center cell lymphoma (**a**) and diffuse large B-cell lymphoma, leg type (**b**), strong CD20 (**c**, **d**) expression is seen for both. While Bcl2 (**e**) and MUM1 (**g**) expression is focal in diffuse follicle center cell lymphoma, diffuse and strong Bcl2 (**f**) and MUM1 (**h**) expression is seen diffuse large B-cell lymphoma, leg type

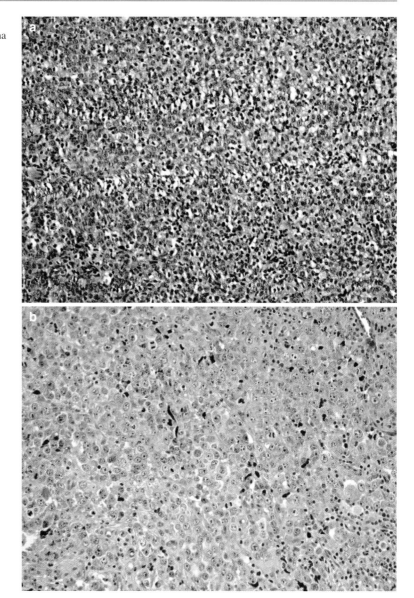

Fig. 3.3 (continued)

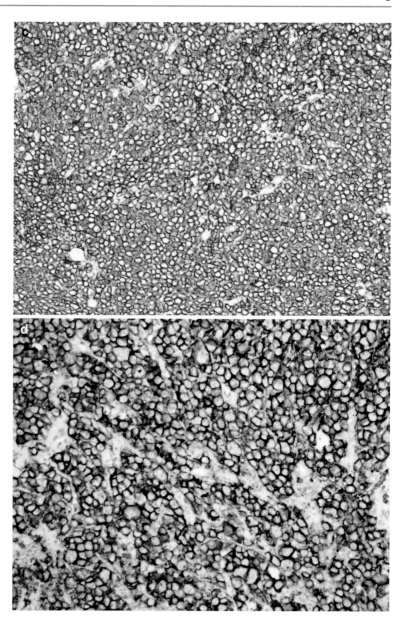

Fig. 3.3 (continued)

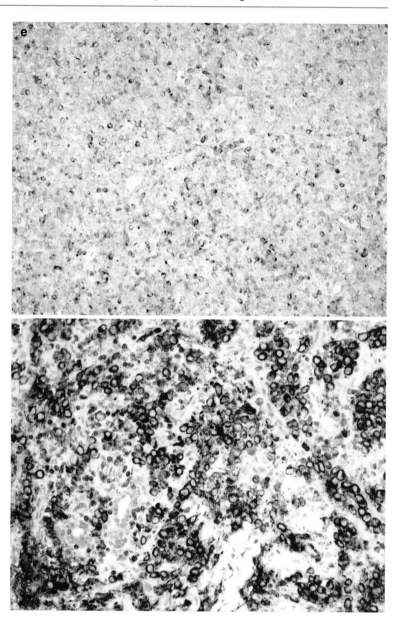

Fig. 3.3 (continued)

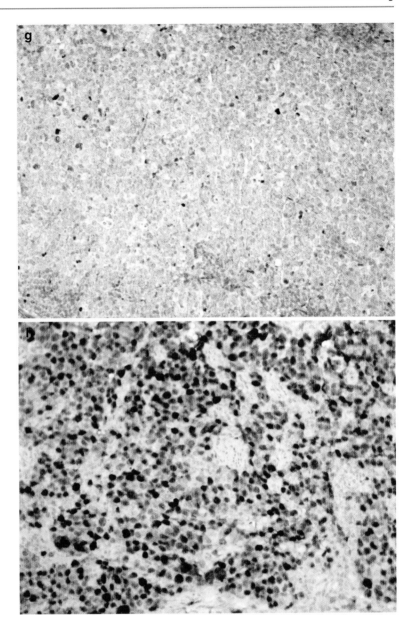

et al. 1998). However, distinguishing these lymphomas through the use of immunohistochemical and molecular markers is of great clinical importance as the 5-year survival of CGD-TCL is much worse than that of SPTCL (11 % versus 82 %, Willemze et al. 2008). Table 3.3 summarizes the immunophenotypes for SPTCL and CGD-TCL. SPTCL expresses a cytotoxic T-cell phenotype: CD3+, CD4−, CD8+, β-F1+, TIA-1+, granzyme B+, and CD56− (Kumar et al. 1998; Hoque et al. 2003; Massone et al. 2004; Willemze et al. 2008; Go and Wester 2004) (Fig. 3.4). While the CD8+ phenotype is vastly predominant for SPTCL, cases of CD4+ CD8− SPTCL have been reported (Kong et al. 2008). CGD-TCL expresses a mature γ/δ T-cell phenotype: CD3+, CD4−, CD8−, β-F1−, TIA-1+, granzyme B+, CD56+ (Massone et al. 2004; Willemze et al. 2005, 2008) (see Fig. 10.36). On frozen section and paraffin (anti-TCR delta) immunohistochemistry, CGD-TCL is positive for TCR gamma-delta, while SPTCL is negative (Willemze et al. 2008; Garcia-Herrera et al.

2011), respectively. TCR gene rearrangement analysis has demonstrated TCR-gamma clonality in approximately 75 % of cases of both SPTCL and CGD-TCL (Willemze et al. 2008). Epstein Barr virus (EBV) testing of either lymphoma is typically negative.

Lupus erythematosus panniculitis also enters into the differential diagnosis. In one-half of the lupus erythematosus panniculitis cases, there are epidermal and dermal changes of discoid lupus erythematosus. In the remaining half there is a predominant subcutaneous pattern with a lymphocytic panniculitis in a lobular pattern with germinal center formation and occasional rimming of adipocytes; thus, in this setting lupus erythematosus panniculitis can mimic the pan-

niculitic lymphomas SPTCL and CGD-TCL (Magro et al. 2001; Aguilera et al. 2007). CD20 is helpful in highlighting clusters or scattered B cells (Massone et al. 2005; Park et al. 2010). The lymphoid infiltrate of lupus erythematosus panniculitis usually comprises a mixture of B and T cells, although a minority of cases (3 of 17 in a study by Park et al.) showed exclusively T-cell infiltrates (Massone et al. 2005; Park et al. 2010). While immunohistochemical studies often show a predominant CD4+ T-cell infiltrate (Park et al. 2010; Massone et al. 2005), others have shown a CD8+ T-cell predominance (Magro et al. 2001) (Table 3.3). Gene rearrangement studies reveal that most lupus erythematosus panniculitis cases exhibit a polyclonal TCR-gamma gene rearrangement, while a small minority of cases showed a monoclonal TCR-gamma gene rearrangement (Park et al. 2010; Magro et al. 2001).

The existence of a borderline diagnosis between lupus erythematosus panniculitis and SPTCL referred to as "atypical lymphocytic lobular panniculitis" and "indeterminate lymphocytic lobular panniculitis" (Magro et al. 2001, 2008) as well as reported cases of SPTCL in patients with systemic lupus erythematosus (Pincus et al. 2009) suggests that there may be a continuous spectrum of disease between lupus erythematosus panniculitis and cutaneous lymphoma. Thus, the integration of clinical findings, histopathologic and immunohisto-

Table 3.2 Immunoprofile of diffuse follicle center cell lymphoma versus cutaneous diffuse large B-cell lymphoma, leg type (Hoefnagel et al. 2003, 2005, 2006; Xie et al. 2008; Senff et al. 2007; Demirkesen et al. 2011; Koens et al. 2010; Pham-Ledard et al. 2010; Kodama et al. 2005)

	Diffuse follicle center cell lymphoma	Cutaneous diffuse large B-cell lymphoma, leg type
CD20	+	+
Bcl2	8–41 %	90–100 %
MUM1	0–50 %	76–100 %
Bcl6	92–100 %	30–100 %
CD10	4–32 %	0–30 %
IgM	0–9 %	100 %
HGAL	88 %	33 %
FOXP1	13 %	100 %

Table 3.3 Immunoprofile of cutaneous γ/δ T-cell lymphoma versus subcutaneous panniculitic T-cell lymphoma versus lupus erythematosus panniculitis (Hoque et al. 2003; Aguilera et al. 2007; Go and Wester 2004; Kong et al. 2008; Massone et al. 2005, 2004, Garcia-Herrera et al. 2011)

	Cutaneous γ/δ T-cell lymphoma	Subcutaneous panniculitic T-cell lymphoma	Lupus erythematosus panniculitis
CD3	+	+	+
CD4	−	−	+
CD8	−	+	− or focally +
CD56	+	−	−
Granzyme B	+	+	−
TIA-1	+	+	− or focally +
βF1	−	+	+
TCRγ	+	−	−
EBER in situ hybridization	−	+ in rare cases (10 %)	−
CD20	−	−	Germinal centers +

Fig. 3.4 In a case of subcutaneous panniculitic T-cell lymphoma (**a**), negative CD4 (**b**) and strong CD8 (**c**) expression is seen

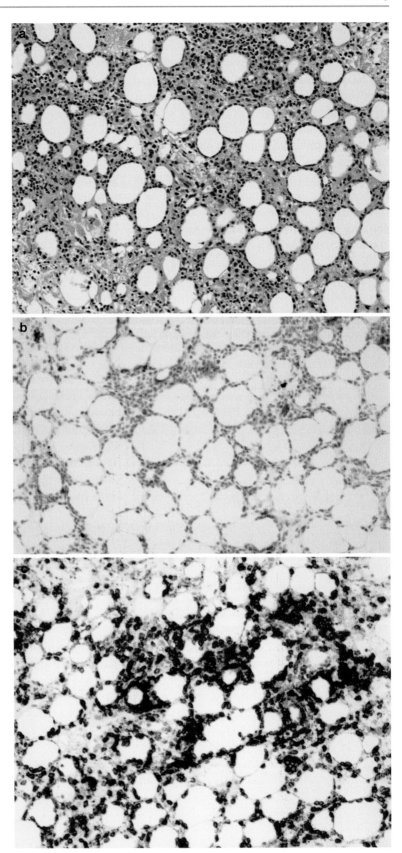

chemical features, and molecular studies are crucial in correctly classifying these entities. In some instances, long-term follow-up is necessary to understand the biologic course of the disease.

Recommended panel (Table 3.3): CD3, CD4, CD8, CD20, CD56, granzyme B, TIA-1, beta F1, TCRγ, TCR delta, and EBER in situ hybridization

CD30+ Lymphoproliferative Disorders Versus Reactive Processes Versus Lymphoma

CD30 is a member of the tumor necrosis factor superfamily (Schwab et al. 1982). Cutaneous infiltrates of CD30-positive lymphocytes can indicate lymphomatoid papulosis (LyP), anaplastic large cell lymphoma (ALCL) (primary or systemic), rare presentations of Hodgkin's disease, large cell transformation of mycosis fungoides, or a range of nonneoplastic reactive processes (Cepeda et al. 2003; Kempf et al. 2012; Werner et al. 2008; Vergier et al. 2000; Kaudewitz et al. 1989).

The use of anaplastic lymphoma kinase-1 (ALK) and epithelial membrane antigen (EMA) immunostains aids in the distinction between systemic anaplastic large cell lymphoma and cutaneous CD30-positive lymphoproliferative diseases. Whereas cases of systemic ALCL possessing a t(2;5)(p23;q35) translocation between nucleophosmin (*NPM*) gene and anaplastic lymphoma kinase (*ALK*) nearly always demonstrate immunohistochemical positivity for ALK (Cataldo et al. 1999; Perkins et al. 2005), primary cutaneous ALCL and LyP have been demonstrated to be almost always negative for ALK by immunohistochemistry (Yamaguchi et al. 2006) (Fig. 3.5). Furthermore, EMA stains the majority of ALK-positive systemic ALCL cases, but does not usually stain primary cutaneous ALCL (ten Berge et al. 2001) (Fig. 3.5). There have been recent isolated cases of cutaneous ALCL without systemic disease and *cytoplasmic* ALK protein expression and variant translocation reported (Kadin et al. 2008; Su et al. 1997; Sasaki et al. 2004). In addition, a series of six children with a single cutaneous ALK+ ALCL, nuclear-cytoplasmic ALK staining characteristic of the t(2;5) chromosomal translocation was reported (Oschlies et al. 2013).

Distinguishing LyP, primary cutaneous ALCL, and nonneoplastic reactive processes requires careful histopathologic evaluation and clinicopathologic correlation. Primary and secondary cutaneous ALCL often express CD30 in greater than 75 % of tumor cells (Kempf et al. 2011; Plaza et al. 2013). Furthermore, the subtype of LyP (A, B, C, or D) can predict different CD30 staining patterns; while most cases of LyP will show CD30 positivity, the small atypical lymphoid cells with cerebriform nuclei seen in type B LyP have been described as CD30 negative (Kempf 2006). However, others have described CD30-positive type B LyP (Saggini et al. 2010). Recently, several markers including TRAF1 (tumor necrosis factor (TNF) receptor-associated factor), MUM1 (multiple myeloma oncogene 1), Bcl2, and CD15 have been evaluated; however, due to overlapping findings, these markers have not been found to be helpful as diagnostic adjuncts in classifying cutaneous CD30-positive lymphoproliferative disorders (Assaf et al. 2007; Kempf et al. 2008; Paulli et al. 1998; Wasco et al. 2008; Benner et al. 2009) (Table 3.4).

Due to advances in antigen retrieval in immunohistochemistry, CD30 positivity can be detected in a variety of nonneoplastic processes in the skin. Scattered CD30+ cells can be seen in insect and spider bites (Smoller et al. 1992); infections including milker's nodule, Herpes simplex virus infection, molluscum contagiosum, scabies infection, leishmaniasis, and syphilis; lymphomatoid drug eruption (Werner et al. 2008); hidradenitis; pityriasis lichenoides et varioliformis acuta (PLEVA); and various other lesions (Cepeda et al. 2003; Kempf et al. 2012) (see Chap. 12 for differential diagnosis). Some authors report that the CD30+ cells of LyP and ALCL tend to be large, atypical, and sometimes arranged in nests or sheets, while the CD30+ cells of reactive processes tend to be smaller, less atypical, and scattered mostly as single cells (Kempf 2006). Other authors reported clusters of CD30-positive large cells with perinuclear staining in reactive

Fig. 3.5 In a cutaneous
anaplastic large cell
lymphoma (**a**), strong CD30
(**b**) expression is seen while
both EMA (**c**) and ALK (**d**)
are negative. On the other
hand, in a systemic
anaplastic large cell
lymphoma involving the skin
(**e**), strong CD30 (**f**), focal
EMA (**g**), and diffuse ALK
(**h**) expression is seen

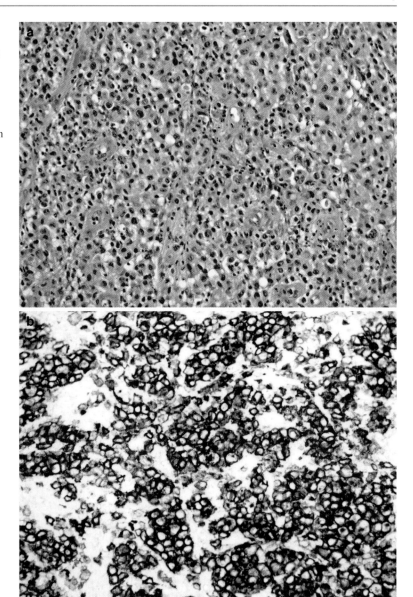

Fig. 3.5 (continued)

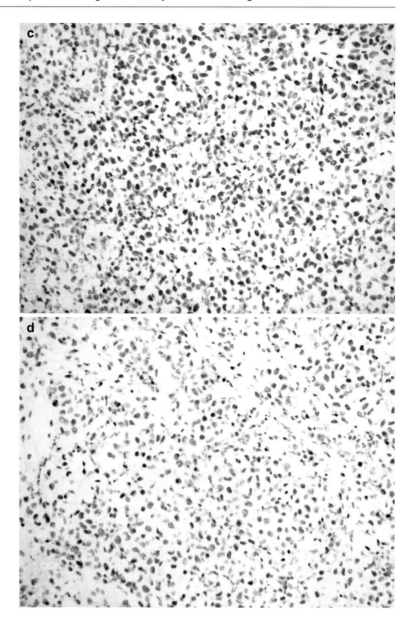

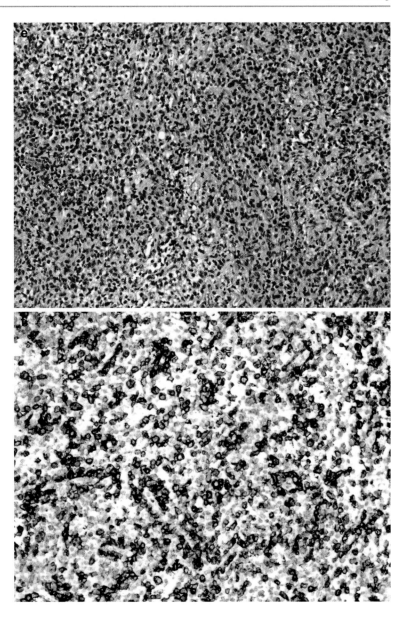

Fig. 3.5 (continued)

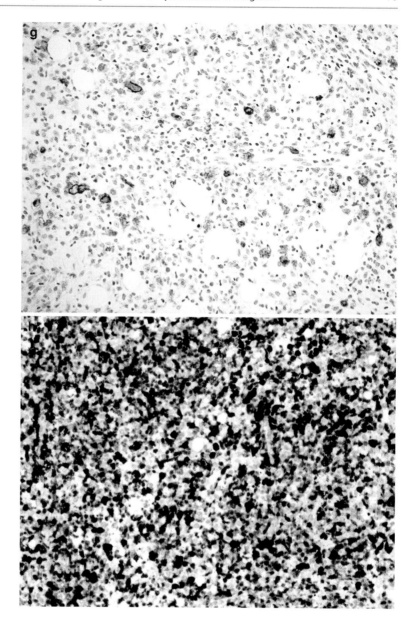

Table 3.4 Immunoprofile of CD30-positive lymphoproliferative disorders versus systemic anaplastic large cell lymphoma versus transformed mycosis fungoides (Kempf et al. 2008; Wasco et al. 2008; Assaf et al. 2007; Benner et al. 2009; Plaza et al. 2013; Kadin et al. 2008)

	Reactive processes	Lymphomatoid papulosis	Cutaneous anaplastic large cell lymphoma	Systemic anaplastic large cell lymphoma	Transformed mycosis fungoides
CD30	Single positive cells	+ <75 %	+ >75 %	+ >75 %	+ >75 %
ALK	–	–	–[a]	+	–
EMA	–	–	–	+	–
MUM1	ND	82–100 %	20–100 %	80–100 %	100 %
TRAF1	ND	84 %	4–87 %	15–50 %	73 %
BCL2	ND	36 %	22 %	38 %	73 %
CD15	ND	18 %	44 %	13 %	9 %

ND not done

[a]Rare cases of cutaneous anaplastic large cell lymphoma with cytoplasmic ALK staining have been reported

processes – a pattern observed in CD30+ lymphoproliferative disorders (Kempf et al. 2008). Cases of PLEVA with CD30-positive cells and monoclonality can be very difficult to distinguish from LyP types B and D (Kempf et al. 2012) (see Chap. 12 for differential diagnosis). Multiple biopsies from lesions with different clinical appearances might be helpful. In the absence of clear differences, histopathologic features diagnostic of a specific reactive process together with clinical correlation may ultimately resolve this diagnostic dilemma.

Recommended panel (Table 3.4): CD30, EMA, and ALK

Follicular Mucinosis Versus Folliculotropic Mycosis Fungoides

In the evaluation of skin biopsies with follicular mucinosis (FM), the distinction between primary follicular mucinosis (PFM) and folliculotropic mycosis fungoides (FMF) with follicular mucin can be challenging and requires attention to clinical information and histopathologic, immunohistochemical, and TCR gene rearrangement studies. Follicular mucinosis can be idiopathic/primary or secondary, occurs mainly in children and young adults, and is not associated with other cutaneous or systemic disorders (Cerroni et al. 2002). These lesions are typically localized and spontaneously regress, though some may be persistent (Gibson et al. 1989; Hempstead and Ackerman 1985; Brown et al. 2002). The secondary form of follicular mucinosis may be an epiphenomenon in a variety of conditions including arthropod assault, lupus erythematosus, eosinophilic folliculitis, as well as cutaneous T-cell lymphoma (Hempstead and Ackerman 1985; Gerami et al. 2008; Cerroni et al. 2002; Rongioletti et al. 2010). Lymphoma-associated follicular mucinosis consists primarily of mycosis fungoides (MF) and its variant folliculotropic mycosis fungoides (FMF) (Gerami et al. 2008; Burg et al. 2005). In some instances, follicular mucinosis may be the first presentation of lymphoma (Cerroni et al. 2002).

The typical immunoprofile of MF is a CD2+, CD3+, CD4+, CD5+, CD45RO+, CD8−, TCRβ+, and CD30− (Burg et al. 2005). Folliculotropic

MF is an uncommon variant of MF with distinctive clinical features, histologic findings, and prognosis, but with identical immunophenotypic and molecular findings as classic MF (Bonta et al. 2000; van Doorn et al. 2002; Gerami et al. 2008). While CD4+ predominance is seen in MF, the majority of cases of primary follicular mucinosis exhibited equivalent numbers of CD4+ and CD8+ lymphocytes (Rongioletti et al. 2010) (Fig. 3.6). Whereas cases of lymphoma-associated follicular mucinosis often exhibit loss of T-cell markers (CD2, CD5), loss of T-cell marker expression would not be expected in the setting of primary follicular mucinosis (Burg et al. 2005; Bonta et al. 2000). Histochemical techniques, including periodic acid-Schiff, colloidal iron, and Alcian blue at pH 2.5 and 0.5, have not been found to be helpful in distinguishing the mucin deposits of PFM and LAFM (Rongioletti et al. 2010). Since clonal TCR gene rearrangement has been detected in a subset of cases of presumed primary follicular mucinosis (Bonta et al. 2000; Brown et al. 2002; Rongioletti et al. 2010; Zelickson et al. 1991; Cerroni et al. 2002), the presence of clonal TCR gene rearrangement does not allow for definitive distinction between primary follicular mucinosis and lymphoma-associated follicular mucinosis. Ultimately, the proper classification of FM as either PFM or FM associated with MF depends on careful consideration of clinical, histopathologic, immunophenotypic, and molecular parameters. Furthermore, some cases of FM may not lend themselves to straightforward classification (see Chap. 4 for discussion of the spectrum of FM, FM dyscrasia, and folliculotropic MF).

Recommended panel: CD2, CD3, CD5, CD4, and CD8

Lymphomatoid Drug Eruption Versus Mycosis Fungoides

In some instances, it is difficult to distinguish mycosis fungoides from lymphomatoid drug reaction, a delayed type hypersensitivity reaction that shares histologic features with MF. One important similarity is involvement of the epidermis by clusters of lymphocytes. This epidermotropism has specifically been noted to target sites of preferential antigen processing, such as the suprapapillary plates, acrosyringea, and hair follicles. Other shared traits may include loss of CD7 on immunohistochemistry and even clonal T-cell receptor gene rearrangements (Magro and Crowson 1996; Murphy et al. 2002; Florell et al. 2006). Since loss of CD7 is commonly seen in a variety of inflammatory disorders (Murphy et al. 2002), partial loss of CD2 or loss of multiple T-cell antigens would be helpful in diagnosing peripheral T-cell lym-

phoma (Michie et al. 1989; Ormsby et al. 2001; Florell et al. 2006). An elevated CD4:CD8 and low CD8:CD3 ratios have been reported to be helpful in diagnosing mycosis fungoides (Florell et al. 2006; Ortonne et al. 2003). In the setting of MF, more CD4+ lymphoid cells are seen in the epidermis. On the contrary, more CD8+ lymphoid cells are seen in the epidermis in the setting of lymphomatoid drug reaction (Fig. 3.7).

Recommended panel: CD2, CD3, CD5, CD4, andCD8

Fig. 3.6 In a case of follicular mucinosis (**a**), the lymphoid infiltrate is positive for CD3 (**b**) and without an increase in the CD4 (**c**) to CD8 (**d**) ratio. On the contrary, in a case of follicular mycosis fungoides (**e**), the lymphoid infiltrate highlighted by CD3 (**f**) is predominantly CD4 positive (**g**) in comparison to CD8 (**h**)

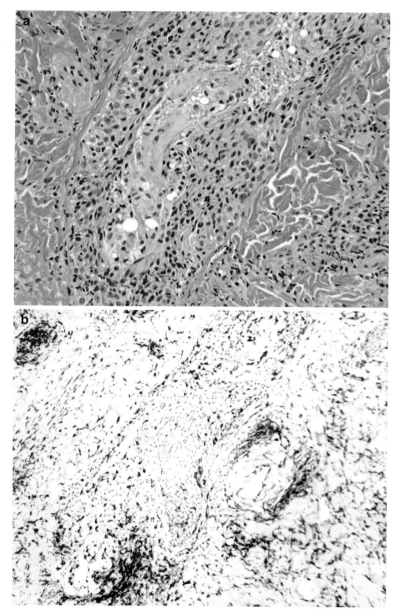

Fig. 3.6 (continued)

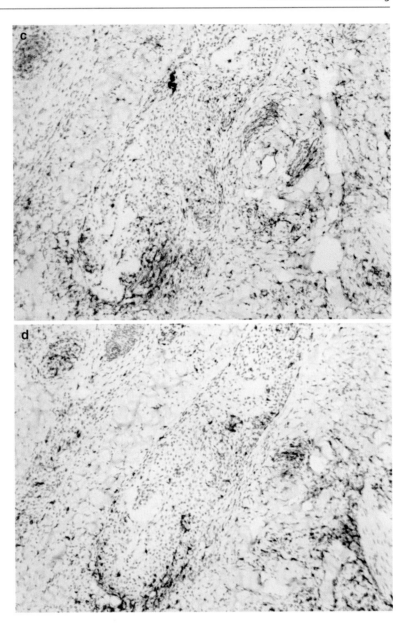

Fig. 3.6   (continued)

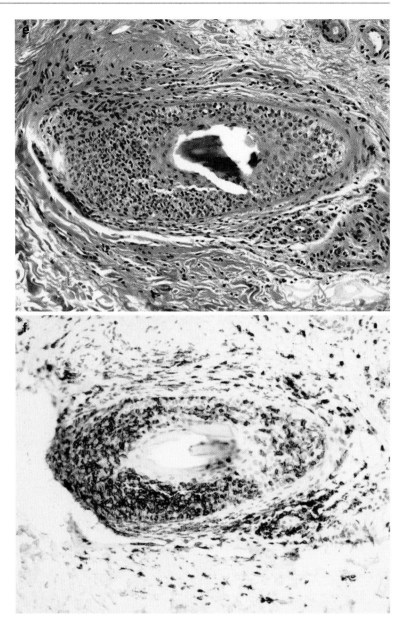

Fig. 3.6 (continued)

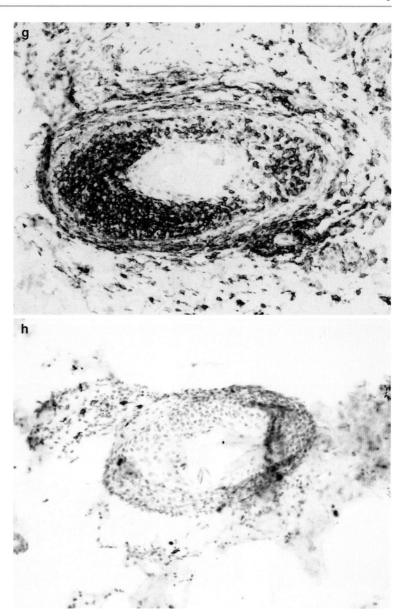

Fig. 3.7 In a case of lymphomatoid drug eruption (**a**), the lymphoid infiltrate within the epidermis is CD3 positive (**b**) and with a decrease in the CD4 (**c**) to CD8 (**d**) ratio. On the other hand, in a case of plaque-stage mycosis fungoides (**e**), the intraepidermal atypical lymphoid cells are CD3 positive (**f**) and predominantly CD4 positive (**g**) in comparison to CD8 (**h**)

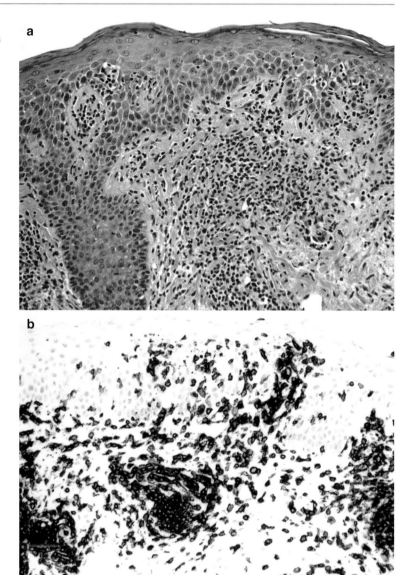

Fig. 3.7 (continued)

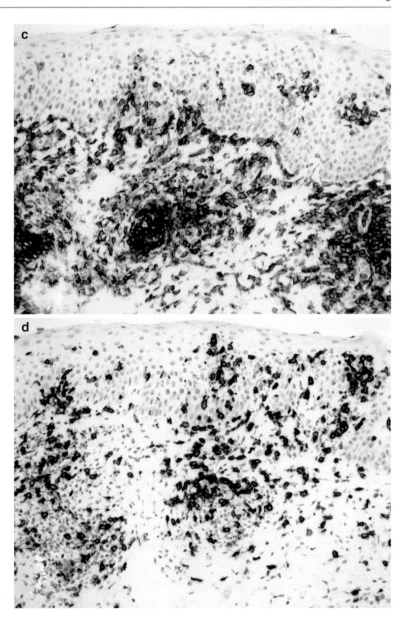

Fig. 3.7 (continued)

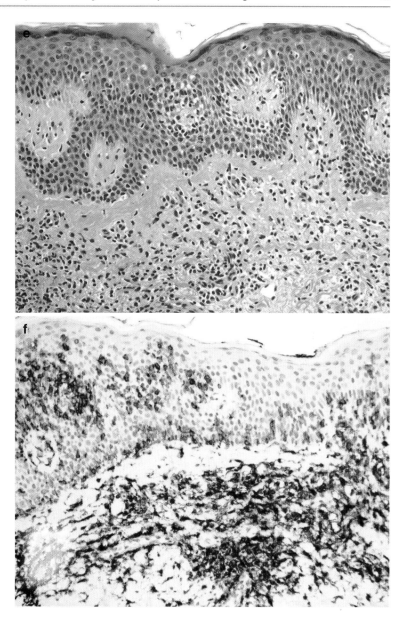

Fig. 3.7 (continued)

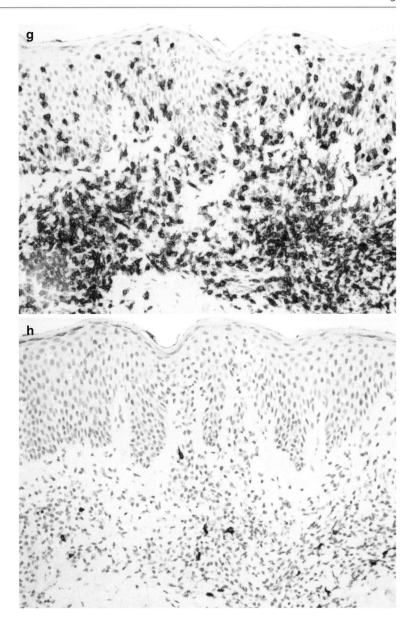

Table 3.5 Selected diagnostic immunohistochemical panels

	Recommended immunohistochemical panel
Reactive lymphoid hyperplasia versus low-grade B-cell lymphoma	CD3, CD20, Bcl2, Bcl6, CD21, kappa, lambda in situ hybridization
Diffuse follicle center cell lymphoma versus cutaneous diffuse large B-cell lymphoma, leg type	CD20, Bcl2, Bcl6, IgM, MUM1
Subcutaneous panniculitic T-cell lymphoma versus cutaneous gamma-delta T-cell lymphoma	CD3, CD4, CD8, CD56, granzyme B, TIA-1, TCR beta F1, TCR gamma
Cutaneous CD30+ lymphoproliferative disorder versus systemic anaplastic large cell lymphoma	CD30, EMA, ALK
Follicular mucinosis versus folliculotropic mycosis fungoides	CD2, CD3, CD4, CD5, CD8
Lymphomatoid drug reaction versus mycosis fungoides	CD2, CD3, CD4, CD5, CD8

TCR T-cell receptor

Summary

In the diagnosis of lymphoid infiltrates, a panel of immunohistochemical markers can be helpful in narrowing the differential diagnoses (Table 3.5). It would be best to establish a differential diagnosis based on clinical and histologic evaluation, order a panel of immunohistochemical stains, and then interpret the stains with the differential diagnosis in mind.

References

Aguilera P, Mascaro JM, Martinez A, Esteve J, Puig S, Campo E, Estrach T. Cutaneous gamma/delta T-cell lymphoma: a histopathologic mimicker of lupus erythematosus profundus (lupus panniculitis). J Am Acad Dermatol. 2007;56(4):643–7.

Assaf C, Hirsch B, Wagner F, Lucka L, Grunbaum M, Gellrich S, et al. Differential expression of TRAF1 aids in the distinction of cutaneous CD30-positive lymphoproliferations. J Invest Dermatol. 2007;127(8):1898–904.

Benner MF, Jansen PM, Meijer CJLM, Willemze R. Diagnostic and prognostic evaluation of phenotypic markers TRAF1, MUM1, BCL2 and CD15 in cutaneous CD30-positive lymphoproliferative disorders. Br J Dermatol. 2009;161(1):121–7. doi:10.1111/j.1365-2133.2009.09147.x.

Bonta MD, Tannous ZS, Demierre M, Gonzalez E, Harris NL, Duncan LM. Rapidly progressing mycosis fungoides presenting as follicular mucinosis. J Am Acad Dermatol. 2000;43(4):635–40.

Brown HA, Gibson LE, Pujol RM, Lust JA, Pittelkow MR. Primary follicular mucinosis: long-term follow-up of patients younger than 40 years with and without clonal T-cell receptor gene rearrangement. J Am Acad Dermatol. 2002;47(6):856–62.

Burg G, Kempf W, Cozzio A, Feit J, Willemze R, Jaffe E, et al. WHO/EORTC classification of cutaneous lymphomas 2005: histological and molecular aspects. J Cutan Pathol. 2005;32(10):647–74.

Cataldo KA, Jalal SM, Law ME, Ansell SM, Inwards DJ, Fine M, et al. Detection of t(2;5) in anaplastic large cell lymphoma: comparison of immunohistochemical studies, FISH, and RT-PCR in paraffin-embedded tissue. Am J Surg Pathol. 1999;23(11):1386–92.

Cepeda LT, Pieretti M, Chapman SF, Horenstein MG. CD30-positive atypical lymphoid cells in common non-neoplastic cutaneous infiltrates rich in neutrophils and eosinophils. Am J Surg Pathol. 2003;27(7):912–8.

Cerroni L, Arzberger E, Putz B, Hofler G, Metze D, Sander CA, et al. Primary cutaneous follicular center cell lymphoma with follicular growth pattern. Blood. 2000;95(12):3922–8.

Cerroni L, Fink-Puches R, Back B, Kerl H. Follicular mucinosis: a critical reappraisal of clinicopathologic features and association with mycosis fungoides and Sezary syndrome. Arch Dermatol. 2002;138(2):182–9.

Cetinozman F, Jansen PM, Willemze R. Expression of programmed death-1 in primary cutaneous CD4-positive small/medium-sized pleomorphic T-cell lymphoma, cutaneous pseudo-T-cell lymphoma, and other types of cutaneous T-cell lymphoma. Am J Surg Pathol. 2012;36(1):109–16. doi:10.1097/PAS.0b013e318230df87.

Child FJ, Russell-Jones R, Woolford AJ, Calonje E, Photiou A, Orchard G, Whittaker SJ. Absence of the t(14;18) chromosomal translocation in primary cutaneous B-cell lymphoma. Br J Dermatol. 2001;144(4):735–44.

Cota C, Vale E, Viana I, Requena L, Ferrara G, Anemona L, et al. Cutaneous manifestations of blastic plasmacytoid dendritic cell neoplasm-morphologic and phenotypic variability in a series of 33 patients. Am J Surg Pathol. 2010;34(1):75–87. doi:10.1097/PAS.0b013e3181c5e26b.

De Leval L, Harris NL, Longtine J, Ferry JA, Duncan LM. Cutaneous B-cell lymphomas of follicular and marginal zone types: Use of Bcl-6, CD10, Bcl-2, and CD21 in differential diagnosis and classification. Am J Surg Pathol. 2001;25(6):732–41.

Demirkesen C, Tuzuner N, Esen T, Lebe B, Ozkal S. The expression of IgM is helpful in the differentiation of primary cutaneous diffuse large B cell lymphoma and follicle center lymphoma. Leuk Res. 2011;35(9): 1269–72. doi:10.1016/j.leukres.2011.06.004.

Dorfman DM, Brown JA, Shahsafaei A, Freeman GJ. Programmed death-1 (PD-1) is a marker of germinal center associated T cells and angioimmunoblastic T-cell lymphoma. Am J Surg Pathol. 2006;30(7):802–10. doi:10.1097/01.pas.0000209855.28282.ce.

Facchetti F, Jones D, Patrella T. Blastic plasmacytoid dendritic cell neoplasm. In: Swerdlow SH, Campo E, Hazzis NL, Jaffe ES, Pileri SA, Stein H, et al., editors. WHO classification of tumors of haematopoietic and lymphoid tissues. Lyon: IARC Press; 2008. p. 145–7.

Feldman AL, Law ME, Inwards DJ, Dogan A, McClure RF, Macon WR. PAX5-positive T-cell anaplastic large cell lymphomas associated with extra copies of the PAX5 gene locus. Mod Pathol. 2010;23(4):593–602. doi:10.1038/modpathol.2010.4.

Florell SR, Cessna M, Lundell RB, Boucher KM, Bowen GM, Harris RM, et al. Usefulness (or lack thereof) of immunophenotyping in atypical cutaneous T-cell infiltrates. Am J Clin Pathol. 2006;125(5):727–36.

Garcia-Herrera A, Song JY, Chuang SS, Villamor N, Colomo L, Pittaluga S, et al. Nonhepatosplenic gammadelta T-cell lymphomas represent a spectrum of aggressive cytotoxic T-cell lymphomas with a mainly extranodal presentation. Am J Surg Pathol. 2011;35(8):1214–25. doi:10.1097/PAS.0b013e31822067d1.

Gerami P, Rosen S, Kuzel T, Boone SL, Guitart J. Folliculotropic mycosis fungoides: an aggressive variant of cutaneous T-cell lymphoma. Arch Dermatol. 2008;144(6):738–46. doi:10.1001/archderm.144.6.738.

Gibson LE, Muller SA, Leiferman KM, Peters MS. Follicular mucinosis: clinical and histopathologic study. J Am Acad Dermatol. 1989;20(3):441–6.

Go RS, Wester SM. Immunophenotypic and molecular features, clinical outcomes, treatments, and prognostic factors associated with subcutaneous panniculitis-like T-cell lymphoma. Cancer. 2004;101(6):1404–13.

Goodlad JR, Krajewski AS, Batstone PJ, McKay P, White JM, Benton EC, et al. Primary cutaneous follicular lymphoma: a clinicopathologic and molecular study of 16 cases in support of a distinct entity. Am J Surg Pathol. 2002;26(6):733–41.

Groh V, Porcelli S, Fabbi M, Lanier LL, Picker LJ, Anderson T, et al. Human lymphocytes bearing T cell receptor gamma/delta are phenotypically diverse and evenly distributed throughout the lymphoid system. J Exp Med. 1989;169(4):1277–94.

Gualco G, Weiss LM, Bacchi CE. MUM1/IRF4: a review. Appl Immunohistochem Mol Morphol. 2010;18(4): 301–10. doi:10.1097/PAI.0b013e3181cf1126.

Hempstead RW, Ackerman AB. Follicular mucinosis. A reaction pattern in follicular epithelium. Am J Dermatopathol. 1985;7(3):245–57.

Hoefnagel JJ, Vermeer MH, Janssen PM, Fleuren GJ, Miejer CJ, Willemze R. Bcl-2, Bcl-6 and CD10 expression in cutaneous B-cell lymphoma: further support for a follicle centre cell origin and differential diagnostic significance. Br J Dermatol. 2003;149(6):1183–91.

Hoefnagel JJ, Dijkman R, Basso K, Jansen PM, Hallermann C, Willemze R, et al. Distinct types of primary cutaneous B-cell lymphoma identified by gene expression profiling. Blood. 2005;105(9):3671–8.

Hoefnagel JJ, Mulder MM, Dreef E, Jansen PM, Pals ST, Meijer CJ, et al. Expression of B-cell transcription factors in primary cutaneous B-cell lymphoma. Mod Pathol. 2006;19(9):1270–6.

Hoque SR, Child FJ, Whittaker SJ, Ferreira S, Orchard G, Jenner K, et al. Subcutaneous panniculitis-like T-cell lymphoma: a clinicopathological, immunophenotypic and molecular analysis of six patients. Br J Dermatol. 2003;148(3):516–25.

Iida S, Rao PH, Butler M, Corradini P, Boccadoro M, Klein B, et al. Deregulation of MUM1/IRF4 by chromosomal translocation in multiple myeloma. Nat Genet. 1997;17(2):226–30.

Ishida Y, Agata Y, Shibahara K, Honjo T. Induced expression of PD-1, a novel member of the immunoglobulin gene superfamily, upon programmed cell death. EMBO J. 1992;11(11):3887–95.

Kadin ME, Pinkus JL, Pinkus GS, Duran IH, Fuller CE, Onciu M, et al. Primary cutaneous ALCL with phosphorylated/activated cytoplasmic ALK and novel phenotype: EMA/MUC1+, cutaneous lymphocyte antigen negative. Am J Surg Pathol. 2008;32(9):1421–6. doi:10.1097/PAS.0b013e3181648d6d.

Kaudewitz P, Stein H, Dallenbach F, Eckert F, Bieber K, Burg G, Braun-Falco O. Primary and secondary cutaneous Ki-1+ (CD30+) anaplastic large cell lymphomas: morphologic, immunohistologic and clinical characteristics. Am J Pathol. 1989;135(2):359–67.

Kempf W. CD30+ lymphoproliferative disorders: histopathology, differential diagnosis, new variants, and simulators. J Cutan Pathol. 2006;33 Suppl 1:58–70.

Kempf W, Kutzner H, Cozzio A, Sander CA, Plaltz MC, Muller B, Plaltz M. MUM1 expression in cutaneous CD30+ lymphoproliferative disorders: a valuable tool for the distinction between lymphomatoid papulosis and primary cutaneous anaplastic large-cell lymphoma. Br J Dermatol. 2008;158(6):1280–7. doi:10.1111/j.1365-2133.2008.08566.x.

Kempf W, Pfaltz K, Vermeer MH, Cozzio A, Ortiz-Romero PL, Bagot M, et al. EORTC, ISCL, and USCLC consensus recommendations for the treatment of primary cutaneous CD30-positive lymphoproliferative disorders: lymphomatoid papulosis and primary cutaneous anaplastic large-cell lymphoma. Blood. 2011;118(15):4024–35. doi:10.1182/blood-2011-05-351346.

Kempf W, Kazakov DV, Palmedo G, Fraitag S, Schaerer L, Kutzner H. Pityriasis lichenoides et varioliformis acuta with numerous CD30(+) cells: a variant mimicking lymphomatoid papulosis and other cutaneous lymphomas. A clinicopathologic, immunohistochemical, and molecular biological study of 13 cases. Am J Surg Pathol. 2012;36(7):1021–9.

Klco JM, Kulkarni S, Kreisel FH, Nguyen T-D T, Hassan A, Fratter JL. Immunohistochemical analysis of monocytic leukemias. Am J Clin Pathol. 2011;135(5):720–30. doi:10.1309/AJCPZ46PMMAWJROT.

Kodama K, Massone C, Chott A, Metze D, Kerl H, Cerroni L. Primary cutaneous large B-cell lymphomas: clinicopathologic features, classification, and prognostic factors in a large series of patients. Blood. 2005;106(7):2491–7.

Koens L, Vermeer MH, Willemze R, Jansen PM. IgM expression on paraffin sections distinguishes primary cutaneous large B-cell lymphoma, leg type from primary cutaneous follicle center lymphoma. Am J Surg Pathol. 2010;34(7):1043–8. doi:10.1097/PAS.0b013e3181e5060a.

Kong YY, Dai B, Kong JC, Zhou XY, Lu HF, Shen L, et al. Subcutaneous panniculitis-like T-cell lymphoma: a clinicopathologic, immunophenotypic, and molecular study of 22 Asian cases according to WHO-EORTC classification. Am J Surg Pathol. 2008;32(10):1495–502. doi:10.1097/PAS.0b013e31817a9081.

Krajewski AS, Myskow MW, Salter DM, Cunningham DS, Ramage EF. Diagnosis of T-cell lymphoma using beta F1, anti-T-cell receptor beta chain antibody. Histopathology. 1989;15(3):239–47. doi:10.1111/j.1365-2559.1989.tb03074.x.

Krenacs L, Himmelmann AW, Quintanilla-Martinez L, Fest T, Riva A, Wellmann A, et al. Transcription factor B cells specific activator protein (BSAP) is differentially expressed in B cells and in subsets of B-cell lymphomas. Blood. 1998;92(4):1308–16.

Kumar S, Krenacs L, Medeiros J, Elenitoba-Johnson KS, Greiner TC, Sorbara L, et al. Subcutaneous panniculitic T-cell lymphoma is a tumor of cytotoxic T lymphocytes. Hum Pathol. 1998;29(4):397–403.

Levy R, Warnke R, Dorfman RF, Haimovich J. The monoclonality of human B-cell lymphomas. J Exp Med. 1977;145(4):1014–28.

Magro CM, Crowson AN. Drug-induced immune dysregulation as a cause of atypical cutaneous lymphoid infiltrates: a hypothesis. Hum Pathol. 1996;27(2):125–32.

Magro CM, Crowson AN, Kovatich AJ, Burns F. Lupus profundus, indeterminate lymphocytic lobular panniculitis and subcutaneous T-cell lymphoma: a spectrum of subcuticular T-cell lymphoid dyscrasia. J Cutan Pathol. 2001;28(5):235–47.

Magro CM, Schaefer JT, Morrison C, Porcu P. Atypical lymphocytic lobular panniculitis: a clonal subcutaneous T-cell dyscrasia. J Cutan Pathol. 2008;35(10):947–54. doi:10.1111/j.1600-0560.2007.00938.x.

Massone C, Chott A, Metze D, Kerl K, Citarella L, Vale E, et al. Subcutaneous, blastic natural killer (NK), NK/T-cell, and other cytotoxic lymphomas of the skin: a morphologic, immunophenotypic, and molecular study of 50 patients. Am J Surg Pathol. 2004;28(6):719–35.

Massone C, Kodama K, Salmhofer W, Abe R, Shimizu H, Parodi A, et al. Lupus erythematosus panniculitis (lupus profundus): clinical, histopathological, and molecular analysis of nine cases. J Cutan Pathol. 2005;32(6):396–404.

Michie SA, Abel EA, Hoppe RT, Warnke RA, Wood GS. Expression of T-cell receptor antigens in mycosis fungoides and inflammatory skin lesions. J Invest Dermatol. 1989;93(1):116–20.

Munoz L, Nomdedeu J, Lopez O, Carnicer MJ, Bellido M, Aventin A, et al. Interleukin-3 receptor alpha chain (CD123) is widely expressed in hematologic malignancies. Haematologica. 2001;86(12):1261–9.

Murphy M, Fullen D, Carlson JA. Low CD7 expression in benign and malignant cutaneous lymphocytic infiltrates: experience with an antibody reactive with paraffin-embedded tissue. Am J Dermatopathol. 2002;24(1):6–16.

Natkunam Y, Warnke RA, Montgomery K, Falini B, van De Rijn M. Analysis of MUM1/IRF4 protein expression using tissue microarrays and immunohistochemistry. Mod Pathol. 2001;14(7):686–94.

Ormsby A, Bergfeld WF, Tubbs RR, Hsi ED. Evaluation of a new paraffin-reactive CD7 T-cell deletion marker and a polymerase chain reaction-based T-cell receptor gene rearrangement assay: implications for diagnosis of mycosis fungoides in community clinical practice. J Am Acad Dermatol. 2001;45(3):405–13.

Ortonne N, Buyukbabani N, Delfau-Larue MH, Bago M, Wechsler J. Value of the CD8-CD3 ratio for the diagnosis of mycosis fungoides. Mod Pathol. 2003;16(9):857–62.

Oschlies I, Lisfeld J, Lamant L, Nakazawa A, d'Amore ES, Hansson U, et al. ALK-positive anaplastic large cell lymphoma limited to the skin: clinical, histopathological and molecular analysis of 6 pediatric cases: a report from the ALCL99 study. Haematological. 2013;98(1):50–6. doi:10.3324/haematol.2012.065664.

Park HS, Choi JW, Kim BK, Cho KH. Lupus erythematosus panniculitis: clinicopathological, immunophenotypic, and molecular studies. Am J Dermatopathol. 2010;32(1):24–30. doi:10.1097/DAD.0b013e3181b4a5ec.

Paulli M, Berti E, Boveri E, Kindl S, Gambini C, Rosso R, et al. Cutaneous CD30+ lymphoproliferative disorders: expression of bcl-2 and proteins of the tumor necrosis factor receptor superfamily. Hum Pathol. 1998;29(11):1223–30.

Perkins SL, Pickering D, Lowe EJ, Zwick D, Abromowitch M, Davenport G, et al. Childhood anaplastic large cell lymphoma has a high incidence of ALK gene rearrangement as determined by immunohistochemical staining and fluorescent in situ hybridization: a genetic and pathological correlation. Br J Haematol. 2005;131(5):624–7.

Pham-Ledard A, Prochazkova-Carlotti M, Vergier B, Petrella T, Grange F, Beylot-Barry M, Merlio JP. IRF4 expression without IRF4 rearrangement is a general feature of primary cutaneous diffuse large B-cell lymphoma, leg type. J Invest Dermatol. 2010;130(5):1470–2.

Pincus LB, LeBoit PE, McCalmont TH, Ricci R, Buzio C, Fox LP, et al. Subcutaneous panniculitis-like T-cell lymphoma with overlapping clinicopathologic features of lupus erythematosus: coexistence of 2 entities? Am J Dermatopathol. 2009;31(6):520–6. doi:10.1097/DAD.0b013e3181a84f32.

Plaza JA, Feldman AL, Magro C. Cutaneous CD30-positive lymphoproliferative disorders with CD8 expression: a clinicopathologic study of 21 cases. J Cutan Pathol. 2013;40(2):236–47. doi:10.1111/cup.12047.

Rodriguez Pinilla SM, Roncador G, Rodriguez-Peralto JL, Mollejo M, Garcia JF, Montes-Moreno S, et al. Primary cutaneous CD4+ small/medium-sized pleomorphic T-cell lymphoma expresses follicular T-cell markers. Am J Surg Pathol. 2009;33(1):81–90. doi:10.1097/PAS.0b013e31818e52fe.

Rodriguez-Pinilla SM, Ortiz-Romera PL, Monsalvez V, Tomas IE, Almagro M, Sevilla A, et al. TCR-gamma expression in primary cutaneous T-cell lymphomas. Am J Surg Pathol. 2013;37(3):375–84. doi:10.1097/PAS.0b013e318275d1a2.

Rojo JM, Bello R, Portoles P. T-cell receptor. Adv Exp Med Biol. 2008;640:1–11. doi:10.1007/978-0-387-09789-3_1.

Rongioletti F, De Lucchi S, Meyes D, Mora M, Rebora A, Zupo S, et al. Follicular mucinosis: a clinicopathologic, histochemical, immunohistochemical and molecular study comparing the primary benign form and the mycosis fungoides-associated follicular mucinosis. J Cutan Pathol. 2010;37(1):15–9. doi:10.1111/j.1600-0560.2009.01338.x.

Saggini A, Gulia A, Argenyi Z, Fink-Puches R, Lissia A, Magana M, et al. A variant of lymphomatoid papulosis simulating primary cutaneous aggressive epidermotropic CD8+ cytotoxic T-cell lymphoma. Description of 9 cases. Am J Surg Pathol. 2010;34(8):1168–75.

Salhany KE, Macon WR, Choi JK, Elenitsas R, Lessin SR, Felgar RE, et al. Subcutaneous panniculitis-like T cell lymphoma: clinicopathologic, immunophenotypic, and genotypic analysis of alpha/beta and gamma/delta subtypes. Am J Surg Pathol. 1998;22(7):881–93.

Sasaki K, Sugaya M, Fujita H, Takeuchi K, Torii H, Asahina A, Tamaki K. A case of primary cutaneous anaplastic large cell lymphoma with variant anaplastic lymphoma kinase translocation. Br J Dermatol. 2004;150(6):1202–7.

Schwab U, Stein H, Gerdes J, Lemke H, Kirchner H, Schaadt M, Diehl V. Production of a monoclonal antibody specific for Hodgkin and Sternberg-Reed cells of Hodgkin's disease and a subset of normal lymphoid cells. Nature. 1982;299(5878):65–7.

Senff NJ, Hoefnagel JJ, Jansen PM, Vermeer MH, van Baarlen J, Blokx WA, et al. Reclassification of 300 primary cutaneous B-cell lymphomas according to the new WHO–EORTC classification for cutaneous lymphomas: comparison with previous classifications and identification of prognostic markers. J Clin Oncol. 2007;25(12):1581–7.

Servitje O, Gallardo F, Estrach T, Pujol RM, Blanco A, Fernandez-Sevilla A, et al. Primary cutaneous marginal zone B-cell lymphoma: a clinical, histopathological, immunophenotypic and molecular genetic study of 22 cases. Br J Dermatol. 2002;147(6):1147–58.

Shinohara T, Taniwaki M, Ishida Y, Kawaichi M, Honjo T. Structure and chromosomal localization of the human PD-1 gene (PDCD1). Genomics. 1995;23(3):704–6. doi:10.1006/geno.1994.1562.

Smoller BR, Longacre TA, Warnke RA. Ki-1 (CD30) expression in differentiation of lymphomatoid papulosis from arthropod bite reactions. Mod Pathol. 1992;5(5):492–6.

Su LD, Schnitzer B, Ross CW, Vasef M, Mori S, Shiota M, et al. The t(2;5)-associated p80 NPM/ALK fusion protein in nodal and cutaneous CD30+ lymphoproliferative disorders. J Cutan Pathol. 1997;24(10):597–603.

Ten Berge RL, Snijdewint FG, von Mensdorff-Pouilly S, Poort-Keesom RJ, Oudejans JJ, Meijer JW, et al. MUC1 (EMA) is preferentially expressed by ALK positive anaplastic large cell lymphoma, in the normally glycosylated or only partly hypoglycosylated form. J Clin Pathol. 2001;54(12):933–9.

Torlakovic E, Torlakovic G, Nguyen PL, Brunning RD, Delabie J. The value of anti-pax5 immunostaining in routinely fixed and paraffin embedded sections: a novel pan-B and B-cell marker. Am J Surg Pathol. 2002;26(10):1343–50.

Tsuboi K, Iida S, Inagaki H, Kato M, Hayami Y, Hanamura I, et al. MUM1/IRF4 expression is a frequent event in mature lymphoid malignancies. Leukemia. 2000;14(3):449–56.

van Doorn R, Scheffer E, Willemze R. Follicular mycosis fungoides, a distinct disease entity with or without associated follicular mucinosis: a clinicopathologic and follow-up study of 51 patients. Arch Dermatol. 2002;138(2):191–8.

Vergier B, de Muret A, Beylot-Barry M, Vaillant L, Ekouevi D, Chene G, et al. Transformation of mycosis fungoides: clinicopathological and prognostic features of 45 cases. Blood. 2000;95(7):2212–8.

Wasco MJ, Fullen D, Su L, Ma L. The expression of MUM1 in cutaneous T-cell lymphoproliferative disorders. Hum Pathol. 2008;39(4):557–63. doi:10.1016/j.humpath.2007.08.013.

Werner B, Massone C, Kerl H, Cerroni L. Large CD30-positive cells in benign, atypical lymphoid infiltrates of the skin. J Cutan Pathol. 2008;35(12):1100–7. doi:10.1111/j.1600-0560.2007.00979.x.

Willemze R. Primary cutaneous B-cell lymphoma: classification and treatment. Curr Opin Oncol. 2006;18(5):425–31.

Willemze R, Jaffe ES, Burg G, Cerroni L, Berti E, Swerdlow SH, et al. WHO-EORTC classification for cutaneous lymphomas. Blood. 2005;105(10):3768–85.

Willemze R, Jansen PM, Cerroni L, Berti E, Santucci M, Assaf C, et al. Subcutaneous panniculitis-like T-cell lymphoma: definition, classification, and prognostic factors: an EORTC Cutaneous Lymphoma Group Study of 83 cases. Blood. 2008;111(2):838–45.

Xie X, Sundram U, Natkunam Y, Kohler S, Hoppe RT, Kim YH, et al. Expression of HGAL in primary cutaneous large B-cell lymphomas: evidence for germinal center derivation of primary cutaneous follicular lymphoma. Mod Pathol. 2008;21(6):653–9. doi:10.1038/modpathol.2008.30.

Yamaguchi T, Oshima K, Karube K, Kawano R, Nakayama J, Suzumiya J, et al. Expression of chemo-

kines and chemokine receptors in cutaneous CD30+ lymphoproliferative disorders. Br J Dermatol. 2006;154(5):904–9.

Zelickson BD, Peters MS, Muller SA, Thibodeau SN, Lust JA, Quam LM, Pittelkow MR. T-cell receptor gene rearrangement analysis: cutaneous T cell lymphoma, peripheral T cell lymphoma, and premalignant and benign cutaneous lymphoproliferative disorders. J Am Acad Dermatol. 1991;25 (5 Pt 1):787–96.

Role of Molecular Genetics and Flow Cytometry Analysis in Cutaneous Hematopathology Including Application in Ten Disease Categories: Using Molecular and Immunophenotyping Techniques in Evaluation of Hyperplasia, Atypical Infiltrates, and Frank Lymphomas

4

Hernani D. Cualing and Marshall E. Kadin

Introduction

Cells derived from neoplastic lymphoid infiltrates usually differ from reactive benign infiltrate by expression of monotypic antigen receptor proteins or clonal deoxyribonucleic acid (DNA) segments of rearranged antigen receptor genes. Ancillary tests such as cell membrane/cytoplasmic light chain restriction, Vbeta T-cell receptor, and killer immunoglobulin receptor (KIR) immunophenotyping by flow cytometry or immunohistochemistry are used to evaluate monotypic antigen protein receptors. In addition, both B- and T-cell genes located in the nucleus are encoding antigen receptors that rearrange as the cell undergoes immunologic and functional maturation. Because cutaneous lymphomas, like those arising in the lymph nodes, show a unique set of rearranged gene segments,

assays for a unique nucleic acid sequence are equivalent to a molecular fingerprint identifying a clone. Hence, neoplasms usually have expanded population of cells possessing this unique DNA sequence. A monoclonal B- or T-cell population may be revealed as a discrete peak or band by polymerase chain reaction (PCR) amplification above a background of polyclonal cell DNA. However, if any lymphoid population is scant with few cells acting as nonspecific templates, owing to an ultrasensitive assay, false positives or pseudoclonal bands may be observed. Similarly, an insufficiently sampled neoplasm may also provide a false-negative result.

In general, the main ancillary tests include cytochemistry, immunophenotyping, and molecular tests. Immunophenotyping includes flow cytometry, immunohistochemistry (IHC), and image cytometry. Cytochemistry is useful for detection of infectious agents, deposits, or intracellular inclusions. Molecular tests consist mainly of in situ hybridization (ISH) and PCR-based tests. ISH tests include detection of restricted immunoglobulin light chains or detection of microorganisms. PCR-based tests consist mainly of detection of B- and T-cell clonality using IgG and T-cell receptor gene rearrangements.

H.D. Cualing, MD (✉)
Department of Hematopathology and Cutaneous Lymphoma, IHCFLOW Diagnostic Laboratory, 18804 Chaville Rd, Lutz, FL 33558, USA
e-mail: ihcflow@verizon.net

M.E. Kadin, MD
Department of Dermatology, Roger Williams Medical Center, Boston University School of Medicine, Providence, RI, USA

H.D. Cualing et al. (eds.), *Cutaneous Hematopathology*,
DOI 10.1007/978-1-4939-0950-6_4, © Springer Science+Business Media New York 2014

Part I. Ancillary Tools to Characterize Cutaneous Infiltrates

Molecular Fingerprint by PCR of Antigen Receptor Genes

Molecular T and B receptor gene rearrangement assays by PCR have a well-defined role in the workup, diagnosis, and monitoring of cutaneous lymphoproliferative diseases. PCR using hetero-duplex and GeneScan capillary electrophoresis has largely replaced Southern blot as a standard in clinical practice and in cutaneous hematopathology (Bruggemann et al. 2007; Gallardo et al. 2008; Langerak et al. 2012; Lukowsky et al. 2010; Morales et al. 2008; Sandberg et al. 2003, 2005). Molecular studies are of critical importance when the histomorphologic and/or clinical presentation of a skin lesion has features that

Table 4.1 Sensitivity and specificity of PCR tests in cutaneous lymphomas and hyperplasias

T cells
MF from reactive dermatitis
TCR gamma 87 %; TCR beta 78 % combining the two: 90 % sensitivity (Lukowsky et al. 2010)
TCR gamma 50–90 %;TCR beta 60–98 %: range of sensitivity (Sproul and Goodlad 2012)
TCR beta or gamma 64 % sensitivity, 84 % specificity BIOMED-2; interpretation subject to use of clinical risk and meaning of oligoclonality (Zhang 2010)
Granulomatous MF (GMF) from reactive granulomas
PCR sensitivity 94 % GMF and 4–14 % in reactive granulomas (Pfaltz et al. 2011; Dabiri et al. 2011)
B cells
IgH PCR 73 % sensitivity and 100 % specificity (Hughes et al. 2001)
CBCL vs. CLH 85 % sensitivity and specificity of 96 % (Morales et al. 2008)
Cutaneous lymphoid hyperplasia (CLH) with clonal dermatitis
4–61 % positive in CLH (Bouloc et al. 1999; Nihal et al. 2003; Boudova et al. 2005)

preclude definitive distinction between a benign process and lymphoma. Although PCR has been mostly used to detect clonality in a cellular specimen, the standardized EuroClonality consensus study elaborates on several PCR amplicon signatures that may be seen in patients with skewed immunity and enhanced immune responses either from transplantation, therapy, inflammation, or infections (Langerak et al. 2012); see Table 4.1. However, judicious use of this test in appropriate cases, with an adequate cellular sample, clinical risk estimation, and a rational algorithm, increases its positive and negative predictive value (Zhang et al. 2010).

The indications for performing this clonality test are dictated by the findings in the biopsy: presumptive morphologic diagnosis with clinical correlation. It is not useful in the following three groups of cases: (1) evidence of "other" infiltrates such as carcinoma, melanoma, sarcoma, or myelomonocytic leukemia, Hodgkin lymphoma; (2) clonal light chain restriction by flow cytometry, image cytometry, IHC, or ISH; and (3) prior diagnostic molecular studies compatible with the working diagnosis; see Table 4.2. In Table 4.2 we present our experience on the applications and indications of molecular tests and their role in cutaneous hematopathology. In that table, molecular tests are not indicated if the histology and IHC results are diagnostic of carcinoma, sarcoma, leukemia, or Hodgkin lymphoma. We also defer these tests if there was a previous diagnostic test on antecedent biopsy. In addition, if clonality has been confirmed by light chain restriction by ISH or by IHC or if the morphology is frankly malignant and dominant markers are diffusely positive that is characteristically that only in neoplasms and not a feature seen in reactive forms, we also do not order the T and B clonality tests.

Of 160 cutaneous lymphohematopoietic cases we saw in consultation in Tampa, FL, from 2010

Table 4.2 Incidence of TCR and BCR clonality assay, $n = 50$ cases (either both, or TCR or IgG only)

A. N tested	TCR+	IgG+	TCR+/IgG+	IgG–; TCR–
50(100 %)	18 (36 %)	10 (20 %)	2 (4 %)	10 (20 %); 18(36 %)

Table 4.3   Cases not requiring PCR clonality assays, $n=110$ cases

	Not indicated morphology	Used instead clonality light chains/		Used instead history of prev tested by PCR
B. Not tested	IHC	tumor marker	Used instead	
Total				
$N=110(100\%)$	$N=14(13\%)$	$N=57(51\%)$	$N=19(17\%)$	$N=20(18\%)$
	12 myeloid sarcoma	Histopathology +	8 by kappa or lambda IHC	TCR or IgG
	1 Merkel cell	Immunostains	7 by CD30-positive pattern	
	1 Hodgkin lymphoma		4 by CD10/BCL6	

to 2013, 50 cases (31 %) had TCR/IgG gene rearrangement studies using GeneScan capillary electrophoresis (BIOMED-2) and 110 cases (69 %) did not have the tests. Frequency of the tests are as follows: both TCR and IgG, 31, 62 %; TCR only, 17, 34 %; IgG only, 2, 4 %. Of these, 11 (22 %) were repeat biopsies/PCR with nine out of 11 cases resulting in a change in diagnosis. Repeat tests were ordered if there was clinical-pathology discordance or doubt of adequate DNA. Four of five with oligoclonal results were from shave biopsies and repeated with excision/punch biopsy which was then adequate. Of the 11, seven atypical hyperplasias with equivocal results were positive leading to diagnosis of five cutaneous B-cell lymphoma (CBCL) and two primary cutaneous small and medium cell T-cell lymphoma (PCSMTCL); two biclonal cases (IgG + TCR+; IgGoligoTCR+) with IgG + TCR- and IgG-TCR + repeat results confirmed CBCL and lymphomatoid papulosis, respectively (Table 4.2).

Overall, we believe that T and B clonality by PCR is indicated/helpful in about a third of cases. Oligoclonal/equivocal results were noted in small usually shave biopsies. Repeat tests are all useful results that need careful correlation with clinical course, histopathology, and immunostaining. In general, no change of original result supports the monoclonal or polyclonal nature. A confirmation may avoid unnecessary expensive treatment or unnecessary staging tests.

It is generally understood that the results of these molecular tests are not the gold standard that equates to a clinical diagnosis considering that these tests do not detect all neoplasms, that there are false-positive and false-negative results,

and that there is a spectrum of skin lesions that evolve from benign cutaneous lymphoid hyperplasia to non-clonal atypical lymphoid hyperplasia, to prelymphomatous " clonal dermatitis," to frank lymphoma as determined by a combined use of clinical behavior, morphological, immunohistochemical, and molecular criteria; see Table 4.3.

Basis of PCR Antigen Receptor Gene Rearrangement Assay

The gene rearrangement sequence as a normal biology of maturing lymphocytes is illustrated in Fig. 4.1. The PCR technique employs unique nucleic acid sequences by generating a set of primers designed to hybridize with and detect family-specific common sequences, so that about seven primers are used instead of the 45 individual primers for the IgH V family or several primers for the possible total of nine variable regions the TCR gamma family.

Examples of assay results and recommended interpretation according to the EuroClonality consortium are shown in Figs. 4.2 and 4.3 (Langerak et al. 2012).

The Concept of Pseudolymphomas (Cutaneous Lymphoid Hyperplasia), Cutaneous Lymphoid Dyscrasias, and Prelymphomatous Infiltrates

Because CTCL and CBCL often evolve over a period of time from an inflammatory background, the precise boundary between

Fig. 4.1 The gene rearrangement sequence as a normal biology of maturing lymphocytes. Mechanism of antigen receptors gene rearrangement to generate a unique sequence detectable by PCR. Germ line to rearrange DNA of T cell receptor beta gene (B cell IgH similar). The diagram illustrates sequence of antigen receptor gene rearrangement to generate codes for receptor diversity (adapted from immuneweb.xxmu.edu) from: (**a**) germ line DNA sequence with variable, diversity, joining, and constant region segments; (**b**, **c**) Tertiary structure altered to place single D segment in close proximity to a single J segment; (**d**) followed by double-stranded DNA break; (**e**) rejoining by RAG (recombination activating gene) proteins (*yellow* bolt); (**f**) excision of intervening DNA; and (**g**) Tdt adds or subtracts random nucleotides (open bolt) to generate a unique rearranged DNA ending with a specific length or base pair that could be assayed by PCR technique

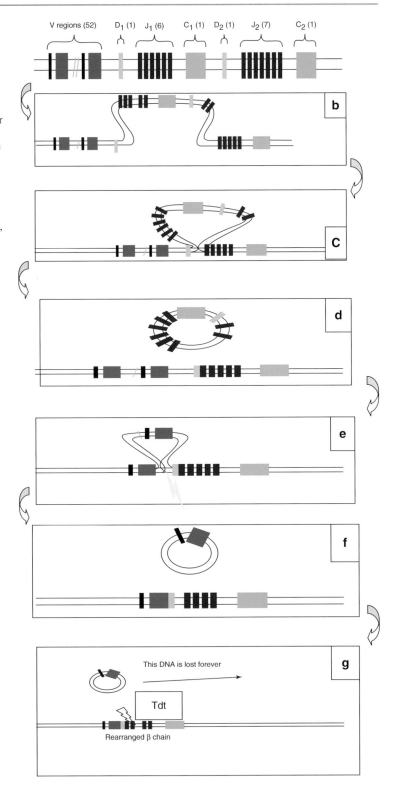

lymphoma and benign could be elusive. In early diseases, cutaneous lymphomas can be difficult to distinguish from benign inflammatory der- matosis or cutaneous lymphoid hyperplasia; hence, it is useful to have descriptors that define histological niches along this continuum. *It*

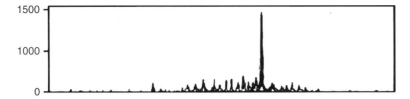

Fig. 4.2 IgH cell peaks and PCR GeneScan interpretation according to the EuroClonality consortium. The above diagram represents typical monoclonal peak with small polyclonal peaks in the background. "Profiles with one or two clear peaks or bands are called 'clonal', with the option to indicate that the intensities are weak or that a polyclonal background is seen." (Langerak 2012). In Sproul and Goodlad (2012), pseudoclonality is also defined as single band/peak or doublet with little if any polyclonal background and rarely reproducible on repeat testing

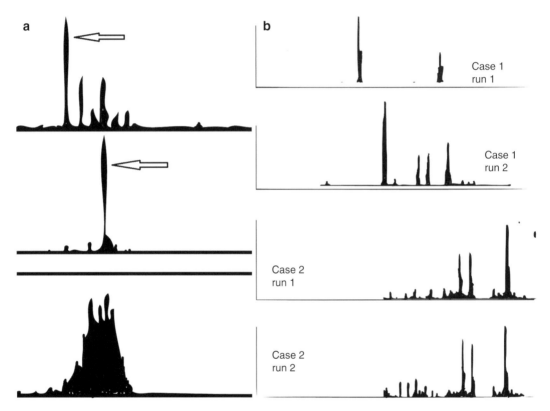

Fig. 4.3 A T beta and gamma gene rearrangement and PCR GeneScan interpretation. (**a**) When one to two peaks or bands are identified that are clearly non-reproducible, this is referred to as "pseudoclonal"; implicit in this description is that clonal signals are seen, but that they differ in size between the duplicates as shown by arrows. The last panel shows a dominant polyclonal population. (**b**) T gamma peaks and recommended interpretations according to the EuroClonality consortium. "Even cases that show a relatively weak clonal peak/band in a polyclonal background can be truly clonal, as long as the pattern is reproducible and preferably seen in multiple targets. Profiles with multiple (defined as three or more) peaks or bands are indicated with the description "multiple products." Such profiles as in case 1 run 1 and 2, are non-reproducible or "pseudoclonal," or in case 2 run 1 and run 2 as reproducible but reflect multiple consistent clones probably due to a dominant immune response" and may be reactive in nature." (Langerak et al. 2012)

should be emphasized that one benign diagnosis in a particular patient does not necessarily evolve to atypical hyperplasia followed by lymphoma. Multiple events required for malignant transformation may not occur for a particular patient.

Definitions

Pseudolymphoma is a nonspecific term for a variety of reactive T- or B-cell infiltrates that simulate cutaneous lymphoma secondary to drugs, immune dysregulation, infection, arthropod bite, or chemical reaction or are idiopathic in origin. Cutaneous lymphoid hyperplasia is a synonymous term, often applied to pseudolymphomas with discrete benign germinal centers. When there is an overlap of clinical and histologic features of hyperplasia or inflammatory dermatosis, with atypical findings, the term pseudolymphoma is often used. A number of classification schemes have been proposed based on etiology, architecture, or immunohistology.

Using immunohistology, B-cell, T-cell, and mixed pseudolymphomas are classified if B or T cells are predominant and mixed if in between. T-cell pseudolymphoma is either epidermotropic and band-like or dermal and nodular in appearance. See Chaps. 5 and 8 for discussion (Rijlaarsdam et al. 1992).

Cutaneous T-cell lymphoid dyscrasias were coined as a unifying term for a group of idiopathic chronic dermatoses with persistent T-cell clones and have uncommon evolution to CTCL; see Table 4.4 (Guitart and Magro 2007).

Prelymphomatous infiltrate includes those skin lesions with a low but defined frequency of progression to cutaneous B- or T-cell lymphoma; see Table 4.6.

Clonality by GeneScan: *monoclonal* pattern is defined as one or two peaks, with a peak height substantially higher than the baseline, with or without a low-level or more prominent smear (polyclonal amplification) pattern in the background; see Figs. 4.2 and 4.3.

An *oligoclonal* pattern is defined as three prominent peaks, with peak height substantially higher than baseline; see Fig. 4.3. The range of analytic sensitivity (assay cannot detect clonality below the given percent of clonal cells over all lymphocytes) of the T-cell receptor gamma and beta PCR assays is 5–10 and 10–15 %, respectively.

Although the presumption is that the infiltrate in pseudolymphoma is benign or reactive, clinicians are often advised that a small percentage of this group can progress to lymphoma, and there-

Table 4.4 Cutaneous pseudolymphomas (or cutaneous lymphoid hyperplasia): histoimmunologic types and clonal pseudolymphomas (citation with clonality studies)

Cutaneous T-cell pseudolymphoma
Lichen planus (Schiller et al. 2000)
PLEVA (Weiss et al. 1987; Weinberg 2002)
Benign lichenoid keratosis (lichen planus like keratosis) (Arai 2007)
Lymphomatoid contact dermatitis (Brady 1999)
Lichen sclerosus (Lukowsky et al. 2000)
Lymphomatoid drug reaction (Brady 1999; Magro 2003)
Cutaneous B-cell pseudolymphoma (Arai et al. 2005; Gilliam and Wood 2000; Nihal et al. 2003)
Borrelia-associated cutaneous lymphoid hyperplasia (CLH) (Tee et al. 2012; Eisendle and Zelger 2009)
Tattoo-associated cutaneous lymphoid hyperplasia (Camilot et al. 2012)
Autoimmune-associated cutaneous lymphoid hyperplasia (Magro et al. 1997)
Atypical CLH (Kulow et al. 2002; Anandasabapathy et al. 2008)
Cutaneous pseudo T/B mixed pseudolymphoma
Mixed nodular pseudolymphoma
Biclonal pseudolymphoma (Kazakov et al. 2006)
Clonal mixed pseudolymphoma of undetermined significance (Melotti et al. 2010; Flaig et al. 2000; Holm et al. 2002; Boer et al. 2008)
Solitary nodular clonal mixed pseudolymphoma of undetermined significance (Beltraminelli et al. 2009)
Cutaneous pseudolymphomatous folliculitis (PF)
PF associated with EGFR antagonist (Kerl 2012; Kakizaki et al. 2012)
Nodular type of PF (Nakamura et al. 2009)
Clonal PF with undetermined significance (Kazakov et al. 2008)
Pseudolymphomatous folliculitis (Fujimura et al. 2012)

Table 4.5 Monoclonal T-cell dyscrasia of undetermined significance (Guitart and Magro 2007)

Hypopigmented interface variant
Pigmented purpuric dermatosis
Atypical lobular lymphocytic panniculitis
Syringolymphoid hyperplasia with alopecia
Idiopathic follicular mucinosis
Pityriasis lichenoides
Parapsoriasis
Clonal erythroderma

fore, long-term follow-up is recommended (Albrecht et al. 2007; Anandasabapathy et al. 2008; Arai et al. 1999, 2005; Bergman 2010). Clinical features are used as a guide to therapy or planning in equivocal cases with "pseudoclonality" (Gilliam and Wood 2000).

The explanation for the foregoing is the well-described pathobiology of cutaneous lymphomas in which cutaneous lymphomas arise from within a population with multiple subclones (Cozzio and French 2008; Ponti et al. 2008) and lymphoid hyperplasias progress with worsening of appearance with or without evidence of a clonal population (Wood 2001; Wood et al. 1989; Kulow et al. 2002). The percentage of clonality detection increases as the lymphoma progresses to a higher stage and as histopathological score increases, especially well documented for mycosis fungoides (MF) (Guitart et al. 2001).

Interpretation of a pseudoclonal result in the face of a normal skin biopsy or discordant skin biopsy findings is interpreted by whether the infiltrate is B or T cell rich or by clinical risk assessment. If there are a small number of discrete bands consistent with oligoclonality, it is often difficult to differentiate lymphoma from a false positive (clonally restricted benign dermatitis). Correlation with immunostains is useful and false positives are often associated with scant infiltrates or infiltrates rich in opposite lineage (T clonality in B cell rich or B clonality in T-cell-rich infiltrate) (Nihal et al. 2000, 2003).

For an excellent introductory review of the role of molecular pathology in cutaneous lymphoma, see Raess and Bagg (2012). Using the heteroduplex assay, in the evaluation of patients suspected of having early MF, Murphy et al. detected identical banded patterns in serial skin biopsies from the same patient. No dominant T-cell clones were found in the inflammatory dermatoses studied (Murphy et al. 2000). In T-cell assay on paraffin-embedded skin tissue using GeneScan capillary electrophoresis (BIOMED-2), performance of both TCR gamma and TCR beta PCR is superior to the use of only one probe, if a risk assessment algorithm is followed (Zhang et al. 2010). Because of these findings and for cost-effective reasons, some centers use this sequential algorithm. For example, if the pretest risk is low-moderate according to clinical criteria and TCR gamma is not detected, TCR beta analysis is not performed. But if TCR gamma rearrangement is found, TCR beta is additionally done, and if both are positive, full support for lymphoma is reported. *If TCR gamma is positive but TCR beta is negative, a repeat test is recommended.* If the risk is moderate-high and a positive TCR gamma is obtained, TCR beta is not performed and the result called positive for lymphoma. If in this case, TCR gamma is initially negative, then TCR beta is performed. If negative, there is no clonal support for lymphoma, but if positive, a diagnosis of lymphoma is supported (Stanford Medical Center esoteric department 2011; Zhang et al. 2010); see Fig. 4.4.

Comparison of Sensitivity and Specificity of PCR of Several Methods

Using the BIOMED-2 method, B-cell clonality technique in formalin-fixed paraffin-embedded tissue is as follows: the DNA from the framework region 3 (FR3) sequence of the IgH genes is amplified to ascertain the presence of a clonal IgH gene rearrangement resulting in 73 % sensitivity and 100 % specificity (Hughes et al. 2001). Similarly, Morales et al. reported IgH clonality can be detected in formalin-fixed samples of CBCL with 85 % sensitivity and specificity of 96 % (Morales et al. 2008). For T cells, BIOMED-2 TCR PCR works well with DNA from paraffin-embedded tissue, in which clonality was detected 90 % on average revealing a high-clonality detection rate in CTCL, and thus is recommended for routine skin biopsy preparations (Hughes et al. 2001; Lukowsky et al. 2010; Luo et al. 2001; Meyer et al. 1997; Morales et al. 2008); see Table 4.1.

Luo et al. compared the capillary electrophoresis (CE) method with the standard denaturing gradient gel electrophoresis (DGGE) method using formalin-fixed specimens. Eleven of 12 (92 %) cases with a definitive diagnosis of T-cell lymphoma were monoclonal by CE, with 100 % concordance with the DGGE method. Of nine specimens morphologically suspicious for T-cell lymphoma, five specimens were positive by CE analysis compared with four specimens

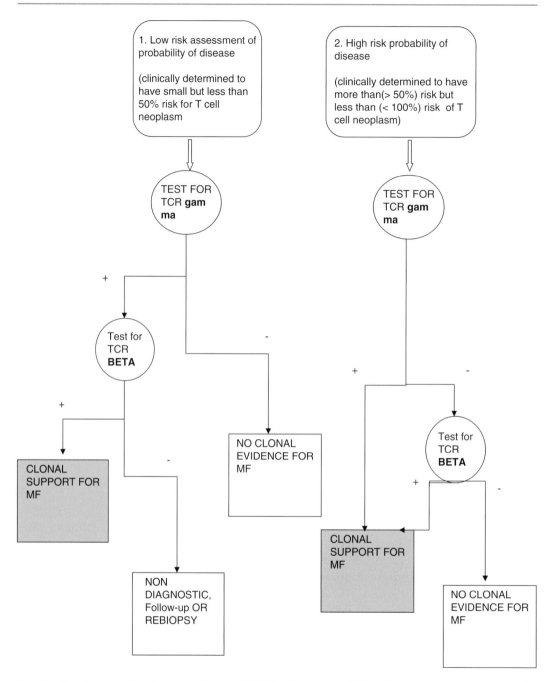

Fig. 4.4 Workflow algorithm for sequential use of PCR for T gamma and T beta for gene rearrangement assay for clonality in assessment in mycosis fungoides (Zhang et al. 2010)

by DGGE. In addition, 14 specimens for staging from patients with known T-cell lymphoma were studied using both the CE and DGGE methods, with a concordance of 86 % (Luo et al. 2001).

Causes of Pseudolymphomas

Atypical lymphocytic infiltrates that mimic cutaneous lymphoma (i.e., pseudolymphomas) are often observed in skin biopsy specimens from

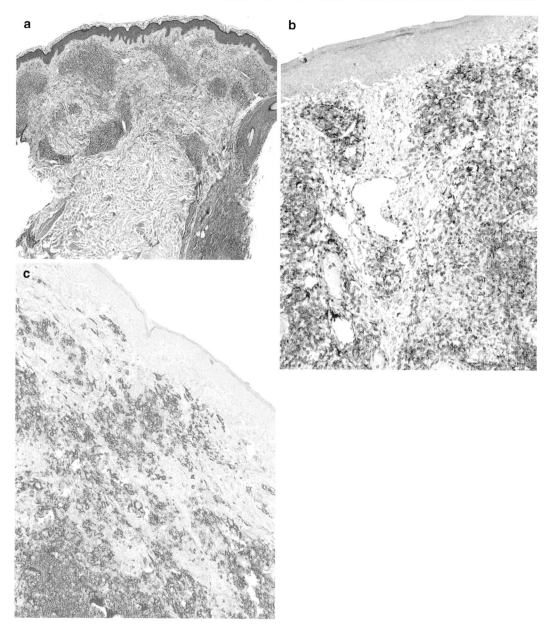

Fig. 4.5 (**a**) Arthropod spider bite from a farmer in Pensacola, Florida, who noted a spider nicked his neck and then complained of persistent nodule for several months which was biopsied. (**b**) shows T-cell reaction in a perivascular nodular pattern in the upper and deep dermis with epitheliotropism in hair and eccrine areas, low power. B.CD3 and (**c**) mixed cell reaction, with similar pattern of CD20 B-cell stains

patients with altered immune function or excessive lymphoid reaction to an antigen. The former may reflect systemic immune dysregulatory states such as collagen vascular disease, and the latter may be secondary to exogenous antigen introduction such vaccination, infection, and arthropod bites; see Fig. 4.5. Among the iatrogenic causes are drug therapy with agents that dysregulate normal lymphocyte function; see Table 4.7 for list of drugs (Brady et al. 1999; Jackson and Nesbit 2012). These drugs encompass those with anti-prefix such as anticonvulsants, antidepressants such as phenothiazines, antibiotics, antihypertensives such as calcium channel blockers, antiinflammatory, antihistamines, and antilipidemic drugs. Chemokines such as interleukins, colony-stimulating factors (CSF), and inhibitors to angiotensin-converting enzyme, tyrosinases and TNF (tumor necrosis factors), are usually given in a short list; see Chap. 15.

The appellation of lymphomatoid hypersensitivity reaction has been applied to cases of drug-associated pseudolymphoma in association with atopy, high IgE, and external contact sensitization such as metals contact reaction; see Fig. 4.6.

As mentioned, two types of T pseudolymphoma that are CTCL mimics include the band-like T and nodular pseudolymphomas. Those with a lichenoid pattern include lymphomatoid contact dermatitis (Fig. 4.7), lichen planus

(Fig. 4.8), and lichen sclerosus (Fig. 4.9). Some examples of idiopathic band-like or nodular/diffuse T-cell pseudolymphoma without T- or B-cell gene rearrangement clonal results are shown in Figs. 4.10 and 4.11, for band-like and nodular/diffuse, respectively. Lichenoid benign lymphomatoid keratosis (Fig. 4.12) may show a nodular pattern and is a differential diagnosis of solitary primary cutaneous small and medium T-cell lymphoma. Many classic dermatitis with lymphoid-rich reaction in epidermis and hair follicles may histologically present as pseudolymphoma such as discoid lupus (Fig. 4.13) and lymphomatoid folliculitis (Fig. 4.14). Pathologically and clinically, distinction of such cases from cutaneous lymphoma is often difficult (Brady et al. 1999). Several unusual and specific entities that may resemble pseudolymphomas include angiolymphoid hyperplasia with eosinophilia (ALHE) or Kimura's disease and Castleman's disease.

Limitation of Molecular Tests

It is important to realize the limitation of molecular assays. Caution is warranted in interpreting results out of context. This is because it has been observed that tumor cells arise from multiple

Table 4.6 Prelymphomatous or MF variants with differences in survival (Agar et al. 2010)

Folliculotropic MF variant 12.6 % of series, median survival 12.2 years, 75 % 5 years and 54 % 10-year survival, 37 % 20-year survival
Hypopigmented MF 3.4 % of series with 98 % 5 and 10-year overall survival
Poikilodermatous MF 20.1 % of series with 89 %,76 %, 50 % 5, 10, 20-year survival, respectively

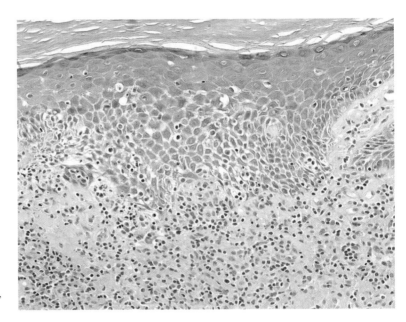

Fig. 4.6 Lymphomatoid drug reaction with dense parakeratosis, spongiosis, and epidermotropic haloed lymphocytes composed of variable sized, small- and medium-sized, non-cerebriform cells (Courtesy of dermatopathologist M. Patel, DermPath Dx Tampa, FL)

Fig. 4.7 Lymphomatoid contact dermatitis with sparse epidermotropic small lymphocytes and a vesicle of Langerhan's cell hyperplasia, basket weave parakeratosis, spongiosis and subepidermal edema, and perivascular infiltrates

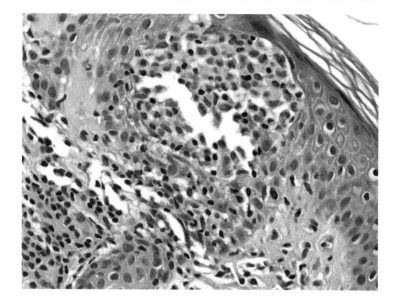

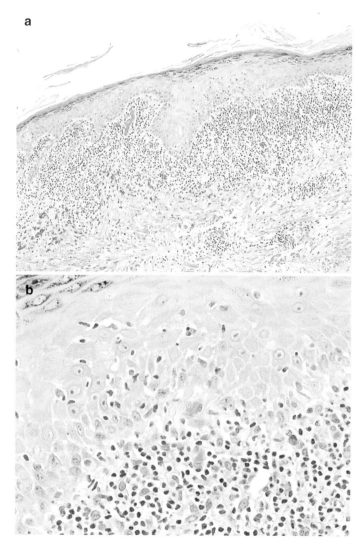

a

b

Fig. 4.8 Lichen planus, (**a**) low power, with lichenoid lymphocytic infiltrate with pigment incontinence and mild acanthosis and epitheliotropism, and (**b**) high power showing atypical small lymphocytes with irregular nuclei with haloes mimicking early MF, but cerebriform cells are difficult to find (Courtesy of dermatopathologist M. Patel, DermPath Dx Tampa, FL)

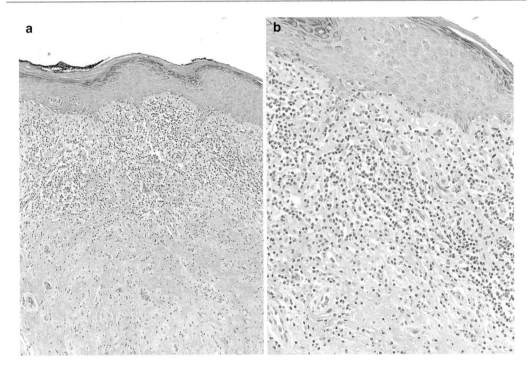

Fig. 4.9 Lichen sclerosus, medium power, (**a**) biopsy from prepuce with sclerotic dense dermal pink paucicellular bottom and a lichenoid lymphocytic infiltrate. In higher power, (**b**) small lymphocytes, some with halo hugging the base of epidermis and tracking upward, sometimes with atypia simulating haloed lymphocytes in mycosis fungoides (Courtesy of dermatopathologist M. Patel, DermPath Dx Tampa, FL)

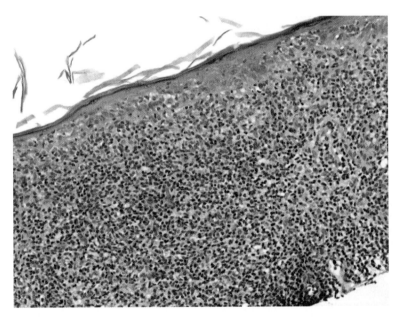

Fig. 4.10 T pseudolymphoma with band-like pattern is among the two common patterns of T-cell pseudolymphoma. This patient has chest nodules with appearance of Grover's disease, lacks T-cell clonality, and has a CD3+ predominant infiltrate with numerous histiocytes and pigmented macrophages. This one may mimic lichenoid or nodular pattern seen in CTCL or that seen secondary to drug hypersensitivity reactions. Other types of patterns seen in hypersensitivity lymphomatoid reactions include interface pattern, psoriasiform dermatitis with lymphoid atypia, nodular lymphoid hyperplasia with B-cell follicular pattern, angiocentric lymphocytic pattern, and finally lymphomatoid follicular mucinosis (Brady et al. 1999)

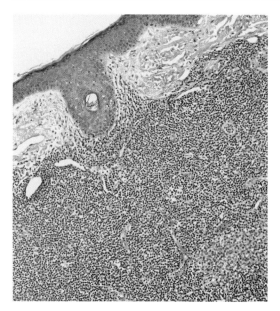

Fig. 4.11 T-cell pseudolymphoma with nodular T pattern, which is distinct from the frequently described B-cell pattern because of the lack of prominent germinal centers, is composed of small- to medium-sized non-atypical lymphocytes admixed with vessels, histiocytes, plasma cells, and occasional atrophic germinal centers characterized as an often solitary nodule, not usually in the head and neck area, by high CD3:CD20 ratio and CD8 predominance, no aberrancy of T antigens, and lack of clonal T cells by PCR. Some lichenoid keratosis with deep nodules overlaps with T-cell pseudolymphoma. Presence of T-cell clonality and atypia raises concern for a solitary primary cutaneous small- to medium-sized T-cell lymphoma

subclones which show instability or clonal heterogeneity, often obscured by a background of reactive cells, in both cutaneous B-cell and T-cell lymphomas (Ponti et al. 2008). Strategies to overcome these limitations include repeat biopsies, duplicate assays in a single biopsy, and correlation of assay results from more than one site. Repeat biopsies are often done for insufficient samples or equivocal results, and in our experience, superficial biopsy or biopsies with scant infiltrates predispose to indeterminate or possibly false-positive or false-negative test results. Equivocal, oligoclonal, or pseudoclonal results may arise as a reflection of the inherent biology and heterogeneity of these lymphoproliferations. Pitfalls include clonal heterogeneity and false negativity due, respectively, to (1) inherent multiband clonal neoplasm or (2) from a limited primer set or ineffective primer annealing due to somatic point mutations. False-positive results may be due to preferential amplification of individual amplicon within a limited pool of polyclonal cells. In specimens submitted for diagnosis, it is also important to keep in mind that detection of clonality is not by itself diagnostic of malignancy as there are many examples of "clonal dermatitis" (Nihal et al. 2000, 2003). In this regard, clinical correlation is of crucial importance: correlative histopathology with

Fig. 4.12 Benign lichenoid keratosis is a T-cell pseudo-lymphoma. Variable epidermal acanthosis with closely apposed band-like dense lichenoid lymphocytic infiltrate. Variable numbers of plasma cells, histiocytes, and eosinophils were identified along with non-atypical small lymphocytes and epidermal parakeratosis, which distinguish these lesions from typical lichen planus. Presence of atypical lymphocytes and prominent epidermotropism raises concern for mycosis fungoides (Courtesy of dermatopathologist M. Patel, DermPath Dx Tampa, FL)

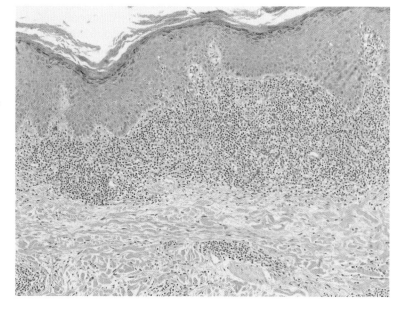

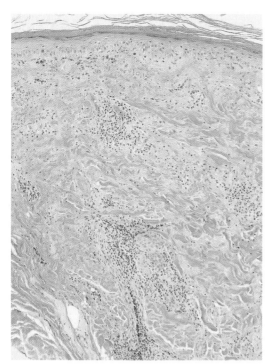

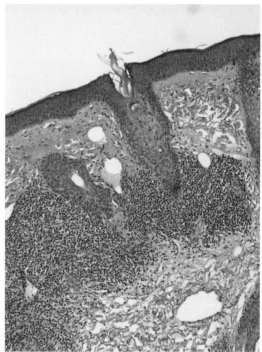

Fig. 4.13 Benign, discoid lupus erythematosus (DLE). Basal layer epithelial vacuolar degeneration, atrophy, parakeratosis, pigment incontinence and thickened basement membrane, deep perivascular and periappendiceal lymphocytic infiltrate, and dermal fibroplasia in this long-standing lesion, with beaded basophilic pale areas positive for dermal mucin (Courtesy of dermatopathologist M. Patel, DermPath Dx Tampa, FL)

Fig. 4.14 Benign lymphomatous folliculitis in a patient with follicular plugging and dermal basophilic-beaded mucinous degeneration (*bottom*) consistent with folliculotropic DLE. Idiopathic pseudolymphomatous folliculitis mimics folliculotropic mycosis fungoides, commonly located on the face as solitary erythematous papules or nodules characterized by regression. Here, a nodular peri-follicular infiltrate of lymphocytes with infiltration of follicular structures and dermis, immunostained as a mixture of B and T cells and lack of clonality by PCR

clinical information, prior history, and/or drug intake. In addition, about 14 % show clonal PCR in well-documented drug-induced pseudolymphoma (Brady et al. 1999). Performance of both tests for TCR gamma or beta gene rearrangement or even better to use a sequential gamma then beta test algorithm incorporating clinically determined low- or high-risk probability of disease, as reported and validated by Zhang et al., tends to maximize predictive value and offer cost-effective and rational workup (Zhang et al. 2010); see Fig. 4.4 for diagram of workflow.

Normal TCR gamma/delta gene segments show a restricted TCR repertoire of only 9–11 rearranged segments when compared with 67 segments for TCR beta rearrangements (van Dongen et al. 2003b). In addition, in some viral infections and after organ transplantation,

immune response of T cells generates only a limited number of TCR gamma-rearranged segments which present a small number of targets for gene rearrangement assays. Hence, the results can show as few oligoclonal or multiple small bands in PCR. Contrary to some notion that this is often a failure of the test, in reality, this multiband peaks could be a reflection of the inherent biology of reactive lymphoid infiltrate in above settings (Kluin-Nelemans et al. 1998; Mariani et al. 2001). Given the highly sensitive PCR, the oligoclones which manifest in these settings are in reality part of a polyclonal response (van Dongen et al. 2003a). In high clinical risk setting, however, oligoclones may indicate a neoplastic population presenting with several dominant or transformed tumor clones (Zhang et al. 2010).

Pseudoclonality and quantity of lymphocytes: In reactive conditions, DNA in cutaneous lymphoid infiltrates produces a polyclonal pattern when amplified by PCR, but when this DNA is serially diluted, a critical level is reached when *an apparent clonal peak appears*. This is paralleled by microdissected lymphocytes from reactive proliferations that give rise to pseudoclonality by PCR. It is estimated that *800–2,000 lymphocytes or 20–40 ng of DNA* is the threshold where pseudoclonality becomes an issue (Sproul and Goodlad 2012).

Role of Flow Cytometry and Image Cytometry

In the past decade, flow cytometric immunophenotyping has proven to be more reliable than morphologic examination in assessing for lymphoma (Sezary cells) in the peripheral blood of patients with mycosis fungoides and Sezary syndrome, as the neoplastic cells have an aberrant immunophenotype (Borowitz et al. 1993; Klemke et al. 2006; Washington et al. 2002; Meyerson 2008).

Although immunohistochemistry is the most convenient immunophenotyping method in office clinical practice, flow cytometry is the preferred method in multiparameter interrogation of cell characteristics. Included in most cutaneous hematopathology reports is the recommendation to the clinician for additional use of flow cytometry in fresh biopsied tissue for confirmation and for further workup. In flow cytometry-equipped centers, 4–8 mm skin biopsies in fresh state appear adequate for the workup of early CTCL and non-MF cutaneous lymphomas (Novelli et al. 2008; Meyerson 2008; Jokinen et al. 2011). Some biopsies may have scant infiltrate and may not yield adequate cells for analysis; however, some centers can analyze as few as 20 cells and find them to be informative (Wood 2006; Finn et al. 1998). In addition, the remaining cellular specimen can be submitted for molecular PCR analysis, after histologic evaluation.

It is also important to know the limitation of flow cytometry. T-cell antigenic alterations are not entirely specific for mycosis fungoides or Sezary syndrome and have been observed in some reactive conditions (Harmon et al. 1996). In addition, in MF there is heterogeneity with a fraction comprised of tumor cells in a background of reactive T cells, averaging 28 % of lymphocytes in skin as malignant. In about half of MF cases, fewer than 10 % are the malignant "cerebriform" component, and therefore judicious *gating* of these malignant cells by skillful use of flow cytometry list-mode data is a well-known strategy (Meyerson 2008; Novelli et al. 2008). Without this added manipulation, the neoplastic cells may be submerged or lost within the cluster of reactive T- or B-cell population. Furthermore, the use of numerical or intensity-based diagnostic criteria may enhance the flow cytometry sensitivity.

Discrete patterns of enumerated cells and their antigen density patterns are useful criteria. Cluster analysis of patterns revolves around three useful flow cytometry applications in skin lymphomas:
1. Enumeration (quantification)
2. Antigen density expression
3. Documenting clonality

The following diagnostic and supportive criteria applied to flow cytometry of skin biopsy are recommended: (Meyerson 2008)
1. Diagnostic evidence:
On CD45 × side scatter gate, discrete cluster of either:
CD4+ CD8–
CD8+ CD4–
CD4+ CD8+
CD4– CD8–
   And presence additionally within this gate of :
Altered or absent CD2, CD3, CD4, CD5, CD7, CD8, or CD26
Aberrant expression of CD10 or CD158k (killer immunoglobulin receptor)
   OR
2. Presence of Clonal population by TCR Vbeta analysis
Supportive, but not diagnostic evidence:
Greater(>) than 50 % CD3+ CD4+ CD7negative (based on CD4 cells)
Greater(>) than 80 % CD3+ CD4+ CD26negative (based on CD4 cells)

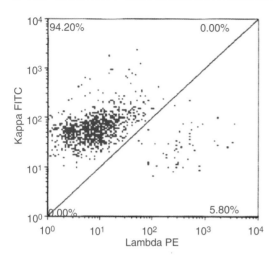

Fig. 4.15 Kappa vs. lambda light chain interrogation of cutaneous lymphoid infiltrate showing skewed distribution on kappa side vs. lambda side indicating presence of a monoclonal kappa B-cell population by flow cytometry light chain analysis

CD4 to CD8 ratio >10:1

CD30 expression

CD25, HLADR, and CD45RA/RO uniform expression

Documenting clonality in a B-cell population is relatively easy by showing a skewed distribution of light chains on B lymphocytes (Fig. 4.15). For T-cell neoplasm, T-cell receptor variable region beta (Vbeta) analysis is used and available in many reference laboratories.

Flow cytometric analysis of T-cell receptor-Vbeta expression is an alternative method to assess and quantify a T-cell clone. Unlike PCR for TCR, *a phenotypic signature of the neoplastic population can be monitored post-therapy by a relatively more accessible flow cytometry technique. Moreover, the flow assay will take hours instead of days, when compared with GeneScan CE PCR.*

For example, a population of polyclonal T cells will express a random relatively equal distribution of Vbeta proteins on the surface. Flow cytometry, in a patient with neutropenia and lymphocytosis, can detect a population with low expression of antigen such CD5 and, using backtracking, follow that population along tubes of different Vbeta probes; see Fig. 4.16. Clonality

can be determined by showing an expansion of cells reacting to a single Vbeta antibody, called direct evidence, or alternatively an absence of reactivity to all panel, called indirect evidence, suggestive of a clone. Lundell et al. directly identified 77 % and indirectly in 23 % of their cases that were PCR confirmed as clonal T cells (Lundell et al. 2005) (Fig. 4.17). Commercially available Vbeta panels (such as Beta Mark TCR repertoire kit by Beckman Coulter) detect about 70 % of the Vbeta families (among a panel directed at 24 markers of Vbeta families). Earlier studies showed concordant results by using a panel covering over 65 % of the T-cell receptor-Vb repertoire. Langerak et al. showed in their study of 47 T-cell lymphoma samples that flow cytometry antibodies detected single Vbeta domain usage in 31 (66 %) and were non-reactive in 16 (34 %), showing 100 % concordance with PCR analysis of the T-cell receptor *beta* gene (Langerak et al. 2001). Morice et al. studied 29 T-cell lymphoproliferative disorders by flow cytometric Vbeta analysis, including ten cases of cutaneous T-cell lymphoma, and showed a good correlation with molecular methods. This group expanded their study to include 11 Sezary syndrome and six mycosis fungoides cases and showed that Vbeta analysis by flow cytometry was helpful for assessing clonality and quantifying the peripheral blood tumor burden (Morice et al. 2006). Feng et al. validated the clinical utility of flow cytometric T-cell receptor-Vbeta analysis in blood staging of mycosis fungoides and Sezary syndrome patients (Feng et al. 2010).

In addition, the promise of monitoring a tumor specific antigen is realized in flow cytometry analysis compared to a PCR. Killer immunoglobulin-like receptors or killer inhibitory receptors (KIR assays) for CD158k have been shown to be useful in detecting clonality in MF and Sezary syndrome. Antibody Q66 and AZ158 in flow cytometry appear to be unique to MF/Sezary and not in reactive T cells, occurring in 88–95 % of circulating cells and in 60 % of skin lesions (Bahler et al. 2008; Lundell et al. 2005; Poszepczynska-Guigne et al. 2004; Wechsler et al. 2003), and additionally useful in large granular lymphocytic leukemia

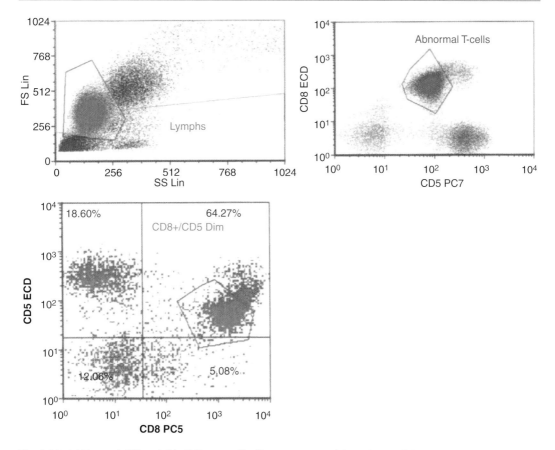

Fig. 4.16 (**a**) Forward (FS) and side (SS) scatter distribution dot plot of small- to medium-sized lymphocytes on *left panel* with backgating selection, on *right panel* using (*red polygon*) choosing the dim CD5 and dim CD8 as the target suspicious cluster of abnormal cells (user labeled as red-colored cluster). (**b**) Dim CD5 and CD8+ (*blue polygon*) dual parameter flow cytometry enumeration, with user-selected backgating strategy as the target population

(Lundell et al. 2005). Application of KIR family of CD158a-k panel or similar lectin-like receptor CD94 was noted to be useful in skin biopsy detection of NK cell lymphomas (Dukers et al. 2001) and by flow cytometry identifying restricted expression of human CD8 KIR subsets (Bjorkstrom et al. 2012).

Commonly seen in clinical practice of cutaneous hematopathology is the infrequent availability of fresh biopsied tissue that is needed by flow cytometry or the less than widespread request for a Vbeta assessment of T-cell clonality; hence, testing using molecular PCR in formalin-fixed paraffin-embedded tissue to supplement flow cytometric findings is recommended by the International Society for Cutaneous Lymphomas (Pimpinelli et al. 2005) and WHO-EORTC and WHO 2008 (Swerdlow et al. 2008).

However, when fresh tissue is not available for flow cytometry specimen, another tissue assay modality or technique may be used. Flow cytometry requires adequately sampled fresh biopsied tissue, which are not available since skin biopsies are often submitted and processed as formalin-fixed paraffin-embedded tissue. In the absence of flow cytometry, alternative strategies for enumeration and clonality analysis may include *image analysis*. Image cytometry is the application of image analysis in immunohistochemistry-stained tissue. These are advanced specialized tools for nuanced counting of tumor

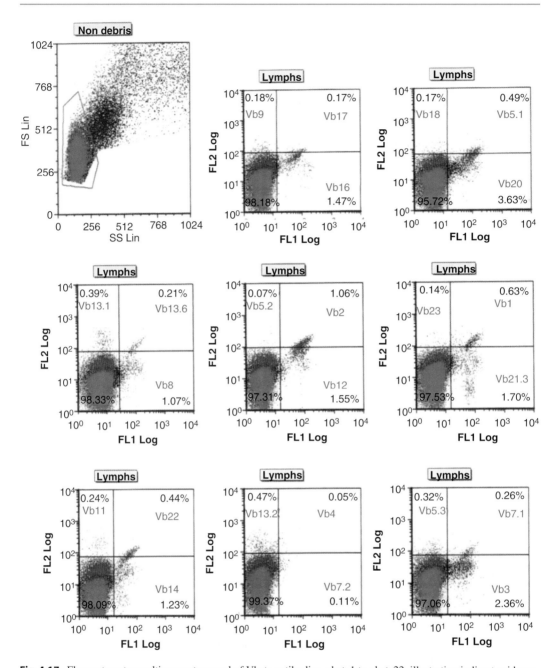

Fig. 4.17 Flow cytometry multiparameter panel of Vbeta antibodies, vbeta1 to vbeta22, illustrating indirect evidence, clone in red cluster in quadrant III, clonality confirmed by T-cell PCR rearrangement

cells especially useful in biopsies already submitted in paraffin-embedded tissue. In the era of whole slide digital pathology and its applications, image cytometry ranks high as a "holy grail" in desired specialized application.

Image Cytometry

Quantitative immunohistochemistry and 2-dimensional image analysis software tools appear to be upward in outlook and poised to be clinically applicable in the distinction between entities in cutaneous hematopathology. Commercially available systems can quantify tissue immunostains. Garcia-Herrera et al. studies documented a group of patients with a histologic picture of primary cutaneous small and medium T-cell lymphoma that, however, behaved aggressively. They noted that this group could be adequately delineated from those that behaved indolently by the use of image cytometry accurately enumerating Ki-67 and CD8+ cells; see Chap. 10 on PCSMTCL discussion (Garcia-Herrera et al. 2008). This technique was successfully applied previously by Carreras et al. who quantified T regulatory cells, CD3, and CD4 T helper cells in whole-tissue sections of follicular lymphoma and reactive follicles using automated scanning microscope and image analysis systems (Ariol 2.1, SL-50; Applied Imaging Corporation, Newcastle on Tyne, United Kingdom) (Carreras et al. 2006). In addition, this technique was successfully implemented in automatically enumerating Ki67 in paraffin-embedded tissue using VirtualFlow method (PC software module provided by IHCFLOW, Inc. Lutz, FL) in Technology and Innovation (Lloyd et al. 2013). The application of the IHCFLOW technology is described in greater detail as follows since this is a relatively new technique.

The number of Ki67-positive T cells was quantified in whole-tissue sections of all samples using an automated scanning microscope and image analysis system (VirtualFlow 10.10; IHCFLOW, Inc, Lutz, FL). Quantification of the Ki67-positive cells was performed with the nuclear Ki67-module using the following strategy. First, the tissue scanning phase was performed with a 4× objective, followed by an automated 20× medium-magnification capture of the field. Subsequently, the optimal evaluation areas, which accounted for 60–100 % of the whole section, were captured by the two observers using DPlan 20× objective and three color charged-coupled device (CCD) with 1,200 × 1,600 pixels. In the next analysis phase, a nuclear high-resolution classifier which was previously trained for all facets and variables in Ki67 nuclear staining was used. The knowledge-domain-based

supervised classifier consisted of a color class definition for the positive and negative nuclei, cytoplasm, and background and a shape-size class definition for the positive and negative nuclei. The color class was defined by the hue, saturation, and intensity parameters, whereas the shape class was defined by the spot width and pixel diameter parameters. The high-throughput classifier was trained in several areas within a tissue sample, often with field with 7,000–10,000 cells in order to avoid miscalculation due to differences in staining and cell composition. The classifier was always trained and recalibrated under the visual supervision of the pathologist. Ki67-positive and Ki67-negative cells were counted independently in the selected compartments. The total number of cells was recorded by adding counts for all compartments. To minimize the heterogeneous distribution of positive cells, a minimum number of ten complete regional areas were selected. Capture to analysis of each image field took 2–10 s in Intel PC, I5, 2.9 mhz CPU. In addition to Ki67, CD8 enumeration of reactive lymphocytes in B-cell lymphomas was performed using VirtualFlow image cytometry in lymph nodal mantle cell lymphomas (Cualing et al. 2007) and a large panel of skin lymphoma-associated antibodies (Fig. 4.19).

Likewise, immunostain enumeration was also applied to CD30+ skin lymphomas. A panel of skin target markers in lymphomatoid papulosis (LyP), cutaneous anaplastic large cell lymphoma (ALCL), and systemic ALCL was studied by Rezania et al. (2008) (Fig. 4.19).The count statistics are shown in Table 4.8. Results with statistical significance data suggested the utility of some antibodies, like TRAF-1 in distinction of primary cutaneous CD30+ skin lymphomas and systemic CD30+ ALCL, which has also been observed by Assaf et al. (2007). EMA has also been useful in this regard with positive anaplastic large cells favoring a systemic form with skin involvement. Another application germane to this field was presented as Oral abstract 088 at 2nd world Congress of Cutaneous Lymphomas, Berlin 2013. Using the NUANCE imaging system, low-level CD30 expression was detected in CTCL and was proffered as an explanation for

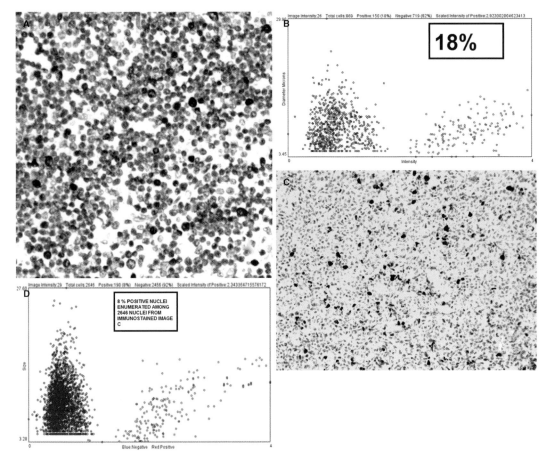

Fig. 4.18 A Ki67 (**a**) positive immunostained lymphocytes in formalin-fixed paraffin-embedded tissue, 20× magnification, and (**b**) corresponding enumerated counts. *Blue dot* plot negative, *Red dots* are positive. Cell size vs. intensity (Lloyd et al. 2013). (**c**) MUM-1 positive lymphocyte nuclear staining in dermal lymphoid infiltrate (**a**) and corresponding enumerated nuclei on the right (**d**). *Blue dot* plot negative, *Red dots* are positive. Cell size vs. intensity (Courtesy of IHCFLOW, Lutz, FL).

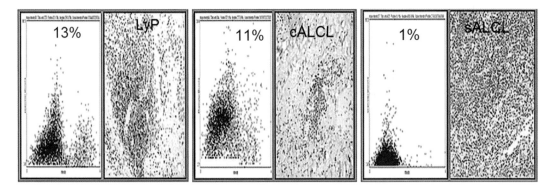

Fig. 4.19 TRAF-1 immunostain on skin biopsy of patients with LyP, cALCL, and sALCL, respectively. The *left panel* with *blue* (negative, hematoxylin only) and *red dot* (positive brown chromogen-decorated cells) plots are the enumeration results with corresponding tissue stains in immediate right of results, respectively. Image cytometry enumeration on alternated panels from left and corresponding immunostains on its right

Table 4.7 List of drugs associated with pseudolymphoma

B-cell pseudolymphoma
Amitriptyline
Fluoxetine
T-cell pseudolymphoma
ACE inhibitors
Allopurinol
Anticonvulsants (carbamazepine, dilantin, phenobarbital)
Antipsychotics
Beta-blockers
Benzodiazepines
Calcium channel blockers
Cyclosporine
Dapsone
Diuretics dyazide
Flexeril
Histamine-2 antagonists
Klonopin
NSAIDs
Nitroprusside
Prozac
Relafen
Sulfa drugs

Table 4.8 Differential expression of image cytometry enumerated antigens in LyP, cALCL, and systemic ALCL

Image cytometry (mean antigen expression (%) ± SD)			
	LyP	pcALCL	sALCL
BCL2	43.2 ± 16.9	26.4 ± 28.5	49.6 ± 35.3
CLA	52.4 ± 25.1	28.6 ± 12.7	6.5 ± 7.6
TRAF-1	25.1 ± 22.4	32.8 ± 22.3	0.9 ± 1.4
NFKB2($p < 0.001$)	0	27.3 ± 29.7	13.8 ± 32.4
CD56 ($p = 0.5283$)	0.2 ± 0.4	0.1 ± 0.3	0
Fascin	16.4 ± 12.7	55.9 ± 12.7	67.1 ± 38.9

There was no significant difference of TRAF-1 staining between LyP and pcALCL ($p > 0.05$)

There were significant differences between LyP and sALCL ($p < 0.01$) and between pcALCL and sALCL ($p < 0.001$)

The tumor cells of all cases of sALCL case were negative for TRAF-1 ($p = 0.0003$)

why anti-CD30 (brentuximab) monoclonal antibody treatment was effective in CTCL. (In Krathen MS, Bashey S, Slava K, Wood G et al., brentuximab vedotin demonstrates clinical activity in mycosis fungoides and Sezary syndrome irrespective of tissue CD30 expression by routine immunohistostaining.)

There has been scant literature in image cytometry application in cutaneous lymphoid infiltrates with few exceptions, despite perceived advantages (Fucich et al. 1999). The direct advantages include optimal use for enumerating the infiltrative areas typical of skin biopsy, which are almost always limited in amount or almost always fixed in formalin. These characteristics lend themselves to tests that are done in situ such as image cytometry, in contrast with a fresh tissue requirement, with disaggregation to single live cells, required in flow cytometry or laser scanning cytometry. The image analysis applications are already commercially available, and its widespread use promises a nuanced distinction between similarly looking entities using tissue-based enumeration. *Definiens* is an image annotation tool which is also commercially available and has wide application of image cytometry in chromogen-immunostained tissue and excels with its annotation technique (Baatz et al. 2009). VirtualFlow image cytometry software tool is similar in function but takes advantage of the already available camera-equipped microscope with microcomputer interface in typical laboratory settings plus provides a flow cytometry-like enumerated statistic with detection sensitivity from low threshold to high level (0–4+ using the 25 % quartile division) (Rezania et al. 2008) (Table 4.8).

Part II. Spectrum of Nonneoplastic Dermatitis, Atypical Phase or Dyscrasia, and Neoplastic Cutaneous Disorders

Spectrum of Dermatitis, Dyscrasia, Prelymphoma to Lymphoma

Although using morphologic criteria alone is neither sensitive nor specific (Lutzner et al. 1971; van der Loo et al. 1981), identification of defined clinical entities is initially approached using histomorphology and, when combined with clinical information and results of ancillary tests, identifies a more precise point along this benign to

Fig. 4.20 Erythroderma, drug induced, showing keratohyaline degeneration, mild perivascular infiltrate, and mild basal spongiosis

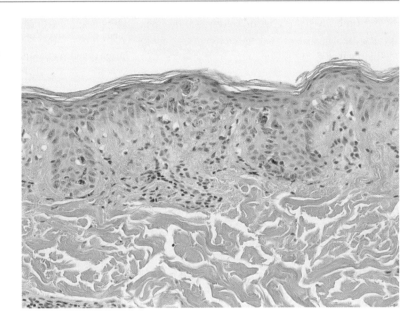

malignant spectrum. Guitart et al. identified eight distinct but idiopathic, clinicopathological conditions characterized by frequent clonal detection, chronic course often resistant to topical treatment, and lack of evidence or potential for CTCL and called them cutaneous T-cell lymphoid dyscrasia (Table 4.5) (Guitart and Magro 2007). We extend the list to ten partners.

Putative Partners Often Cited as a Clinical and Pathological Differential with a Continuous Spectrum of Lymphoproliferative T and B Entities from Benign to Malignant

1. *Benign erythroderma to clonal erythroderma dyscrasia to erythrodermic MF/ Sezary syndrome*
2. *Vitiligo to hypopigmented interface variant to hypopigmented MF*
3. *Pityriasis lichenoides to pityriasis lichenoides dyscrasia to MF, variant possibly CD8 type*
4. *Parapsoriasis to parapsoriasis dyscrasia to parapsoriasis grand plaque to MF*
5. *Syringolymphoid hyperplasia with alopecia to syringolymphoid MF*
6. *Benign follicular mucinosis to follicular mucinosis dyscrasia to follicular MF*
7. *Lupus profundus to atypical lobular lymphocytic panniculitis to indolent subcutaneous*

lymphoma to subcutaneous panniculitic lymphoma
8. *Benign granulomatous lesions to granulomatous dyscrasia to granulomatous MF*
9. *Cutaneous B-cell hyperplasia to atypical cutaneous B-cell hyperplasia to cutaneous B-cell lymphoma*
10. *Solitary pseudo T-cell lymphoma to solitary T-cell nodule of uncertain significance to primary cutaneous small and medium T-cell lymphoma*

Benign Erythroderma to Clonal Erythroderma Dyscrasia to Erythrodermic MF/Sezary Syndrome

Erythroderma is an inflammatory skin reaction affecting greater than 90 % of body, with an annual incidence of one per 100,000 population (Sigurdsson et al. 2001). Benign causes include eczemas, psoriasis, and drug reaction, but idiopathic erythroderma, which accounts for 15–30 %, appears to have potential to progress to MF (Akhyani et al. 2005; Botella-Estrada et al. 1994; Sigurdsson et al. 1997) (Fig. 4.20).

Chronic idiopathic erythroderma or "red man syndrome" is recalcitrant to therapy, and about 5–12 % from this group may progress to MF/Sezary syndrome (Sigurdsson et al. 1997; Vonderheid 2006). The group that developed MF fulfilled the criteria of pre-Sezary syndrome: chronic erythroderma, Sezary count less than 1,000/ul, lymphadenopathy, and increased IgE (Buechner and Winkelmann 1983; Winkelmann et al. 1984).

Another group that appears to be similar to pre-Sezary syndrome, with clonal expansion of T cells with CD4+ CD7–CD26– but which has not yet developed CTCL after 4 years follow-up, is called monoclonal T-cell dyscrasia of undetermined significance (Gniadecki and Lukowsky 2005). Of 30 patients studied, Gniadecki et al. described ten patients with idiopathic erythroderma, and five showed clonal idiopathic recalcitrant erythroderma which did not fulfill criteria for MF or Sezary syndrome. These five patients had circulating clonal T cells; one of five had both clonal skin and blood findings, with a phenotype of CD4+ CD7–CD26–, and was called clonal erythroderma dyscrasia. The following are characteristics of chronic recalcitrant erythroderma in the elderly labeled as monoclonal T-cell dyscrasia of undetermined significance: (1) symptoms persisting more than 6 months without any response to local or systemic glucocorticoid treatment; (2) monoclonal T cells with a CD7-CD45RO+ phenotype in 37–86 % of cells in the blood, Sezary count less than 5 % or less than 1,000/ul, and a low CD4/CD8 ratio; (3) no lymphadenopathy or bone marrow involvement; (4) blood with increased IgE or eosinophils; and (5) morphologically the CD7– and CD4+ cells are small lymphocytes and not cytologically typical Sezary cells. Skin biopsy shows a superficial perivascular lymphocytic infiltrate which also may be seen in true Sezary syndrome (see Chap. 6).

Non-cerebriform lymphocytes may show a monoclonal CD4+ CD7-CD45RO+ in patients with autoimmune and inflammatory diseases. Rheumatoid arthritis is a typical example (Schmidt et al. 1996). Finding clones of T cells in blood in random studies of patients without T lymphomas may indicate a group called T-cell clones of undetermined significance (Muche et al. 2003). Clonal T-cell populations of undetermined significance are more commonly found in elderly individuals, which is the age group affected by Sezary syndrome (Clambey et al. 2005). However, these clonal T cells of the elderly are derived from CD8+ memory cells which are different from the CD4+ Sezary cell phenotype.

Erythrodermic MF/Sezary Syndrome criteria are well described and include finding clonal T cells and Sezary cell counts of more than 1,000/ul in blood (Olsen et al. 2007; Pimpinelli et al. 2005; Swerdlow et al. 2008) (Fig. 4.21).

Vitiligo to Hypopigmented Interface Variant to Hypopigmented MF

Early inflammatory lesions of vitiligo show epidermotropic features mimicking hypopigmented MF. Exocytosis of lymphocytes into the lower epidermis, and lichenoid pseudolymphomatous lesions in inflammatory vitiligo, and absence of both clinical features of MF and clonality favor vitiligo over MF but sometimes the border between these disorders remains obscure. The most often cited differential diagnosis is benign vitiligo, pityriasis alba, tinea versicolor, and others (El-Darouti et al. 2006).

Guitart et al. described a *hypopigmented interface variant* that does not fulfill the criteria for hypopigmented MF (Guitart and Magro 2007; Pimpinelli et al. 2005) and is often asymmetric, with minimal scale and no atopic diathesis. Biopsies show basally located epidermotropic CD8+ lymphocytes; these cases respond well to phototherapy with repigmentation (Lambroza et al. 1995; Stone et al. 2001).

However, true hypopigmented lymphomas arising from patients with erythrodermic MF and Sezary syndrome are documented (Bouloc et al. 2000).

Hypopigmented MF characteristics: An overrepresentation of the hypopigmented variant of MF has been described in dark-skinned children of mostly of Asian and African-Caribbean descent although Caucasian patients are also reported

Fig. 4.21 Palmar erythema
with scaly excoriations in a
patient with long-standing
Sezary syndrome

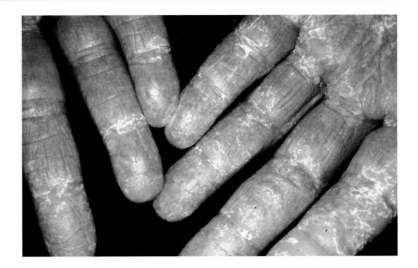

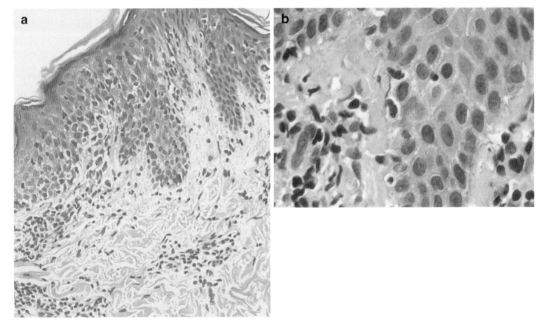

Fig. 4.22 (**a**) Hypopigmented interface variant of T-cell
dyscrasia, biopsied from a mulatto teen from Ascension
Is. (see Chap. 6 for clinic picture); low-power histopathology shows hypopigmented epidermis with small to intermediate cells along basal layer and perivascular upper
dermal infiltrate. (**b**) High-power view with basal localized haloed atypical lymphocytes, which on PCR demonstrated oligoclonal T gamma bands

(Ardigo et al. 2003). Most patients with childhood-onset hypopigmented disease have experienced no progression beyond stage IB disease
(Neuhaus et al. 2000; Whittam et al. 2000), and
this subgroup of hypopigmented childhood-onset
MF appears to have an excellent prognosis
(Fig. 4.22). See Chap. 6 for clinic picture.

Clonality: Both presence (Ardigo et al. 2003)
and absence of T-cell clones have been reported,
and those without clones were called mimics of
hypopigmented MF (Petit et al. 2003; Werner
et al. 2005). All seven Caucasian patients
reported by Ardigo et al. have had PCR detected
T-cell clones. In general, clonality favors CTCL

over inflammation. Clonality was demonstrated in 83.5 % of CTCL and in 2.3 % of benign inflammatory disease using heteroduplex PCR ($p<0.001$) (Ponti et al. 2008).

Pityriasis Lichenoides to Pityriasis Lichenoides Dyscrasia to Cytotoxic Variant MF

Pityriasis lichenoides is an interface dermatitis with necrotic keratinocytes, migration of lymphocytes into all layers of the epidermis, and extravasated red cells. Pityriasis lichenoides lesions frequently contain clonal T cells. Progression to malignant lymphoma (mycosis fungoides) is rare (Boccara et al. 2012; Magro et al. 2007). The rare pityriasis lichenoides cases that progress include those reported to evolve to a CD8+ type of MF (Tomasini et al. 2002; Wenzel et al. 2005).

PLEVA (pityriasis lichenoides et varioliformis acuta) is the acute form, and *PLC* (pityriasis lichenoides chronica) is the chronic type, with the former showing predilection for younger patients and the latter for older patients. Clinically, hemorrhagic flares with scarring are seen in the acute form which has been described as predominantly CD8+ cytotoxic in contrast to the predominantly CD4 infiltrate in the chronic form. Phenotypic aberrancy with loss of CD7 is seen in both forms, and despite frequent demonstration of T-cell clonality by PCR, from 57 % (Weinberg et al. 2002) to 67 % (Dereure et al. 2000), most do not progress to clinical MF (Dereure et al. 2000; Kadin 2002; Weinberg et al. 2002; Ko et al. 2000; Magro et al. 2002, 2007). See Chap. 6 for figures and discussion of these cases.

CD8+ MF is a rare variant of MF occurring in less than 5 % of all MF and is associated with an indolent course and frequent poikilodermatous presentation (hypo- or hyperpigmented) (Nikolaou et al. 2009) or junctional localization (Dummer et al 2002). These could arise de novo or in association with LyP or pityriasis lichenoides or follicular MF (Diwan and Ivan 2009; Nikolaou et al. 2009; Tomasini et al. 2002; Dummer et al. 2002). These cases have to be dif-

ferentiated from aggressive CD8 epidermotropic T-cell lymphoma (Agnarsson et al. 1990; Diwan and Ivan 2009; Nofal et al. 2012; Berti et al. 1999) and from the CD8+ nodular variant of PCSMTCL with predilection to the ear and nose. See Chap. 10 for discussion.

Parapsoriasis to Parapsoriasis Dyscrasia to Parapsoriasis Digitate, "En Grande" Plaque, MF

Parapsoriasis is a group of chronic dermatoses with scaly erythematous patches resembling psoriasis. It has been stated that most MF belong to the conceptual group of parapsoriasis lichenoides (Wolf et al. 2009), and those not fulfilling the MF criteria may be part of the group of parapsoriasis dyscrasias (Guitart and Magro 2007).

For those not fulfilling the criteria for a diagnosis of MF and those cases with a clinical picture of parapsoriasis with minimal epidermotropism, perivascular and interstitial small lymphocytes with insignificant atypia, and lacking Pautrier's microabscesses but showing clonal T cells on PCR, may belong in the spectrum of *parapsoriasis-lymphoid T-cell dyscrasia* (Guitart and Magro 2007).

Pre-mycosis fungoides: Although controversial, some evidence indicates that "digitate and large plaque" parapsoriasis may be pre-mycosis fungoides or clinical manifestations of MF, respectively. In small "plaque" (digitate patch) type with patchy lesions, the size and shape of fingerprints have a low frequency of clonal T cells, but 10 % of cases evolve to MF (Vakeva et al. 2005; Burg and Dummer 1995; Hu and Winkelmann 1973; Haeffner et al. 1995; Muche et al. 1999). Some authors believe that cases evolve into CTCL and hence are part of the MF spectrum, but it must be stressed that such instances appear to be rare (Burg et al. 1996, 2002; Belousova et al. 2008). Conservative management is therefore recommended (Cerroni et al. 2009).

A comparison of clonality in early MF and large plaque parapsoriasis showed reproducible results by GeneScan method implying true clones instead of pseudoclonality. A monoclonal

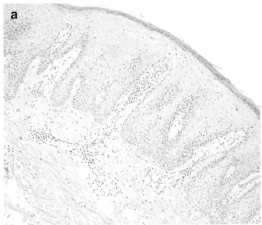
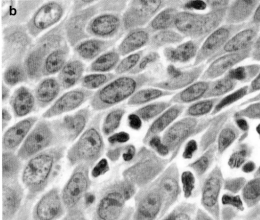

Fig. 4.23 Parapsoriasis dyscrasia, showing (**a**) epidermis with psoriasiform hyperplasia, keratinized stratum corneum, superficial perivascular, and interstitial lymphoid infiltrate, with (**b**) mild atypia on high-power view show- ing clusters of irregular hyperchromatic lymphocytes around haloes of Langerhan's cells. This patient's biopsy, taken from isolated large plaques, showed T-cell clonality by PCR

T-cell infiltrate was demonstrated by repeated TCR-gamma-PCR in lesional skin specimens in 19.2 % of parapsoriasis patients and in 66.6 % of early-stage MF cases ($p=0.013$) (Klemke et al. 2002). Many, therefore, consider "large plaque psoriasis" to a be part of the early presentation of classic MF (Cerroni et al. 2009, Costa et al. 2003; Tamagawa et al. 2005). Some studies document 50 % of "large plaque psoriasis" to contain clonal T cells (Simon et al. 2000) (Fig. 4.23).

Syringolymphoid Hyperplasia with Alopecia to Syringolymphoid Dyscrasia to Syringolymphoid MF

Syringolymphoid hyperplasia with alopecia has been originally described in patients with hyperplastic lymphoid lesions centered on eccrine glands with syringometaplasia (Hobbs et al. 2003; Sarkany 1969). These cases are sometimes associated with MF or follicular mucinosis (Tannous et al. 1999; Thein et al. 2004) and similar histologically to the lymphoepithelial lesions seen in Sjogren's syndrome (Fig. 4.24). Finding atypical to cerebriform lymphoid cell infiltrate with epidermotropism and eccrinotropism in a case with syringolymphoid hyperplasia raises concern for a *syringotropic cutaneous T-cell lymphoma* (Burg and Schmockel 1992). Scant molecular clonality data are described (Thein et al. 2004; Tannous et al. 1999).

Some patients *with syringolymphoid hyperplasia with alopecia* may be asymptomatic or may have pruritic skin lesions, may not respond to corticosteroids, and may have an associated Sjogren's syndrome (Huang et al. 1996). The clinical differential includes alopecia areata, keratosis pilaris, exanthema, and eczema and, if atypical morphology is lacking, raises a diagnostic dilemma between benign eccrinotropic pseudolymphoma and if with clonality the differential is between adnexotropic dyscrasia or syringotropic mycosis fungoides (Guitart and Magro 2007).

This group with syringolymphoid MF overlaps with some cases of folliculotropic mycosis fungoides, which is generally considered to be a variant of MF. Hobbs described two patients (Hobbs et al. 2003), Thein et al. five cases, (Thein et al. 2004) and Pileri et al. 14 cases, the largest among these series. The clinicopathologic features of these 14 patients with syringotropic MF showed a M:F of 1:4, with a median age of 59 (range, 33–83 years). Eight patients had multiple generalized lesions, and six patients had large, solitary patches or plaques in the extremities,

Fig. 4.24 Syringolymphoid hyperplasia, benign, with small lymphocytic infiltrate in the eccrine coil with hyperplasia of the eccrine epithelium in a patient with alopecia, but without associated folliculotropic lymphoid infiltrate or clonal T cells

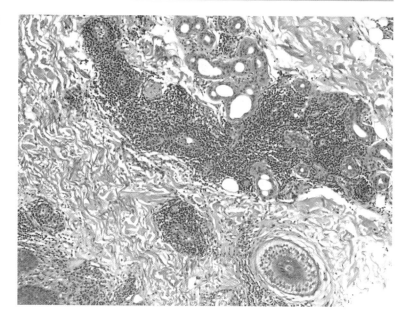

trunk, and eyebrows. Four of these eight patients had existing MF. Histologically, these show prominent involvement of the eccrine glands, some syringometaplasia of glands surrounded by dense lymphoid infiltrates with prominent epitheliotropism. Frequent overlap with typical MF is seen since the epidermis, and hair follicles are described to be involved in 13 and 8 biopsies, respectively (Pileri et al. 2011).

Benign Follicular Mucinosis to Follicular Mucinosis Dyscrasia to Follicular MF

Follicular mucinosis refers to both benign and chronic idiopathic dermatosis in children and lymphoma-related follicular mycosis fungoides or *folliculotropic MF (F-MF)* in adults with associated follicular mucinosis. Clinical presentations of this MF variant of F-MF include reddish plaques with follicular accentuation, often in the head, scalp, and neck areas in contrast to the often body-suit-localized distribution of typical mycosis fungoides. *Pilotropic MF* is the term applied to cerebriform infiltrate in hair follicles without mucinosis.

Idiopathic follicular mucinosis was first described in 1957 by Pinkus with follow-up descriptions (Pinkus 1983) and Jablonska et al. who proposed the term "follicular mucinosis" (FM). The histology of juvenile idiopathic form of FM is characterized by follicular retention and follicular hyperkeratosis accompanied by lymphocytic infiltration with an eosinophilic component (Jablonska et al. 1959).

Role of clonal assessment: Consequently, in these cases, T-cell gene rearrangement is often ordered. Absence of clonality along with known etiology favors benign FM, but its absence with a clinically suspected lesion does not rule out follicular MF, since false-negative results occur in early or equivocal cases. However, the presence of clonality, although it favors follicular MF, does not always portend an ominous course, in a setting of follicular mucinosis. For example, Brown et al. reported a 10-year follow-up of seven patients younger than 40 years with primary FM without evidence of associated dermatoses or lymphoma of whom five had clonal T-cell receptor (TCR) gene rearrangements. After follow-up ranging from 5 to 23 years, no patient showed progression to cutaneous T-cell lymphoma and although some patients had persistent manifestations of FM despite various treatments (Brown et al. 2002). It is important to distinguish benign FM from FM associated with mycosis fungoides because the latter carries a grave prognosis (Olsen et al. 2007; van Doorn et al. 2000).

Cerroni et al. 2002 reviewed data from 44 patients with FM divided into two groups, ("idiopathic" FM; mean age 37·5 years) comprised 15 patients. Group 2 included 28 patients (mean age 52·2 years) with FM associated with mycosis fungoides (MF) or Sézary syndrome. The mean age of patients with "idiopathic" FM was lower, but there were three areas of overlap between the two groups: (1) both appear to localize on the head and neck; (2) the histopathological findings were similar; and (3) about 50 % of tested patients of each group show a monoclonal rearrangement of the TCR γ gene. Differences: One difference is 11/16 (69 %) with "idiopathic" FM had solitary lesions at presentation versus only 2/28 (7 %) with lymphoma-associated FM. Moreover, the lymphoma-associated FM shows lesions in other body sites including body-suit areas. Therefore, the authors proposed that despite overlapping criteria to differentiate "idiopathic" from lymphoma-associated FM, they suggest that "idiopathic" FM might be a localized form of T-cell lymphoma with excellent prognosis but requiring long-term follow-up. Despite and according to these results, it seems idiopathic follicular mucinosis and follicular MF may be distinguishable. For cases that are not clear-cut, it may be useful to recommend long-term follow-up for emergence of MF and similar to the recommendations for the localized variant of pagetoid reticulosis (Woringer–Kolopp disease), solitary MF, and parapsoriasis en plaque. Therefore, long-term follow-up is necessary in patients with so-called "idiopathic" FM (Cerroni et al. 2002). Other authors concur (Boer and Ackerman 2004; Boer et al. 2004). Meanwhile, true benign forms of follicular mucinosis are common in clinical practice.

Benign or reactive follicular mucinosis, when seen in adults, in contrast to the idiopathic variety common in children, may be associated with other clinical conditions such as eczema, discoid lupus erythematosus, or drug induced associated with antidepressant therapy (Magro and Crowson

1996). If the histology is mainly pilotropic, without mucinosis, a suspicion for pilotropic MF without FM is warranted especially if the infiltrate is atypical and clinically shows a body-suit distribution and a clinical picture typical of MF. Lacking atypia or typical MF appearance, *pilotropic or follicular mucinosis dyscrasia* is the recommended terminology by Magro et al. (Guitart and Magro 2007). In addition, patients with follicular MF are usually older than 40 years, defined histologically with perifollicular and follicular localization of atypical and cerebriform small lymphocytes with or without mucin or hyaluronic acid deposits in hair follicles (colloidal Fe or Alcian blue detection of follicular mucinosis) (Fig. 4.25).

Lupus Profundus to Atypical Lobular Lymphocytic Panniculitis to Indolent Subcutaneous Lymphoma to Subcutaneous Panniculitic Lymphoma

In addition, *subcutaneous lymphoid dyscrasia* was also referred by Guitart et al. to a group that includes *lupus profundus to atypical lymphocytic lobular panniculitis to indolent panniculitic lymphomas* (Magro et al. 2001, 2004, 2008; Magro and Wang 2012). The discussion below suggests that clonal T cells in a biopsy of a patient with lobular panniculitis do not necessarily equate to a lymphoma.

Lupus profundus or lupus panniculitis is characterized by multiple nodules, plaques, ulceration, and histology of discoid lupus or not with lipoatrophy and septal and lobular panniculitis, along with karyorrhexis, lymphocytic infiltrates with plasma cells and vasculopathy, as well as mucin deposits (Fig. 4.26). These cases show no clonal T cells (Massone et al. 2005). It is a chronic disease, frequently in adult women with or without lupus epidermal changes, presence of hyaline fat necrosis and hyalinization of lobules and septa, and frequent lymphocytic infiltrates at the periphery of fat lobules, in contrast to the typical findings of rimming of lymphocytes in fat lobules and clonal T cells in subcutaneous pan-

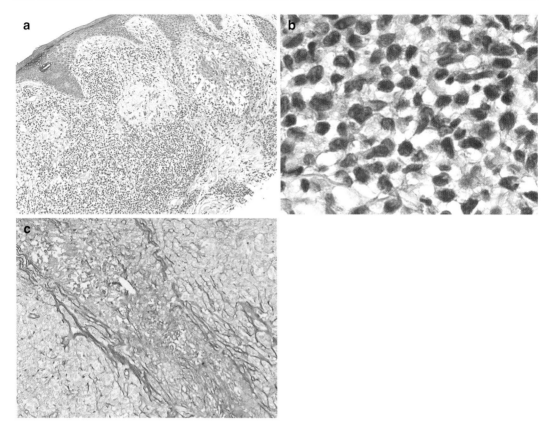

Fig. 4.25 (**a**) Follicular mucinosis, low-power view, with folliculotropic lymphocytes in outer root sheath and expanded root with mucinous degeneration on *right* of the picture. (**b**) Oil power magnification view of the atypical hyperchromatic small- to medium-sized lymphocytes on *middle panel*. (**c**) Colloidal Fe stain with bluish red mucinous vacuoles inside follicular spaces

niculitic T-cell lymphoma. In a setting of immunosuppression or organ transplant, infection-related panniculitis is a differential diagnosis characterized by frequent neutrophil-rich infiltrate and granulomatous inflammation, in contrast to the lymphoid-rich infiltrate of lupus panniculitis. Alcohol or chronic pancreatitis-related panniculitis may be considered within the contextual setting, in a male patient with an elevated lipase serology, and presents with painful panniculitis in extremities. Biopsy usually shows presence of ghost necrotic adipocytes.

Atypical lymphocytic lobular panniculitis (ALLP) is a subcutaneous lymphoid dyscrasia often in young male patients with painless nodules in the extremities (Magro et al. 2004), *unrelated to lupus panniculitis*, histologically with eccrinotropic and lymphohistiocytic infiltrate, nuclear atypia, and focal necrosis associated with clonal T cells (Fig. 4.27). Constitutional symptoms herald overlap with subcutaneous panniculitic T-cell lymphoma(SPTCL) (Guitart and Magro 2007). Both conditions have persistent clonal T cells, small-intermediate size atypical lymphocytes, and aberrant loss of T antigens. However, several differences are seen. SPTCL has a severe angiodestructive pattern with vessel thrombosis, karyorrhectic debris, rimming of hyperchromatic lymphocytes, and fat necrosis, but not seen in ALLP; with less lymphocytic infiltration in ALLP; and with inconspicuous hemophagocytosis in ALLP. Mixed CD4:CD8 with decreased ratio is seen more in ALLP compared to the CD8 predominance in SPTCL or

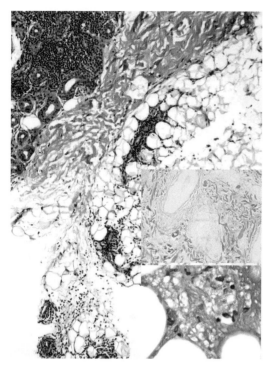

phages with phagocytosed erythrocytes and leucocytes bulging the cytoplasm – and lobular panniculitis. Most CHP are possibly the clinical harbinger of SPTCL.

There is an overlap between clonal ALLP and clonal CHP, and some of these cases may be part of the early SPTCL. In both CHP and SPTCL, T lymphocytes and histiocytes infiltrate the lobules in sheets or lacelike pattern. A CD4-secreted phagocytic-inducing factor (PIF) may account for the cytophagic properties of the benign histiocytes in CHP. A mixed CD4 CD8 population may be seen in early SPTCL simulating ALLP. Although bone marrow may not show T-cell lymphoma, hemophagocytic syndrome may be seen. Presence of an atypical aggressive clinical presentation with T-cell clonality, CD8 cytotoxic infiltrates, and fatal hemophagocytic syndrome suggests a diagnosis of subcutaneous panniculitic T-cell lymphoma (Gonzalez et al. 1991; Salhany et al. 1998).

Fig. 4.26 Lupus panniculitis, low power, and on high power in other areas of the biopsy, hyalinosis of fat lobules (*lower inset*), and mucin deposition (*upper inset*)

Benign Granulomatous Lesions to Granulomatous Dyscrasia to Granulomatous MF

double CD4 and CD8 loss in gamma delta T-cell lymphoma, another cytotoxic lymphoma with frequent panniculitic localization. In addition, presence of germinal centers, prominent mucin deposits, and hyalinosis of fat lobules is more in favor of lupus panniculitis and not ALLP or SPTCL.

Additionally, histologically finding "beanbag" cytophagic histiocytes in panniculus raises the differential diagnosis of cytophagic histiocytic panniculitis, especially in a setting with fever and hemorrhagic diathesis (Fig. 4.28) (Requena and Sanchez 2001; Winkelmann 1980; Craig et al. 1998). Cytophagic histiocytic panniculitis (CHP) is a reactive process secondary to a variety of diseases (neoplastic and nonneoplastic) associated with cytophagocytosis, "beanbag" histiocytes – composed of macro-

Granulomas are seen in about 2 % of either B-cell or T-cell lymphomas of skin (Scarabello et al. 2002). Histiocytic infiltrates of single cells and clusters are a common component of pseudolymphomas and in the presence of a pseudoclone may lead to a false diagnosis of granulomatous cutaneous lymphoma (Fig. 4.29) (Boer et al. 2008). Significant granulomatous infiltrates comprise at least 25 % of the skin biopsy (Scarabello et al 2002). Giant cells may accompany these clusters or be part of an epithelioid granulomatous infiltrate. Lymphocyte-poor epithelioid granulomas in skin raise sarcoidosis as the primary diagnosis, but lymphoid-rich epithelioid granulomas are most concerning for lymphomaassociated granulomas.

In a setting of mycosis fungoides with granulomas, granulomatous MF and granulomatous slack skin disease are considerations. The histology of these two types is overlapping, but clini-

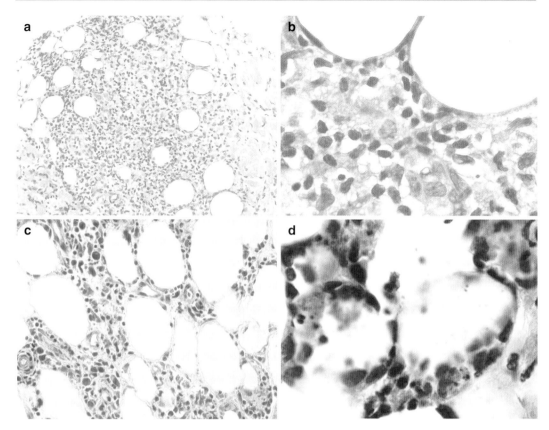

Fig. 4.27 Atypical lobular lymphocytic panniculitis, (**a**) with lymphoid-rich lobular panniculitis, and on molecular test, the lymphocytes are monoclonal T cells by GeneScan PCR but clinically presented with a solitary nodule with no evidence of lymphoma over the years. (**b**) High-power view with atypical hyperchromatic lymphocytes, permeating interstitial spaces, without rimming of fat spaces. (**c**) Subcutaneous panniculitic T-cell lymphoma, T alpha–beta cell phenotype, with lobular and septal panniculitis, and minimal dermal involvement, medium-power view. (**d**) High-power view showing rimming of fat cells with hyperchromatic pleomorphic small- and medium-sized lymphocytes and mixed with cytophagic histiocytes with karyorrhexis and cytophagic granular debris

cally bulky skin folds in intertriginous (groins, scrotal, and axillary) areas favor granulomatous slack skin disease, which tends to have a more favorable long-term course. Recently, a t(3:9)(q12p24) karyotypic marker has been described in GSS (Ikonomou et al. 2007).

A diffuse, nodular, and perivascular pattern is seen in granulomatous MF, and in one of five patients, CD30+ transformed nodules of large MF cells were associated with granulomatous MF. Granulomatous MF typically presents with hyperpigmented or reddish plaques or nodules in an adult male with a 1.5M:F ratio and median age of 46 years (22–71). Histologically, a granuloma annulare-like pattern is not seen and most cases are CD4+ and CD8 negative, similar to MF. Unlike typical MF, epidermotropism in granulomatous MF is absent in half of the cases. Distinction is important because the granulomatous MF variant shows increased extracutaneous spread, therapy resistance, and associated transformed MF and hence shows a decreased disease-specific survival rate of 66 % compared to non-granulomatous Alibert–Bazin MF (Kempf et al. 2008). Large vessel infiltration and multinucleated giant cells are noted in one-third of

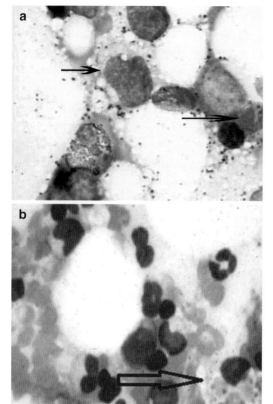

Most cases (87 %) of granulomatous MF contain clonal T cells, which is a useful distinction from cutaneous sarcoidosis (Kempf et al. 2008). However, finding clonal T cells in a granulomatous dermal lesion is not always diagnostic of granulomatous MF. In a setting of known treatments, a drug-induced granulomatous dyscrasia is a consideration, given that antigen loss and clonal T cells are also present in this group. "Drug-induced lymphoid and granulomatous lymphoid dyscrasia" were recently described in ten patients with reversible lesions by Magro et al. as belonging to the group with persistent T-cell clonal granulomatous dermatitis that resemble granulomatous MF histologically (Magro et al. 2003, 2010).

Cutaneous B-Cell Hyperplasia to Atypical Cutaneous B-Cell Hyperplasia to Cutaneous B-Cell Lymphoma

A cutaneous B-cell hyperplastic pattern with clonal population by PCR was well described (Nihal et al. 2000, 2003) suggesting a continuum of hyperplasia to lymphoma, perhaps analogous to the concept of dyscrasia. We have observed this in practice on repeated biopsies of patients with long-standing cutaneous lymphoid hyperplasia that show slowly progressive histoimmunologic changes that evolve to a B-cell lymphoma (Kulow et al. 2002). We observed an intervening period we call atypical cutaneous lymphoid hyperplasia where histology shows disorganized germinal centers, haphazard mixture of Bcl6+ centroblast clusters with interfollicular T cells, increasing CD20 positive clusters, and deep localization of nodules (Fig. 4.31).The concept of progression from premalignant to malignant B-cell disorder is already well accepted in plasma cell dyscrasia as in the MGUS to myeloma spectrum and in blood lymphocytosis with monoclonal lymphocytosis of uncertain significance to CLL.

Fig. 4.28 (a) Cytophagic histiocytic panniculitis, high-power view, of angiocentric lymphoid infiltrate with admixed erythro-cytophagic histiocytes (*arrow*), and mostly non-atypical small round lymphocytes clustered on vessels and in between fat cells, in a patient with hemophagocytic syndrome, and (b) Giemsa-stained bone marrow imprint with a histiocyte (*arrow*) with red cell and platelets phagocytosis

cases (LeBoit et al. 1988) (Fig. 4.30). Sarcoid-like granulomas are seen in most of the dermis. A juvenile granulomatous variant with onset in childhood appears to have a higher risk for development of another lymphoma.

Fig.4.29 Lymphohistiocytic clusters on right lower area and on left, (**a**) Langhans multinucleated giant cell; findings frequently seen in pseudolymphomas

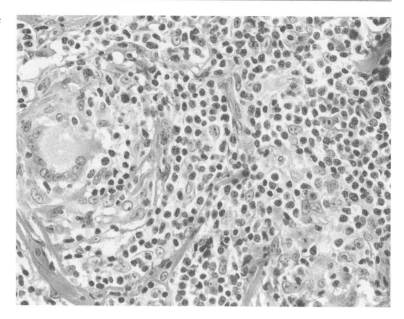

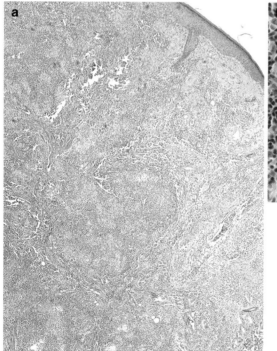

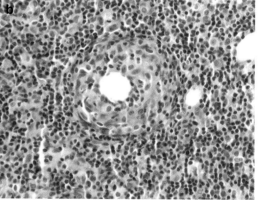

Fig. 4.30 (**a**) Granulomatous MF with nodules of lymphoid aggregates mixed with paler epithelioid granulomas in dermis and minimal epidermotropism. (**b**) Perivascular granuloma in granulomatous MF, with surrounding lymphohistiocytic clusters

Solitary Pseudo T-Cell Lymphoma to Solitary T-Cell Nodule of Uncertain Significance to Primary Cutaneous Small and Medium T-Cell Lymphoma

In a study of a large group of PCSMTCL, with many showing clonal T cells, the same group of Beltraminelli et al. upon review of 136 and Leinweber et al. in 26 patients proposed the term "solitary T-cell nodule of uncertain significance" because it appears in both studies to show very rare progression to skin malignancy or skin recurrence in solitary cases. In the group of 136 patients with (male to female = 1:1; median age: 53 years, age range: 3–90 years) cutaneous lesions classified as small-/medium-sized pleomorphic T-cell lymphoma, all but three patients presented with solitary nodules located mostly on the head and neck area . Histopathologic features showed nodular or diffuse infiltrates of small- to medium-sized pleomorphic T lymphocytes, and monoclonal T-cell receptor gamma gene was found in 60 % of tested cases (Fig. 4.32). Follow-up data of 45 patients revealed that 41 patients were alive without lymphoma after a median time of 63 months (range: 1–357 months), whereas four were alive with cutaneous disease (range: 2–16 months). Because of these findings, "cutaneous nodular proliferation of pleomorphic T lymphocytes of undetermined significance" was recommended as properly descriptive of these cases, akin to monoclonal lymphocytosis of uncertain significance and monoclonal gammopathy of uncertain significance in the B-CLL-group and myeloma

spectrum, respectively (Beltraminelli et al. 2009; Leinweber et al. 2009)

Conclusion

Despite the judicious use of molecular genetics and flow cytometry, the distinction of benign dermatitis from malignant lymphoma may not be possible in a select few cases, because of the prevailing widely held notion that lymphoid clones may be found in cutaneous biopsies along the clinical spectrum from benign dermatitis to frank lymphoma. Detected clones may be small but because of the ultrasensitive PCR technique are easily recovered from a reactive milieu. Several approaches to clarify an equivocal molecular result in the face of clinical and immunopathological findings may be employed, as we have found useful in cutaneous hematopathology community practice.

We noted in general that this approach is welcome and encouraged by practicing dermatologists who refer challenging biopsies. Hence, confirmation of "true" monoclonality versus clonality in pseudolymphoma is important, and the following strategy and/or recommendations are made:

1. Search for monoclonal gene rearrangements showing identical results from multiple skin biopsy sites, if there are multiple lesions, concurrently or on follow-up.
2. Look for monoclonal identical bands or peaks noted from GeneScan histograms in skin and extracutaneous tissues, such as lymph node or blood.

Fig. 4.31 Atypical cutaneous lymphoid hyperplasia (ACLH). (**a**) Large multinodular infiltrate with a top heavy pattern extending to the border of subcutaneous tissue, with fragmented and disorganized germinal centers surrounded by darker mantle zone. The loss of typical biphasic pattern of a normal germinal center (*arrow*) is often the harbinger of atypical cutaneous B-cell hyperplasia. The figure immediately below A shows atypical pleomorphic cells within a germinal center, a cytologic feature

of atypical cutaneous lymphoid hyperplasia. (**b**) Bcl6-disorganized pattern in ACLH reflective of histology. (**c**) Similarly, change in Ki67 polarized normal pattern to a haphazard or disorganized pattern is also seen in both ACLH and cutaneous lymphoma. (**d**). Normal medium-power histology of cutaneous hyperplastic germinal center favoring a benign pattern with the, (**e**), corresponding polarized Ki67 normal staining with organized polarity of high and low gradation

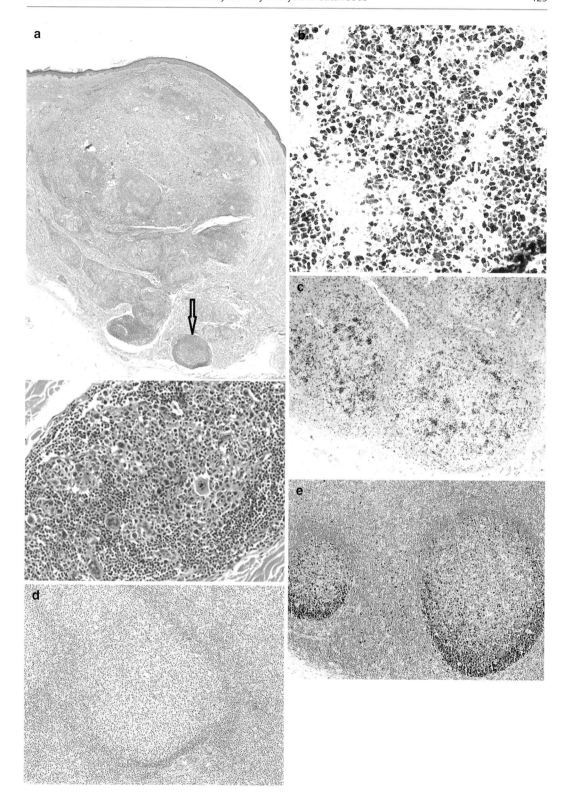

Fig. 4.32 Solitary CD3+
T-cell pseudolymphoma
showing a dense nodular and
perivascular and eccrinotropic infiltrate extending deep
and hugging the dermoepi-
dermal junction

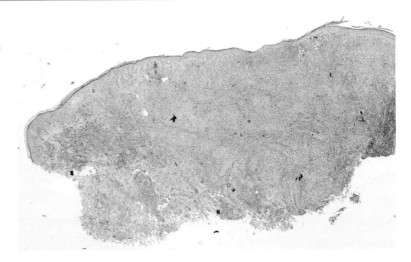

3. When confronted with suspiciously insufficient DNA from unrepresentative samples, request repeat or excisional biopsy of
the entire lesion, or a larger lesion may be a
clinically important confirmatory approach.
Shave and punch biopsy of a large lesion is
often performed to minimize cutaneous
morbidity, but if the biopsy turns out to be
lymphohematopoietic, a more representative excision or excision of the mass may
be a more representative specimen.

4. On repeated T or B-cell gene rearrangements, change in status of clonality and
change of status from negative to positive,
from biclonal to monoclonal, and from
monoclonal to polyclonal are all useful
results that require correlation with the clinical course, histopathology, and immunophenotyping. In general, no change of original
result supports the monoclonal or polyclonal
nature. Confirmation may avoid unnecessary expensive treatment or unneeded
expensive laboratory or staging workup
(Cualing and Morgan 2013).

5. Clonal identity or persistence of identical
monoclonal band clone from dual sites
concurrently or from sequential biopsy of
different or same sites provides firm evidence of a stable clone of T cells favoring
neoplasm over reactive clonal dermatitis
(Mahalingam 2003; Thurber et al. 2007;
Wood 2001; Zhang et al. 2010) and may

reveal transformation of a cutaneous lymphoid hyperplasia to a frank lymphoma in
B-cell neoplasm (Kulow et al. 2002).

In those cases with a benign clinical course
or a solitary long-standing lesion, despite the
finding of confirmed clonality, the positive
result may not necessarily be diagnostic of lymphoma, especially when the lesion has disap-
peared, regressed, or did not progress over
several months or years of follow-up. An example may be because of very indolent and unpro-
gressive behavior of some of the cases diagnosed
as PCSMTCL; these cases, especially if they are
solitary or not monoclonal, may be called "cutaneous nodular proliferation of pleomorphic T
lymphocytes of undetermined significance" or
"solitary small- to medium-sized pleomorphic
T-cell nodules of undetermined significance" as
a tenable interpretation (Beltraminelli et al.
2009; Leinweber et al. 2009).

The concept that there is a spectrum of
findings between frank reactive inflammatory
mimics of lymphoma to clonal dermatitis to
frank lymphoma is not new, as we and other
authors have reported. However, very few of
the persistent clonal but reactive cases progress to lymphoma, and conservative but
watchful management appears to be the best
plan (Wood 2001; Kulow et al. 2002;
Gniadecki 2004; Gniadecki and Lukowsky
2005; Burg et al. 2001, 2005; Guitart and
Magro 2007).

References

Agar NS, Wedgeworth E, Crichton S, Mitchell TJ, Cox M, Ferreira S, Robson A, Calonje E, Stefanato CM, Wain EM, Wilkins B, Fields PA, Dean A, Webb K, Scarisbrick J, Morris S, Whittaker SJ. Survival outcomes and prognostic factors in mycosis fungoides/Sezary syndrome: validation of the revised International Society for Cutaneous Lymphomas/European Organisation for Research and Treatment of Cancer staging proposal. J Clin Oncol. 2010;28(31):4730–9.

Agnarsson BA, Vonderheid EC, Kadin ME. Cutaneous T cell lymphoma with suppressor/cytotoxic (CD8) phenotype: identification of rapidly progressive and chronic subtypes. J Am Acad Dermatol. 1990;22(4):569–77.

Akhyani M, Ghodsi ZS, Toosi S, Dabbaghian H. Erythroderma: a clinical study of 97 cases. BMC Dermatol. 2005;5:5.

Albrecht J, Fine LA, Piette W. Drug-associated lymphoma and pseudolymphoma: recognition and management. Dermatol Clin. 2007;25(2):233–44, vi.

Anandasabapathy N, Pulitzer M, Epstein W, Rosenman K, Latkowski JA. Pseudolymphoma evolving into diffuse large B-cell lymphoma. Dermatol Online J. 2008;14(5):22.

Arai E, Okubo H, Tsuchida T, Kitamura K, Katayama I. Pseudolymphomatous folliculitis: a clinicopathologic study of 15 cases of cutaneous pseudolymphoma with follicular invasion. Am J Surg Pathol. 1999;23(11): 1313–9.

Arai E, Shimizu M, Hirose T. A review of 55 cases of cutaneous lymphoid hyperplasia: reassessment of the histopathologic findings leading to reclassification of 4 lesions as cutaneous marginal zone lymphoma and 19 as pseudolymphomatous folliculitis. Hum Pathol. 2005;36(5):505–11.

Arai E, Shimizu M, Tsuchida T, Izaki S, Ogawa F, Hirose T. Lymphomatoid keratosis: an epidermotropic type of cutaneous lymphoid hyperplasia: clinicopathological, immunohistochemical, and molecular biological study of 6 cases. Arch Dermatol 2007;143:53–9.

Ardigo M, Borroni G, Muscardin L, Kerl H, Cerroni L. Hypopigmented mycosis fungoides in Caucasian patients: a clinicopathologic study of 7 cases. J Am Acad Dermatol 2003;49:264–70.

Assaf C, Hirsch B, Wagner F, Lucka L, Grunbaum M, Gellrich S, Lukowsky A, Sterry W, Stein H, Durkop H. Differential expression of TRAF1 aids in the distinction of cutaneous CD30-positive lymphoproliferations. J Invest Dermatol. 2007;127(8):1898–904.

Baatz M, Zimmermann J, Blackmore CG. Automated analysis and detailed quantification of biomedical images using Definiens Cognition Network Technology. Comb Chem High Throughput Screen. 2009;12(9):908–16.

Bahler DW, Hartung L, Hill S, Bowen GM, Vonderheid EC. CD158k/KIR3DL2 is a useful marker for identifying neoplastic T-cells in Sezary syndrome by flow cytometry. Cytometry B Clin Cytom. 2008;74(3):156–62.

Belousova IE, Vanecek T, Samtsov AV, Michal M, Kazakov DV. A patient with clinicopathologic features

of small plaque parapsoriasis presenting later with plaque-stage mycosis fungoides: report of a case and comparative retrospective study of 27 cases of "non-progressive" small plaque parapsoriasis. J Am Acad Dermatol. 2008;59(3):474–82.

Beltraminelli H, Leinweber B, Kerl H, Cerroni L. Primary cutaneous CD4+ small-/medium-sized pleomorphic T-cell lymphoma: a cutaneous nodular proliferation of pleomorphic T lymphocytes of undetermined significance? A study of 136 cases. Am J Dermatopathol. 2009;31(4):317–22.

Bergman R. Pseudolymphoma and cutaneous lymphoma: facts and controversies. Clin Dermatol. 2010;28(5): 568–74.

Berti E, Tomasini D, Vermeer MH, Meijer CJ, Alessi E, Willemze R. Primary cutaneous CD8-positive epidermotropic cytotoxic T cell lymphomas. A distinct clinicopathological entity with an aggressive clinical behavior. Am J Pathol. 1999;155(2):483–92.

Bjorkstrom NK, Beziat V, Cichocki F, Liu LL, Levine J, Larsson S, Koup RA, Anderson SK, Ljunggren HG, Malmberg KJ. CD8 T cells express randomly selected KIRs with distinct specificities compared with NK cells. Blood. 2012;120(17):3455–65.

Boccara O, Blanche S, de PY, Brousse N, Bodemer C, Fraitag S. Cutaneous hematologic disorders in children. Pediatr Blood Cancer 2012;58:226–32.

Boer A, Ackerman AB. Alopecia mucinosa or follicular mucinosis – the problem is terminology! J Cutan Pathol. 2004;31(2):210–1.

Boer A, Guo Y, Ackerman AB. Alopecia mucinosa is mycosis fungoides. Am J Dermatopathol. 2004;26(1): 33–52.

Boer A, Tirumalae R, Bresch M, Falk TM. Pseudoclonality in cutaneous pseudolymphomas: a pitfall in interpretation of rearrangement studies. Br J Dermatol. 2008; 159(2):394–402.

Borowitz MJ, Weidner A, Olsen EA, Picker LJ. Abnormalities of circulating T-cell subpopulations in patients with cutaneous T-cell lymphoma: cutaneous lymphocyte-associated antigen expression on T cells correlates with extent of disease. Leukemia. 1993;7(6):859–63.

Botella-Estrada R, Sanmartin O, Oliver V, Febrer I, Aliaga A. Erythroderma. A clinicopathological study of 56 cases. Arch Dermatol. 1994;130(12):1503–7.

Boudova L, Kazakov DV, Sima R, Vanecek T, Torlakovic E, Lamovec J, et al. Cutaneous lymphoid hyperplasia and other lymphoid infiltrates of the breast nipple: a retrospective clinicopathologic study of fifty-six patients. Am J Dermatopathol. 2005;27(5):375–86.

Bouloc A, Fau-Larue MH, Lenormand B, Meunier F, Wechsler J, Thomine E, et al. Polymerase chain reaction analysis of immunoglobulin gene rearrangement in cutaneous lymphoid hyperplasias. French Study Group for Cutaneous Lymphomas. Arch Dermatol. 1999;135(2):168–72.

Bouloc A, Grange F, fau-Larue MH, Dieng MT, Tortel MC, Avril MF, Revuz J, Bagot M, Wechsler J. Leucoderma associated with flares of erythrodermic cutaneous T-cell lymphomas: four cases. The French Study Group of Cutaneous Lymphomas. Br J Dermatol. 2000;143(4):832–6.

Brady SP, Magro CM, az-Cano SJ, Wolfe HJ. Analysis of clonality of atypical cutaneous lymphoid infiltrates associated with drug therapy by PCR/DGGE. Hum Pathol. 1999;30(2):130–6.

Brown HA, Gibson LE, Pujol RM, Lust JA, Pittelkow MR. Primary follicular mucinosis: long-term follow-up of patients younger than 40 years with and without clonal T-cell receptor gene rearrangement. J Am Acad Dermatol. 2002;47(6):856–62.

Bruggemann M, White H, Gaulard P, Garcia-Sanz R, Gameiro P, Oeschger S, Jasani B, Ott M, Delsol G, Orfao A, Tiemann M, Herbst H, Langerak AW, Spaargaren M, Moreau E, Groenen PJ, Sambade C, Foroni L, Carter GI, Hummel M, Bastard C, Davi F, fau-Larue MH, Kneba M, van Dongen JJ, Beldjord K, Molina TJ. Powerful strategy for polymerase chain reaction-based clonality assessment in T-cell malignancies Report of the BIOMED-2 Concerted Action BHM4 CT98-3936. Leukemia. 2007;21(2):215–21.

Buechner SA, Winkelmann RK. Pre-Sezary erythroderma evolving to Sezary syndrome. A report of seven cases. Arch Dermatol. 1983;119(4):285–91.

Burg G, Dummer R. Small plaque (digitate) parapsoriasis is an 'abortive cutaneous T-cell lymphoma' and is not mycosis fungoides. Arch Dermatol. 1995;131(3):336–8.

Burg G, Dummer R, Haeffner A, Kempf W, Kadin M. From inflammation to neoplasia: mycosis fungoides evolves from reactive inflammatory conditions (lymphoid infiltrates) transforming into neoplastic plaques and tumors. Arch Dermatol 2001;137:949–52.

Burg G, Dummer R, Kempf W. Dyscrasias with "undetermined significance". Arch Dermatol. 2005;141(3): 382–4.

Burg G, Dummer R, Nestle FO, Doebbeling U, Haeffner A. Cutaneous lymphomas consist of a spectrum of nosologically different entities including mycosis fungoides and small plaque parapsoriasis. Arch Dermatol. 1996;132(5):567–72.

Burg G, Kempf W, Haeffner A, Dobbeling U, Nestle FO, Boni R, Kadin M, Dummer R. From inflammation to neoplasia: new concepts in the pathogenesis of cutaneous lymphomas. Recent Results Cancer Res. 2002; 160:271–80.

Burg G, Schmockel C. Syringolymphoid hyperplasia with alopecia–a syringotropic cutaneous T-cell lymphoma? Dermatology. 1992;184(4):306–7.

Camilot D, Arnez ZM, Luzar B, Pizem J, Zgavec B, Falconieri G. Cutaneous pseudolymphoma following tattoo application: report of two new cases of a potential lymphoma mimicker. Int J Surg Pathol. 2012;20(3):311–5.

Carreras J, Lopez-Guillermo A, Fox BC, Colomo L, Martinez A, Roncador G, Montserrat E, Campo E, Banham AH. High numbers of tumor-infiltrating FOXP3-positive regulatory T cells are associated with improved overall survival in follicular lymphoma. Blood. 2006;108(9):2957–64.

Cerroni L, Fink-Puches R, Back B, Kerl H. Follicular mucinosis: a critical reappraisal of clinicopathologic features and association with mycosis fungoides and Sezary syndrome. Arch Dermatol. 2002;138(2):182–9.

Cerroni L, Gatter K, Kerl H. Skin lymphoma: the illustrated guide. 3rd ed. Hoboken, NJ, USA: Wiley-Blackwell; 2009.

Clambey ET, van Dyk LF, Kappler JW, Marrack P. Non-malignant clonal expansions of CD8+ memory T cells in aged individuals. Immunol Rev. 2005;205: 170–89.

Costa C, Gallardo F, Bellosillo B, Espinet B, Pujol RM, Barranco C, Serrano S, Sole F. Analysis of T-cell receptor gamma gene rearrangements by PCR-Genescan and PCR-polyacrylamide gel electrophoresis in early-stage mycosis fungoides/large-plaque parapsoriasis. Dermatology. 2003;207(4):418–9.

Cozzio A, French LE. T-cell clonality assays: how do they compare? J Invest Dermatol. 2008;128(4):771–3.

Craig AJ, Cualing H, Thomas G, Lamerson C, Smith R. Cytophagic histiocytic panniculitis – a syndrome associated with benign and malignant panniculitis: case comparison and review of the literature. J Am Acad Dermatol. 1998;39(5 Pt 1):721–36.

Cualing HD, Morgan MB. Experience and lessons from use of molecular clonality PCR tests in cutaneous hematopathology practice. Arch Pathol Lab Med. Archives of Pathology & Laboratory Medicine: October 2013, Vol. 137, No. 10, pp. 1343–1526. doi: http://dx.doi.org/10.5858/arpa.2013-0354-AB)

Cualing HD, Zhong E, Moscinski L. "Virtual flow cytometry" of immunostained lymphocytes on microscopic tissue slides: iHCFlow tissue cytometry. Cytometry B Clin Cytom. 2007;72(1):63–76.

Dabiri S, Morales A, Ma L, Sundram U, Kim YH, Arber DA, et al. The frequency of dual TCR-PCR clonality in granulomatous disorders. J Cutan Pathol. 2011; 38(9):704–9.

Dereure O, Levi E, Kadin ME. T-Cell clonality in pityriasis lichenoides et varioliformis acuta: a heteroduplex analysis of 20 cases. Arch Dermatol. 2000;136(12): 1483–6.

Diwan H, Ivan D. CD8-positive mycosis fungoides and primary cutaneous aggressive epidermotropic CD8-positive cytotoxic T-cell lymphoma. J Cutan Pathol. 2009;36(3):390–2.

Dukers DF, Vermeer MH, Jaspars LH, Sander CA, Flaig MJ, Vos W, Willemze R, Meijer CJ. Expression of killer cell inhibitory receptors is restricted to true NK cell lymphomas and a subset of intestinal enteropathy-type T cell lymphomas with a cytotoxic phenotype. J Clin Pathol. 2001;54(3):224–8.

Dummer R, Kamarashev J, Kempf W, Haffner AC, Hess-Schmid M, Burg G. Junctional CD8+ cutaneous lymphomas with nonaggressive clinical behavior: a CD8+ variant of mycosis fungoides? Arch Dermatol. 2002;138(2):199–203.

Eisendle K, Zelger B. The expanding spectrum of cutaneous borreliosis. G Ital Dermatol Venereol. 2009; 144(2):157–71.

El-Darouti MA, Marzouk SA, Azzam O, Fawzi MM, bdel-Halim MR, Zayed AA, Leheta TM. Vitiligo vs. hypopigmented mycosis fungoides (histopathological and immunohistochemical study, univariate analysis). Eur J Dermatol. 2006;16(1):17–22.

Feng B, Jorgensen JL, Jones D, Chen SS, Hu Y, Medeiros LJ, Wang SA. Flow cytometric detection of peripheral blood involvement by mycosis fungoides and Sezary syndrome using T-cell receptor Vbeta chain antibodies and its application in blood staging. Mod Pathol. 2010;23(2):284–95.

Finn WG, Peterson LC, James C, Goolsby CL. Enhanced detection of malignant lymphoma in cerebrospinal fluid by multiparameter flow cytometry. Am J Clin Pathol. 1998;110(3):341–6.

Flaig MJ, Schuhmann K, Sander CA. Impact of molecular analysis in the diagnosis of cutaneous lymphoid infiltrates. Semin Cutan Med Surg. 2000;19(2):87–90.

Fucich LF, Freeman SF, Boh EE, McBurney E, Marrogi AJ. Atypical cutaneous lymphocytic infiltrate and a role for quantitative immunohistochemistry and gene rearrangement studies. Int J Dermatol. 1999;38(10): 749–56.

Fujimura T, Hidaka T, Hashimoto A, Aiba S. Dermoscopy findings of pseudolymphomatous folliculitis. Case Rep Dermatol. 2012;4(2):154–7.

Gallardo F, Bellosillo B, Serrano S, Pujol RM. Genotypic analysis in primary cutaneous lymphomas using the standardized BIOMED-2 polymerase chain reaction protocols. Actas Dermosifiliogr. 2008;99(8):608–20.

Garcia-Herrera A, Colomo L, Camos M, Carreras J, Balague O, Martinez A, Lopez-Guillermo A, Estrach T, Campo E. Primary cutaneous small/medium CD4+ T-cell lymphomas: a heterogeneous group of tumors with different clinicopathologic features and outcome. J Clin Oncol. 2008;26(20):3364–71.

Gilliam AC, Wood GS. Cutaneous lymphoid hyperplasias. Semin Cutan Med Surg. 2000;19(2):133–41.

Gniadecki R. Neoplastic stem cells in cutaneous lymphomas: evidence and clinical implications. Arch Dermatol. 2004;140(9):1156–60.

Gniadecki R, Lukowsky A. Monoclonal T-cell dyscrasia of undetermined significance associated with recalcitrant erythroderma. Arch Dermatol. 2005;141(3): 361–7.

Gonzalez CL, Medeiros LJ, Braziel RM, Jaffe ES. T-cell lymphoma involving subcutaneous tissue. A clinicopathologic entity commonly associated with hemophagocytic syndrome. Am J Surg Pathol. 1991;15(1):17–27.

Guitart J, Magro C. Cutaneous T-cell lymphoid dyscrasia: a unifying term for idiopathic chronic dermatoses with persistent T-cell clones. Arch Dermatol. 2007;143(7): 921–32.

Guitart J, Kennedy J, Ronan S, Chmiel JS, Hsiegh YC, Variakojis D. Histologic criteria for the diagnosis of mycosis fungoides: proposal for a grading system to standardize pathology reporting. J Cutan Pathol. 2001;28(4):174–83.

Haeffner AC, Smoller BR, Zepter K, Wood GS. Differentiation and clonality of lesional lymphocytes in small plaque parapsoriasis. Arch Dermatol. 1995; 131(3):321–4.

Harmon CB, Witzig TE, Katzmann JA, Pittelkow MR. Detection of circulating T cells with CD4+ CD7- immunophenotype in patients with benign and malignant lymphoproliferative dermatoses. J Am Acad Dermatol. 1996;35(3 Pt 1):404–10.

Hobbs JL, Chaffins ML, Douglass MC. Syringolymphoid hyperplasia with alopecia: two case reports and review of the literature. J Am Acad Dermatol. 2003;49(6): 1177–80.

Holm N, Flaig MJ, Yazdi AS, Sander CA. The value of molecular analysis by PCR in the diagnosis of cutaneous lymphocytic infiltrates. J Cutan Pathol. 2002; 29(8):447–52.

Hu CH, Winkelmann RK. Digitate dermatosis. A new look at symmetrical, small plaque parapsoriasis. Arch Dermatol. 1973;107(1):65–9.

Huang CL, Kuo TT, Chan HL. Acquired generalized hypohidrosis/anhidrosis with subclinical Sjogren's syndrome: report of a case with diffuse syringolymphoid hyperplasia and lymphocytic sialadenitis. J Am Acad Dermatol. 1996;35(2 Pt 2):350–2.

Hughes J, Weston S, Bennetts B, Prasad M, Angulo R, Jaworskit R, Jolles S, Kossard S, Fox S, Benson E. The application of a PCR technique for the detection of immunoglobulin heavy chain gene rearrangements in fresh or paraffin-embedded skin tissue. Pathology. 2001;33(2):222–5.

Ikonomou IM, Aamot HV, Heim S, Fossa A, Delabie J. Granulomatous slack skin with a translocation t(3;9) (q12;p24). Am J Surg Pathol. 2007;31(5):803–6.

Jablonska S, Chorzelski T, LANCUCKI J. Mucinosis follicularis. Hautarzt. 1959;10:27–33.

Jackson S, and Nesbit L. Differential diagnosis for the dermatologist. 2nd ed. New York: Springer; 2012.

Jokinen CH, Fromm JR, Argenyi ZB, Olerud J, Wood BL, Greisman HA. Flow cytometric evaluation of skin biopsies for mycosis fungoides. Am J Dermatopathol. 2011;33(5):483–91.

Kadin ME. T-cell clonality in pityriasis lichenoides: evidence for a premalignant or reactive immune disorder? Arch Dermatol. 2002;138(8):1089–90.

Kakizaki A, Fujimura T, Numata I, Hashimoto A, Aiba S. Pseudolymphomatous folliculitis on the nose. Case Rep Dermatol. 2012;4(1):27–30.

Kazakov DV, Kutzner H, Palmedo G, Boudova L, Michaelis S, Michal M, et al. Primary cutaneous lymphoproliferative disorders with dual lineage rearrangement. Am J Dermatopathol. 2006;28(5):399–409.

Kazakov DV, Belousova IE, Kacerovska D, Sima R, Vanecek T, Vazmitel M, et al. Hyperplasia of hair follicles and other adnexal structures in cutaneous lymphoproliferative disorders: a study of 53 cases, including so-called pseudolymphomatous folliculitis and overt lymphomas. Am J Surg Pathol. 2008;32(10):1468–78.

Kempf W, Levi E, Kamarashev J, et al. Fascin expression in CD30-positive cutaneous lymphoproliferative disorders. J Cutan Pathol. 2002;29:295–300.

Kempf W, Ostheeren-Michaelis S, Paulli M, Lucioni M, Wechsler J, Audring H, Assaf C, Rudiger T, Willemze R, Meijer CJ, Berti E, Cerroni L, Santucci M, Hallermann C, Berneburg M, Chimenti S, Robson A, Marschalko M, Kazakov DV, Petrella T, Fraitag S, Carlotti A, Courville P, Laeng H, Knobler R, Golling P, Dummer R, Burg G. Granulomatous mycosis fungoides and granulomatous slack skin: a multicenter study of the Cutaneous Lymphoma Histopathology Task Force Group of the European Organization For Research and Treatment of Cancer (EORTC). Arch Dermatol. 2008;144(12):1609–17.

Kerl K. Histopathological patterns indicative of distinct adverse drug reactions. Chem Immunol Allergy. 2012;97:61–78.

Klemke CD, Dippel E, Dembinski A, Ponitz N, Assaf C, Hummel M, Stein H, Goerdt S. Clonal T cell receptor gamma-chain gene rearrangement by PCR-based GeneScan analysis in the skin and blood of patients with parapsoriasis and early-stage mycosis fungoides. J Pathol. 2002;197(3):348–54.

Klemke CD, Fritzsching B, Franz B, Kleinmann EV, Oberle N, Poenitz N, Sykora J, Banham AH, Roncador G, Kuhn A, Goerdt S, Krammer PH, Suri-Payer E. Paucity of FOXP3+ cells in skin and peripheral blood distinguishes Sezary syndrome from other cutaneous T-cell lymphomas. Leukemia. 2006;20(6):1123–9.

Kluin-Nelemans HC, Kester MG, van deCorput L, Boor PP, Landegent JE, van Dongen JJ, Willemze R, Falkenburg JH. Correction of abnormal T-cell receptor repertoire during interferon-alpha therapy in patients with hairy cell leukemia. Blood. 1998;91(11): 4224–31.

Ko JW, Seong JY, Suh KS, Kim ST. Pityriasis lichenoides-like mycosis fungoides in children. Br J Dermatol. 2000;142(2):347–52.

Kulow BF, Cualing H, Steele P, VanHorn J, Breneman JC, Mutasim DF, Breneman DL. Progression of cutaneous B-cell pseudolymphoma to cutaneous B-cell lymphoma. J Cutan Med Surg. 2002;6(6):519–28.

Lambroza E, Cohen SR, Phelps R, Lebwohl M, Braverman IM, DiCostanzo D. Hypopigmented variant of mycosis fungoides: demography, histopathology, and treatment of seven cases. J Am Acad Dermatol. 1995;32(6): 987–93.

Langerak AW, van Den BR, Wolvers-Tettero IL, Boor PP, van Lochem EG, Hooijkaas H, van Dongen JJ. Molecular and flow cytometric analysis of the Vbeta repertoire for clonality assessment in mature TCRalphabeta T-cell proliferations. Blood. 2001;98(1):165–73.

Langerak AW, Groenen PJ, Bruggemann M, Beldjord K, Bellan C, Bonello L, Boone E, Carter GI, Catherwood M, Davi F, fau-Laure MH, Diss T, Evans PA, Gameiro P, Garcia SR, Gonzalez D, Grand D, Hakansson A, Hummel M, Liu H, Lombardia L, Macintyre EA, Milner BJ, Montes-Moreno S, Schuuring E, Spaargaren M, Hodges E, van Dongen JJ. EuroClonality/BIOMED-2 guidelines for interpretation and reporting of Ig/TCR clonality testing in suspected lymphoprolif-erations. Leukemia. 2012;26(10):2159–71.

LeBoit PE, Zackheim HS, White Jr CR. Granulomatous variants of cutaneous T-cell lymphoma. The histopathology of granulomatous mycosis fungoides and granulomatous slack skin. Am J Surg Pathol. 1988;12(2):83–95.

Leinweber B, Beltraminelli H, Kerl H, Cerroni L. Solitary small- to medium-sized pleomorphic T-cell nodules of undetermined significance: clinical, histopathological, immunohistochemical and molecular analysis of 26 cases. Dermatology. 2009;219(1):42–7.

Lloyd M, Burke N, Kalantapour F, Niesen M, Hall A, Pennypacker K, Citron B, Chiam P, Vernard A, Mohasweta D, Mohapatra S, Cualing H, Blanck G. Quantitative morphological and molecular pathology 1 of the human thymus correlate with infant cause of death. Technology and Innovation – Proceedings of the National Academy of Inventors™, Tampa, University of South Florida (in press).

Lukowsky A, Muche JM, Sterry W, Audring H. Detection of expanded T cell clones in skin biopsy samples of patients with lichen sclerosus et atrophicus by T cell receptor-gamma polymerase chain reaction assays. J Invest Dermatol. 2000;115(2):254–9.

Lukowsky A, Muche JM, Mobs M, Assaf C, Humme D, Hummel M, Sterry W, Steinhoff M. Evaluation of T-cell clonality in archival skin biopsy samples of cutaneous T-cell lymphomas using the biomed-2 PCR protocol. Diagn Mol Pathol. 2010;19(2):70–7.

Lundell R, Hartung L, Hill S, Perkins SL, Bahler DW. T-cell large granular lymphocyte leukemias have multiple phenotypic abnormalities involving pan-T-cell antigens and receptors for MHC molecules. Am J Clin Pathol. 2005;124(6):937–46.

Luo V, Lessin SR, Wilson RB, Rennert H, Tozer C, Benoit B, Leonard DG. Detection of clonal T-cell receptor gamma gene rearrangements using fluorescent-based PCR and automated high-resolution capillary electro-phoresis. Mol Diagn. 2001;6(3):169–79.

Lutzner MA, Hobbs JW, Horvath P. Ultrastructure of abnormal cells in Sezary syndrome, mycosis fungoi-des, and parapsoriasis en plaque. Arch Dermatol. 1971;103(4):375–86.

Magro CM, Crowson AN. Drug-induced immune dys-regulation as a cause of atypical cutaneous lymphoid infiltrates: a hypothesis. Hum Pathol. 1996;27(2): 125–32.

Magro CM, Wang X. Indolent primary cutaneous gamma/delta T-cell lymphoma localized to the subcutaneous panniculus and its association with atypical lympho-cytic lobular panniculitis. Am J Clin Pathol. 2012; 138(1):50–6.

Magro CM, Crowson AN, Harrist TJ. Atypical lymphoid infiltrates arising in cutaneous lesions of connective tissue disease. Am J Dermatopathol. 1997;19(5): 446–55.

Magro CM, Crowson AN, Kovatich AJ, Burns F. Lupus profundus, indeterminate lymphocytic lobular pan-niculitis and subcutaneous T-cell lymphoma: a spec-trum of subcuticular T-cell lymphoid dyscrasia. J Cutan Pathol. 2001;28(5):235–47.

Magro C, Crowson AN, Kovatich A, Burns F. Pityriasis lichenoides: a clonal T-cell lymphoproliferative disorder. Hum Pathol. 2002;33(8):788–95.

Magro CM, Crowson AN, Kovatich AJ, Burns F. Drug-induced reversible lymphoid dyscrasia: a clonal lymphomatoid dermatitis of memory and activated T cells. Hum Pathol. 2003;34(2):119–29.

Magro CM, Crowson AN, Byrd JC, Soleymani AD, Shendrik I. Atypical lymphocytic lobular panniculitis. J Cutan Pathol. 2004;31(4):300–6.

Magro CM, Crowson AN, Morrison C, Li J. Pityriasis lichenoides chronica: stratification by molecular and phenotypic profile. Hum Pathol 2007;38:479–90.

Magro CM, Schaefer JT, Morrison C, Porcu P. Atypical lymphocytic lobular panniculitis: a clonal subcutaneous T-cell dyscrasia. J Cutan Pathol. 2008;35(10): 947–54.

Magro CM, Cruz-Inigo AE, Votava H, Jacobs M, Wolfe D, Crowson AN. Drug-associated reversible granulomatous T cell dyscrasia: a distinct subset of the interstitial granulomatous drug reaction. J Cutan Pathol. 2010;37 Suppl 1:96–111.

Mahalingam M. Atypical cutaneous lymphocytic infiltrate--aucicellularity and 'pseudo'clonality. J Cutan Pathol. 2003;30(8):521.

Mariani S, Coscia M, Even J, Peola S, Foglietta M, Boccadoro M, Sbaiz L, Restagno G, Pileri A, Massaia M. Severe and long-lasting disruption of T-cell receptor diversity in human myeloma after high-dose chemotherapy and autologous peripheral blood progenitor cell infusion. Br J Haematol. 2001;113(4):1051–9.

Massone C, Kodama K, Salmhofer W, Abe R, Shimizu H, Parodi A, Kerl H, Cerroni L. Lupus erythematosus panniculitis (lupus profundus): clinical, histopathological, and molecular analysis of nine cases. J Cutan Pathol. 2005;32(6):396–404.

Melotti CZ, Amary MF, Sotto MN, Diss T, Sanches JA. Polymerase chain reaction-based clonality analysis of cutaneous B-cell lymphoproliferative processes. Clinics (Sao Paulo). 2010;65(1):53–60.

Meyer JC, Hassam S, Dummer R, Muletta S, Dobbeling U, Dommann SN, Burg G. A realistic approach to the sensitivity of PCR-DGGE and its application as a sensitive tool for the detection of clonality in cutaneous T-cell proliferations. Exp Dermatol. 1997;6(3):122–7.

Meyerson HJ. Flow cytometry for the diagnosis of mycosis fungoides. G Ital Dermatol Venereol. 2008;143(1): 21–41.

Morales AV, Arber DA, Seo K, Kohler S, Kim YH, Sundram UN. Evaluation of B-cell clonality using the BIOMED-2 PCR method effectively distinguishes cutaneous B-cell lymphoma from benign lymphoid infiltrates. Am J Dermatopathol. 2008;30(5):425–30.

Morice WG, Katzmann JA, Pittelkow MR, El-Azhary RA, Gibson LE, Hanson CA. A comparison of morphologic features, flow cytometry, TCR-Vbeta analysis, and TCR-PCR in qualitative and quantitative assessment of peripheral blood involvement by Sezary syndrome. Am J Clin Pathol. 2006;125(3):364–74.

Muche JM, Lukowsky A, Heim J, Friedrich M, Audring H, Sterry W. Demonstration of frequent occurrence of clonal T cells in the peripheral blood but not in the skin of patients with small plaque parapsoriasis. Blood. 1999;94(4):1409–17.

Muche JM, Sterry W, Gellrich S, Rzany B, Audring H, Lukowsky A. Peripheral blood T-cell clonality in mycosis fungoides and nonlymphoma controls. Diagn Mol Pathol. 2003;12(3):142–50.

Murphy M, Signoretti S, Kadin ME, Loda M. Detection of TCR-gamma gene rearrangements in early mycosis fungoides by non-radioactive PCR-SSCP. J Cutan Pathol 2000;27:228-34.

Nakamura M, Kabashima K, Tokura Y. Pseudolymphomatous folliculitis presenting with multiple nodules. Eur J Dermatol. 2009;19(3):263–4.

Neuhaus IM, Ramos-Caro FA, Hassanein AM. Hypopigmented mycosis fungoides in childhood and adolescence. Pediatr Dermatol. 2000;17(5):403–6.

Nihal M, Mikkola D, Wood GS. Detection of clonally restricted immunoglobulin heavy chain gene rearrangements in normal and lesional skin: analysis of the B cell component of the skin-associated lymphoid tissue and implications for the molecular diagnosis of cutaneous B cell lymphomas. J Mol Diagn. 2000; 2(1):5–10.

Nihal M, Mikkola D, Horvath N, Gilliam AC, Stevens SR, Spiro TP, Cooper KD, Wood GS. Cutaneous lymphoid hyperplasia: a lymphoproliferative continuum with lymphomatous potential. Hum Pathol. 2003;34(6): 617–22.

Nikolaou VA, Papadavid E, Katsambas A, Stratigos AJ, Marinos L, Anagnostou D, Antoniou C. Clinical characteristics and course of CD8+ cytotoxic variant of mycosis fungoides: a case series of seven patients. Br J Dermatol. 2009;161(4):826–30.

Nofal A, bdel-Mawla MY, Assaf M, Salah E. Primary cutaneous aggressive epidermotropic CD8(+) T-cell lymphoma: Proposed diagnostic criteria and therapeutic evaluation. J Am Acad Dermatol. 2012;67(4): 748–59.

Novelli M, Fierro MT, Quaglino P, Comessatti A, Lisa F, Ponti R, Savoia P, Bernengo MG. Flow cytometry immunophenotyping in mycosis fungoides. J Am Acad Dermatol. 2008;59(3):533–4.

Olsen E, Vonderheid E, Pimpinelli N, Willemze R, Kim Y, Knobler R, Zackheim H, Duvic M, Estrach T, Lamberg S, Wood G, Dummer R, Ranki A, Burg G, Heald P, Pittelkow M, Bernengo MG, Sterry W, Laroche L, Trautinger F, Whittaker S. Revisions to the staging and classification of mycosis fungoides and Sezary syndrome: a proposal of the International Society for Cutaneous Lymphomas (ISCL) and the cutaneous lymphoma task force of the European Organization of Research and Treatment of Cancer (EORTC). Blood. 2007;110(6):1713–22.

Petit T, Cribier B, Bagot M, Wechsler J. Inflammatory vitiligo-like macules that simulate hypopigmented mycosis fungoides. Eur J Dermatol. 2003;13(4): 410–2.

Pfaltz K, Kerl K, Palmedo G, Kutzner H, Kempf W. Clonality in sarcoidosis, granuloma annulare, and granulomatous mycosis fungoides. Am J Dermatopathol. 2011;33(7):659–62.

Pileri A, Facchetti F, Rutten A, Zumiani G, Boi S, Fink-Puches R, Cerroni L. Syringotropic mycosis fungoides: a rare variant of the disease with peculiar clinicopathologic features. Am J Surg Pathol. 2011; 35(1):100–9.

Pimpinelli N, Olsen EA, Santucci M, Vonderheid E, Haeffner AC, Stevens S, Burg G, Cerroni L, Dreno B, Glusac E, Guitart J, Heald PW, Kempf W, Knobler R, Lessin S, Sander C, Smoller BS, Telang G, Whittaker S, Iwatsuki K, Obitz E, Takigawa M, Turner ML, Wood GS. Defining early mycosis fungoides. J Am Acad Dermatol. 2005;53(6):1053–63.

Pinkus H. Alopecia mucinosa. Additional data in 1983. Arch Dermatol. 1983;119(8):698–9.

Ponti R, Fierro MT, Quaglino P, Lisa B, Paola FC, Michela O, Paolo F, Comessatti A, Novelli M, Bernengo MG. TCRgamma-chain gene rearrangement by PCR-based GeneScan: diagnostic accuracy improvement and clonal heterogeneity analysis in multiple cutaneous T-cell lymphoma samples. J Invest Dermatol. 2008;128(4):1030–8.

Poszepczynska-Guigne E, Schiavon V, D'Incan M, Echchakir H, Musette P, Ortonne N, Boumsell L, Moretta A, Bensussan A, Bagot M. CD158k/KIR3DL2 is a new phenotypic marker of Sezary cells: relevance for the diagnosis and follow-up of Sezary syndrome. J Invest Dermatol. 2004;122(3):820–3.

Raess PW, Bagg A. The role of molecular pathology in the diagnosis of cutaneous lymphomas. Patholog Res Int. 2012;2012:913523.

Requena L, Sanchez YE. Panniculitis. Part II. Mostly lobular panniculitis. J Am Acad Dermatol. 2001; 45(3):325–61.

Rezania D, Sagatys E, Glass F, Kadin M, Cualing H. Cutaneous lymphocyte antigen and TRAF-1 are useful in differentiating lymphomatoid papulosis, cutaneous ALCL and systemic ALCL. Am Soc Hematol, Abstracts 50th annual meeting. San Francisco, CA 2008

Rijlaarsdam JU, Scheffer E, Meijer CJ, Willemze R. Cutaneous pseudo-T-cell lymphomas. A clinicopathologic study of 20 patients. Cancer. 1992;69(3):717–24.

Salhany KE, Macon WR, Choi JK, Elenitsas R, Lessin SR, Felgar RE, Wilson DM, Przybylski GK, Lister J, Wasik MA, Swerdlow SH. Subcutaneous panniculitis-like T-cell lymphoma: clinicopathologic, immunophenotypic, and genotypic analysis of alpha/beta and gamma/delta subtypes. Am J Surg Pathol. 1998;22(7):881–93.

Sandberg Y, Heule F, Lam K, Lugtenburg PJ, Wolvers-Tettero IL, van Dongen JJ, Langerak AW. Molecular immunoglobulin/T- cell receptor clonality analysis in cutaneous lymphoproliferations. Experience with the BIOMED-2 standardized polymerase chain reaction protocol. Haematologica. 2003;88(6):659–70.

Sandberg Y, van Gastel-Mol EJ, Verhaaf B, Lam KH, van Dongen JJ, Langerak AW. BIOMED-2 multiplex immunoglobulin/T-cell receptor polymerase chain reaction protocols can reliably replace Southern blot analysis in routine clonality diagnostics. J Mol Diagn. 2005;7(4):495–503.

Sarkany I. Patchy alopecia, anhidrosis, eccrine gland wall hypertrophy and vasculitis. Proc R Soc Med. 1969;62(2):157–9.

Scarabello A, Leinweber B, Ardigo M, Rutten A, Feller AC, Kerl H, Cerroni L. Cutaneous lymphomas with prominent granulomatous reaction: a potential pitfall in the histopathologic diagnosis of cutaneous T- and B-cell lymphomas. Am J Surg Pathol. 2002;26(10): 1259–68.

Schiller PI, Flaig MJ, Puchta U, Kind P, Sander CA. Detection of clonal T cells in lichen planus. Arch Dermatol Res. 2000;292(11):568–9.

Schmidt D, Goronzy JJ, Weyand CM. CD4+ CD7-CD28- T cells are expanded in Rheumatoid Arthritis and are characterized by autoreactivity. J Clin Invest. 1996;97(9):2027–37.

Sigurdsson V, Toonstra J, van Vloten WA. Idiopathic erythroderma: a follow-up study of 28 patients. Dermatology. 1997;194(2):98–101.

Sigurdsson V, Steegmans PH, van Vloten WA. The incidence of erythroderma: a survey among all dermatologists in The Netherlands. J Am Acad Dermatol. 2001;45(5):675–8.

Simon M, Flaig MJ, Kind P, Sander CA, Kaudewitz P. Large plaque parapsoriasis: clinical and genotypic correlations. J Cutan Pathol. 2000;27(2):57–60.

Sproul A, Goodlad JR. Clonality Testing of cutaneous lymphoid infiltrates: practicalities, pitfalls and potential uses. J Haematopathol. 2012;5(1):69–82.

Stone ML, Styles AR, Cockerell CJ, Pandya AG. Hypopigmented mycosis fungoides: a report of 7 cases and review of the literature. Cutis. 2001;67(2):133–8.

Swerdlow SJ, Campo E, Harris NL, Jaffe ES, Pileri S, Stein H, Thiele J, Vardiman JW (eds) WHO classification of tumors of haematopoieitic and lymphoid tissues. 4th ed. Geneva, Switzerland: Who Press; 2008.

Tamagawa R, Katoh N, Shimazaki C, Okano A, Yamada S, Ichihashi K, Masuda K, Kishimoto S. Lymphoma with large-plaque parapsoriasis treated with PUVA. Eur J Dermatol. 2005;15(4):265–7.

Tannous Z, Baldassano MF, Li VW, Kvedar J, Duncan LM. Syringolymphoid hyperplasia and follicular mucinosis in a patient with cutaneous T-cell lymphoma. J Am Acad Dermatol. 1999;41(2 Pt 2):303–8.

Tee SI, Martinez-Escaname M, Zuriel D, Fried I, Wolf I, Massone C, et al. Acrodermatitis chronica atrophicans with pseudolymphomatous infiltrates. Am J Dermatopathol. 2013;35(3):338–42. doi: 10.1097/DAD.0b013e31826b7487.

Thein M, Ravat F, Orchard G, Calonje E, Russell-Jones R. Syringotropic cutaneous T-cell lymphoma: an immunophenotypic and genotypic study of five cases. Br J Dermatol. 2004;151(1):216–26.

Thurber SE, Zhang B, Kim YH, Schrijver I, Zehnder J, Kohler S. T-cell clonality analysis in biopsy specimens from two different skin sites shows high specificity in the diagnosis of patients with suggested mycosis fungoides. J Am Acad Dermatol. 2007;57(5):782–90.

Tomasini D, Zampatti C, Palmedo G, Bonfacini V, Sangalli G, Kutzner H. Cytotoxic mycosis fungoides evolving from pityriasis lichenoides chronica in a seventeen-year-old girl. Report of a case. Dermatology. 2002;205(2):176–9.

Vakeva L, Sarna S, Vaalasti A, Pukkala E, Kariniemi AL, Ranki A. A retrospective study of the probability of the evolution of parapsoriasis en plaques into mycosis fungoides. Acta Derm Venereol. 2005;85(4):318–23.

van der Loo EM, Cnossen J, Meijer CJ. Morphological aspects of T cell subpopulations in human blood: characterization of the cerebriform mononuclear cells in healthy individuals. Clin Exp Immunol. 1981;43(3):506–16.

van Dongen JJ, Langerak AW, Bruggemann M, Evans PA, Hummel M, Lavender FL, Delabesse E, Davi F, Schuuring E, Garcia-Sanz R, van Krieken JH, Droese J, Gonzalez D, Bastard C, White HE, Spaargaren M, Gonzalez M, Parreira A, Smith JL, Morgan GJ, Kneba M, Macintyre EA. Design and standardization of PCR primers and protocols for detection of clonal immunoglobulin and T-cell receptor gene recombinations in suspect lymphoproliferations: report of the BIOMED-2 Concerted Action BMH4-CT98-3936. Leukemia. 2003;17(12):2257–317.

van Doorn R, Van Haselen CW, van V, V et al. Mycosis fungoides: disease evolution and prognosis of 309 Dutch patients. Arch Dermatol 2000;136:504–10.

Vonderheid EC. On the diagnosis of erythrodermic cutaneous T-cell lymphoma. J Cutan Pathol. 2006;33 Suppl 1:27–42.

Washington LT, Huh YO, Powers LC, Duvic M, Jones D. A stable aberrant immunophenotype characterizes nearly all cases of cutaneous T-cell lymphoma in blood and can be used to monitor response to therapy. BMC Clin Pathol. 2002;2(1):5.

Wechsler J, Bagot M, Nikolova M, Parolini S, Martin-Garcia N, Boumsell L, Moretta A, Bensussan A. Killer cell immunoglobulin-like receptor expression delineates in situ Sezary syndrome lymphocytes. J Pathol. 2003;199(1):77–83.

Weinberg JM, Kristal L, Chooback L, Honig PJ, Kramer EM, Lessin SR. The clonal nature of pityriasis lichenoides. Arch Dermatol. 2002;138(8):1063–7.

Weiss LM, Wood GS, Ellisen LW, Reynolds TC, Sklar J. Clonal T-cell populations in pityriasis lichenoides et varioliformis acuta (Mucha-Habermann disease). Am J Pathol. 1987;126(3):417–21.

Wenzel J, Gutgemann I, Distelmaier M, Uerlich M, Mikus S, Bieber T, Tuting T. The role of cytotoxic skin-homing CD8+ lymphocytes in cutaneous cytotoxic T-cell lymphoma and pityriasis lichenoides. J Am Acad Dermatol. 2005;53(3):422–7.

Werner B, Brown S, Ackerman AB. "Hypopigmented mycosis fungoides" is not always mycosis fungoides! Am J Dermatopathol. 2005;27(1):56–67.

Whittam LR, Calonje E, Orchard G, Fraser-Andrews EA, Woolford A, Russell-Jones R. CD8-positive juvenile onset mycosis fungoides: an immunohistochemical and genotypic analysis of six cases. Br J Dermatol. 2000;143(6):1199–204.

Winkelmann RK. Panniculitis with cellular phagocytosis. Chronic form of histiocytic panniculitis with fever, pancytopenia, polyserositis and lethal hemorrhagic diathesis. Hautarzt. 1980;31(11):588–94.

Winkelmann RK, Buechner SA, az-Perez JL. Pre-Sezary syndrome. J Am Acad Dermatol. 1984;10(6):992–9.

Wolf IH, Kerl K, Cerroni L, Kerl H. Parapsoriasis lichenoides/parapsoriasis variegata–a new concept. J Dtsch Dermatol Ges. 2009;7(11):993–5.

Wood GS. Analysis of clonality in cutaneous T cell lymphoma and associated diseases. Ann N Y Acad Sci. 2001;941:26–30.

Wood B. 9-color and 10-color flow cytometry in the clinical laboratory. Arch Pathol Lab Med. 2006;130(5):680–90.

Wood GS, Ngan BY, Tung R, Hoffman TE, Abel EA, Hoppe RT, Warnke RA, Cleary ML, Sklar J. Clonal rearrangements of immunoglobulin genes and progression to B cell lymphoma in cutaneous lymphoid hyperplasia. Am J Pathol. 1989;135(1):13–9.

Zhang B, Beck AH, Taube JM, Kohler S, Seo K, Zwerner J, Viakhereva N, Sundram U, Kim YH, Schrijver I, Arber DA, Zehnder JL. Combined use of PCR-based TCRG and TCRB clonality tests on paraffin-embedded skin tissue in the differential diagnosis of mycosis fungoides and inflammatory dermatoses. J Mol Diagn. 2010;12(3):320–7.

Uma N. Sundram

Atopic Dermatitis

Introduction and Clinical Features

Atopic dermatitis is an inflammatory disease of the skin which occurs in individuals with a personal or family history of atopy (Weedon 2010). It is a common disorder, and the diagnosis is made on the basis of a constellation of clinical features. The major criteria for its diagnosis include the presence of pruritus, chronicity, and a history of atopy (Williams et al. 1994). In young children, there is an erythematous papulovesicular rash with erosions involving the face, arms, and legs (Heskel and Lobitz 1983). Adults often have lichenified lesions involving the flexures (Ozkaya 2005).

Histopathology and Immunophenotype

The histopathology of atopic dermatitis falls into the category of spongiotic dermatitis. One can see acute, subacute, and chronic forms of this disease (White 1983). There can be significant overlap

U.N. Sundram, MD, PhD
Department of Pathology, Stanford Hospital and Clinics, 300 Pasteur Drive, Room H2110, Stanford, CA 94305, USA
e-mail: sundram@stanford.edu

between the findings of atopic dermatitis and other entities within the category of spongiotic dermatitis. In acute lesions, there is spongiosis within the epidermis, accompanied in some cases by vesiculation. Exocytosis of lymphocytes is present, and when significant spongiosis is also present, the diagnosis of mycosis fungoides can be excluded. Langerhans' cells microabscesses are present in acute lesions. In subacute lesions, there is acanthosis of the epidermis with irregular psoriasiform hyperplasia. These findings are more pronounced in chronic atopic dermatitis, in which there can be significant psoriasiform hyperplasia with only mild spongiosis. In both the subacute and chronic forms, there can be overlying lichen simplex chronicus, which leads to hypergranulosis, hyperkeratosis, and papillary dermal fibrosis. Since spongiosis is decreased in subacute and chronic forms, hence in such cases, the presence of exocytosis can sometimes be mistaken for the epidermotropism of mycosis fungoides. In addition, Langerhans cell "microabscesses" or microvesicles can mimic Pautrier's microabscesses, particularly on low power examination. The presence of eosinophils is a useful clue pointing to the diagnosis of atopic dermatitis, as significant numbers of eosinophils are not present in mycosis fungoides (Dalton et al. 2012). In addition, Langerhans cells are larger than cerebriform cells, show grooved vesicular pale ovoid histiocytic nuclei, and with thin nuclear membrane and moderate amount of cytoplasm. The lymphocytes

H.D. Cualing et al. (eds.), *Cutaneous Hematopathology*,
DOI 10.1007/978-1-4939-0950-6_5, © Springer Science+Business Media New York 2014

of atopic dermatitis are primarily T cells that express CD3 and CD4; this is also the immunophenotype of mycosis fungoides and other CD4-expressing cutaneous T-cell lymphoma, but one difference is that the collection of Langerhans cells expresses S100, CD1a, and Langerin, which are not true of cells of mycosis fungoides.

Interestingly, expression of adhesion molecules has been shown to be important in demonstrating the exocytosis/epidermotropism features of atopic dermatitis (Jung et al. 1997). In a study by Jung et al., α6 integrin was shown to be dramatically upregulated on endothelial cells and in the epidermis after exposure to atopic antigens. The authors speculate that α6 integrin may play a crucial role in the exocytosis of T cells in atopic dermatitis.

Genetics and Molecular Findings

Genetics probably plays a role in the pathogenesis of atopic dermatitis, given the usual presence of a family history of atopy and high twin concordance (Cookson 2001). Allelic associations have been described with chromosomes 11q13, 13q12-q14, and 5q31-q33 (Coleman et al. 1997; Beyer et al. 2000). Genes encoding GATA3, IL-4R, CTLA4, eotaxin, filaggrin, and portions of the receptors for IgE have all been implicated (Weedon 2010).

Prognosis and Clinical Course

The course of atopic dermatitis is one of remissions and exacerbations, and as the patient ages, there are increased symptom-free periods (Weedon 2010). The mainstay of treatment has been a combination of emollients and topical corticosteroids. Topical calcineurin inhibitors can also be used as second-line therapy for head and neck disease (Rustin 2007).

Differential Diagnosis

As noted above, atopic dermatitis shares nearly identical histologic features with other members

Table 5.1 Clinical and morphologic comparisons between atopic dermatitis and mycosis fungoides

	Atopic dermatitis	Mycosis fungoides
Common in children	Yes	No
Involvement of flexures	Yes	No
Spongiosis is present	Yes	No
Microabscesses	Langerhans cell	Pautrier's (tumor cells)
Cytologic atypia within T cells	No	Yes
Phenotype of T cells	CD4	CD4

of the "spongiotic dermatitis family," including contact dermatitis, id reaction, drug hypersensitivity reactions, nummular dermatitis, and arthropod hypersensitivity reactions. Cutaneous dermatophytosis can give similar findings, so a periodic acid-Schiff stain with diastase (PASD) or other fungal stain should always be done in these cases to exclude a fungal infection. Fungal infections can also give rise to a "mycosis fungoides"-like histologic picture. Careful correlation with clinical findings is important in arriving at the correct diagnosis (Table 5.1).

Lymphomatoid Contact Dermatitis

Introduction and Clinical Features

Allergic contact dermatitis is an inflammatory condition caused by contact exposure to an allergen (Weedon 2010). Importantly, contact dermatitis is often seen in the context of an occupation, such as hairdressing or veterinary medicine (Sajjachareonpong 2002; Bulcke and Devos 2007). Clinically there may be papules, small vesicles, or plaques, which are pruritic. The lesions develop 12–48 h after exposure to the antigen. In 1976, Orbaneja et al. described four patients with skin lesions clinically and histologically compatible with mycosis fungoides (Orbaneja et al. 1976). The lesions first appeared on the anterior thighs before appearing on the face and arms and were accompanied by intense burning and pruritus. Interestingly, these patients gave a positive patch test with the striker part of a matchbox which was often stored in the trouser

Table 5.2 Clinical and morphologic comparisons between lymphomatoid contact dermatitis and mycosis fungoides

	Lymphomatoid contact dermatitis	Mycosis fungoides
Distribution	Extremities, face	Usually sun-protected areas (bathing trunk distribution)
Association with occupation	Yes	No
Pruritus is present	Yes, extensive	Sometimes
Temporal association with contactant	Yes	No
Spongiosis is present	Yes	No
Eosinophils are present	Yes, sometimes extensive	Yes, limited
Cytologic atypia within T cells	Yes	Yes
Phenotype of T cells	CD4	CD4
Positive clonality assays	No	Yes

pockets; a standard patch test was negative. The lesions resolved completely when contact with the substance (phosphorus sesquisulfide) was removed. Such lesions have also been described by Ackerman et al. as a stimulant of mycosis fungoides (Ackerman et al. 1974) and have been described in association with a variety of agents (Table 5.2).

Histopathology and Immunophenotype

On histology, these lesions demonstrate a band-like infiltrate of T cells with epidermotropism. In the study of lymphomatoid contact dermatitis by Gomez-Orbaneja et al., the band-like infiltrate contains histiocytes and eosinophils, as well as lymphocytes (Orbaneja et al. 1976). In chronic lesions, the epidermis may be acanthotic. Some epidermal spongiosis may be present, which can help to distinguish these lesions from mycosis fungoides. In most cases, however, it can be quite difficult to differentiate the intraepidermal

collections of mononuclear cells in lymphomatoid contact dermatitis from the Pautrier's microabscesses of mycosis fungoides (Orbaneja et al. 1976; Ayala 1987). In addition, the cells on high power may show nuclear hyperchromasia, similar to mycosis fungoides. Detailed immunohistochemical studies have not been performed on these rare cases; however, it is known from the limited published immunohistochemical findings that the infiltrate in lymphomatoid contact dermatitis is composed of T cells that express CD4 (Smolle et al. 1990).

Prognosis and Clinical Course

In most cases described in the literature, these lesions have resolved when the offending agent is removed. This differs from lesions of mycosis fungoides, which do not demonstrate association with an offending agent. Interestingly, in at least one case, the patient developed T-cell prolymphocytic leukemia with involvement of the skin by malignant infiltrates after being initially diagnosed with lymphomatoid contact dermatitis (Braun et al. 2000; Abraham et al. 2006). It is the authors' supposition that the initial biopsy and diagnosis probably represented very early involvement of the skin by T-cell leukemia and emphasizes the necessity in these cases for careful long-term follow-up to ensure that the appropriate diagnosis has been made initially.

Differential Diagnosis

Similar to atopic dermatitis, contact dermatitis belongs to the "spongiotic dermatitis" family, and therefore the differential diagnosis includes atopic dermatitis, id reaction, drug hypersensitivity reactions, arthropod hypersensitivity reactions, and nummular dermatitis. If the patients have a more generalized eruption, and the eruption does not clear with avoidance of offending agents, one could also consider chronic photosensitivity dermatitis or actinic reticuloid within the differential (Ecker and Winkelmann et al. 1981). The presence of atypical T cells within the epidermis necessitates inclusion of mycosis

Table 5.3 Agents that cause lymphomatoid contact dermatitis

Agent	Reference
Para tertiary butyl phenol formaldehyde resin	Evans et al. (2003)
p-Phenylenediamine	Calzavara-Pinton et al. (2002)
Ethylenediamine dihydrochloride	Wall (1982)
Nickel	Danese and Bertazzoni (1995), Houck et al. (1997)
Cobalt naphthenate	Schena et al. (1995)
Gold	Conde-Taboada et al. (2007)
Isopropyldiphenylenediamine	Marlière et al. (1998), Martínez-Morán et al. (2009)

fungoides within the differential (Table 5.3), but a careful search for offending agents may help confirm the diagnosis of contact dermatitis.

Lymphomatoid Lichenoid Keratosis

Introduction and Clinical Features

Lichenoid keratosis is a common clinical entity with a differential diagnosis that includes basal cell or squamous cell carcinoma, actinic keratosis, verruca, and atypical nevi. Lymphomatoid lichenoid keratosis was originally proposed in 1997 to describe an entity which was clinically similar (a solitary erythematous patch) but showed the histologic features of mycosis fungoides (Al Hoqail and Crawford 2002; Arai et al. 2007; Kossard 1997; Evans et al. 1997; Choi et al. 2010; Morgan et al. 2005; Cerroni et al. 1999). The main differential diagnosis for this entity was unilesional mycosis fungoides, and indeed, on many occasions such a lesion has been misdiagnosed as mycosis fungoides (Kossard 1997). Al Hoqail and Crawford described a series of 15 patients who had solitary lesions, usually on the upper trunk, with a mean lesional size of around 0.6 cm (Al Hoqail and Crawford 2002). The lesions were biopsied or excised because of a clinical concern for cutaneous cancer, with

basal cell carcinoma being the most common concern. Similarly, Arai and coworkers studied six cases which they defined narrowly as patients presenting with a solitary scaly plaque which demonstrated the histologic features of mycosis fungoides on microscopic examination (Arai et al. 2007). The patients were adults, the lesions were usually around 0.8 cm in size and demonstrated a predilection for the face. Clinically the lesions were thought to be either large actinic keratoses or seborrheic keratoses. None of these cases (in either study) were thought to clinically be mycosis fungoides.

Histopathology

On histology, the lesions demonstrate a striking resemblance to mycosis fungoides (Al Hoqail and Crawford 2002; Arai et al. 2007; Evans et al. 1997; Choi et al. 2010; Morgan et al. 2005) (Fig. 5.1). Al Hoqail and Crawford looked specifically for different specific findings of mycosis fungoides and found them to be represented in different percentages in these lesions. For example, Pautrier's microabscesses were present in 93 % of cases, epidermotropism in 80 %, basal alignment of lymphocytes in 93 %, atypical cytologic features in lymphocytes in 47 % (Figs. 5.2 and 5.3), and papillary dermal fibrosis in 40 % (Al Hoqail and Crawford 2002). Plasma cells were present in 60 % of cases, but no eosinophils were found. In the study of Arai et al., all cases demonstrated a band-like infiltrate of lymphocytes, epidermal involvement of lymphocytes out of proportion to accompanying spongiosis, basilar lymphocytes, and formation of Pautrier's microabscesses (Arai et al. 2007). No atypical keratinocytes or atypical lymphocytes were observed in this study, and lesions demonstrating the typical features of lichenoid keratosis were not studied. Within the lesions, there were plasma cells, eosinophils, and melanophages. Al Hoqail and Crawford documented the presence of typical findings of lichenoid keratosis such as hypergranulosis (53 % of cases), necrotic keratinocytes (73 % of cases), solar lentigo and seborrheic keratosis adjacent to the lesion

Fig. 5.1 Lymphomatoid lichenoid keratosis. There is a dense band-like infiltrate of small and large lymphocytes within the dermis with epidermal involvement (H + E, 10×)

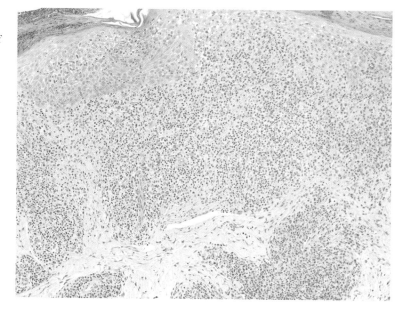

Fig. 5.2 Lymphomatoid lichenoid keratosis. Large atypical lymphocytes populate the lower half of the epidermis, and there are angulated forms (H + E, 20×)

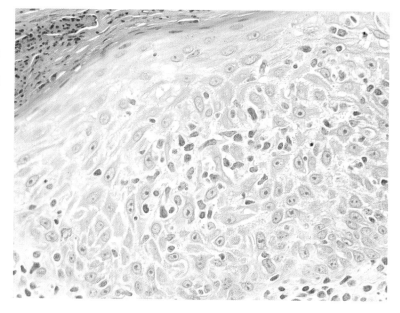

(60 % of cases), and pointed contours of rete ridges (73 % of cases) (Al Hoqail and Crawford 2002). While the cases of Arai et al. were more narrowly defined, they still found parakeratosis and acanthosis, which are more typical findings of lichenoid keratosis (Arai et al. 2007). Both studies noted the presence of hypergranulosis and plasma cells, which are unusual findings in mycosis fungoides. However, it is important to note that in both studies, many if not all of the cases lacked characteristic findings of lichenoid keratosis, which would make the distinction from mycosis fungoides on morphologic grounds difficult (Arai et al. 2007).

Fig. 5.3 Lymphomatoid lichenoid keratosis. Basal vacuolar alteration accompanies the infiltrate (H + E, 20×)

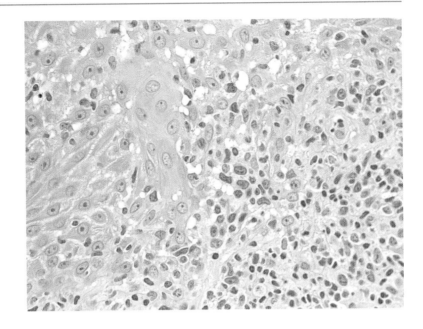

Fig. 5.4 Lymphomatoid lichenoid keratosis. The infiltrate is composed primarily of CD4-expressing T cells (20×)

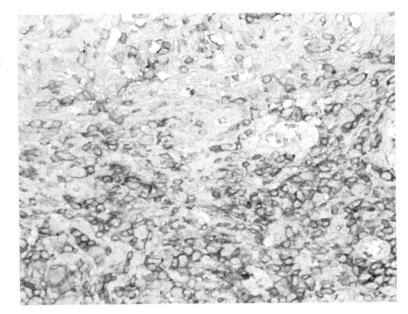

Immunophenotype

Interestingly, in the study of Arai et al., numerous B cells were admixed with T cells within the infiltrate, and in some cases, B cells formed Pautrier's microabscesses (Arai et al. 2007). CD4-expressing T cells predominated over CD8-expressing T cells, and epidermotropism of CD3-expressing cells was seen (Fig. 5.4). Interdigitating and Langerhans cells were present within the epidermis and expressed S100 and CD1a, respectively. The presence of B-cell-predominant Pautrier's microabscesses and CD1a and S100 expressing cells within the epidermis are both thought to be unusual findings in mycosis fungoides (Igisu et al. 1983).

Table 5.4 Clinical and morphologic comparisons between lymphomatoid lichenoid keratosis and mycosis fungoides

	Lymphomatoid lichenoid keratosis	Mycosis fungoides (unilesional)	Mycosis fungoides (classic)
Solitary lesion	Yes	Yes	No
Distribution	Truncal and face	Truncal (Cerroni et al. 1999)	Buttocks, trunk, inner arms, upper thighs
Clinical suspicion for mycosis fungoides	Low	Intermediate to high (Arai et al. 2007)	High
Presence of parakeratosis, hypergranulosis, acanthosis, and plasma cells	Yes	No	No
Presence of saw tooth rete ridges	Yes (Al Hoqail and Crawford 2002)	No	No
Adjacent typical solar lentigo or seborrheic keratosis	Yes (Al Hoqail and Crawford 2002)	No	No
Cytologic atypia within T cells	Yes	Yes	Yes
Phenotype of T cells	CD4	CD4	CD4
Phenotype of epidermotropic cells	Admixed CD20+ B cells (Arai et al. 2007)	CD4+ T cells only	CD4+ T cells only

Genetics and Molecular Findings

T-cell receptor gene rearrangement and IgH clonality assays were both performed in the cases of Arai et al. (2007). IgH clonality assays were negative in all cases, but in two cases, T-cell receptor gene rearrangements were seen. Interestingly, T-cell receptor (TCR) gamma and TCR beta chains were both rearranged in one case.

Prognosis and Clinical Course

Complete excisions are curative in these cases. Although follow-up is limited, no patient to date has developed widespread lesions of mycosis fungoides.

Differential Diagnosis

The major differential diagnostic considerations include unilesional mycosis fungoides, lichenoid actinic keratosis, and lichenoid lymphomatoid drug eruption. In classic mycosis fungoides, the lesions consist of erythematous patches in sun-protected sites (bathing trunk distribution). The buttocks, inner arms, and trunk are often affected. In cases of unilesional mycosis fungoides, there is a single lesion, often truncal, with a size range

between 1 and 2 cm. This entity is thought to be distinct from pagetoid reticulosis (Cerroni et al. 1999; Jones and Chu 1981). The distinction between unilesional mycosis fungoides and lymphomatoid lichenoid keratosis (as defined by Arai et al.) can be very difficult (Arai et al. 2007; Cerroni et al. 1999; Oliver and Winkelmann 1989). Histologic and immunohistochemical features can sometimes be helpful in making this distinction (Table 5.4). Lymphomatoid drug eruptions have a temporal connection to offending medications and other agents.

Mycosis Fungoides-Like Lymphomatoid Drug Eruption

Introduction and Clinical Features

Lymphomatoid drug eruption (also known as lymphomatoid hypersensitivity reaction (Gilliam and Wood 2000)) is a rash caused by certain medications (Navarro et al. 2011; Choi et al. 2003; Miranda-Romero et al. 2001; Fitzpatrick 1992; Welykyj et al. 1990). Lymphomatoid drug eruptions that mimic mycosis fungoides will be discussed in this section and are primarily caused by anticonvulsants (such as carbamazepine), but other drugs can cause this condition as well (Ploysangam et al.

Fig. 5.5 Lymphomatoid drug eruption. There is a dense deep and diffuse infiltrate of atypical lymphocytes with involvement of the epidermis and hair follicle (H + E, 4×)

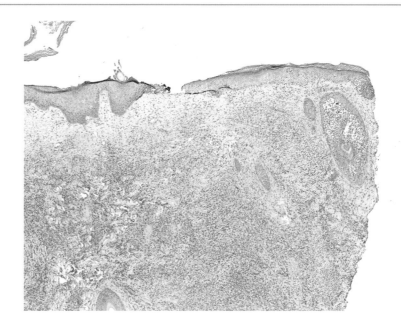

1998). Phenytoin- and carbamazepine-induced hypersensitivity is associated with a classic triad of fever, rash, and lymphadenopathy, as well as peripheral blood abnormalities, and these findings resolve after the agent is discontinued (Ploysangam et al. 1998). The syndrome can occur shortly after the drug is ingested, and skin lesions can be single or multiple and generalized. Rarely, a Sézary syndrome-like erythrodermic eruption can take place (Ploysangam et al. 1998). Drugs other than anticonvulsants can also give rise to pseudolymphomas. These too are temporally connected to the offending agent and can give rise to single or multiple lesions or a Sézary syndrome-like erythroderma.

Histopathology and Immunophenotype

On histology, the findings can be identical to mycosis fungoides (Fig. 5.5) (Souteyrand and d'Incan 1990). There can be a band-like infiltrate of lymphocytes, many of them atypical. They can demonstrate epidermotropism with formation of Pautrier's-like microabscesses, and follicular mucinosis has been documented (Fig. 5.6) (Navarro et al. 2011). On immunophenotyping, the atypical cells are usually of T-cell origin (Miranda-Romero et al. 2001), and CD30 expression can be seen (Fig. 5.7a, b) (Pulitzer et al. 2013).

Genetics and Molecular Findings

In a study by Brady et al., the skin lesions of 14 patients with known lymphomatoid drug eruptions were tested via T-cell receptor gene rearrangement studies and IgH clonality assays for the presence of a clone (Brady et al. 1999). Two of 14 patients were found to have TCR clones, but none had IgH clones. Both the skin rash and monoclonal population of T cells resolved upon discontinuation of the drug.

Differential Diagnosis

The main differential diagnosis is with mycosis fungoides, which can be excluded on the basis of good clinical information and resolution of the rash and other systemic findings upon discontinuation of the drug (Table 5.5).

Fig. 5.6 Lymphomatoid drug eruption. Higher power view shows formation of Pautrier's-like microabscesses and basal lining by large atypical lymphocytes (H + E, 20×)

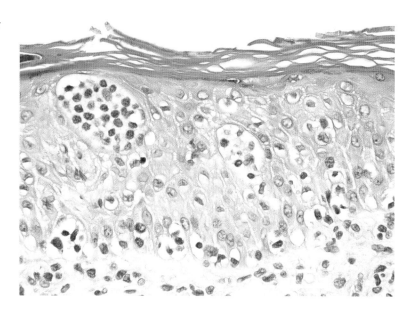

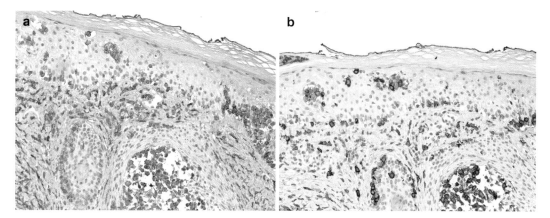

Fig. 5.7 Lymphomatoid drug eruption. The lymphocytes express both CD4 (**a**) and CD30 (**b**) (20× for both)

Table 5.5 Clinical and morphologic comparisons between mycosis fungoides-like lymphomatoid drug eruptions and mycosis fungoides

	Mycosis fungoides-like lymphomatoid drug eruption	Mycosis fungoides
Clinical findings	Widespread morbilliform eruption	Patches and plaques involving sun protected areas
Systemic symptoms	Yes, lymphadenopathy, fever, hepatosplenomegaly, eosinophilia	No
Resolution of lesions upon removal of offending agent	Yes	No
Microabscesses	Pautrier's like	Pautrier's (tumor cells)
Cytologic atypia within T cells	Yes	Yes
TCR clonality	Positive sometimes (Brady et al. 1999)	Usually positive

Table 5.6 Clinical and morphologic comparisons between lichenoid drug eruptions, lichen planus, and mycosis fungoides

	Lichenoid drug eruptions	Lichen planus	Lichenoid mycosis fungoides
Clinical distribution	Extremities, trunk, oral	Extremities (flexors), trunk, genitals, oral	No
Clinical appearance	Small flat-topped papules, pruritic	Small flat topped papules, pruritic	Erythematous patches, sun-protected areas
Resolution upon removal of drug	Yes	No	No
Eosinophils are present	Yes	Minor feature	Minor feature
Clusters of necrotic keratinocytes	Yes, high percentage	Yes, low percentage	Yes, very low percentage
Cytologic atypia within T cells	No	No	Yes

Lichenoid Drug Eruptions

Introduction and Clinical Features

Lichenoid drug eruptions clinically mimic lichen planus but are caused by a variety of medications, such as gold (Penneys 1979), methyldopa (Burry 1976), β-adrenergic blocking agents (Hawk 1980), penicillamine (Van Hecke et al. 1981), synthetic antimalarials (Bauer 1981), and ethambutol (Grossman et al. 1995). Newer drugs to cause this effect include imatinib (Kuraishi et al. 2010) and tumor necrosis factor-α antagonists (Asarch et al. 2009). The eruption clears when the offending agent is withdrawn (Weedon 1998). The lesions consist of flat-topped pruritic papules occurring on the limbs, chest, and back. More pronounced hyperpigmentation has been reported with lichenoid drug eruptions than with lichen planus. Oral lichen planus may also occur with ingestion of certain drugs and can take time to resolve even after the drug is removed (Weedon 1998).

Histopathology and Immunophenotype

On histopathology, there is hyperkeratosis, hypergranulosis, and acanthosis of the epidermis. A band-like infiltrate of lymphocytes is present and partially obscures the dermal epidermal junction; however, this infiltrate is thought to be less dense in lichenoid drug eruptions than in lichen planus and tends to involve the deeper reticular dermis. Necrotic keratinocytes, Civatte bodies,

and Max Joseph spaces are seen, and there is usually more pigment dropout noted with lichenoid drug eruptions than with lichen planus (Weedon 1998). The presence of eosinophils is a good clue to the diagnosis (Lage et al. 2012).

Differential Diagnosis

The primary differential diagnosis is with lichen planus, and the distinction can be difficult as the clinical and histologic features of these two entities overlap significantly (Lage et al. 2012) (Table 5.6). A recent paper has suggested that the presence of clusters of apoptotic cells and eosinophils are both statistically significant findings in distinguishing between these two entities; lichenoid drug eruptions tend to have both findings more than lichen planus (Lage et al. 2012). Removal of any new drugs may shed light on the diagnosis, as idiopathic lichen planus is not associated with drug ingestion. Lichenoid mycosis fungoides is also a differential diagnostic consideration (Guitart et al. 1997). Rarely, a lichenoid drug eruption may mimic mycosis fungoides histologically, but the clinical presentation is usually that of a drug eruption (Wu et al. 2010). Other studies have demonstrated that paucity of intraepidermal Foxp3-positive T cells may be used to confirm the diagnosis of a lichenoid mycosis fungoides and argue against lichen planus or a lichenoid drug eruption (Wada et al. 2010). Molecular studies on lichenoid drug eruptions are very limited, but clonal reactive infiltrates in the skin have been documented (Zhang et al. 2010), and lesions

Fig. 5.8 Pigmented purpuric dermatosis. There is a dense band-like infiltrate of lymphocytes at the dermal epidermal junction with accompanying extravasation of erythrocytes. The infiltrate extends into the deeper reticular dermis in a wedge-shaped fashion (H + E, 10×)

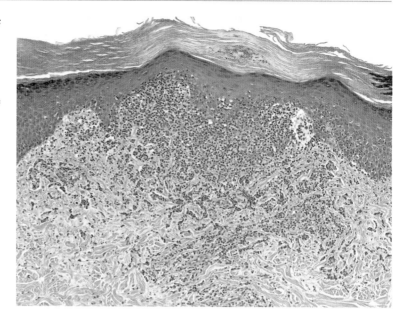

of lichen planus are known to harbor clones (Holm et al. 2002). Removal of any new medication should first be initiated to determine if the agent is the cause of the eruption; this may be the most effective way of confirming that the eruption is related to a drug.

Pigmented Purpuric Dermatosis

Introduction and Clinical Features

Pigmented purpuric dermatosis (PPD) constitutes a group of diseases consisting of purpuric lesions, usually on the legs, with variable pigmentation due to extravasation of erythrocytes (Weedon 1998). The different clinical categories of PPD include Schamberg's disease, purpura annularis telangiectodes of Majocchi, pigmented purpuric lichenoid dermatosis of Gougerot and Blum, and lichen aureus. Schamberg's disease is the most common and is characterized by minute purpuric macules on the lower extremities which coalesce into patches. The lesions of purpura annularis telangiectodes of Majocchi are composed of annular patches with perifollicular punctate lesions and telangiectasias (Newton and Raimer 1985). The lesions of pigmented purpuric lichenoid dermatosis of Gougerot and Blum are composed of lichenoid papules which may coalesce to give plaque-like lesions, also primarily on the lower legs (Newton and Raimer 1985). The lesions of lichen aureus are a distinctive golden brown color and are usually annular. While they are often found on the lower legs, they can also involve the back and upper extremities. Some systemic diseases, such as lupus erythematosus and liver disease, have been associated with PPD, as well as numerous drugs, such as lipid-lowering drugs and angiotensin-converting enzyme (ACE) inhibitors (Sarantopoulous et al. 2013).

Histopathology and Immunophenotype

All entities in the category of PPD have similar histologic findings. They are composed of a mild to moderately dense infiltrate of lymphocytes at the dermal epidermal junction which extends to involve the superficial vascular plexus (Fig. 5.8). The lymphocytic infiltrate in Schamberg's disease may be mild, but it may be dense and band-like in lichen aureus (Weedon 1998). An overall lichenoid pattern has been described in the pigmented purpuric lichenoid dermatosis of Gougerot and

Fig. 5.9 Pigmented purpuric
dermatosis. Sawtooth
changes are noted within the
rete pegs, and there is basal
vacuolar change with
intraepidermal extravasated
erythrocytes (H + E, 40×)

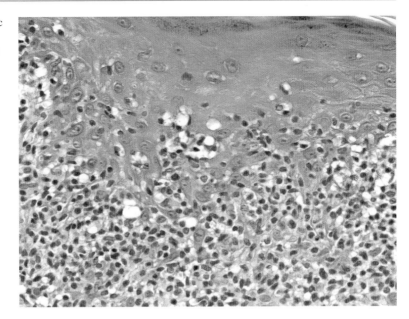

Fig. 5.10 Pigmented
purpuric dermatosis. High
power examination shows the
presence of a small
Pautrier's-like microabscess
(H + E, 90×)

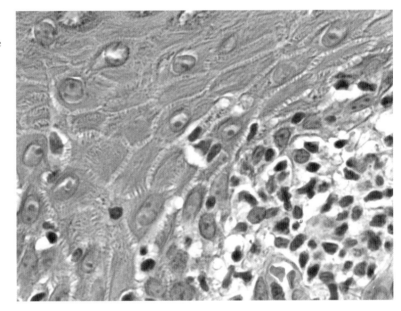

Blum, and in lichen aureus, there is usually a thin grenz zone (Sarantopoulous et al. 2013). The overlying epidermis may demonstrate orthokeratotic hyperkeratosis or demonstrate parakeratosis. The lymphocytes extend into the epidermis, and there is usually associated spongiosis. Sometimes basal vacuolar alteration and necrotic keratinocytes can be observed (Fig. 5.9). Extravasated erythrocytes are almost always present, and sometimes the erythrocytes are within the epidermis. Rarely one may see Pautrier's-like microabscesses (Fig. 5.10). In older lesions, hemosiderin deposition may be observed free in the dermis or within histiocytes, and these deposits are highlighted by a Prussian blue stain. Immunophenotyping of lesions of PPD shows these to be composed of T cells that express CD4 (Smoller and Kamel 1991; Harvell et al. 2003).

Table 5.7 Clinical and morphologic comparisons between pigmented purpuric dermatosis and pigmented purpuric dermatosis-like mycosis fungoides

	Pigmented purpuric dermatosis	Pigmented purpuric dermatosis-like mycosis fungoides
Purpuric lesions	Yes	Yes
Location of lymphocytic infiltrate	Mostly superficial dermis	Superficial and mid dermis
Extravasation of erythrocytes and hemosiderin deposition	Yes	Yes
Microabscesses	Pautrier's-like lymphocytic collections (Magro et al. 2007a, b)	Pautrier's (tumor cells)
Cytologic atypia within T cells	Yes, mild	Yes
Phenotype of T cells	Primarily CD4 (Sarantopoulos et al. 2013)	Primarily CD4
T-cell clonality assays	Sometimes positive	Usually positive

Genetics and Molecular Findings

PPD has been reported numerous times to harbor clones, and some authors consider this entity to be a precursor of mycosis fungoides (Sarantopoulous et al. 2013; Crowson et al. 1999; Toro et al. 1997; Magro et al. 2007b; Chen et al. 2004). Indeed, several reports exist documenting transformation of PPD into mycosis fungoides after several years (Georgala et al. 2001; Viseux et al. 2003).

Prognosis and Clinical Course

Although the condition is a benign one, in general, the course is chronic, with exacerbations and remissions of disease (Tristani Firouzi et al. 2001). Rarely, PPD may undergo spontaneous resolution. Treatment courses are generally ineffective, although topical corticosteroids, PUVA, and systemic steroids have been used.

Differential Diagnosis

Given the mild spongiosis accompanying this entity, one could also consider spongiotic dermatitis in the differential diagnosis, which would include atopic dermatitis, contact dermatitis, nummular dermatitis, drug hypersensitivity reactions, arthropod hypersensitivity reactions, and id reactions. This would be a particular problem if the clinical scenario is not well described and the biopsy does not show findings of extravasated erythrocytes or hemosiderin deposition. An eczematous lesion on the lower extremities would pose a particular problem if clinical descriptions of the lesions are not provided, as there is often a background of stasis changes. Other entities to consider include fixed drug eruption (which is usually not as extensive and has numerous well-formed necrotic keratinocytes) and a leukocytoclastic vasculitis (which would demonstrate a true vasculitis with neutrophils, leukocytoclasis, necrosis of vessel walls, and fibrin deposition) (Tristani Firouzi et al. 2001). There can also be significant overlap with the so-called pigmented purpuric dermatitis-like mycosis fungoides (PPD-like mycosis fungoides), a very rare variant of mycosis fungoides (Toro et al. 1997; Georgala et al. 2001; Lipsker 2003) (Table 5.7). These lesions clinically present similarly as those of PPD, but the lesions tend to be more extensive, with extension beyond the typical areas of involvement of PPD. Histologically they appear similar as well, but the lesions of PPD-like mycosis fungoides tend to have a much deeper infiltrate of lymphocytes (Reddy and Bhawan 2007). Both express CD4 (Magro et al. 2007a, b; Sardana et al. 2004), and both can demonstrate T-cell clonality (Zhang et al. 2010; Crowson et al. 1999; Toro et al. 1997; Magro et al. 2007a, b; Fink Puches et al. 2008; Thurber et al. 2007; Plaza et al. 2008). Close clinical follow-up is recommended of cases that seem suspicious for mycosis fungoides, as currently there are no good immunohistochemical or molecular

Fig. 5.11 Lichen sclerosus. There is a band-like infiltrate of lymphocytes with follicular plugging in an early inflammatory lesion. Focal involvement of the epidermis by lymphocytes is seen (H + E, 10×)

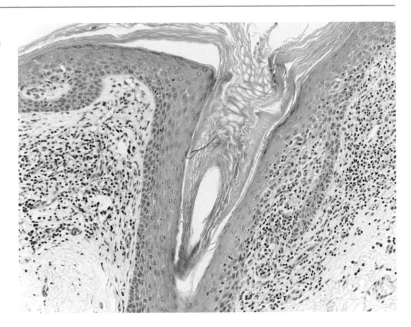

methods for differentiation between cases of very unusual PPD and PPD-like mycosis fungoides.

Lichen Sclerosus

Introduction and Clinical Features

Lichen sclerosus (previously known as lichen sclerosus et atrophicus) is a chronic condition that primarily affects postmenopausal women in the anogenital area, although premenopausal women and children can also be affected. Extragenital lesions of lichen sclerosus can occur and are often truncal or involve the upper extremities. Males are affected less commonly (known as balanitis xerotica obliterans), are usually children or young adults when affected, and the lesions in severe cases can result in phimosis (Weedon 1998). Clinically, these are ivory-colored papules that coalesce to form plaques. Follicular accentuation is often seen, and the lesions can undergo atrophy leading to a wrinkled and depressed scar ("cigarette paper atrophy"). The lesions in the genital area have a higher propensity to develop dysplasia and squamous cell carcinoma and should be carefully screened for malignancy.

Histopathology and Immunophenotype

On histology, the lesions demonstrate epidermal acanthosis, hyperkeratosis, and follicular plugging (Fig. 5.11). There can be superimposed hypergranulosis and fibrotic changes within the dermis which may be a result of superimposed scratching and lichenification. In early lesions, there is a band-like infiltrate of lymphocytes at the dermal epidermal junction, subtle basal vacuolar alteration, rare necrotic keratinocytes, and infiltration of the epidermis by lymphocytes. In later lesions, there are pale changes within the upper collagen (homogenization) that are bordered inferiorly by an infiltrate of lymphocytes. The overlying epidermis is flattened and atrophic with loss of rete pegs. Pigment dropout may be seen within the upper dermis. The upper vascular plexus is composed of dilated and ectatic vessels, and surrounding mild hemorrhage can be seen. Appendages appear normal and undisplaced, and there is no loss of perieccrine fat. Moderate cytologic atypia may be seen in some cases (Fig. 5.12), and Pautrier's-like microabscesses have been observed (Fig. 5.13). In some cases, there can be extensive colonization of the epidermis by lymphocytes

Fig. 5.12 Lichen sclerosus. Basilar lining by atypical lymphocytes is seen (H + E, 20×)

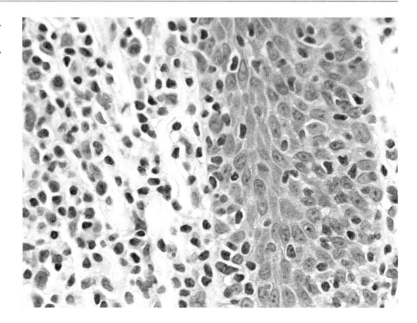

Fig. 5.13 Lichen sclerosus. High power view shows formation of a Pautrier's-like microabscess with moderately atypical lymphocytes (H + E, 20×)

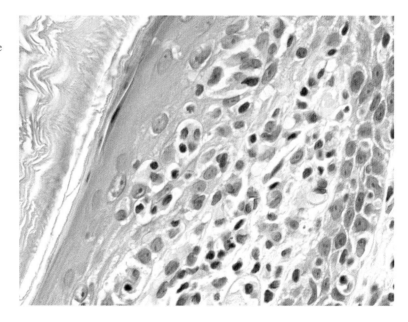

without associated spongiosis (Fig. 5.14). On immunophenotyping, equivalent number of CD4- and CD8-expressing T cells are seen in the infiltrate; the number of B cells is much less (Smoller and Kamel 1991; Terlou et al. 2012; Regauer and Beham-Schmid 2006; Ben Hur et al. 2001; Gross et al. 2001; Carlson et al. 2000; Scrimin et al. 2000; Farrell et al. 1999; Hinchliffe et al. 1994).

Genetics and Molecular Findings

A correlation has been found between certain HLA subtypes and the development of lichen sclerosus, especially in children (Tilly et al. 2004), and lichen sclerosus has been described in twins (Meyrick Thomas and Kennedy 1986) and in sisters (Sahn et al. 1994), suggesting, at least in some cases, a genetic predisposition to the disease. In addition,

Fig. 5.14 Lichen sclerosus. In another case, extensive colonization of the overlying epidermis with lymphocytes is seen (H + E, 10×)

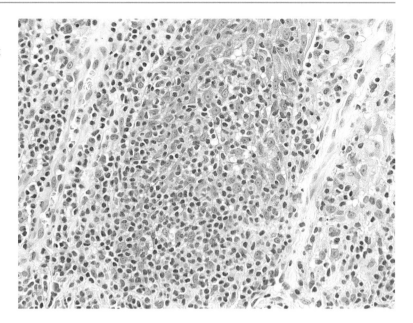

T-cell receptor clonality assays have been reported to show a monoclonal band in 50–60 % of cases of lichen sclerosus in some series (Regauer and Beham-Schmid 2006) and in a much smaller population of cases in others (Citarella et al. 2003).

Prognosis and Clinical Course

Unfortunately, hormonal interventions are largely ineffective, and the current treatment approaches usually involve the use of high-potency steroids on a scheduled basis to prevent steroid atrophy (Tilly et al. 2004). Surgical intervention may be necessary for treatment of highly advanced cases of phimosis or fused labial mucosae. There is a risk of development of squamous cell carcinoma, and the connection with the presence of high-risk subtypes of human papillomavirus is uncertain (McCluggage 2013). These cases are followed closely clinically to ensure that early lesions of dysplasia and carcinoma are adequately treated.

Differential Diagnosis

In early lesions, the differential diagnostic considerations include lichen planus, contact dermatitis, or atopic dermatitis, and many lesions of lichen sclerosus often have superimposed lichen simplex chronicus. Lichen planus and spongiotic entities do not usually demonstrate the characteristic changes of collagen seen in lichen sclerosus nor do they tend to have atrophic epidermal changes (unless there is coexisting steroid atrophy). Eosinophils are more common in atrophic and contact dermatitis than in either lichen planus or lichen sclerosus. The early lesions of lichen planus of the vulva and lichen sclerosus can be quite difficult to distinguish from each other. Early lesions of lichen sclerosus can also mimic mycosis fungoides (Citarella et al. 2003; Suchak et al. 2010) and can be clonal (Regauer and Beham-Schmid 2004) (Table 5.8). In such cases, it may be worthwhile to repeat the biopsy in a

Table 5.8 Clinical and morphologic comparisons between lichen sclerosus and mycosis fungoides

	Lichen sclerosus	Mycosis fungoides
Anogenital involvement	Yes	Yes
Ivory-colored coalescing papules with follicular accentuation	Yes	No, tend to be erythematous patches and plaques
Hyperkeratosis, follicular plugging, and epidermal atrophy	Yes, common	Yes, rare
Homogenization of collagen	Yes, but not in early lesions	No
Cytologic atypia within T cells	No	Yes
Phenotype of T cells	Mixture of CD4 and CD8	CD4
T-cell clonality	Positive sometimes	Usually positive

few months' time to determine if the lesions evolve to demonstrate the characteristic findings of lichen sclerosus (Suchak et al. 2010). Late lesions of lichen sclerosus, especially at extragenital sites, can mimic morphea. Clues that point to lichen sclerosus include the presence of pigment dropout, basal vacuolar alteration, necrotic keratinocytes, and preservation of appendages.

Annular Lichenoid Dermatitis of Youth

Introduction and Clinical Features

Annular lichenoid dermatitis of youth is a clinical entity which was first described by Annessi et al. in 2003 (Kleikamp et al. 2008; Tsoitis et al. 2009; Cesinaro et al. 2009; Leger et al. 2013; Huh and Kanitakis 2010). They observed 23 patients in whom they described red macules and annular lesions with central hypopigmentation. The lesions are bordered by lichenoid papules. These lesions are usually found on the flanks and groins of children (Tsoitis et al. 2009) and adolescents, but adults have been described with the condition (Cesinaro et al. 2009). Older lesions have hyperpigmented borders (Annessi et al. 2003).

Histopathology and Immunophenotype

On histology, a band-like infiltrate is noted at the dermal epidermal junction concentrated at the tips of rete pegs with associated necrotic keratinocytes (Kleikamp et al. 2008). In older lesions, there is flattening of the rete pegs with clusters of necrotic keratinocytes. Immunohistochemical analysis showed that the infiltrate was composed of a mixture of CD4- and CD8-positive T cells, with the intraepidermal T cells being primarily CD8 positive. The CD8-positive T cells co-expressed TIA-1 (Kleikamp et al. 2008).

Genetics and Molecular Findings

T-cell receptor gene rearrangements and IgH clonality assays are negative, as are polymerase chain reaction (PCR) testing for Borrelia DNA and parvovirus B19 DNA (Kleikamp et al. 2008).

Prognosis and Clinical Course

In the original report by Annessi et al., treatment with potent topical steroids cleared the lesions, but they recurred over a 5-year period with a chronic clinical course (Annessi et al. 2003). Psoralen and ultraviolet A (PUVA) and systemic steroids have also been tried with similar results (Tsoitis et al. 2009). Interestingly, in the case report of Kleikamp et al., the patient's lesions resolve with topical tacrolimus without pigmentary changes, and there was no recurrence after a 2-year follow-up period (Kleikamp et al. 2008). Spontaneous resolutions of lesions have been described (Cesinaro et al. 2009).

Table 5.9 Clinical and morphologic comparisons between annular lichenoid dermatitis of youth and mycosis fungoides

	Annular lichenoid dermatitis of youth	Mycosis fungoides, hypopigmented variant
Primarily described in children	Yes	Yes
Involvement of sun-spared areas	Yes	Yes
Lichenoid infiltrate with colloid bodies	Yes	No, but present in lichenoid mycosis fungoides
Cytologic atypia within T cells	No	Yes
Phenotype of T cells	CD8	CD8
Positive T-cell clonality assays	No	Yes

Differential Diagnosis

The differential diagnosis includes pediatric annular erythema, inflammatory morphea, inflammatory vitiligo, and mycosis fungoides (and other CD8+ epidermotropic lymphomas) (Kleikamp et al. 2008) (Table 5.9). A lichenoid infiltrate would be unusual for both morphea and annular erythemas, and its presence would strongly argue against those diagnoses. The clinical distribution of vitiligo is different from annular lichenoid dermatitis of youth, and loss of melanocytes is seen (Cesinaro et al. 2009). The hypopigmented variant of mycosis fungoides poses a particular problem (Figs. 5.15 and 5.16) (Zackheim et al. 1982; Neuhaus et al. 2000). In general, mycosis fungoides is composed primarily of CD4-expressing T cells, whereas annular lichenoid dermatitis of youth shows a mixture of CD4- and CD8-expressing T cells in the dermis, and where intraepidermal lymphocytes are present, they express CD8 (Kleikamp et al. 2008). However, hypopigmented mycosis fungoides also expresses CD8 (Fig. 5.17) and is present in young people, similar to annular lichenoid dermatitis of youth. T-cell clonality assays can be useful, as they are usually positive in hypopigmented mycosis

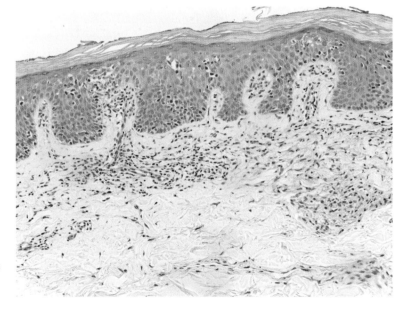

Fig. 5.15 Hypopigmented mycosis fungoides. A band-like infiltrate of highly atypical lymphocytes is noted at the dermal epidermal junction, and there is significant epidermotropism (H + E, 10×)

Fig. 5.16 Hypopigmented mycosis fungoides. There is lining of the basal layer by highly atypical lymphocytes and small Pautrier's microabscesses (H +E, 20×)

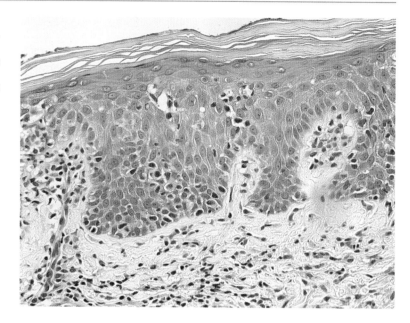

Fig. 5.17 Hypopigmented mycosis fungoides. The epidermotropic cells express CD8 (H + E, 20×)

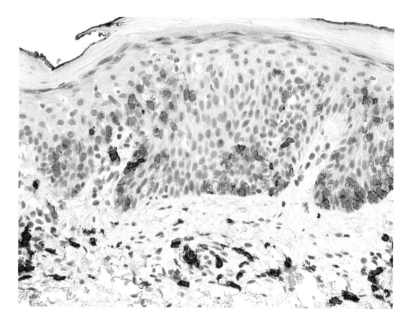

fungoides but negative in annular lichenoid dermatitis of youth (Annessi et al. 2003; Kleikamp et al. 2008; Tsoitis et al. 2009). These findings do not overlap with CD8+ aggressive epidermotropic cytotoxic T-cell lymphoma, as those are highly aggressive nodular lymphoma lesions that do not usually occur in the pediatric population. Moreover, on histology, pronounced epidermotropism is seen. Similarly, while cutaneous gamma delta T-cell lymphoma can be CD8+ on occasion, and these are also rare, highly aggressive lymphomas that show pronounced epidermotropism and are uncommon in children.

Table 5.10 Clinical and morphologic comparisons between inflammatory vitiligo-like macules and hypopigmented mycosis fungoides

	Inflammatory vitiligo-like macules	Hypopigmented mycosis fungoides
Limited to the trunk	Yes	No
Dense lichenoid infiltrate	Yes	Yes, in lichenoid mycosis fungoides
Epidermotropism	Less common	More common (Koorse et al. 2012)
Cytologic atypia within T cells	No	Yes
Loss of melanocytes	Yes, complete	Yes, partial
Loss of pigment	Yes, total	Yes, partial
Wiry dermal collagen	No	Yes
Thickening of basement membrane	Yes	No
Phenotype of T cells	CD8	CD8
TCR clonality assays	Negative	Positive

Inflammatory Vitiligo Like Macules

Introduction and Clinical Features

In this condition, patients develop irregular symmetrical hypopigmented macules and patches on the trunk with no known antecedents, but the histopathologic findings resemble mycosis fungoides (Petit et al. 2003; El Darouti et al. 2006). The lesions contain an erythematous and papular border and can be quite large. Clinically they resemble vitiligo.

Histopathology and Immunophenotype

On histopathology, on a biopsy taken from an erythematous border, a dense band-like infiltrate is seen at the dermal epidermal junction with extensive involvement of the overlying epidermis (Petit et al. 2003). On immunohistochemistry, the lesional cells overwhelmingly express CD8, especially the intraepidermal lymphocytes. HMB-45 staining shows complete lack of melanocytes in the affected skin.

Genetics and Molecular Findings

PCR clonality assays using denaturing gradient gel electrophoresis performed on DNA isolated from the erythematous border of the lesion are negative (Petit et al. 2003).

Prognosis and Clinical Course

No changes were observed with the lesions when they were treated with PUVA; however, application of topical steroids stopped extension of the lesions and led to their diminution (Petit et al. 2003). Rebiopsy of the lesions poststeroid therapy showed regression of the infiltrate. Sun exposure did not repigment the lesions.

Differential Diagnosis

These lesions are thought to represent inflammatory vitiligo, given the loss of melanocytes and lack of preceding exposure to toxins or chemicals (Petit et al. 2003). The main differential diagnosis is hypopigmented mycosis fungoides (Tables 5.10 and 5.11) (El Darouti et al. 2006; Singh et al. 2006; Ranawaka et al. 2011; Koorse et al. 2012; Fink Puches et al. 2004). The presence of an erythematous, raised border surrounding the hypopigmented patches is an unusual finding for mycosis fungoides (Petit et al. 2003). In addition, while CD8+ T cells can be seen in both entities, T-cell clonality assays are negative in inflammatory vitiligo and positive in mycosis fungoides. Other features found to be helpful in distinguishing vitiligo from hypopigmented

Table 5.11 The differential diagnosis of hypopigmented patches in children and adolescents

	Pityriasis alba	Vitiligo	Lichen sclerosus	Hypopigmented mycosis fungoides
Common in children	Yes (Werner et al. 2005)	No	No	Yes
Distribution	Face primarily	Face, distal extremities	Primarily genitals, truncal	Sun-spared areas; in some cases, involvement of lower legs (Ngo et al. 2009)
Pigmentary status	Hypopigmented	Depigmented	Hypopigmented	Hypopigmented
Spongiosis is present	Yes, mild	Yes, mild	No, usually lichenoid	No
Cytologic atypia within T cells	No	No	No	Yes
TCR clonality assays	Negative	Negative	Positive, sometimes	Positive

mycosis fungoides include fibrosis of the papillary collagen, partial loss of pigment, and preservation of some melanocytes (all seen more commonly in mycosis fungoides). In vitiligo, complete loss of pigment, total loss of melanocytes, and thickening of the basement membrane are more common than in mycosis fungoides (El Darouti et al. 2006).

Human Immunodeficiency Virus (HIV)-Related CD8+ Atypical Skin Infiltrates

Introduction and Clinical Features

Patients with the human immunodeficiency virus (HIV) infection may suffer from a wide variety of immunologic disorders due to their profound immunosuppression (Guitart et al. 1999; Zhang et al. 1995; Weedon 1998). While many of them also develop aggressive lymphomas, a small percentage is thought to develop mycosis fungoides (Guitart et al. 1999). These have been reported to have a chronic course, similar to immunocompetent patients who develop mycosis fungoides (Burns and Cooper 1993). In addition, many develop cutaneous infiltrates that are CD8 + and mimic mycosis fungoides histologically (Zhang et al. 1995; Weedon 1998). These patients clinically can develop patches, plaques, and nodules, some of them in a photodistributed fashion, or erythroderma (Zhang et al. 1995; Weedon 1998).

Bone marrow and lymph node involvement may be noted clinically (Zhang et al. 1995). Skin involvement may be widespread (Zhang et al. 1995).

Histopathology and Immunophenotype

On histology, there is a band-like infiltrate of lymphocytes at the dermal epidermal junction with epidermal involvement by lymphocytes (Fig. 5.18). In some cases, true interface activity can be seen as well as basilar lining by lymphocytes (Fig. 5.19). Follicular involvement by lymphocytes can also be seen, with focal follicular mucinosis. Some cases demonstrate syringeal involvement (Fig. 5.20). Eosinophils and dermal fibroplasia are also seen. Small Pautrier's-like microabscesses can be seen, and there is mild atypia within the lymphocytes (Fig. 5.21). The infiltrating cells were CD8 predominant in many of the cases tested, while a minority had a mixture of CD4- and CD8-expressing cells (Zhang et al. 1995; Weedon 1998). CD7 loss was seen in these cases, similar to mycosis fungoides.

Genetics and Molecular Findings

T-cell receptor gene rearrangement studies were performed in nine cases in two separate studies, and none were positive.

Fig. 5.18 HIV-related dermatitis. There is a band-like infiltrate of lymphocytes at the dermal epidermal junction with involvement of the overlying epidermis. There is mild hyperkeratosis of the stratum corneum (H + E, 4×)

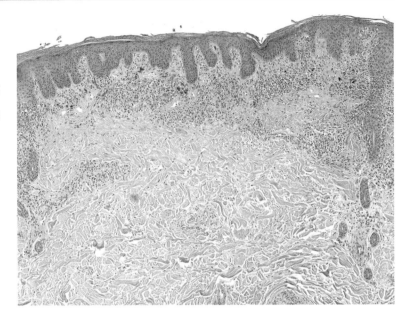

Fig. 5.19 HIV-related dermatitis. The papillary dermis is fibrotic and there is pigment dropout (H + E, 10×)

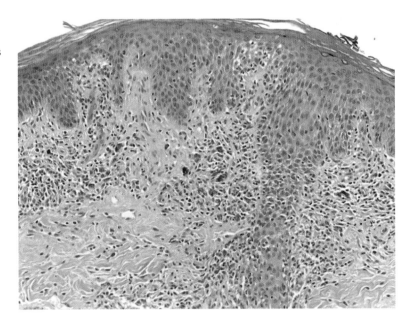

Prognosis and Clinical Course

In one well-documented study, eight of nine patients died, but this was primarily due to acquired immunodeficiency syndrome (AIDS) wasting syndrome or infection (Zhang et al. 1995). Their clinical lesions were treated with PUVA, chemotherapy, or topical steroids with partial to no response.

Differential Diagnosis

The primary differential diagnostic consideration in these cases is true mycosis fungoides, as this entity can mimic mycosis fungoides closely on histology (Table 5.12). Complicating the story is the fact that indolent mycosis fungoides can occur in patients with HIV (Guitart et al. 1999). These infiltrates differ from classic mycosis fungoides in

Fig. 5.20 HIV-related dermatitis. There is infiltration of the sweat duct by atypical lymphocytes (H + E, 20×)

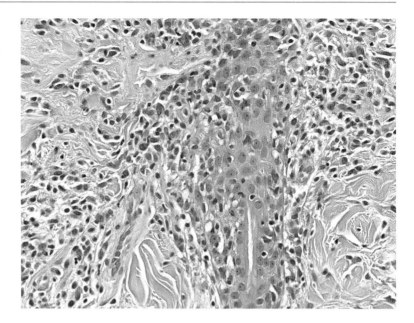

Fig. 5.21 HIV-related dermatitis. Higher power view of the lymphocytes shows nuclear hyperchromasia and small nuclear notches (H + E, 40×)

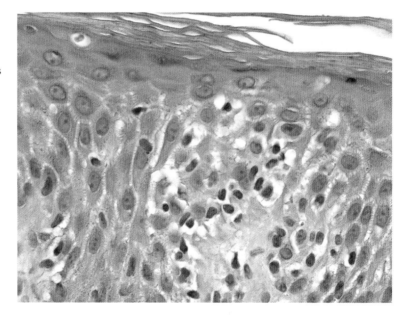

the fact that they express CD8 and do not demonstrate the presence of a T-cell clone. Another entity to consider in the differential diagnosis, given the photodistributed nature of the process in some cases, is chronic actinic dermatitis or actinic reticuloid, which is also predominantly of CD8 origin. In photodistributed cases, the distinction between HIV-related skin infiltrates and chronic actinic dermatitis may not be possible, and indeed they may represent the same entity.

Lichenoid Lupus Erythematosus

Introduction and Clinical Features

Cutaneous lupus erythematosus may be skin limited or linked to systemic lupus erythematosus (Weedon 1998). Typically, the lesions are photodistributed (head and neck, V of chest, arms), and the face is often involved (malar rash). The lesions can be large and are indurated,

Table 5.12 Clinical and morphologic comparisons between HIV-related CD8+ dermatitis and mycosis fungoides

	HIV-related CD8± dermatitis	Mycosis fungoides
Distribution	Erythroderma, extensive involvement by patches, plaques, and nodules	In advanced cases, erythroderma, extensive involvement by patches, plaques, and nodules
Photodistributed	Yes, sometimes	No
Interface dermatitis	Yes	Yes, in lichenoid mycosis fungoides
Microabscesses	Pautrier's like	Pautrier's (tumor cells)
Cytologic atypia within T cells	Yes, mild	Yes
Eosinophils	Yes	Rare
Phenotype of T cells	CD8	CD4 (except in cases of CD8-expressing MF)
T-cell receptor gene rearrangement	No	Yes

erythematous, scaly plaques. They can also present as subcutaneous nodules with little surface change (lupus panniculitis) as well as oral lesions. Serologic abnormalities can be present, and in systemic disease, the kidneys can be affected. The scalp can be affected, and a scarring alopecia can ensue. In lesions that show overlap with lichen planus (lichenoid lupus erythematosus), the lesions are large, atrophic plaques with a red to violet color, mild hyperpigmentation at the borders, and telangiectasias (Romero et al. 1977). No flat-topped papules are seen and follicular plugging is minimal. Photosensitivity is not usually seen. The lesions tend to involve the acral extremities with nail involvement being quite common.

Histopathology and Immunophenotype

On histopathology, there can be a variety of different patterns that can be present. Typically the lesions have a superficial and deep infiltrate of lymphocytes with periadnexal and perivascular accentuation. Interface activity is present and there is pigment dropout. In chronic lesions, the basement membrane is thickened and can be detected using a PASD stain. In the lichenoid variant, the infiltrate is quite dense with overlying compact hyperkeratosis, hypergranulosis, acanthosis, and necrotic keratinocytes. Necrotic keratinocytes are present within the dermis (Oliver et al. 1989), and dermal mucin is present. These areas comingled with areas that were lymphocyte

poor with perivascular accentuation and little involvement of the epidermis (Romero et al. 1977; Oliver et al. 1989; Crowson and Magro 1999). Both eosinophils and plasma cells are seen. In oral lesions, the infiltrate is again band-like with numerous lymphocytes, and plasma cells are prominent. On immunohistochemistry, there is a mixture of CD4- and CD8-expressing T cells (Harvell et al. 2003). On direct immunofluorescence of involved skin, these cases tend to show both linear and granular deposition of antibody at the dermal epidermal junction of C3, IgG, IgM, and IgA.

Genetics, Molecular Findings, and Serologic Studies

While lichenoid lupus erythematosus has not been extensively studied via current molecular techniques, limited analysis of lupus erythematosus cases by T-cell receptor gene rearrangements using BIOMED 2 primers does not demonstrate a detectable clone (Zhang et al. 2010). On serology, in general, patients have a high titer of antinuclear antibodies (ANA), antibodies to DNA, and low to high titers of anti-Ro/SSA antibodies, even in skin-limited disease.

Prognosis and Clinical Course

This version of lupus erythematosus tends to be extremely long term with poor response to therapy, which includes topical and systemic

Table 5.13 The differential diagnosis of lichenoid lupus erythematosus

	Lichenoid lupus erythematosus	Chronic graft-versus-host disease	Lupus-like drug eruption	Mycosis fungoides
Acral and nail involvement	Yes	No	No	No
Necrotic keratinocytes within hair follicles	No	Yes	No	No
Dermal mucin	Yes	No	Yes	No
Microabscesses	Pautrier's like	No	No	Pautrier's (tumor cells)
Cytologic atypia within T cells	Yes	No	No	Yes
Phenotype of T cells	CD4	Mixture of CD4 and CD8	N/A	CD4
TCR clonality assays	Negative	Negative	N/A	Positive

corticosteroids, antimalarials, and immunosuppressive drugs (Romero et al. 1977).

Differential Diagnosis

The primary differential diagnosis includes lichen planus (Romero et al. 1977; Oliver et al. 1989), chronic graft-versus-host disease (Hu et al. 2012; Goiriz et al. 2008), drug eruptions (Crowson and Magro 1999), and lichenoid mycosis fungoides (Friss et al. 1995) (Table 5.13). In typical cases, lichen planus has an infiltrate limited to the dermal epidermal junction, with accompanying cytoid body formation and Max Joseph clefts. In contrast, in lupus erythematosus, the infiltrate tends to be more sparse with individual necrotic keratinocytes rather than cytoid body formation. No cleft formation is usually seen. However, there can be significant overlap between lichen planus and lichenoid lupus erythematosus in certain circumstances (Romero et al. 1977; Oliver et al. 1989), and careful clinical correlation with clinical follow-up may be the only way to distinguish between the two entities. Chronic graft-versus-host disease can have a lichenoid pattern and can rarely mimic lupus (Hu et al. 2012; Goiriz et al. 2008). The clinical setting can help distinguish between the two entities; in addition, dermal mucin deposition is not seen in lichenoid graft-versus-host disease (Goiriz et al. 2008). Drug eruptions resolve when an offending agent is removed, and this may be a good way to distinguish between a drug-related event and idiopathic lupus erythematosus (Crowson and Magro 1999). Finally, lichenoid mycosis fungoides remains within the differential. There are rare cases of cutaneous lupus pathologically mimicking mycosis fungoides reported in the literature. In these cases, atypical lymphocytes can involve the overlying epidermis with collections of Pautrier's-like microabscesses. Immunophenotypic analysis can show an overwhelming CD4 to CD8 ratio (20:1) (Friss et al. 1995). Direct immunofluorescence studies and serologic studies can help distinguish between these two entities, and TCR gene rearrangement studies should be negative in lupus and positive in mycosis fungoides (Weedon 1998).

Lichen Simplex Chronicus

Introduction and Clinical Features

Lichen simplex chronicus occurs in the context of chronic pruritus and usually overlies other inflammatory conditions such as atopic dermatitis and lichen sclerosus (Weedon 1998). Clinically, these are symmetric thick erythematous plaques with lichenification and are associated with other signs of pruritus (i.e., excoriations).

Histopathology and Immunophenotype

On histology, the epidermis is acanthotic with overlying hyperkeratosis and sometimes mild parakeratosis, usually patchy rather than diffuse. A very mild lymphocytic infiltrate usually infiltrates the epidermis, and there is underlying mild perivascular infiltrates of lymphocytes with papillary dermal fibrosis. The collagen can demonstrate scar-like changes with vertically oriented collagen bundles and horizontally oriented vessels.

Prognosis and Clinical Course

The changes of lichenification can decrease if pruritus is controlled with emoliation and/or topical steroids.

Differential Diagnosis

The important differential diagnosis is with chronic spongiotic dermatitides, which include atopic dermatitis, contact dermatitis, id reaction, drug hypersensitivity reactions, nummular dermatitis, and arthropod hypersensitivity reactions. Cutaneous dermatophytosis can demonstrate similar findings (chronic tinea infection), and a PASD stain should be performed to exclude this possibility. Partially treated psoriasis may also show similar findings and may not demonstrate Munro's microabscesses or neutrophil transmigration; correlation with clinical findings may be necessary to exclude psoriasis. Rarely, partially treated mycosis fungoides may show overlap with lichen simplex chronicus; T-cell receptor PCR analysis, especially comparing analysis from more than one site, may help confirm the diagnosis of mycosis fungoides (Table 5.14). It is important to note that lichen simplex chronicus

Table 5.14 Clinical and morphologic comparisons between lichen simplex chronicus and mycosis fungoides

	Lichen simplex chronicus	Mycosis fungoides
Lichenification	Present	Usually absent, unless lesions are extremely pruritic
Epidermal acanthosis	Yes	No, unless chronic, pruritic lesion
Spongiosis is present	Yes, mild	No
Cytologic atypia within T cells	No	Yes

may be superimposed on all of the conditions listed in the differential diagnosis.

Actinic Reticuloid

Introduction and Clinical Features

Actinic reticuloid is a chronic persistent photosensitive dermatosis that primarily affects older men and is part of the chronic actinic dermatosis group of disorders (Ploysangam et al. 1998; Ive et al. 1969; Frain-Bell and Johnson 1979; Johnson et al. 1979). It is thought to be caused by persistent exposure to sunlight, is extremely pruritic, and is often occupational in origin. The lesions are usually on the head and neck and other sun-exposed areas and are red purple, scaly, lichenoid infiltrative papules, plaques, and nodules (Ploysangam et al. 1998). Extension into areas of sun protection can be seen in severe cases. Chronic rubbing of the scalp can cause alopecia. Patients can develop lymphadenopathy, leonine facies, and erythroderma, and the findings may be difficult to distinguish from lymphoma (Neild et al. 1982; Thomsen 1977). There is evidence to suggest that actinic reticuloid may be in part due to contact allergy to plants and synthetic chemicals (Frain-Bell and Johnson 1979). Sensitivities have been demonstrated to UVB, UVA, fluorescent light, and visible light (Ploysangam et al. 1998).

Histopathology and Immunophenotype

On histology, there is psoriasiform hyperplasia and minimal spongiosis with involvement of the epidermis by lymphocytes (Ploysangam et al. 1998). On high power examination the lymphocytes are atypical with nuclear hyperchromasia and hyperconvolution, and Pautrier's-like microabscesses can be seen. The papillary dermal collagen is thickened, and there are vertically oriented collagen bundles and horizontally oriented blood vessels, similar to lichen simplex chronicus. The blood vessels have thickened walls, and plump fibroblasts are present within the dermis. Immunophenotyping shows the infiltrate to be composed of CD8-expressing T cells (Bakels et al. 1998).

Genetics and Molecular Findings

Analysis of cases of actinic reticuloid and cases of Sézary syndrome showed that T-cell receptor clonality assays were positive in the skin and peripheral blood of patients with Sézary syndrome but not in patients with actinic reticuloid (Bakels et al. 1998).

Prognosis and Clinical Course

In general, actinic reticuloid runs a chronic clinical course and does not respond to typical therapies of photosensitive disorders (Ploysangam et al. 1998). Strict photorestriction is paramount as is avoidance of all possible responsible contactants, and patients are encouraged to regularly apply topical sun protection or wear protective clothing and hats. Combinations of photochemotherapy, topical and systemic corticosteroids, azathioprine, and cyclosporine have been reported to be beneficial. Rarely patients with actinic reticuloid have developed lymphoma, and it is unclear whether these cases represent true lymphomas that were initially misdiagnosed as actinic reticuloid or actinic reticuloid undergoing malignant transformation (Neild et al. 1982; Thomsen 1977; De Silva et al. 2000). In one study of two patients, over a period of years after the initial diagnosis of actinic reticuloid, the patients developed what appeared to be erythroderma, patches and plaques consistent clinically with mycosis fungoides (De Silva et al. 2000). They also acquired a TCR clone in their skin biopsies, but peripheral blood remained negative for TCR clonality assays. The dermal infiltrates continued to be CD8+, however. Both patients developed lymphadenopathy which showed dermatopathic changes and had a negative clone. The authors speculate that these two cases may

Table 5.15 Clinical and morphologic comparisons between actinic reticuloid and mycosis fungoides

	Actinic reticuloid	Mycosis fungoides
Sun-exposed areas	Yes	No
Gender and age restricted	Yes, older males	No
Spongiosis is present	Yes, very mild	No
Microabscesses	Pautrier's microabscess-like collections	Pautrier's (tumor cells)
Cytologic atypia within T cells	Yes	Yes
Phenotype of T cells	CD8	CD4
TCR clonality assays	Negative	Positive

represent either extensive actinic reticuloid or so-called photosensitive mycosis fungoides.

Differential Diagnosis

The most important differential diagnostic consideration is with mycosis fungoides, and indeed, there is controversy in the literature regarding whether photosensitive mycosis fungoides exists or if it represents a clone positive version of actinic reticuloid (Table 5.15). The cases described in the literature of photosensitive mycosis fungoides arising in the context of actinic reticuloid are particularly interesting, as they are of CD8 origin, which is unlike 95 % of all cases of mycosis fungoides described (De Silva et al. 2000). Therefore, one could surmise that immunophenotyping and T-cell clonality assays may help distinguish actinic reticuloid from mycosis fungoides and Sézary syndrome in nearly all cases, as mycosis fungoides/Sézary syndrome should be of CD4 origin and harbor a T-cell clone, and actinic reticuloid should be of CD8 origin and be negative in a TCR clonality assay (Bakels et al. 1998). Very rare cases of actinic reticuloid that develop a widespread eruption may either be unusual clone positive versions of actinic reticuloid or true photosensitive mycosis fungoides, initially misdiagnosed as actinic reticuloid.

Fig. 5.22 Pityriasis lichenoides chronica. A patchy lymphocytic infiltrate is present in the papillary dermis with involvement of the overlying epidermis (H + E, 4×)

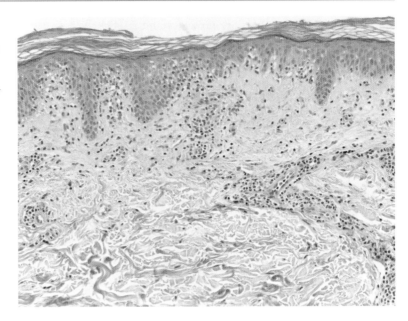

Pityriasis Lichenoides Chronica/ Pityriasis Lichenoides et Varioliformis Acuta

Introduction and Clinical Features

Pityriasis lichenoides chronica (PLC) shares a spectrum of findings with its acute clinical counterpart, pityriasis lichenoides et varioliformis acuta (PLEVA) (Weedon 1998). This papulosquamous eruption can affect all ages, involves the trunk and extremities, is primarily asymptomatic, and resolves without treatment, leaving behind an atrophic or varioliform scar (Magro et al. 2002). The crops of papules form continuously and last weeks to months before resolution. It is not unusual to see many lesions in different stages of evolution on the patient at one time. The lesions have a red-brown color upon initial formation and an adherent mica-like scale (Magro et al. 2002). The disease process itself may persist for years. PLEVA is more common in children, and the lesions are erythematous, variably purpuric papules with crusting and ulceration (Magro et al. 2002). In patients who eventually developed mycosis fungoides, a second clinical population of larger arcuate plaques was also present.

Histopathology and Immunophenotype

On histology, pityriasis lichenoides tends to show both a lichenoid and a spongiotic pattern (Sarantopoulos et al. 2013; Weedon 1998). The overlying stratum corneum shows mounds of parakeratosis, and there can be extensive lymphocyte involvement of the epidermis (Fig. 5.22). Extravasation of erythrocytes is often seen and can be present within the epidermis. There is basal vacuolar alteration and necrotic keratinocytes at the dermal epidermal junction, as well as intraepidermal collections of Langerhans cells as well as Pautrier's microabscess-like collections of lymphocytes (Fig. 5.23). A band-like infiltrate is present within the dermis. Lesions of PLEVA tend to have a deeper and dense infiltrate with ulceration. On immunophenotyping, the infiltrating lymphocytes have been reported to be predominantly CD4+ (Magro et al. 2002) and CD8+ (Fig. 5.24), in different series. In a series studied by Magro et al., small CD8+ T cells accompanied larger CD4+ intraepidermal T cells, and these smaller cells co-expressed CD56. Large atypical cells, often CD30+, can accompany the lesions of PLEVA.

Fig. 5.23 Pityriasis lichenoides chronica. High power examination shows intraepidermal involvement by atypical lymphocytes with nuclear hyperchromasia, ovoid nuclei, and some notched nuclei (H + E, 40×)

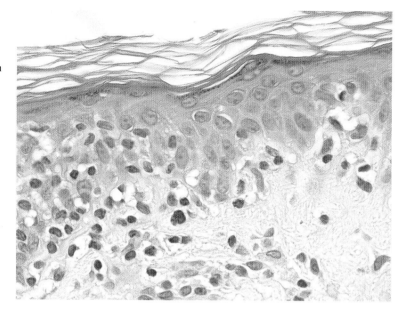

Fig. 5.24 Pityriasis lichenoides chronica. The infiltrate strongly expresses CD8 (H + E, 20×)

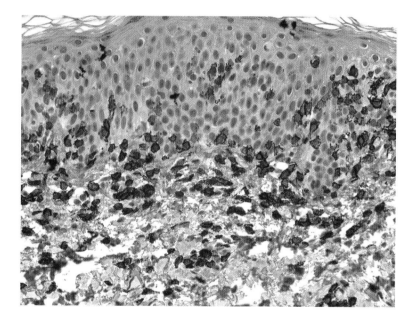

Genetics and Molecular Findings

Significant research has been done on the molecular characteristics of pityriasis lichenoides (Magro et al. 2002, 2007a, b; Panhans et al. 1996; Weiss et al. 1987; Dereure et al. 2000; Wang et al. 2007; Ko et al. 2000; Shieh et al. 2001; Weinberg et al. 2002). In the study of Magro et al., 25 of 27 cases of PLEVA and PLC in which amplifiable DNA could be found yielded a T-cell receptor clone. In addition, the authors detected the same clone in three different sites in at least one patient, which offers some evidence that PLC/PLEVA may (at least in some cases) represent a pre-lymphoma state (Magro et al. 2002). These findings were subsequently duplicated in a follow-up prospective study which used current BIOMED 2 protocols for TCR β analysis (Magro et al. 2007a, b). In smaller studies of PLC in an adult and in three children, TCR clonality assays yielded a positive clone (Wang et al. 2007; Ko et al. 2000).

Prognosis and Clinical Course

By and large, the lesions of PLC and PLEVA have a chronic clinical course but remit over time. They show responsiveness to potent topical corticosteroids (Wang et al. 2007), PUVA (Ko et al. 2000) and chemotherapeutic agents such as methotrexate. In many studies of PLC and PLEVA, a proportion of patients have developed mycosis fungoides (Magro et al. 2002, 2007a, b; Ko et al. 2000; Boccara et al. 2012; Fortson et al. 1990). In some studies, there is some doubt as to whether the lesions studied are actually those of mycosis fungoides, since the lesions seem to have the clinical features of PLC but the histologic features of mycosis fungoides (Wang et al. 2007; Ko et al. 2000; Boccara et al. 2012). However, in the studies of Magro et al., the authors do have patients that develop the more characteristic patches of mycosis fungoides (Magro et al. 2002, 2007a, b). Therefore, it does seem prudent to follow all PLC/PLEVA patients over time, to ensure that they do not develop mycosis fungoides (Shieh et al. 2001; Pileri et al. 2012; Fraitag et al. 2012).

Differential Diagnosis

Given the lichenoid pattern of the infiltrate, entities within the lichenoid/interface differential diagnosis should also be considered, such as lichen planus, erythema multiforme, lichenoid/interface drug eruption, connective tissue disease, graft-versus-host disease, and fixed drug eruption. The clinical findings in lichen planus, erythema multiforme, fixed drug eruption, and connective tissue disease are quite distinctive and will serve to exclude these possibilities. In addition, the lack of preexisting

transplantation and a careful search for offending drug agents should result in excluding graft-versus-host disease and drug eruptions, respectively. Spongiotic processes also enter into the differential, but can usually be excluded if extravasation of erythrocytes is prominent. Entities such as pityriasis rosea and pigmented purpuric dermatoses are harder to exclude, but their characteristic clinical findings should help place them further down on the differential. The distinction between lymphomatoid papulosis (Lyp) and PLEVA is particularly challenging, especially as both demonstrate expression of CD30 (Kempf et al. 2012). However, lesions of Lyp have a polymorphous population of cells, including neutrophils, eosinophils, and plasma cells, and lesions of PLEVA are often quite monomorphous and composed primarily of lymphocytes (Magro et al. 2002). Many lesions of PLC can closely mimic mycosis fungoides histologically, and T-cell receptor gene rearrangements can be positive, even on multiple biopsies (Table 5.16). The clinical setting would be very useful, as lesions of mycosis fungoides are usually patches, plaques, or tumors, and lesions of PLC tend to be regressing papules (an unusual presentation for mycosis fungoides). Also, intraepidermal lymphocytes in PLC tend to be a combination of CD4- and CD8-expressing T cells, whereas the intraepidermal lymphocytes in mycosis fungoides tend to be almost purely of CD4 origin. However, it is important to remember that at least in some cases, patients with PLC do develop mycosis fungoides, and as such, cases of PLC would benefit from long-term clinical follow-up.

Langerhans Cell Hyperplasia

Introduction and Clinical Features

Langerhans cells are important members of the skin immune system and are known to play a role during the induction phase of adaptive immune responses (Pigozzi et al. 2006). Langerhans cells and dermal dendritic cells are professional antigen-processing and antigen-presenting cells and express CD1a in high quantities. CD1-expressing cells primarily present lipid antigens for recognition by T cells

Table 5.16 Clinical and morphologic comparisons between pityriasis lichenoides chronica, pityriasis lichenoides et varioliformis acuta, and mycosis fungoides

	Pityriasis lichenoides chronica	Pityriasis lichenoides et varioliformis acuta	Mycosis fungoides
Common in children	No	Yes	No
Appearing and resolving in crops	Yes	Yes	No
Ulcerating, hemorrhagic lesions	No	Yes	No
Morphology of lesions	Papules, some plaques	Ulcerating hemorrhagic nodules	Patches, plaques, tumors
Lichenoid pattern	Yes	Yes	Yes, in lichenoid MF
Microabscesses	Pautrier's-like microabscesses, Langerhans' cell microabscesses	Pautrier's-like microabscesses, Langerhans' cell microabscesses	Pautrier's (tumor cells)
Lymphocytic involvement of epidermis	Yes, mild spongiosis	Yes, mild spongiosis	Yes, mild spongiosis
Extravasation of erythrocytes	Yes	Yes	Yes, in PPE-like MF
Cytologic atypia within T cells	Yes	Yes	Yes
Phenotype of T cells	Mixture of CD4 and CD8, in some cases CD8 predominates (Magro et al. 2002, 2007a, b)	Mixture of CD4 and CD8, in some cases CD8 predominates	CD4
Loss of CD5	Yes, subpopulation of cases (Magro et al. 2002)	Yes, subpopulation of cases	Yes
TCR clonality assays	Positive, especially in cases with atypical T cells	Positive, especially in cases with atypical T cells	Positive

and often populate infiltrates that are T-cell rich (McClain et al. 2004). Langerhans cell hyperplasia can be seen in many T-cell rich reactive entities, such as scabies (Bhattacharjee and Glusac 2007), contact dermatitis (Drut et al. 2010), lichen planus, psoriasis, atopic dermatitis, and pityriasis lichenoides chronica. It can also be seen in mycosis fungoides (Christie et al. 2006) and lymphomatoid papulosis (Jokinen et al. 2007).

Histopathology and Immunophenotype

On histology, numerous Langerhans cells are noted within the dermis and the epidermis. The Langerhans cells form microabscesses within the epidermis. Depending on the associated disorder, the epidermis can also show acanthosis, hyperkeratosis, and spongiosis. There can be a band-like infiltrate within the dermis, and the infiltrate can extend to involve the deeper reticular dermis. The infiltrate can be composed of lymphocytes, eosinophils, and plasma cells, as well as Langerhans cells and dermal dendritic cells. Scabetic mites may be identifiable in lesions of scabies.

Prognosis and Clinical Course

The prognosis and clinical course of the lesions depend on the underlying etiology. If treated appropriately, the lesions (such as those associated with scabies) resolve and do not persist, unlike lesions of mycosis fungoides. Lesions of lymphomatoid papulosis have a relapsing and remitting course but will respond to methotrexate.

Differential Diagnosis

The important differential diagnostic considerations include both Langerhans cell histiocytosis (LCH) and mycosis fungoides (Table 5.17). There

Table 5.17 Clinical and morphologic comparisons between Langerhans cell hyperplasia and mycosis fungoides

	Langerhans cell hyperplasia	Mycosis fungoides
Associated with scabies	Yes	No
Associated with CD1a + Langerhans cells	Yes	Yes, seldom
Spongiosis is present	Yes	No
Microabscesses	Langerhans cell	Pautrier's (tumor cells)
Cytologic atypia within T cells	No	Yes

is debate within the literature as to the benign or malignant nature of Langerhans cell histiocytosis, which renders more difficult our ability to distinguish between Langerhans cell hyperplasia seen in association with other entities and Langerhans cell histiocytosis (McClain et al. 2004; Murphy 1985). An underlying etiology should always be searched for histologically, including scabetic mites, the band-like infiltrate of lichen planus, Munro's microabscesses of psoriasis, significant epidermal spongiosis, and red blood cell extravasation. Careful clinical correlation is crucial to ensure that the lesion being treated is that of LCH and not a hyperplastic process. Children with LCH have a characteristic clinical setting: the lesions are composed of yellow-brown papules which appear on the face, trunk, and buttocks and can coalesce to form an eruption that resembles seborrheic dermatitis. Involvement of the bone and systemic symptoms can both be present. Histologically Langerhans cell hyperplasia can also resemble mycosis fungoides, especially when it is present in the context of lichen planus, psoriasis, and atopic dermatitis. Correlation with clinical findings and histologic examination of the cytology of the T cells can both be very helpful in excluding mycosis fungoides.

Reactive Erythroderma

Introduction and Clinical Features

Erythroderma (exfoliative dermatitis) is characterized by near complete erythema of the skin (over 90 %) accompanied by scaling (Sigurdsson et al. 1996; Yuan et al. 2010; Vonderheid 2006). The patients often have intractable pruritus and can sometimes have fever, lymphadenopathy, peripheral blood changes, alopecia, palmar hyperkeratosis, pitting edema, and nail changes. In one study of 82 patients, erythroderma was most often reactive in nature (95 %) and psoriasis was a common culprit (48 %) (Yuan et al. 2010; Vonderheid 2006). Reactive erythroderma can also be caused by seborrheic dermatitis (12 %), atopic dermatitis (22 %), contact dermatitis (9 %), id reaction, pityriasis rubra pilaris (4 %), drug eruptions (14 %), and photoreactions (such as chronic actinic dermatitis or actinic reticuloid (3 %). Less common reactive causes include dermatomyositis, sarcoidosis, hypereosinophilic syndrome, congenital ichthyosiform erythroderma, pemphigus foliaceus, and stasis dermatitis (Yuan et al. 2010; Vonderheid 2006). Erythroderma can also be paraneoplastic or caused by mycosis fungoides/Sézary syndrome or leukemia cutis (chronic lymphocytic leukemia). The patients are commonly men (Sigurdsson et al. 1996), and serum IgE levels were often elevated. In most instances, distinction between patients involved by reactive erythroderma and erythroderma caused by a malignancy was not possible by routine clinical examination, unless patients also have superimposed tumors and infiltrative plaques and leonine facies, which would favor lymphoma.

Histopathology and Immunophenotype

The histopathology can be very variable and reflect the underlying pathophysiology. For example, patients with erythrodermic psoriasis, seborrheic dermatitis, and pityriasis rubra pilaris often have psoriasiform epidermal hyperplasia, diffuse or alternating parakeratosis, and neutrophilic transmigration (in the case of psoriasis). Erythroderma due to contact or atopic dermatitis, drug hypersensitivity reaction, and id hypersensitivity reaction can also show psoriasiform changes but may have accompanying mild spongiosis and eosinophils. Erythroderma due to a paraneoplastic syndrome may have very nonspecific findings, similar to that described above. While erythroderma due to advanced erythrodermic mycosis fungoides and Sézary syndrome may be easily diagnosed on histopathology due to the presence of atypical T cells, early lesions can be extremely difficult and show significant overlap histopathologically with reactive erythroderma (Vonderheid 2006). The histologic findings in chronic actinic dermatitis may show significant overlap with other entities in the reactive erythroderma group, and those of actinic reticuloid will show overlap with mycosis fungoides/Sézary syndrome. On immunophenotyping, T cells in many of the entities listed above (except actinic reticuloid) can show a CD4+ T-cell predominance, and cells of mycosis fungoides and Sézary syndrome will show an aberrant T-cell phenotype, such as loss of CD5 and CD2. The T cells in actinic reticuloid are of CD8 origin. In general, however, use of histology and immunohistochemistry to distinguish between early lesions of mycosis fungoides/Sézary syndrome in an erythrodermic patient and reactive erythroderma was not found to be useful by Vonderheid (2006). The lymph node biopsy often shows dermatopathic changes in reactive cases and can also show involvement by lymphoma if the cause of erythema is mycosis fungoides or Sézary syndrome.

Genetics, Molecular Findings, and Peripheral Blood Analysis

Examination of the peripheral blood is crucial in cases of erythroderma, which can often show an elevated erythrocyte sedimentation rate (ESR), increased white blood cell count, high level of C-reactive protein, and eosinophilia (Sigurdsson et al. 1996; Yuan et al. 2010). Atypical cerebriform lymphocytes (Sézary cells) may be present even in cases of reactive erythroderma. However, >20 % of the lymphocyte population or an absolute count of >1.0 K/uL can both indicate involvement by leukemia. Rarely, a high count of Sézary cells can be seen in reactive erythroderma (Vonderheid 2006), and the diagnosis should be confirmed to be reactive based on clinical findings. In addition, patients with Sézary syndrome have other abnormal blood findings. They may have a CD4/CD8 ratio >10, loss of CD7, evidence of a T-cell receptor gene rearrangement clone, or a chromosomally abnormal T-cell clone, and these would all be very unusual findings in reactive erythroderma. In addition, flow cytometry is used often to distinguish between reactive and malignant erythroderma. Malignant Sézary cells often have diminishment or loss of CD3, CD4, CD2, and CD5. In addition, loss of CD7 and CD26 has both been found to be present more often in malignant Sézary cells, and expansion of this group of atypical lymphocytes to amounts greater than 30–40 % of total number of lymphocytes is a significant finding that points to leukemia. Flow cytometric analysis of expression of Vβ proteins can also be performed, as restricted Vβ expression has been linked to Sézary syndrome; however, this finding is not thought to be specific (Vonderheid 2006; Russell Jones and Whittaker 1999). Molecular analysis of both skin and blood has been extensively studied in Sézary syndrome. Southern blot analysis was the approach of choice for analysis of the peripheral blood for T-cell receptor clones and was quite useful, as the detection threshold was relatively high (1–5 %). Using this method, detection of clones in reactive erythroderma was rare (Vonderheid 2006). PCR methodologies are used more commonly now; as these techniques are more sensitive, both reactive erythroderma and Sézary syndrome have been shown to demonstrate clones (Vonderheid 2006). In the skin, Southern blot detection of T-cell receptor clones is virtually diagnostic of Sézary syndrome, as this method does not usually detect clones in skin biopsies of reactive erythroderma. However, as in blood, PCR analysis for T-cell receptor gene rearrangement clones has replaced Southern blotting, primarily due to the fact that a lot of material is needed for Southern blot analysis and skin biopsies are small. However, given increased sensitivity with PCR analysis, false-positive results are often encountered (up to 25 %), as are false-negative results (Vonderheid 2006; Zhang et al. 2010). For this reason, clones detected in the skin are often compared to those in blood and vice versa for the most specific results in excluding reactive erythroderma. If matching clones are found, the results are indicative of Sézary syndrome, but it is important to note that such findings

Table 5.18 Clinical and morphologic comparisons between reactive erythroderma and erythrodermic mycosis fungoides/Sézary syndrome

	Reactive erythroderma	Erythrodermic mycosis fungoides/Sézary syndrome
Ectropion	No	Yes
Alopecia	Yes	Yes
Associated skin lesions such as tumors, infiltrative plaques, and/or leonine facies	No	Yes
Spongiosis is present	Yes, mild	Yes, mild
Necrotic keratinocytes	Yes	Yes
Microabscesses	Langerhans cell	Pautrier's (tumor cells)
Cytologic atypia within T cells	No	Yes, but can be mild
Phenotype of T cells	CD4 (except in cases of actinic reticuloid)	CD4
Abnormalities in peripheral blood	Yes, low percentage of patients	Yes, high percentage of patients
Matching clones in the skin and blood	Very rare	Common

can also be seen in reactive erythroderma about 5 % of the time (Vonderheid 2006).

Prognosis and Clinical Course

While the prognosis of patients with reactive erythroderma is generally good, interestingly, men with reactive erythroderma were found to have a statistically significant shorter survival rate than age-matched men in the general population (Sigurdsson et al. 1996). The reason for this finding is unclear. Most patients with reactive erythroderma improved when their symptoms were treated and causes for the erythroderma removed (i.e., via drug withdrawal or sun protection) (Sigurdsson et al. 1996; Yuan et al. 2010).

Differential Diagnosis

The main differential diagnostic consideration is with erythrodermic mycosis fungoides and Sézary syndrome (Table 5.18). Patients with lymphoma or leukemia often have other skin lesions that would not be seen in reactive processes, such as tumors or leonine facies. Ectropion is also a good indicator of Sézary syndrome. In advanced cases, large atypical cells are seen in skin biopsies and peripheral blood of patients with Sézary syndrome. However, in early cases,

the distinction between Sézary syndrome and reactive erythroderma is still quite difficult. Factors that favor Sézary syndrome include abnormalities in the peripheral blood demonstrated via morphology and flow cytometry of the T-cell population and matching T-cell receptor clones between skin and blood or skin, blood, and involved lymph nodes. Matching clones found over time in various synchronous or serially biopsied skin can also be helpful in confirming the diagnosis of Sézary syndrome.

References

Abraham S, Braun RP, Matthes T, Saurat JH. A follow up: previously reported apparent lymphomatoid contact dermatitis, now followed by T cell prolymphocytic leukemia. Br J Dermatol. 2006;155(3):633–4.

Ackerman AB, Breza TS, Capland L. Spongiotic simulants of mycosis fungoides. Arch Dermatol. 1974;109(2):218–20.

Al Hoqail IA, Crawford RI. Benign lichenoid keratoses with histologic features of mycosis fungoides: clinicopathologic description of a clinically significant histologic pattern. J Cutan Pathol. 2002;29(5):291–4.

Annessi G, Paradisi M, Angelo C, Perez M, Puddu P, Girolomoni G. Annular lichenoid dermatitis of youth. J Am Acad Dermatol. 2003;49(6):1029–36.

Arai E, Shimizu M, Tsuchida T, Izaki S, Ogawa F, Hirose T. Lymphomatoid keratosis. An epidermotropic type of cutaneous lymphoid hyperplasia: clinicopathological, immunohistochemical, and molecular biological study of 6 cases. Arch Dermatol. 2007;143(1):53–9.

Asarch A, Gottlieb AB, Lee J, Masterpol KS, Scheinman PL, Stadecker MJ, et al. Lichen planus-like eruptions: an emerging side effect of tumor necrosis factor-alpha antagonists. J Am Acad Dermatol. 2009;61(1):104–11. doi:10.1016/j.jaad.2008.09.032.

Ayala F, Balato N, Nappa P, De Rosa G, Lembo G. Lymphomatoid contact dermatitis. Contact Dermatitis. 1987;17(5):311–3.

Bakels V, van Oostveen JW, Preesman AH, Meijer CJ, Willemze R. Differentiation between actinic reticuloid and cutaneous T cell lymphoma by T cell receptor gamma gene rearrangement analysis and immunophenotyping. J Clin Pathol. 1998;51(2):154–8.

Bauer F. Quinacrine hydrochloride drug eruption (tropical lichenoid dermatitis). J Am Acad Dermatol. 1981;4(2):239–48.

Ben Hur H, Ashkenazi M, Huszar M, Gurevich P, Zusman I. Lymphoid elements and apoptosis related proteins (Fas, Fas ligand, p53 and bcl-2) in lichen sclerosus and carcinoma of the vulva. Eur J Gynaecol Oncol. 2001;22(2):104–9.

Beyer K, Nickel R, Freidhoff L, Bjorksten B, Huang SK, Barnes KC, et al. Association and linkage of atopic dermatitis with chromosome 13q12-14 and 5q31-33 markers. J Invest Dermatol. 2000;115(5):906–8.

Bhattacharjee P, Glusac EJ. Langerhans cell hyperplasia in scabies: a mimic of Langerhans cell histiocytosis. J Cutan Pathol. 2007;34(9):716–20.

Boccara O, Blanche S, de Prost Y, Brousse N, Bodemar C, Fraitag S. Cutaneous hematologic disorders in children. Pediatr Blood Cancer. 2012;58(2):226–32. doi:10.1002/pbc.23103.

Brady SP, Magro CM, Diaz-Cano SJ, Wolfe HJ. Analysis of clonality of atypical cutaneous lymphoid infiltrates associated with drug therapy by PCR/DGGE. Hum Pathol. 1999;30(2):130–6.

Braun RP, French LE, Feldmann R, Chavaz P, Saurat JH. Cutaneous pseudolymphoma, lymphomatoid contact dermatitis type, as an unusual cause of symmetrical upper eyelid nodules. Br J Dermatol. 2000;143(2):411–4.

Bulcke DM, Devos SA. Hand and forearm dermatoses among veterinarians. J Eur Acad Dermatol Venereol. 2007;21(3):360–3.

Burns MK, Cooper KD. Cutaneous T cell lymphoma associated with HIV infection. J Am Acad Dermatol. 1993;29(3):394–9.

Burry JN. Ulcerative lichenoid eruption from methyldopa. Arch Dermatol. 1976;112(6):880.

Calzavara-Pinton P, Capezzera R, Zane C, Brezzi A, Pasolini G, Ubiali A, Facchetti F. Lymphomatoid allergic contact dermatitis from para-phenylenediamine. Contact Dermatitis. 2002;47(3):173–4.

Carlson JA, Grabowski R, Chichester P, Paunovich E, Malfetano J. Comparative immunophenotypic study of lichen sclerosus: epidermotropic CD57+ lymphocytes are numerous – implications for pathogenesis. Am J Dermatopathol. 2000;22(1):7–16.

Cerroni L, Fink Puches R, El Shabrawi CL, Soyer HP, LeBoit PE, Kerl H. Solitary skin lesions with histopathologic features of early mycosis fungoides. Am J Dermatopathol. 1999;21(6):518–24.

Cesinaro AM, Sighinolfi P, Greco A, Garagnani L, Conti A, Fantini F. Annular lichenoid dermatitis of youth…. and beyond: a series of six cases. Am J Dermatopathol. 2009;31(3):263–7.

Chen M, Deng A, Crowson AN, Srinivasan M, Yearsley KH, Jewell S, et al. Assessment of T cell clonality via T cell receptor gamma rearrangements in cutaneous T cell dominant infiltrates using polymerase chain reaction and single stranded DNA conformational polymorphism assay. Appl Immunohistochem Mol Morphol. 2004;12(4):373–9.

Choi MJ, Kim HS, Kim HO, Song KY, Park YM. A case of lymphomatoid keratosis. Ann Dermatol. 2010;22(2):219–22. doi:10.5021/ad.2010.22.2.219.

Choi TS, Doh KS, Kim SH, Jang MS, Suh KS, Kim ST. Clinicopathological and genotypic aspects of anticonvulsant induced pseudolymphoma syndrome. Br J Dermatol. 2003;148(4):730–6.

Christie LJ, Evans AT, Bray SE, Smith ME, Kernohan NM, Levison DA, Goodlad JR. Lesions resembling Langerhans cell histiocytosis in association with other lymphoproliferative disorders: a reactive or neoplastic phenomenon? Hum Pathol. 2006;37(1):32–9.

Citarella L, Massone C, Kerl H, Cerroni L. Lichen sclerosus with histopathologic features simulating early mycosis fungoides. Am J Dermatopathol. 2003;25(6):463–5.

Coleman R, Trebath RC, Harper JI. Genetic studies of atopy and atopic dermatitis. Br J Dermatol. 1997;136(1):1–5.

Conde-Taboada A, Róson E, Fernández-Redondo V, García-Doval I, De La Torre C, Cruces M. Lymphomatoid contact dermatitis induced by gold earrings. Contact Dermatitis. 2007;56(3):179–81.

Cookson WO. The genetics of atopic dermatitis: strategies, candidate genes, and genome screens. J Am Acad Dermatol. 2001;45(1 Suppl):S7–9.

Crowson AN, Magro CM. Lichenoid and subacute cutaneous lupus erythematosus-like dermatitis associated with antihistamine therapy. J Cutan Pathol. 1999;26(2):95–9.

Crowson AN, Magro CM, Zahorchak R. Atypical pigmentary purpura: a clinical, histopathologic, and genotypic study. Hum Pathol. 1999;30(9):1004–12.

Dalton SR, Chandler WM, Abuzeid M, Hossler EW, Ferringer T, Elston DM, LeBoit PE. Eosinophils in mycosis fungoides: an uncommon finding in the patch and plaque stages. Am J Dermatopathol. 2012;34(6):586–91. doi:10.1097/DAD.0b013e31823d921b.

Danese P, Bertazzoni MG. Lymphomatoid contact dermatitis due to nickel. Contact Dermatitis. 1995;33(4):268–9.

De Silva BD, McLaren K, Kavanagh GM. Photosensitive mycosis fungoides or actinic reticuloid? Br J Dermatol. 2000;142(6):1221–7.

Dereure O, Levi E, Kadin M. T cell clonality in pityriasis lichenoides et varioliformis acuta. A heteroduplex analysis of 20 cases. Arch Dermatol. 2000;136(12):1483–6.

Drut R, Peral CG, Garone A, Rositto A. Fetal Pediatr Pathol. 2010;29(4):231–8. doi:10.3109/15513811003789610.

Ecker RI, Winkelmann RK. Lymphomatoid contact dermatitis. Contact Dermatitis. 1981;7(2):84–93.

El Darouti MA, Marzouk SA, Azzam O, et al. Vitiligo vs. hypopigmented mycosis fungoides (histopathological and immunohistochemical study, univariate analysis). Eur J Dermatol. 2006;16(1):17–22.

Evans AV, Banerjee P, McFadden JP, Calonje E. Lymphomatoid contact dermatitis to para tertyl butyl phenol resin. Clin Exp Dermatol. 2003;28(3):272–3.

Evans L, Mackey SL, Vidmar DA. An asymptomatic scaly plaque: unilesional mycosis fungoides (MF). Arch Dermatol. 1997;133(2):231–4.

Farrell AM, Marren P, Dean D, Wojnarowska F. Lichen sclerosus: evidence that immunological changes occur at all levels of the skin. Br J Dermatol. 1999;140(6):1087–92.

Fink Puches R, Chott A, Ardigó M, Simonitsch I, Ferrara G, Kerl H, Cerroni L. The spectrum of cutaneous lymphomas in patients less than 20 years of age. Pediatr Dermatol. 2004;21(5):525–33.

Fink Puches R, Wolf P, Kerl H, Cerroni L. Lichen aureus: clinicopathologic features, natural history, and relationship to mycosis fungoides. Arch Dermatol. 2008;144(9):1169–73. doi:10.1001/archderm.144.9.1169.

Fitzpatrick JE. New histopathologic findings in drug eruptions. Dermatol Clin. 1992;10(1):19–36.

Fortson JS, Schroeter AL, Esterly NB. Cutaneous T cell lymphoma (parapsoriasis en plaque): an association with pityriasis lichenoides et varioliformis acuta in young children. Arch Dermatol. 1990;126(11):1449–53.

Frain-Bell W, Johnson BE. Contact allergic sensitivity to plants and the photosensitivity dermatitis and actinic reticuloid syndrome. Br J Dermatol. 1979;101(5):503–12.

Fraitag S, Boccara O, Brousse N, Bodemer C. Mycosis fungoides following pityriasis lichenoides: an exceptional event or a potential evolution? Pediatr Blood Cancer. 2012;58(2):307. doi:10.1002/pbc.23288.

Friss AB, Cohen PR, Bruce S, Duvic M. Chronic cutaneous lupus erythematosus mimicking mycosis fungoides. J Am Acad Dermatol. 1995;33(5 Pt 2):891–5.

Georgala S, Katoulis AC, Symeonidou S, Georgala C, Vavopoulos G. Persistent pigmented purpuric eruption associated with mycosis fungoides: a case report and review of the literature. J Eur Acad Dermatol Venereol. 2001;15(1):62–4.

Gilliam AC, Wood GS. Cutaneous lymphoid hyperplasia. Semin Cutan Med Surg. 2000;19(2):133–41.

Goiriz R, Peñas PF, Delgado-Jiménez Y, Fernández-Herrara J, Aragüés-Montañés M, Fraga J, García-Díez A. Cutaneous lichenoid graft versus host disease mimicking lupus erythematosus. Lupus. 2008;17(6):591–5. doi:10.1177/0961203307087874.

Gross T, Wagner A, Ugurel S, Tilgen W, Reinhold U. Identification of TIA-1+ and granzyme B + cytotoxic T cells in lichen sclerosus et atrophicus. Dermatology. 2001;202(3):198–202.

Grossman ME, Warren K, Mady A, Satra KH. Lichenoid eruption associated with ethambutol. J Am Acad Dermatol. 1995;33(4):675–6.

Guitart J, Peduto M, Caro WA, Roenigk HH. Lichenoid changes in mycosis fungoides. J Am Acad Dermatol. 1997;36(3 Pt 1):417–22.

Guitart J, Variakojis D, Kuzel T, Rosen S. Cutaneous CD8+ T cell infiltrates in advanced HIV infection. J Am Acad Dermatol. 1999;41(5 Pt 1):722–77.

Harvell JD, Nowfar Rad M, Sundram U. An immunohistochemical study of CD4, CD8, TIA-1, and CD56 subsets in inflammatory skin disease. J Cutan Pathol. 2003;30(2):108–13.

Hawk JLM. Lichenoid drug eruption induced by propranolol. Clin Exp Dermatol. 1980;5(1):93–6.

Heskel N, Lobitz Jr WC. Atopic dermatitis in children: clinical features and management. Semin Dermatol. 1983;2:39–44.

Hinchliffe SA Ciftci AO, Khine MM, Rickwood AM, Ashwood J, McGill F, et al. Composition of the inflammatory infiltrate in pediatric penile lichen sclerosus et atrophicus (balanitis xerotica obliterans): a prospective, comparative immunophenotyping study. Pediatr Pathol. 1994;14(2):223–33.

Holm N, Flaig MJ, Yazdi AS, Sander CA. The value of molecular analysis by PCR in the diagnosis of cutaneous lymphocytic infiltrates. J Cutan Pathol. 2002;29(8):447–52.

Houck HE, Wirth FA, Kauffman CL. Lymphomatoid contact dermatitis caused by nickel. Am J Contact Dermat. 1997;8(3):175–6.

Hu SW, Myskowski PL, Papadopoulos EB, Busam KJ. Chronic cutaneous graft versus host disease simulating hypertrophic lupus erythematosus – a case report of a new morphologic variant of graft versus host disease. Am J Dermatopathol. 2012;34(6):e81–3. doi:10.1097/DAD.0b013e31823395f0.

Huh W, Kanitakis J. Annular lichenoid dermatitis of youth: report of the first Japanese case and published work review. J Dermatol. 2010;37(6):531–3. doi:10.1111/j.1346-8138.2009.00740.x.

Igisu K, Watanabe S, Shimosato Y, Kukita A. Langerhans cells and their precursors with S100 protein in mycosis fungoides. Jpn J Clin Oncol. 1983;13(4):693–702.

Ive FA, Magnus IA, Warin RP, Jones EW. "Actinic reticuloid": a chronic dermatosis associated with severe photosensitivity and the histological resemblance to lymphoma. Br J Dermatol. 1969;81(7):469–85.

Johnson SC, Cripps DJ, Norback DH. Actinic reticuloid: a clinical, pathologic, and action spectrum study. Arch Dermatol. 1979;115(9):1078–83.

Jokinen CH, Wolgamot GM, Wood BL, Olerud J, Argenyi ZB. Lymphomatoid papulosis with CD1a + dendritic cell hyperplasia, mimicking Langerhans cell histiocytosis. J Cutan Pathol. 2007;34(7):584–7.

Jones RR, Chu A. Pagetoid reticulosis and solitary mycosis fungoides: distinct clinicopathological entities. J Cutan Pathol. 1981;8(1):40–51.

Jung K, Imhof BA, Linse R, Wollina U, Neumann C. Adhesion molecules in atopic dermatitis: upregulation of α6 integrin expression in spontaneous lesional skin as well as in atopen, antigen and irritative induced patch test reactions. Int Arch Allergy Immunol. 1997;113(4):495–504.

Kempf W, Kazakov DV, Palmedo G, Fraitag S, Schaerer L, Kutzner H. Pityriasis lichenoides et varioliformis acuta with numerous CD30(+) cells; a variant mimicking lymphomatoid papulosis and other cutaneous lymphomas. A clinicopathologic, immunohistochemical, and molecular biological study of 13 cases. Am J Surg Pathol. 2012;36(7):1021–9.

Kleikamp S, Kutzner H, Frosch PJ. Annular lichenoid dermatitis of youth-a further case in a 12 year old girl. J Dtsch Dermatol Ges. 2008;6(8):653–6. doi:10.1111/j.1610-0387.2008.06575.x.

Ko JW, Seong JY, Suh KS, Kim ST. Pityriasis lichenoides-like mycosis fungoides in children. Br J Dermatol. 2000;142(2):347–52.

Koorse S, Tirumalae R, Yeliur IK, Jayaseelan E. Clinicopathologic profile of hypopigmented mycosis fungoides in India. Am J Dermatopathol. 2012;34(2):161–4. doi:10.1097/DAD.0b013e31822e6877.

Kossard S. Unilesional mycosis fungoides or lymphomatoid keratosis? Arch Dermatol. 1997;133(10):1312–3.

Kuraishi N, Nagai Y, Hasegawa M, Ishikawa O. Lichenoid drug eruption with palmoplantar hyperkeratosis due to imatinib mesylate: a case report and a review of the literature. Acta Derm Venereol. 2010;90(1):73–6. doi:10.2340/00015555-0758.

Lage D, Juliano PB, Metze K, de Souza EM, Cintra ML. Lichen planus and lichenoid drug induced eruption: a histological and immunohistochemical study. Int J Dermatol. 2012;51(10):1199–205. doi:10.1111/j.1365-4632.2011.05113.x.

Leger MC, Gonzalez ME, Meehan S, Schaffer JV. Annular lichenoid dermatitis of youth in an American boy. J Am Acad Dermatol. 2013;68(5):e155–6. doi:10.1016/j.jaad.2012.01.030.

Lipsker D. The pigmented and purpuric dermatitis and the many faces of mycosis fungoides. Dermatology. 2003;207(3):246–7.

Magro C, Crowson AN, Kovatich A, Burns F. Pityriasis lichenoides: a clonal T cell lymphoproliferative disorder. Hum Pathol. 2002;33(8):788–95.

Magro CM, Crowson AN, Morrison C, Li J. Pityriasis lichenoides chronica: stratification by molecular and phenotypic profile. Hum Pathol. 2007a;38(3):479–90.

Magro CM, Schaefer JT, Crowson AN, Li J, Morrison C. Pigmented purpuric dermatosis: classification by phenotypic and molecular profiles. Am J Clin Pathol. 2007b;128(2):218–29.

Marlière V, Beylot-Barry M, Doutre MS, Furioli M, Vergier B, Dubus P, et al. Lymphomatoid contact dermatitis caused by isopropyldiphenylenediamine: two cases. J Allergy Clin Immunol. 1998;102(1):152–3.

Martínez-Morán C, Sanz-Muñoz C, Morales-Callaghan AM, Garrido-Ríos AA, Torrero V, Miranda-Romero A. Lymphomatoid contact dermatitis. Contact Dermatitis. 2009;60(1):53–5.

McClain KL, Natkunam Y, Swerdlow SH. Atypical cellular disorders. Hematol Am Soc Hematol Educ Program. 2004;2004:283–96.

McCluggage WG. Premalignant lesions of the lower female genital tract: cervix, vagina and vulva. Pathology. 2013;45(3):214–28. doi:10.1097/PAT.0b013e32835f21b1.

Meyrick Thomas RH, Kennedy CT. The development of lichen sclerosus and atrophicus in monozygotic twin girls. Br J Dermatol. 1986;114(3):377–9.

Miranda-Romero A, Pérez-Oliva N, Aragoneses H, Bastida J, Raya C, González-Lopez A, García-Muñoz M. Carbamazepine hypersensitivity reaction mimicking mycosis fungoides. Cutis. 2001;67(1):47–51.

Morgan MB, Stevens GL, Switlyk S. Benign lichenoid keratosis: a clinical and pathologic reappraisal of 1040 cases. Am J Dermatopathol. 2005;27(5):387–92.

Murphy GF. Cell membrane glycoproteins and Langerhans cells. Hum Pathol. 1985;16(2):103–12.

Navarro R, Llamas M, Gallo E, Sánchez-Pérez J, Fraga J, García-Diez A. Follicular mucinosis in a mycosis fungoides like hypersensitivity syndrome induced by oxcarbamazepine. J Cutan Pathol. 2011;38(12):1009–11. doi:10.1111/j.1600-0560.2011.01791.x.

Neild VS, Hawk JL, Eady RA, Cream JJ. Actinic reticuloid with Sézary cells. Clin Exp Dermatol. 1982;7(2):143–8.

Neuhaus IM, Ramos-Caro FA, Hassanein AM. Hypopigmented mycosis fungoides in childhood and adolescence. Pediatr Dermatol. 2000;17(5):403–6.

Newton RC, Raimer SS. Pigmented purpuric eruptions. Dermatol Clin. 1985;3(1):165–9.

Ngo JT, Trotter MJ, Haber RM. Juvenile onset hypopigmented mycosis fungoides mimicking vitiligo. J Cutan Med Surg. 2009;13(4):230–3.

Oliver GF, Winkelmann RK. Unilesional mycosis fungoides: a distinct entity. J Am Acad Dermatol. 1989;20(1):63–70.

Oliver GF, Winkelmann RK, Muller SA. Lichenoid dermatitis: a clinicopathologic and immunopathologic review of sixty two cases. J Am Acad Dermatol. 1989;21(2 Pt 1):284–92.

Orbaneja JG, Diez LI, Lozano JLS, Salazar LC. Lymphomatoid contact dermatitis: a syndrome produced by epicutaneous hypersensitivity with clinical features and a histopathologic picture similar to that of mycosis fungoides. Contact Dermatitis. 1976;2(3):139–43.

Ozkaya E. Adult onset atopic dermatitis. J Am Acad Dermatol. 2005;52(4):579–82.

Panhans A, Bodemar C, Macinthyre E, Fraitag S, Paul C, de Prost Y. Pityriasis lichenoides of childhood with atypical CD30 positive cells and clonal T cell receptor gene rearrangements. J Am Acad Dermatol. 1996;35(3 Pt 1):489–90.

Penneys NS. Gold therapy: dermatologic uses and toxicities. J Am Acad Dermatol. 1979;1(4):315–20.

Petit T, Cribier B, Bagot M, Wechsler J. Inflammatory vitiligo like macules that simulate hypopigmented mycosis fungoides. Eur J Dermatol. 2003;13(4):410–2.

Pigozzi B, Bordignon M, Belloni Fortina A, Michelotto G, Alaibac M. Expression of the CD1a molecule in B and T cell lymphoproliferative skin conditions. Oncol Rep. 2006;15(2):347–51.

Pileri A, Neri I, Raone B, Ciabatti S, Bellini F, Patrizi A. Mycosis fungoides following pityriasis lichenoides: an exceptional event or a potential evolution? Pediatr Blood Cancer. 2012;58(2):306. doi:10.1002/pbc.23260.

Plaza JA, Morrison C, Magro CM. Assessment of TCR beta clonality in a diverse group of cutaneous T cell infiltrates. J Cutan Pathol. 2008;35(4):358–65.

Ploysangam T, Breneman DL, Mutasim DF. Cutaneous pseudolymphomas. J Am Acad Dermatol. 1998;38(6 Pt 1):877–905.

Pulitzer MP, Nolan KA, Oshman RG, Phelps RG. CD30+ lymphomatoid drug reactions. Am J Dermatopathol. 2013;35(3):343–50. doi:10.1097/DAD.0b013e31826bc1e5.

Ranawaka RR, Abeygunasekara PH, de Silva MVC. Hypopigmented mycosis fungoides in type V skin: a report of 5 cases. Case Rep Dermatol Med. 2011;2011:190572. doi:10.1155/2011/190572.

Reddy K, Bhawan J. Histologic mimickers of mycosis fungoides; a review. J Cutan Pathol. 2007;34(7):519–25.

Regauer S, Beham-Schmid C. Monoclonally rearranged gamma T cell receptor in lichen sclerosus – a finding of clinical significance? Am J Dermatopathol. 2004;26(4):349–50.

Regauer S, Beham-Schmid C. Detailed analysis of the T cell lymphocytic infiltrate in penile lichen sclerosus: an immunohistochemical and molecular investigation. Histopathology. 2006;48(6):730–5.

Romero RW, Nesbitt LT, Reed RJ. Unusual variant of lupus erythematosus or lichen planus. Clinical, histopathologic, and immunofluorescent studies. Arch Dermatol. 1977;113(6):741–8.

Russell Jones R, Whittaker S. T cell receptor gene rearrangement in the diagnosis of Sézary syndrome. J Am Acad Dermatol. 1999;41(2 Pt 1):254–9.

Rustin MHA. The safety of tacrolimus ointment for the treatment of atopic dermatitis: a review. Br J Dermatol. 2007;157(5):862–73.

Sahn EE, Bluestein EL, Oliva S. Familial lichen sclerosus et atrophicus in childhood. Pediatr Dermatol. 1994;11(2):160–3.

Sajjachareonpong P, Lee A, Nixon R. Immediate type latex hypersensitivity in a hairdresser. Australas J Dermatol. 2002;43(2):150–1.

Sarantopoulos GP, Palla B, Said J, Kinney MC, Swerdlow SM, Willemze R, Binder SW. Mimics of cutaneous lymphoma: report of the 2011 Society for Hematopathology/European Association for Haematopathology workshop. Am J Clin Pathol. 2013;139(4):536–51. doi:10.1309/AJCPX4BXTP2QBRKO.

Sardana K, Sarkar R, Sehgal VN. Pigmented purpuric dermatoses: an overview. Int J Dermatol. 2004;43(7):482–8.

Schena D, Rosina P, Chieregato C, Colombari R. Lymphomatoid like contact dermatitis from cobalt naphthenate. Contact Dermatitis. 1995;33(3):197–8.

Scrimin F, Rustja S, Radillo O, Volpe C, Abrami R, Guaschino S. Vulvar lichen sclerosus: an immunologic study. Obstet Gynecol. 2000;95(1):147–50.

Shieh S, Mikkola DL, Wood GS. Differentiation and clonality of lesional lymphocytes in pityriasis lichenoides chronica. Arch Dermatol. 2001;137(3):305–8.

Sigurdsson V, Toonstra J, Hezemans-Boer M, van Vloten WA. Erythroderma: a clinical and follow up of 102 patients, with special emphasis on survival. J Am Acad Dermatol. 1996;35(1):53–7.

Singh ZN, Tretiakova MS, Shea CR, Pertonic-Rosic VM. Decreased CD117 expression in hypopigmented mycosis fungoides correlates with hypomelanosis: lessons learned from vitiligo. Mod Pathol. 2006;19(9):1255–60.

Smolle J, Torne R, Soyer HP, Kerl H. Immunohistochemical classification of cutaneous pseudolymphomas: delineation of distinct patterns. J Cutan Pathol. 1990;17(3):149–59.

Smoller BR, Kamel OW. Pigmented purpuric eruptions: immunopathologic studies supportive of a common immunophenotype. J Cutan Pathol. 1991;18(6):423–7.

Souteyrand P, d'Incan M. Drug induced mycosis fungoides like lesions. Curr Probl Dermatol. 1990;19:176–82.

Suchak R, Verdolini R, Robson A, Stefanato CM. Extragenital lichen sclerosus et atrophicus mimicking cutaneous T cell lymphoma: report of a case. J Cutan Pathol. 2010;37(9):982–6. doi:10.1111/j.1600-0560.2009.01452.x.

Terlou A, Santegoets LA, van der Meijden WI, Heijmans-Antonissen C, Swagemakers SM, van der Spek PJ, et al. An autoimmune phenotype in vulvar lichen sclerosus and lichen planus: a Th1 response and high levels of microRNA-155. J Invest Dermatol. 2012;132(3 Pt 1):658–66.

Thomsen K. The development of Hodgkin's disease in a patient with actinic reticuloid. Clin Exp Dermatol. 1977;2(2):109–13.

Thurber SE, Zhang B, Kim YH, Schrijver I, Zehnder J, Kohler S. T cell clonality analysis in biopsy specimens from two different skin sites shows high specificity in the diagnosis of patients with suggested mycosis fungoides. J Am Acad Dermatol. 2007;57(5):783–90.

Tilly JJ, Drolet BA, Esterly NB. Lichenoid eruptions in children. J Am Acad Dermatol. 2004;51(4):606–24.

Toro JR, Sander CA, LeBoit PE. Persistent pigmented purpuric dermatitis and mycosis fungoides: stimulant, precursor, or both? A study by light microscopy and molecular methods. Am J Dermatopathol. 1997;19(2):108–18.

Tristani Firouzi P, Meadows KP, Vanderhooft S. Pigmented purpuric eruptions of childhood: a series of cases and review of the literature. Pediatr Dermatol. 2001;18(4):299–304.

Tsoitis G, Kanitakis J, Kyamidis K, Asvesti K, Lefaki I. Annular lichenoid dermatitis of youth. J Eur Acad Dermatol Venereol. 2009;23(11):1339–40. doi:10.1111/j.1468-3083.2009.03213.x.

Van Hecke E, Kint A, Temmerman L. A lichenoid eruption induced by penicillamine. Arch Dermatol. 1981;117(10):676–7.

Viseux V, Schoenlaub P, Cnudde F, Le Roux P, Leroy JP, Plantin P. Pigmented purpuric dermatitis preceding the diagnosis of mycosis fungoides by 24 years. Dermatology. 2003;207(3):331–2.

Vonderheid EC. On the diagnosis of erythrodermic cutaneous T cell lymphoma. J Cutan Pathol. 2006;33 Suppl 1:27–42.

Wada DA, Wilcox RA, Weenig RH, Gibson LE. Paucity of intraepidermal Foxp3-positive T cells in cutaneous T-cell lymphoma in contrast to spongiotic and lichenoid dermatitis. J Cutan Pathol. 2010;37(5):535–41. doi:10.1111/j.1600-0560.2009.01381.x.

Wall LM. Lymphomatoid contact dermatitis due to ethylenediamine dihydrochloride. Contact Dermatitis. 1982;8(1):51–4.

Wang SH, Hsiao CH, Hsiao PF, Chu CY. Adult pityriasis lichenoides like mycosis fungoides with high density of CD8 positive T lymphocytic infiltration. J Eur Acad Dermatol Venereol. 2007;21(3):401–2.

Weedon D. Weedon's skin pathology. 1st ed. Edinburgh: Churchill Livingstone/Elsevier; 1998.

Weedon D. Weedon's skin pathology. 3rd ed. Edinburgh: Churchill Livingstone/Elsevier; 2010.

Weinberg JM, Kristal L, Chooback L, Honig PJ, Kramer EM, Lessin SR. The clonal nature of pityriasis lichenoides. Arch Dermatol. 2002;138(8):1063–7.

Weiss LM, Wood GS, Ellisen LW, Reynolds TC, Sklar J. Clonal T cell populations in pityriasis lichenoides et varioliformis acuta (Mucha Habermann disease). Am J Pathol. 1987;121(3):417–21.

Welykyj S, Gradinin R, Nakao J, Massa M. Carbamazepine induced eruption histologically mimicking mycosis fungoides. J Cutan Pathol. 1990;17(2):111–6.

Werner B, Brown S, Ackerman AB. "Hypopigmented mycosis fungoides" is not always mycosis fungoides! Am J Dermatopathol. 2005;27(1):56–67.

White Jr CR. Histopathology of atopic dermatitis. Semin Dermatol. 1983;2:34–8.

Williams HC, Burney PG, Hay RJ, Archer CB, Shipley MJ, Hunter JJ, et al. The UK working party's diagnostic criteria for atopic dermatitis. I. Derivation of a minimum set of discriminators for atopic dermatitis. Br J Dermatol. 1994;131(3):383–96.

Wu J, Vender R, Jambrosic J. Drug induced lichenoid dermatitis with histopathologic features of mycosis fungoides in a patient with psoriasis. J Cutan Med Surg. 2010;14(6):307–9. doi:10.2310/7750.2010. 09073.

Yuan XY, Guo JY, Dang YP, Qiao L, Liu W. Erythroderma: a clinical etiological study of 82 cases. Eur J Dermatol. 2010;20(3):373–7. doi:10.1684/ejd.2010.0943.

Zackheim HS, Epstein EH, Grekin DA, McNutt NS. Mycosis fungoides presenting as areas of hypopigmentation. J Am Acad Dermatol. 1982;6(3): 340–5.

Zhang B, Beck AH, Taube JM, Kohler S, Seo K, Zwerner J, et al. Combined use of PCR based TCRG and TCRB clonality tests on paraffin embedded skin tissue in the differential diagnosis of mycosis fungoides and inflammatory dermatoses. J Mol Diagn. 2010;12(3):320–7. doi:10.2353/jmoldx. 2010.090123.

Zhang P, Chiriboga L, Jacobson M, Marsh E, Hennessey P, Schinella R, Feiner H. Mycosis fungoides like T cell cutaneous lymphoid infiltrates in patients with HIV infection. Am J Dermatopathol. 1995;17(1):29–35.

Neoplastic Epidermotropic Diseases

6

Marshall E. Kadin and Hernani D. Cualing

Mycosis Fungoides

Definition

Mycosis fungoides is an epidermotropic primary cutaneous T-cell lymphoma derived from mature (memory) CD4+ T cells in 95 % of cases; the remaining cases have a CD8 phenotype. Neoplastic cells typically comprise a minority of the cellular infiltrate in early disease in which Th1 cells predominate, whereas disease progression with increased neoplastic cells shifts to a Th2 signature (Vowels et al. 1994).

Epidemiology

Most patients are adults, but children are also affected, often with a hypopigmented variant. The male/female ratio is 2:1. Blacks are affected at a higher rate. For further details, refer to Chap. 10.

M.E. Kadin, MD (✉)
Department of Dermatology, Roger Williams
Medical Center, Boston University School of Medicine,
50 Maude Street, Elmhurst Bldg,
Providence, RI 02908, USA
e-mail: mkadin@chartercare.org

H.D. Cualing, MD
Department of Hematopathology and Cutaneous
Lymphoma, IHCFLOW Diagnostic Laboratory,
18804 Chaville Rd, Lutz, FL 33558, USA

Clinical Appearance of Lesions

Initial lesions are often very (paper-)thin and slightly erythematous, possibly with overlying silvery scale, and tumor cells confined to the epidermis and superficial dermis (Fig. 6.1a, b). These lesions are often referred to as patches or parapsoriasis en plaque. As neoplastic cell infiltration of the dermis becomes more extensive, clinical lesions become thicker and manifest as indurated plaques (Fig. 6.1c, d). The final stage of progression is a tumor, a raised nodule >1.5 cm in diameter which may become ulcerated. The progression to tumors is due to infiltration of the deeper portions of the dermis often with extension into the subcutis (Fig. 6.1e, f).

Pattern of Infiltration

The hallmark histologic feature of MF is epidermotropism (infiltration of the epidermis) by medium-sized atypical lymphocytes with highly irregular, convoluted, or cerebriform (brain-like) nuclear outlines (Fig. 6.2). In one-third or more MF patients, aggregates of three or more atypical lymphocytes are found within the epidermis, often in association with Langerhans cells (LC) which are antigen-presenting cells with abundant pale-staining cytoplasm and elongated irregular nuclei. These intraepidermal aggregates of atypical lymphocytes and Langerhans cells are referred to as a Pautrier microabscess and are considered to be unique to

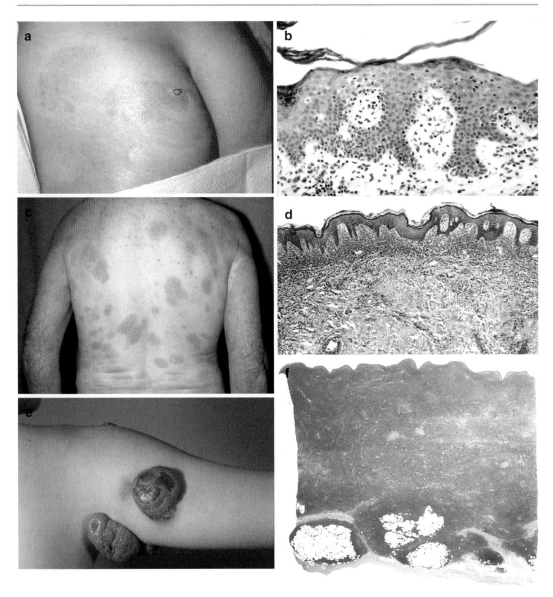

Fig. 6.1 Different mycosis fungoides lesions and corresponding histologies are shown. (**a**) Early patch lesions on the buttock of a patient. Site of a punch biopsy is shown in an inked circle. The lesion was shown to be clonal by TCR gene rearrangement analysis. (**b**) Histology of patch lesion. (**c**) Multiple red plaque lesions of MF. (**d**) Band-like dermal-epidermal lymphocytic infiltrate of plaque lesion. (This image was originally published in ASH Image Bank. Marshall Kadin. Mycosis Fungoides. ASH Image Bank. 2005; 0000438 © the American Society of Hematology.) (**e**) Mycosis fungoides tumors on arm. (**f**) Full-thickness dermal lymphocyte infiltrate extending into subcutis of mycosis fungoides tumor

mycosis fungoides (and Sézary syndrome) and therefore virtually diagnostic histologic features of MF (Fig. 6.3). Initially, these atypical lymphocytes tend to line up at the junction of the dermal-epidermal junction (Fig. 6.4). As progression to tumor stage occurs, there is commonly loss of epidermotropism. This may be due to a loss of surface molecules required for neoplastic cells to bind to epidermal keratinocytes (Fig. 6.5).

Fig. 6.2 Epidermotropism of atypical lymphocytes with highly convoluted "cerebriform" nuclei in mycosis fungoides (This image was originally published in ASH Image Bank. Marshall Kadin. Mycosis Fungoides - 3. ASH Image Bank. 2005; 00003006 © the American Society of Hematology)

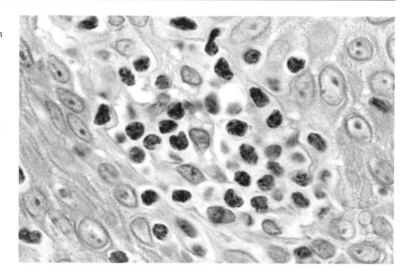

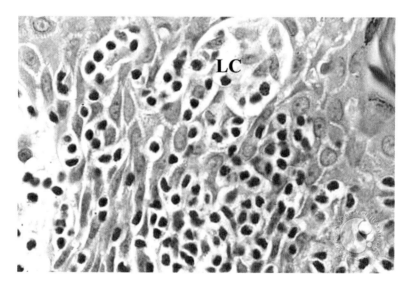

Fig. 6.3 Pautrier microabscess in epidermis of mycosis fungoides skin lesion. Some lymphocytes have a clear space (halo) around them which is a characteristic of tumor cells in mycosis fungoides. In one area near the top of the image, the lymphocytes are in contact with a collection of Langerhans cells (*LC*) which are antigen-presenting cells in the epidermis and are thought to be involved in the pathogenesis of mycosis fungoides. They are distinguished from mycosis fungoides lymphocytes by their pale-staining nuclei and abundant cytoplasm (This image was originally published in ASH Image Bank. Marshall Kadin. Mycosis Fungoides - 4. ASH Image Bank. 2005; 00003007 © the American Society of Hematology)

It can be difficult to make a definitive histopathologic diagnosis of early MF (Santucci et al. 2000). An algorithm for the diagnosis of early MF is presented in Table 6.1. It can be difficult to establish a diagnosis of erythrodermic MF because of the frequent predominance of inflammatory cells (Vonderheid 2006). Multiple skin biopsies may be necessary to establish a firm diagnosis. A definitive diagnosis may require additional blood studies and/or biopsy of an enlarged lymph node. For patients presenting with tumors, it is important to

Fig. 6.4 Lining up of
lymphocytes with haloes in
basal layer of epidermis in
"early" patch lesion of
mycosis fungoides

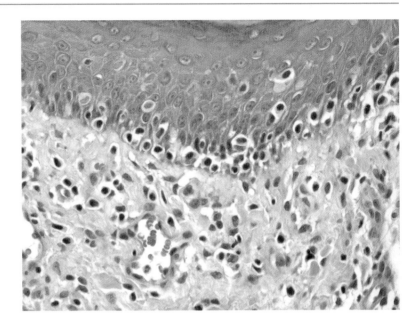

Fig. 6.5 Mechanism of
epidermotropism of
neoplastic lymphocytes.
Lymphocytes expressing
surface LFA-1 and chemo-
kine receptor CXCR3 are
attracted to epidermal
keratinocytes by chemokine
IFN-inducible protein
(CXCL10) and bind to
ICAM-1 expressed on
keratinocytes

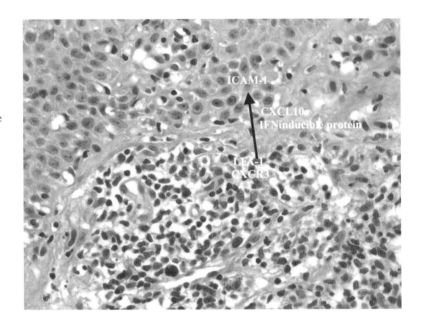

differentiate tumor-stage MF from non-MF
subtypes of CTCL, e.g., de novo anaplastic
large-cell lymphoma or peripheral T-cell lymphoma, NOS. In classic MF, tumors generally
develop in the presence of patch or plaque disease and not de novo.

Cytomorphology

The Dutch cutaneous lymphoma group uses the
diameter (>7.5 μm) of the nuclei of cerebriform
mononuclear cells to define abnormal (neoplastic) cells (Fig. 6.6). Large-cell transformation

Table 6.1 Algorithm for the diagnosis of early MF

Criteria	Major (2 points)	Minor (1 point)
Clinical		
Persistent and/or progressive patches and plaques plus	Any 2	Any 1
Non-sun-exposed location		
Size/shape variation		
Poikiloderma		
Histopathologic		
Superficial lymphoid infiltrate plus	Both	Either
Epidermotropism without spongiosis		
Lymphoid atypia (enlarged hyperchromatic, cerebriform, irregular nuclear contours)		
Molecular/biologic: clonal TCR gene rearrangement	Not applicable	Present
Immunopathologic		
CD2, CD3, and CD5 less than 50 % of T cells	Not applicable	Any 1
CD7 less than 10 % of T cells		
Epidermal discordance from expression of CD2, CD3, CD5, or CD7 on dermal T cells		

Adapted from Pimpinelli et al. (2005), with permission from Elsevier

Fig. 6.6 Typical cerebriform lymphocytes with nuclear diameter of >7 µm

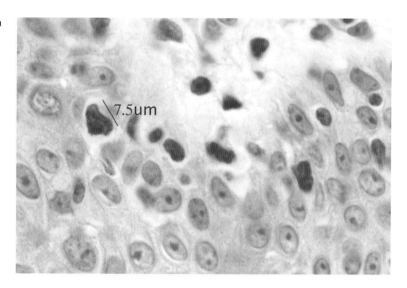

(LCT) is defined as showing large cells (≥4 times the size of a small lymphocyte) in 25 % or more of the dermal infiltrate or forming microscopic nodules (Fig. 6.7). These large cells may or may not be CD30+. Benner reported that CD30 expression is associated with an improved survival in LCT of MF (Benner et al. 2012). The possibility that a patient with CD30+ nodules might have primary cutaneous CD30+ anaplastic large-cell lymphoma coexisting with MF is important to consider. The coexistence of typical patches and plaques of MF is regarded as evidence that such lesions represent large-cell transformation (CD30+) of MF rather than a separate primary cutaneous anaplastic large-cell lymphoma. LCT is a poor prognostic sign, seen most

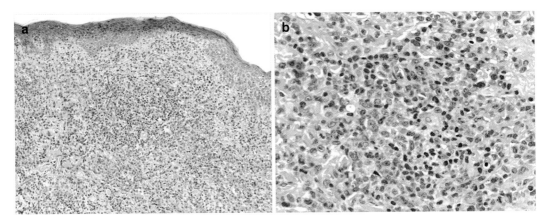

Fig. 6.7 Large-cell transformation of mycosis fungoides. (**a**) Extensive dermal infiltration with focal epidermotropism of tumor cells. (**b**) A spectrum of cells is seen; neoplastic cells are >4 times larger than normal lymphocytes

commonly in tumor-stage MF and less commonly in plaque-stage and erythrodermic MF. Clinical tumors often occur in concert with LCT (Vergier et al. 2000). Based on molecular analysis, large-cell transformation in MF/SS represents evolution of the original malignant clone (Wolfe et al. 1995).

Folliculotropic MF

Folliculotropic MF is characterized by atypical CD4+ T lymphocytes that surround and infiltrate the hair follicles (folliculotropism), usually without evidence of epidermotropism and with frequent concomitant follicular mucinosis (Fig. 6.8). Clinically, folliculotropic MF is typically classified under the T1 or T2 skin ratings even though the infiltrate extends histologically along hair follicles deeper than is typical for a plaque-stage disease. Folliculotropic MF has been shown to be associated with a worse prognosis than expected for the same clinical stage (Benner et al. 2012).

Poikilodermatous MF

A variant found more often in elderly patients. Lesions have an atrophic variegated appear-ance. Histology reveals prominent dilated blood vessels and paucicellular lymphoid infiltrate (Fig. 6.9).

Papular MF

Kodama et al. described six patients with early manifestations of MF characterized by the sole presence of papules which, unlike the papules of lymphomatoid papulosis (LyP), did not show a tendency for spontaneous resolution (Kodama et al. 2005). Histologic examination confirmed the diagnosis of MF in all cases. Immunohistochemical staining for CD30 was negative in all cases distinguishing these cases from LyP. Follow-up data showed nonaggressive behavior of the disease, confirming that the lesions were not manifestations of advanced MF. The authors concluded that papular MF is a variant of early MF characterized by papules in the absence of conventional early lesions (patches) of the disease.

Hypopigmented MF

The diagnosis of hypopigmented MF should be considered in patients with persistent hypochromic patches. Rizzo et al. described six children

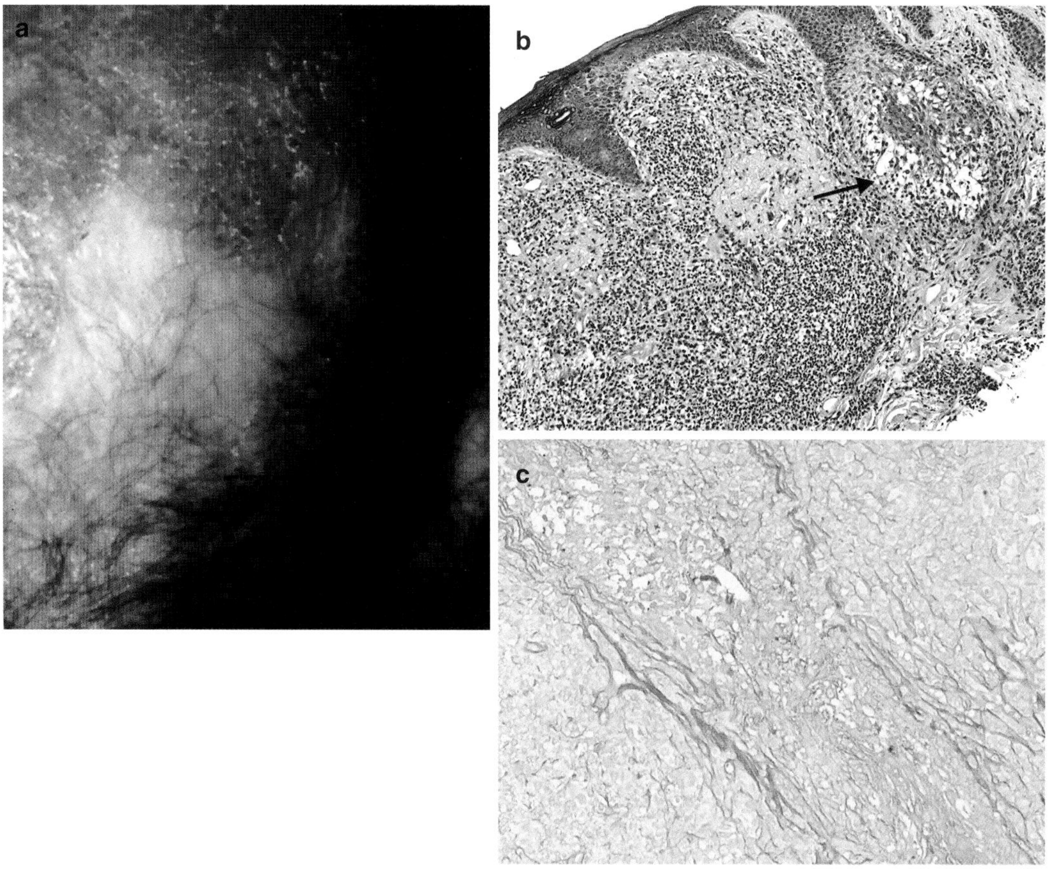

Fig. 6.8 Folliculotropic mycosis fungoides with mucinous change. (**a**) Clinical appearance of alopecia resulting from destruction of hair follicles. (**b**) Histology of MF with diffuse lymphocytic infiltrate and destruction of hair follicles (*arrow*). (**c**) Colloidal iron stain of mucinous change

and adolescents between 5 and 19 years of age who had dark skin and presented with a hypopigmented variant of MF (Fig. 6.10); some lesions expressed the T-cell CD8+ phenotype (Rizzo et al. 2012). The main histopathologic findings were basilar lymphocytes, Pautrier microabscesses, eccrine infiltration, and dermal fibrosis (Fig. 6.11).

Granulomatous MF and Slack Skin

Granulomatous slack skin (GSS) is a rare cutaneous disorder characterized by evolution of circumscribed erythematous loose skin masses, especially in the body folds, and histologically by a loss of elastic fibers and granulomatous T-cell infiltrates (Fig. 6.12). Patients with granulomatous MF and GSS have overlapping histologic features and differ only clinically by the development of bulky skin folds in GSS. Development of hanging skin folds is restricted to the intertriginous body regions. Histologically, epidermotropism of lymphocytes is not a prominent feature (Kempf et al. 2008). GSS is associated with a monomorphous T-helper cell immunophenotype and clonal rearrangement of the T-cell receptor beta gene. The histologic discrimination of granulomatous cutaneous T-cell lymphomas (CTCLs) from reactive granulomatous disorders such as sarcoidosis and granuloma annulare (GA) may be difficult due to overlapping histologic features. The presence of clonal T cells argues in

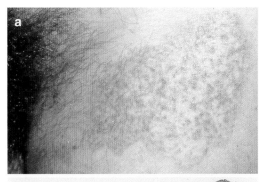

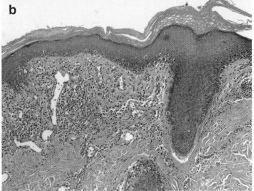

Fig. 6.9 Poikilodermatous mycosis fungoides. (**a**) Clinical appearance shows atrophy and dilated blood vessels. (**b**) Neoplastic lymphocytes tagging epidermis and surrounding dilated blood vessels

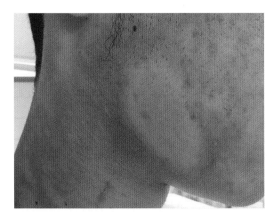

Fig. 6.10 Hypopigmented mycosis fungoides with oligoclonal TCR gene rearrangement on cheek of a dark-skinned boy from Ascension Island

favor of a granulomatous CTCL, while a polyclonal T-cell population makes the presence of a sarcoidosis or granuloma annulare more likely. Mycosis fungoides with reactive lymphoid folli-

cles may represent an early histopathologic picture of granulomatous slack skin. Granulomatous CTCLs have a therapy-resistant, slowly progressive course. The prognosis of GMF appears worse than that of classic non-granulomatous mycosis (Kempf et al. 2008).

Pagetoid Reticulosis

Pagetoid skin lesions are localized, often to distal extremities (Fig. 6.13a). Neoplastic cells show marked epidermotropism (Fig. 6.13b). They are medium- to large-sized, often cerebriform, and can have hyperchromatic chromatin. The phenotype can be CD4+ or CD8+ (Fig. 6.13b, c), and neoplastic cells may co-express CD30, but not ALK. Dissemination does not occur. Patient survival is excellent.

Sézary Syndrome

Sézary syndrome (SS) is a triad of generalized erythroderma, lymphadenopathy, and leukemic neoplastic cells (Fig. 6.14). Consistent with its relationship to mycosis fungoides, leukemic Sézary cells have convoluted nuclei. The diagnosis of SS requires 1,000 neoplastic cells/ml of blood. The skin of SS patients may show some degree of clinically apparent infiltration caused by tumor cells or an inflammatory reaction with or without edema.

Immunophenotype

Most cutaneous malignant T cells originate from memory T cells expressing CD45R0 of either CD4 or CD8 subsets. A stepwise differential antigen expression profile indicates that early on, CTCL may show a high level of cutaneous lymphocyte antigen (CLA), high density of surface antigen expression of chemokine and integrin receptors, and increased density of pan-T-cell markers such as CD3 along with CD5, CD7, and CD26. As the disease progresses and there is an increase number of large transformed cells, a

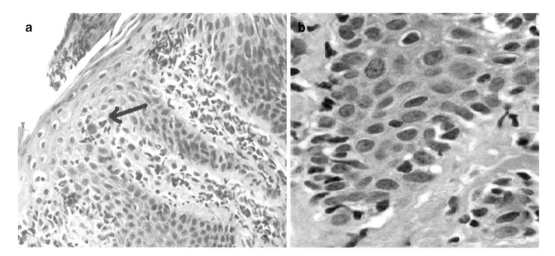

Fig. 6.11 Histopathology of hypopigmented mycosis fungoides. (**a**) Atypical lymphocytes forming collections of three or more (Pautrier microabscess), *arrow*. (**b**) Atypical haloed lymphocytes show tagging of basal layer of epidermis with vacuolar change and hypopigmentation

variable decrease in many of these surface antigens is also observed.

In approximately 95 % of MF, the neoplastic cells are derived from CD4+ T cells and the remainder from CD8+ T cells. In early stages, neoplastic cells generally express T-cell antigens CD3, CD2 and CD5; CD7 is absent in one-third of cases (Fig. 6.15). Tumor stage often shows loss of CD2, CD3, and/or CD5; large-cell transformation is frequently CD30+. Sézary cells are phenotyped by flow cytometry (Sokolowska-Wojdylo et al. 2005). They are CD4+, CD26−, and usually CD7− (Jones et al. 2001). The blood of elderly individuals and some patients with benign inflammatory dermatoses may also show CD7 deletion. Loss of CD26 may be more specific for the neoplastic lymphocytes (Bernengo et al. 2001). Identification of neoplastic cells by flow cytometry is complicated, however, by the fact that all neoplastic lymphocytes may not have the same phenotypic features and several clones may be present in a given patient with SS (Jackow et al. 1997).

The malignant T cells of mycosis fungoides and Sézary syndrome appear to be each derived from different sets of memory T cells, the former home to the skin while the latter have surface molecules favoring circulation in the blood (Campbell et al. 2010). Cutaneous MF cells express cutaneous lymphocyte antigen (CLA) and CCR4. The T-helper subset of Th2-like cells additionally expresses CD4 but lacks CCR7. In contrast to epidermotropic MF cells, circulating Sézary cells express CCR7, a marker of central or lymph node memory T cells. These key differences in phenotype enable MF cells to reside in the skin while imbuing Sézary cells with systemic or circulation-tropic localization. Addressins enable homing to specific organs. Skin-homing addressins include CLA, an adhesion protein molecule that allows recognition of E-selectin, which is expressed on post-capillary venules in the dermis (Borowitz et al. 1993). This receptor is upregulated in inflammation-promoting transmigration of homing cells to skin. Other chemokines such as CCR4 and CCR8 also promote skin homing of lymphocytes. In contrast, T cells destined elsewhere, such as intestinal mucosa, express CCR9.

Cytogenetics and Molecular Findings

Mao et al. detected oncogene copy number gains of RAF1 (3p25), CTSB (8p22), PAK1 (11q13), and JUNB (19p13) in five of seven cases of

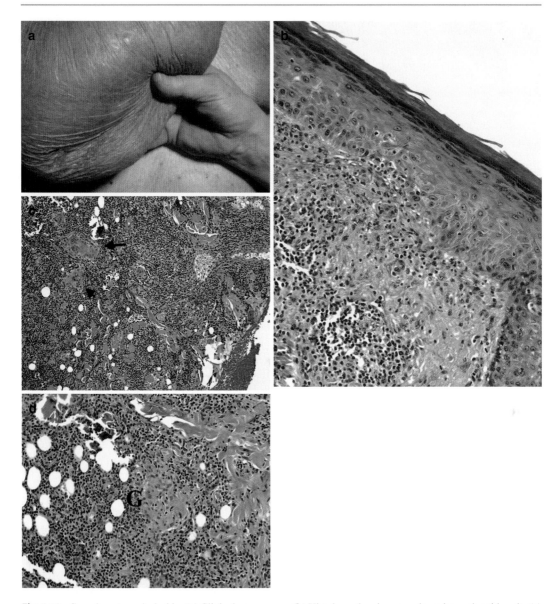

Fig. 6.12 Granulomatous slack skin. (**a**) Clinical appearance. (**b**) Histology showing granuloma beneath epidermis. (**c**) Multiple granulomas in dermal lymphoid infiltrate (*arrows*). (**d**) Granuloma without necrosis designated "G"

mycosis fungoides (MF)/Sézary syndrome (SS) (71 %); gains of FGFR1 (8p11), PTPN (20q13), and BCR (22q11) in four cases (57 %); and gains of MYCL1 (1p34), PIK3CA (3q26), HRAS (11p15), MYBL2 (20q13), and ZNF217 (20q13) in three cases (43 %). Nuclear expression of JUNB by neoplastic cells shows that JUNB may be critical in the pathogenesis of primary cutaneous T-cell lymphomas (Mao et al. 2003). In a

study of patients with MF and SS, Karenko found that aberrations of chromosomes 1, 6, and 11 seem to be a hallmark of the disease, detectable even in remission, and increase with disease activity. Aberrations of chromosomes 8 and 17 were associated with active or progressive disease (Karenko et al. 2003).

Zhang et al. compared genes expressed in early MF with those expressed in chronic derma-

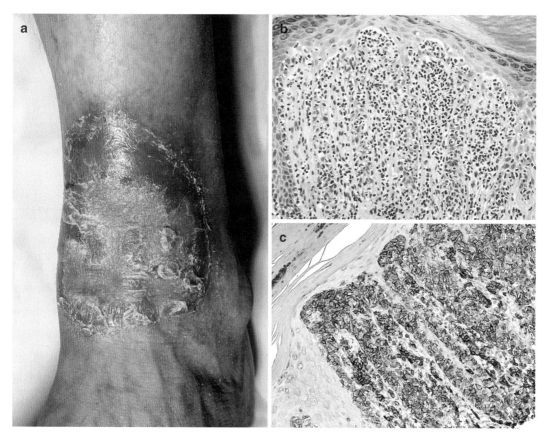

Fig. 6.13 (a) Pagetoid reticulosis localized to lower leg. (b) Pagetoid infiltration pattern in epidermis. (c) Neoplastic cells stain for CD8

titis. They identified nine genes specifically increased in early MF lesions that showed no significant upregulation in chronic dermatitis. Two of these genes, TOX and PDCD1, showed high discriminating power between early MF lesions and biopsies from benign dermatitis determined by RNA expression. TOX demonstrated highly specific staining of MF cells in early MF skin biopsies detected by immunohistochemistry and immunofluorescence, including the early epidermotropic cells in Pautrier microabscesses (Zhang et al. 2012).

Demonstration of identical clonal gene rearrangements in multiple skin biopsy specimens is recommended to confirm a diagnosis of early MF in challenging cases. Identical banded patterns were demonstrated by Murphy et al. in serial skin biopsies from the same patient. No dominant T-cell clones were found in the inflammatory dermatoses (Murphy et al. 2000). However, because PCR is sensitive enough to detect dominant TCR-gamma gene rearrangements in a subset of patients with chronic dermatitis, it cannot be used as the sole criterion for establishing a diagnosis of T-cell lymphoma (Wood et al. 1994). As with other molecular biologic clonality assays, clinicopathologic correlation is essential. Nevertheless, the detection of dominant clonality in some cases of histologically nonspecific dermatitis allows the identification of a previously unrecognized subset of patients, i.e., those with "clonal dermatitis" (Wood et al. 1994). Wood suggested that it will be important to determine the long-term risk of MF/SS among these patients because MF/SS can sometimes present with lesions indistinguishable from clonal dermatitis.

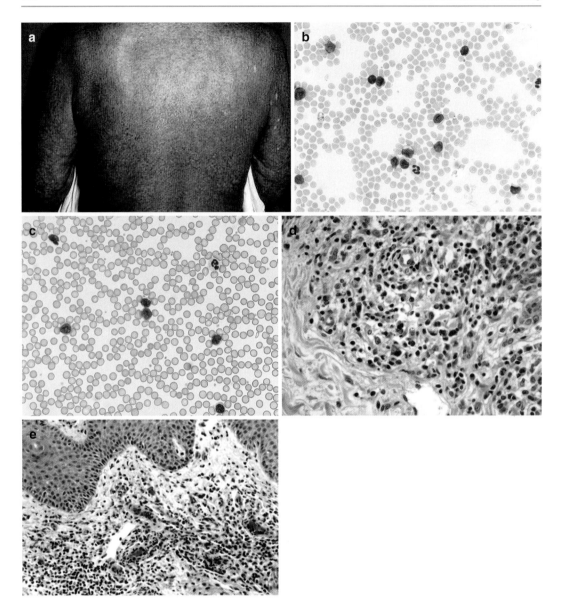

Fig. 6.14 Sézary syndrome. (**a**) Generalized erythro-derma in a patient with triad of erythroderma, lymphade-nopathy, and circulating neoplastic lymphocytes. Patients often experience intense itching and loss of body heat through skin. (**b**, **c**) Sézary cells with convoluted nuclei in the blood. (**d**) Dermal infiltrate of neoplastic cells. (**e**) Skin with inflammatory appearance in SS patient

Clinical Behavior

The prognosis of CTCL is clearly related to the stage of the disease, the nomenclature of which has recently undergone revision (Olsen et al. 2007). The stage of a patient with MF/SS refers to the overall tumor burden at time of initial diag-nosis. Changes in the tumor burden in patients with MF/SS often occur during the course of the disease, which affects treatment choices and response to treatment.

Skin: A T1 skin rating is defined as papules, patches, and/or plaques covering less than 10 % body surface area (BSA). A T2 skin rating is

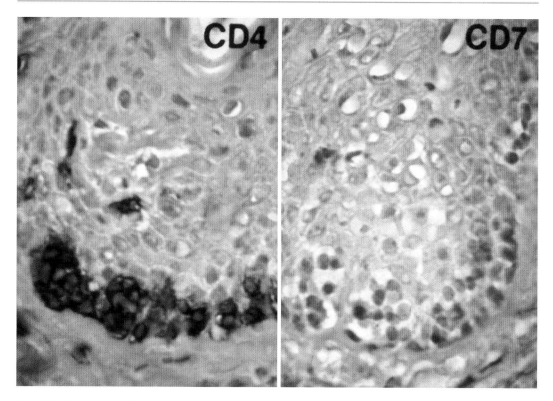

Fig. 6.15 Immunoperoxidase stain of skin of mycosis fungoides patient showing tumor cells in basal layer of epidermis expressing CD4 but not CD7

defined as patches and/or plaques covering 10 % or more BSA. T3 refers to one or more skin tumors >1 cm in diameter. T4 is the confluence of erythema covering >80 % of body area.

Lymph Nodes: The presence or absence of nodal involvement is designated by N staging. The prognosis in MF/SS is clearly related to partially or completely effaced nodal architecture as defined by either the NCI-VA (LN1 to LN4) or Dutch (grade 3/4) grading system (Vonderheid et al. 1994). The NCI grading system defines LN1 to LN2 as not involved (Dutch N1) and LN3 and LN4 as involved in CTCL; LN3 denotes clusters of cerebriform cells without effacement, and LN4 shows effacement by tumor cells corresponding to N3 and N4 of the Dutch grading system, respectively (Sausville et al. 1985; Olsen et al. 2007). Figure 6.16 illustrates varying degrees of involvement of lymph nodes of patients with mycosis fungoides. In addition to

routine histologic examination, a portion of the lymph node should be processed for immunohistochemistry, flow cytometry, and/or molecular genetic or cytogenetic analysis. A novel approach to identify occult tumor cells in lymph nodes is by the use of immunohistochemistry employing monoclonal antibodies against tumor-specific variable regions of the TCR. Figure 6.17 illustrates detection of occult tumor cells and highlighting of their nuclear irregularity by immunoperoxidase staining with a monoclonal antibody against Vbeta8 that was the variable region used during rearrangement of the TCR gene in this case of MF. The identification of a tissue immunostained detectable clone, i.e., Vbeta8 used by neoplastic cells in this particular case, can also be detected by flow cytometry on cell suspensions of lymph node (see Chap. 4). Because excisional lymph node biopsies put the patient at risk for sepsis, especially in erythrodermic

Fig. 6.16 Lymph nodes of MF patients. (**a**) Lymph node is partially effaced by infiltrate of mycosis fungoides cells highlighted by the *rectangle*. A residual germinal center and lymph node sinuses are seen. (**b**) Dermatopathic lymphade- nopathy, grade 1 (Dutch) and NCI grade LN1–LN2 with pale dermatopathic low-power appearance. (**c**) Dermatopathic lymph node with numerous pale-staining Langerhans cells and melanophages containing melanin pigment

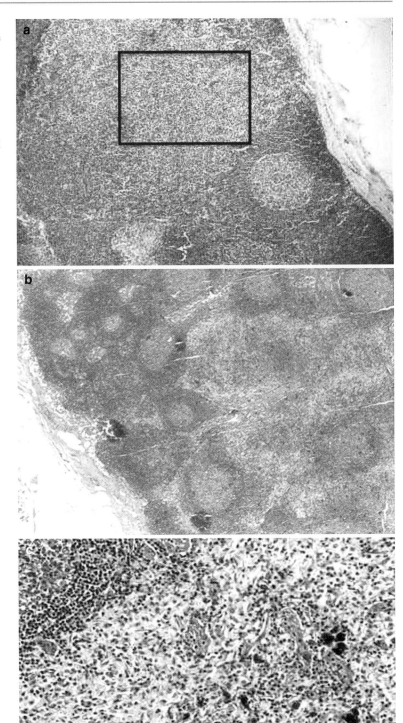

Fig.6.17 Immunoperoxidase stain revealing occult tumor cells with convoluted nuclei whose DNA had undergone rearrangement of the TCR using V*beta*8 in an N1 lymph node of MF patient

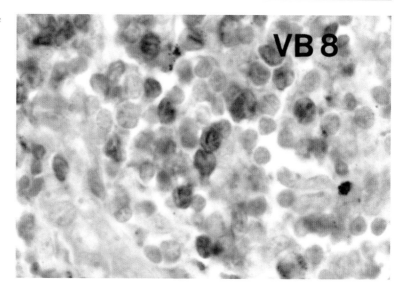

patients whose skin is often colonized with *Staphylococcus*, alternative methods to obtain nodal tissue (core biopsy or fine needle aspiration [FNA]) have been suggested as potential substitutes, particularly if combined with flow cytometry (Galindo et al. 2000). FNA can be facilitated by imaging methods (Pappa et al. 1996) but does *not* provide the histopathologic assessment of nodal architecture necessary for grading of nodal involvement.

Blood: The assessment of blood tumor burden in CTCL, based on morphologic features of the neoplastic cells alone (e.g., Sézary cell counts), is subject to interobserver variability, although absolute counts of Sézary cells continue to be used in staging at centers where such counts are routinely performed (Vonderheid et al. 2006). *B0* indicates absence of significant blood involvement; <5 % of peripheral blood lymphocytes are Sézary cells. *B1* indicates low tumor burden; >5 % of peripheral blood lymphocytes are typical Sézary cells but insufficient to meet criteria for B2. *B2* is high blood tumor burden, >1,000 Sézary cells in the blood with positive clone. The designation "a" or "b" following B0 or B1 indicates whether the clone is absent or present, respectively. The presence of a peripheral blood clone

in MF patients, if the same as that in the skin, has been found to have prognostic significance independent of the skin stage (Fraser-Andrews et al. 2000).

Other Laboratory Prognostic Biomarkers: We evaluated histologic and laboratory biomarkers to predict progression of early MF. We measured serum soluble CD30 (sCD30) in 96 patients with early MF followed up to 20 years. Patient serum levels were compared with those of healthy control subjects. Above normal serum sCD30 identified MF patients with worse survival (Kadin et al. 2012; Vonderheid et al. 2013).

To identify other prognostic markers for early MF patients, a cohort of 33 patients with MF at stages I to IIA who had subsequent progression of disease were compared against 70 stage-matched MF cases without observed progression. Significant factors that correlated with both disease progression and overall survival were (1) the presence of large Pautrier microabscesses (ten or more atypical lymphocytes) (Fig. 6.18), (2) the presence of atypical lymphocytes with hyperchromatic or vesicular nuclei in the dermal infiltrate (Fig. 6.19), (3) less than 20 % CD8+ cells in the dermal infiltrate, and (4) above normal (>122 U/ml) serum IgE level (Vonderheid et al. 2013) (see Table 6.2).

MF/SS cells express receptors for T-cell growth factor IL-2. The serum concentration of soluble alpha-chain receptor for interleukin-2 (sIL-2R) was determined in 101 patients with cutaneous T-cell lymphoma (CTCL). Serum concentration of sIL-2R correlated positively with CTCL tumor burden as determined by several clinical parameters (i.e., clinical subtype of disease, extent of skin involvement, T rating, and stage), serum lactate dehydrogenase concentration, and Sézary cell counts in

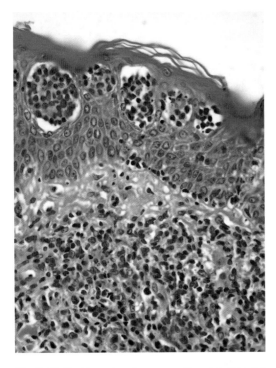

Fig. 6.18 Pautrier microabscesses with more than ten neoplastic lymphocytes are associated with a poor prognosis of patients with early MF (stages I to IIA)

Table 6.2 Independent prognostic factors in mycosis fungoides (Agar et al. 2010; Vonderheid et al. 2013)

Risk for disease progression
Large-cell transformation
Tumor distribution
Large Pautrier microabscesses (10 or more atypical lymphocytes)
Atypical lymphocytes with hyperchromatic or vesicular nuclei in the dermal infiltrate
Less than 20 % CD8+ cells in the dermal infiltrate
Above normal (>122 U/ml) serum IgE level
Poor survival
Advanced skin T stage
Peripheral blood T-cell clone without Sézary cells
Folliculotropic MF
Increased lactic dehydrogenase (LDH)
Improved survival
MF with lymphomatoid papulosis
MF, poikilodermatous subtype
Hypopigmented MF

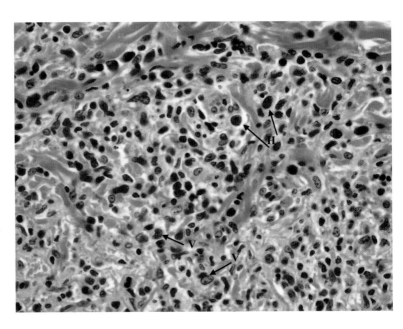

Fig. 6.19 Atypical lymphocytes with hyperchromatic (*H*) or vesicular (*V*) nuclei in the dermal infiltrate shown here are associated with a poor prognosis of patients with early MF (stages I to II)

erythrodermic disease (Wasik et al. 1996). The median value of sIL-2R in erythrodermic CTCL was more than threefold higher than that of classic MF. The proportion of patients with elevated sIL-2R concentration (>1,000 U/mL) also increased in CTCL in a similar fashion according to the clinical type of disease (MF patch phase, 15 %; MF plaque phase, 33 %; MF tumor phase, 47 %; and erythrodermic variants, 90 %).

Demonstration of T-cell clonality at the time of diagnosis provides prognostic information related to disease progression. Vega compared TCR gene rearrangements in separate disease sites (Vega et al. 2002). Patients who had the same gene rearrangement detected in multiple concurrent biopsy specimens at the time of diagnosis were more likely to have progressive disease than those who had different TCR gene rearrangements ($p = 0.04$).

Differential Diagnosis of Mycosis Fungoides

A current concept is that mycosis fungoides evolves from reactive inflammatory conditions (lymphoid infiltrates) transforming into neoplastic plaques and tumors (Burg et al. 2001). The latent time for diagnosis of MF decreased from about 5–6 years to about 3 years after the introduction of modern ancillary tools such as immunohistochemistry and molecular detection of TCR gene rearrangements (Reddy and Bhawan 1994). The presence of cerebriform cells and Pautrier microabscesses and absence of spongiosis strongly support a diagnosis of MF/SS. An abnormal immunophenotype and demonstration of T-cell clonality are useful adjuncts. However, sensitive PCR methods have revealed some cases of histologically nonspecific dermatitis to be consistent with "clonal dermatitis" (Wood et al. 1994). The pathologist may help the clinician by clearly indicating the level of certainty of the diagnosis as (1) suspicious for MF/SS, (2) consistent with MF/SS, and (3) diagnostic of MF/SS.

Smoller retrospectively reviewed histologic sections from 64 patients with mycosis fungoides (MF+) and compared the findings with sections from 47 patients who were biopsied to exclude

MF and were shown not to have the disease (MF−) (Smoller et al. 1995). Patients were selected as MF + or MF− independent of histologic findings based on the clinical course with at least 3 years of follow-up and immunophenotyping results. Following patient selection, at least two observers reviewed each slide without knowledge of final diagnosis and graded the intensity of approximately 25 histologic parameters. On univariate analysis, the following parameters were significant at beyond the $p = 0.01$ level: Pautrier abscesses, haloed lymphocytes, exocytosis, disproportionate epidermotropism, epidermal lymphocytes larger than dermal lymphocytes, hyperconvoluted intraepidermal lymphocytes, and lymphocytes aligned within the basal layer. Haloed lymphocytes (Figs. 6.3 and 6.4) proved to be the most robust discriminator of MF from non-MF on multivariate analysis. Few cases demonstrated all histologic features. Pautrier microabscesses were seen in only 37.5 % of their cases. The authors concluded that a combination of specific histologic parameters can be used to establish a microscopic diagnosis of MF without the necessity of confirmatory immunophenotyping in the vast majority of cases.

Table 6.3 lists the most common benign entities in the differential diagnosis of mycosis fungoides and Sézary syndrome. These and other nonmalignant epidermotropic T-cell disorders are discussed in greater detail below and further expanded into other entities in Chap. 5.

Inflammation/Nonspecific Dermatitis

A number of cutaneous inflammatory conditions can mimic early MF. Inchara and Rajalakshmi focused on the distinction of inflammatory conditions and early MF (Inchara and Rajalakshmi 2008). They performed a double-blind retrospective review of 50 cases clinically/histologically suspicious for MF. The diagnoses were established based on the response to treatment and follow-up. The slides were analyzed double-blinded by two observers independently. Twenty-eight histologic criteria were assessed and each criterion was graded. Univariate analysis was

Table 6.3 Benign conditions with epidermotropism mimicking MF/SS

Disorder	Distinguishing clinical features	Distinguishing pathologic features
Inflammation Chronic dermatitis	Eczema, contact allergens	Eosinophils, mast cells
Psoriasis	Extensor surfaces, elbows, knees, arthritis	Neutrophil abscesses, acanthosis
Lymphomatoid drug eruption	Drug history	Spongiosis Intraepidermal CD8+ T cells
Other interface dermatitides	Oral lesions in lichen planus; hemorrhagic papules in PLEVA, viral inclusions in infections	Lichenoid features: hydropic change and keratinocyte necrosis in basal layer
Benign erythroderma	Absence of nail dystrophy Uncommonly clonal by TCR gene analysis	Absence of band-like infiltrate and cerebriform cells
Lichen aureus	Asymmetric involvement of lower extremities Clonal in ½ cases	Lichenoid papules and plaques with a golden to purplish color

performed on the results. Of the 28 criteria used, the following 15 achieved significance on univariate analysis: disproportionate epidermotropism, tagging of lymphocytes along the basal layer, haloed lymphocytes, convoluted lymphocytes, Pautrier abscesses, larger epidermal lymphocytes, wiry dermal collagen, absence of edema, eccrine infiltration, folliculotropism, follicular mucin, involvement of papillary and reticular dermis, monomorphous infiltrates, and atypia of dermal lymphocytes. The criteria that were 100 % specific for MF included convoluted lymphocytes, eccrine infiltration, and follicular mucin. Absence of edema was 100 % sensitive and specific in distinguishing MF from its inflammatory mimics.

Interface Dermatitis

Interface dermatitis is characterized by a prominent mixed mononuclear cell infiltrate which obscures the dermal-epidermal junction. Epidermal cell damage with keratinocyte death and hydropic changes is seen which is most pronounced at the basal cell layer. Civatte bodies representing damaged keratinocytes are formed in the epidermis and colloid bodies in dermis (Fig. 6.20). Cytotoxic lymphocytes with a Th1 cytokine profile secreting interferon (IFN) predominate. Benign disorders with an interface pat-

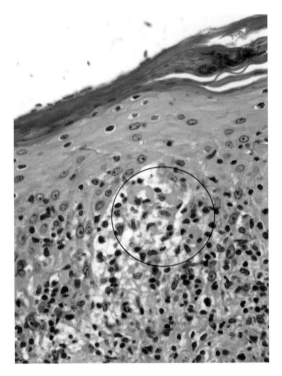

Fig. 6.20 Interface dermatitis with pink colloid bodies (*circled*) at the dermal-epidermal junction

tern include lichen planus, pityriasis lichenoides et varioliformis acuta (PLEVA) and pityriasis lichenoides chronica (PLC), fixed drug eruption, lichen aureus, cutaneous lupus, toxic epidermal necrosis/Stevens-Johnson syndrome, and lymphomatoid drug reaction (Fig. 6.21). It should be

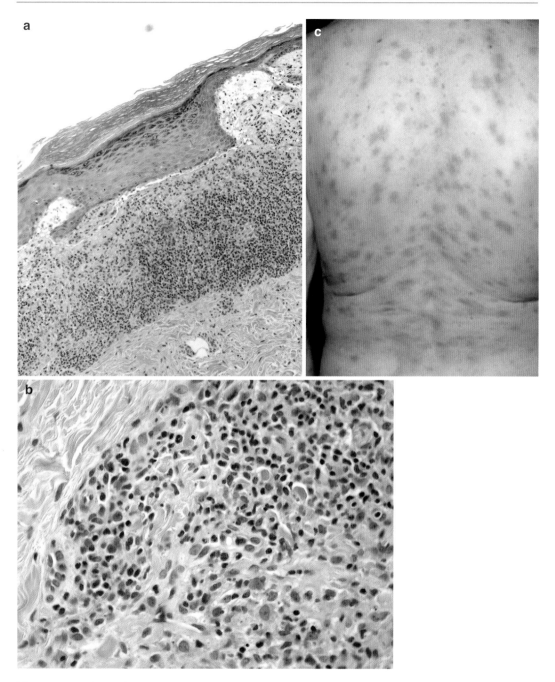

Fig. 6.21 Lymphomatoid drug reaction. (**a**) Dense band-like subepidermal lymphocytic infiltrate. (**b**) Polymorphous infiltrate with eosinophils. (**c**) Clinical picture

appreciated that a subset of patients with MF can present with lichenoid changes (Guitart et al. 1997). The pathologic features of lichenoid MF may have a striking resemblance to lichen planus and other lichenoid dermatitides (see Chap. 5). Lymphocyte atypia and prominent basal cell layer epidermotropism distinguish lichenoid MF from lichen planus.

Psoriasis

A common condition affecting approximately three million persons in the United States. Psoriasis is an immune-mediated disorder involving Th1, Th17, and Th22 cells which attract neutrophils and inhibit terminal differentiation of keratinocytes, leading to marked acanthosis and neutrophilic abscesses. There are five types of psoriasis: plaque, guttate, inverse, pustular, and erythrodermic. The most common form, plaque psoriasis, is commonly seen as red and white hues of scaly patches appearing on the top layer of the epidermis. They are most prominent on extensor surfaces, e.g., elbows and knees, but can affect any area, including the scalp, palms of hands and soles of feet, genitals, and scalp. Local psoriatic changes can be triggered by an injury to the skin known as the Koebner phenomenon. Fingernails and toenails are frequently affected (psoriatic nail dystrophy) and can be seen as an isolated sign. Psoriasis can also cause inflammation of the joints, i.e., psoriatic arthritis. Itching is characteristic. Severe cases are treated with biologicals that block tumor necrosis factor (TNF) and other cytokine receptors. Psoriatic lesions lack the nuclear atypia of MF; Pautrier microabscesses are not seen.

Anaplastic Large-Cell Lymphoma

For patients presenting with tumors (T3), it is important to differentiate large-cell transformation in MF (LCT-MF) from cutaneous ALCL (cALCL) and other non-MF subtypes of CTCL. In classic MF, tumor lesions generally develop in the presence of a patch or plaque disease. cALCL lack cerebriform cells and a spectrum of cell sizes, features typical of tumor-stage MF (see Figs. 6.8 and 12.12). Epidermotropism is more common in tumor-stage MF than in ALCL. Most cases of LCT-MF can be distinguished from cALCL because the typical LCT-MF does not meet combined cytologic and immunologic criteria for cALCL, i.e., most large-cell tumors arising in MF do not exhibit >75 % anaplastic CD30+ large cells. Only about 40 % have >75 % CD30+ cells and

most of those display much more heterogeneous cytology than typical cALCL. Among two series of 100 and 45 patients with LCT, the proportion of cases with >75 % CD30+ large cells was 39 and 16 %, respectively (Benner et al. 2012; Vergier et al. 2000). These cases would be difficult to distinguish from cALCL. Overall, the LCT-MF cases that truly overlap with cALCL based on combined cytologic/CD30 features amount to <10 % of MF patients with large-cell tumors.

Benign Erythroderma

Benign erythroderma can closely resemble Sézary syndrome in clinical appearance. Histopathology is helpful in making the distinction. Sentis et al. reviewed histologic sections from 11 patients with Sézary syndrome and compared them with those from four patients with erythrodermic mycosis fungoides and 24 patients with a benign form of erythroderma, including 15 patients with chronic dermatitis, four with a generalized drug eruption, and five with an erythrodermic psoriasis. The most important discriminating histologic feature in patients with Sézary syndrome was the presence of a monotonous band-like or perivascular infiltrate in the papillary dermis, mainly composed of large cerebriform mononuclear cells, as seen in 7 of 11 Sézary syndrome patients (Sentis et al. 1986). Pautrier microabscesses were observed in 7 of 11 Sézary syndrome patients and two of four patients with erythrodermic mycosis fungoides, but not in any of the patients with a benign form of erythroderma; their presence was therefore considered a reliable criterion in differentiating erythrodermic cutaneous T-cell lymphoma from benign forms of erythroderma. TCR beta gene rearrangement analysis on peripheral blood lymphocytes (PBL) is a sensitive and highly specific technique, that may contribute significantly to the differential diagnosis of patients with erythroderma. Bakels performed T-cell receptor beta (TCR beta) gene rearrangement analysis on PBL from 32 patients with erythroderma, including ten patients with SS, three patients with another type of cutaneous T-cell lymphoma, and 19 patients with a benign erythroderma (Bakels et al. 1991). Clonal TCR beta gene rearrangements were found in eight of ten patients with SS, one T-cell chronic lymphocytic leukemia (T-CLL) patient, one of two patients with erythrodermic mycosis fungoides, and only 1 of 19 patients from the benign erythroderma group. In the two "false-negative" cases of SS, clonal TCR beta gene rearrangements were detected in PBL obtained during follow-up. Because both "false-positive" and "false-negative" results may occur, the results of gene rearrangement analysis should always be considered in conjunction with clinical, histologic, and immunophenotypical data (Bakels et al. 1991).

Lichen Aureus (Pigmented Purpura Dermatoses)

Lichen aureus is a localized variant of pigmented purpuric dermatitis (PPD). It occurs in adults and children in whom there is a tendency for slow, spontaneous improvement and resolution (Gelmetti et al. 1991). Association with MF is controversial. The eruption consists of lichenoid papules and plaques with a golden to purplish color, and the histology reveals a dense and band-like infiltrate hugging the epidermis (Fig. 6.22). It consists of lymphocytes and histiocytes, commonly with extravasation of erythrocytes. The eruption is asymptomatic and has a prolonged course. Fink-Puches et al. reviewed clinicopathologic features of 23 patients with lichen aureus. Lesions were asymmetrically localized on one area of the body (mostly one extremity) and were characterized histologically by dense, band-like lymphocytic infiltrates. A monoclonal T-cell population was detected in half of the cases. There was no relationship between the presence or absence of monoclonality and patient status at follow-up assessments (Fink-Puches et al. 2008).

Epidermotropic T-Cell Neoplasms Simulating MF and SS

Table 6.4 lists the epidermotropic T-cell neoplasms in the differential diagnosis with mycosis

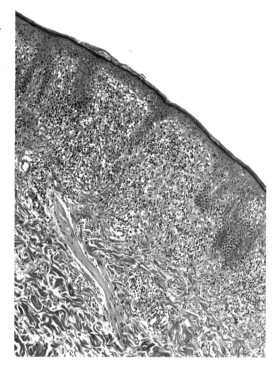

Fig. 6.22 Lichen aureus—a band-like lymphocytic infiltrate with extravasated erythrocytes hugging the epidermis

fungoides and Sézary syndrome. Lymphomatoid papulosis (LyP) is a clonal CD30+ primary cutaneous lymphoproliferative disorders and therefore is included in the discussion of epidermotropic T-cell malignancies.

Lymphomatoid Papulosis (LyP) Type B

LyP type B is characterized by epidermotropic atypical medium-sized lymphocytes which may have cerebriform nuclei (Fig. 6.23). There is some controversy as to whether the atypical cells can be CD30+. Willemze states that LyP type B is CD30 negative, whereas in our experience, some cases are CD30+. Lesions are very difficult to distinguish from patch or papular lesions of MF. The distinction of MF and LyP type B is mainly clinical; LyP lesions are papules that regress spontaneously. LyP type B can also be difficult to distinguish from pityriasis lichenoides chronica (PLC). Necrotic keratinocytes and

Table 6.4 Comparison of neoplastic epidermotropic diseases

Entity	Clinical	Pathology	Immunophenotype	Genetics/molecular
Mycosis fungoides	Generalized patches, plaques, tumors	Cerebriform cells. Pautrier microabscesses in one-third	CD4+ (95 %)	Multiple chromosomal aberrations. Clonal TCR, may be oligoclonal, JunB overexpressed
Sézary syndrome	Triad of erythroderma, lymphadenopathy, and leukemic cells (>1,000/ml³)	Inflammation, may not be diagnostic Sézary cells in peripheral blood	CD4+, CD7–	Multiple chromosomal aberrations. Clonal TCR in contrast to benign erythroderma
Pagetoid reticulosis	Localized lesions, often acral	Extensive epidermal infiltration	CD4 or CD8+, may be CD30+	Data not available
Cutaneous lesions of HTLV-1 adult T-cell leukemia/lymphoma	Rash, papules, or nodules; "flower" cells in blood	Epidermal and dermal infiltrates, multilobated nuclei	FoxP3, CD25, CD4+, may be CD30+	Clonal integration of HTLV-1
Aggressive CD8+ epidermotropic T-cell lymphoma	Nodulo-eruptive cutaneous and mucosal lesions	Band-like infiltrates of immunoblasts, showing a diffuse infiltration of an acanthotic epidermis with variable degrees of spongiosis, intraepidermal blistering, and necrosis	CD8+, CD7+, TIA-1+, CD2–	Clonal TCR
Lymphomatoid papulosis, type B	Self-healing papules	Cerebriform cells in epidermis and dermis	CD4+, CD30 often weak or absent	No data
Lymphomatoid papulosis associated with 6p25.3 rearrangement	Elderly patients with self-healing papules	Biphasic epidermal LyP type B and dermal type C pattern	CD3+, may be double negative for CD4 and CD8 Biphasic CD30, weaker in epidermis	Rearrangement of locus at 6p25.3 involving IRF4 and DUSP22

Fig. 6.23 Lymphomatoid papulosis type B. (**a**) LyP type B with epidermotropic cerebriform cells closely resembles MF histologically. (**b**) The distinction is made by the clinical appearance of regressing papules as shown here

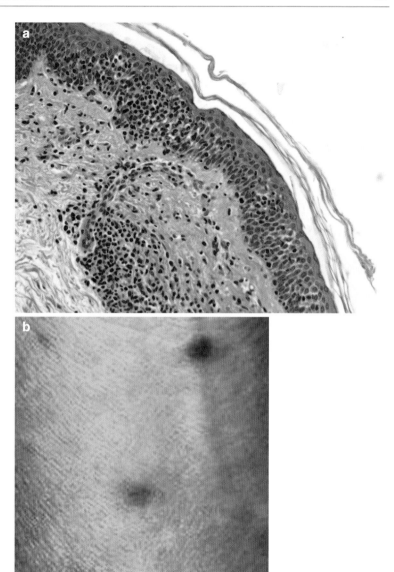

extravasation of erythrocytes seen in PLC are uncommon in LyP type B. PLC tends to affect younger patients than LyP and is unlikely to coexist with lesions of LyP type A which frequently occur together with LyP type B.

Lymphomatoid Papulosis Associated with 6p25.3 Rearrangement

This recently recognized subtype of LyP has a dual epidermal and dermal component. This LyP subtype is illustrated in Chap. 12. A characteristic and reproducible finding is the presence of an extensive atypical lymphoid infiltrate in the epidermis simulating lesions of pagetoid reticulosis and LyP type D (illustrated in Chap. 12). The intraepidermal component is largely confined to the area directly overlying the dermal nodule. The atypical cells in the dermis are medium- to large-sized and contained abundant, finely granular cytoplasm. Cells with reniform nuclei reminiscent of the "hallmark" cells of ALCL (Benharroch et al. 1998), are seen in all cases, but are rare (Karai et al. 2013). Most dermal tumor cells are smaller and have more hyperchromatic nuclei than those typically seen in ALCL. CD30 staining shows an unusual, biphasic pattern in most cases, with strong diffuse staining in the dermis and weaker staining in the epidermis. Most patients described to date are over age 50 with a male predominance.

Primary Cutaneous CD8-Positive Aggressive Epidermotropic Cytotoxic T-Cell Lymphoma

This is a clinically striking lymphoma which has features of multiple eruptive papules, nodules, and tumor, often showing central necrosis and ulceration. We described five patients who had rapidly progressive disease characterized by distinctive papulonodular skin lesions (four patients), involvement of palms or soles (four patients) or oral cavity (two patients), and poor response to standard topical therapy (four patients) (Agnarsson et al. 1990). Histologic examination showed extensive epidermotropism associated with pagetoid features (Fig. 6.24). Immunoperoxidase studies revealed a novel aberrant T-cell phenotype characterized by CD8 and lack of expression of CD4 and CD2 but positive staining for CD3 and CD7. In contrast, the neoplastic cells from four patients with clinically more chronic CD8+ cutaneous T-cell lymphoma, although also commonly epidermotropic, had a different aberrant T-cell phenotype similar to that often seen in CD4+ mycosis fungoides; that is, there was lack of

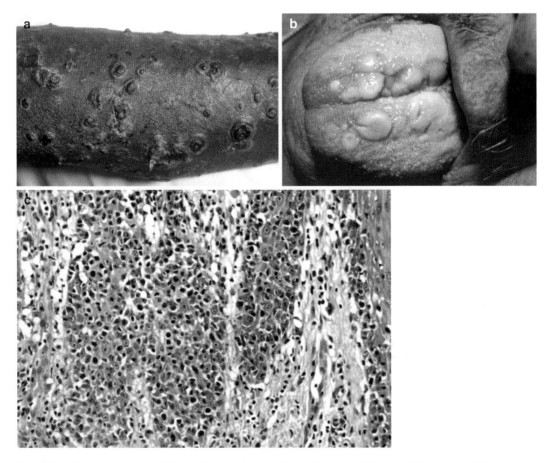

Fig. 6.24 Primary cutaneous CD8-positive aggressive epidermotropic cytotoxic T-cell lymphoma. (**a**) Nodular eruptions on arm. (**b**) Nodular lesions on tongue. (**c**) Pagetoid pattern. (**d**) Immunoblastic cells. (**e**) Mitoses and karyorrhexis (Reprinted from Agnarsson et al. (1990) with permission from Elsevier)

Fig. 6.24 (continued)

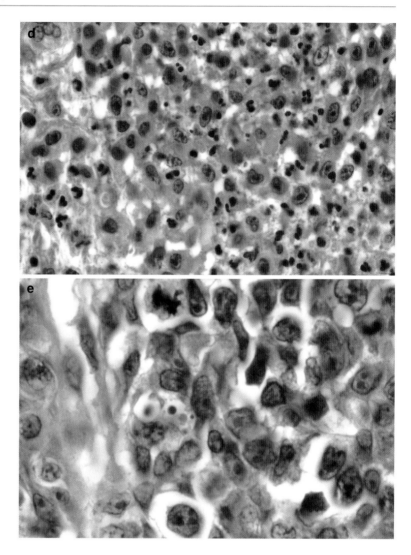

expression of CD7 but a positive reaction to staining for CD2. In two cases the tumor cells acquired the CD7 antigen or lost the CD2 antigen with progression of the disease (Agnarsson et al. 1990). Our findings have been extended by Berti et al. who reported eight patients whose clinical characteristics included presentation with generalized patches, plaques, papulonodules, and tumors mimicking disseminated pagetoid reticulosis; metastatic spread to unusual sites, such as the lung, testis, central nervous system, and oral cavity, but not to the lymph nodes; and an aggressive course (median survival of 32 months). Histologically, these lymphomas were characterized by band-like infiltrates consisting of pleomorphic T cells or immunoblasts, showing a diffuse infiltration of an acanthotic epidermis with variable degrees of spongiosis, intraepidermal blistering, and necrosis. The neoplastic cells showed a high Ki-67 proliferation index and expression of CD3, CD8, CD7, CD45RA, TCR betaF1, and TIA-1 markers, whereas CD2 and CD5 were frequently lost. Expression of TIA-1 pointed out that these lymphomas are derived from a cytotoxic T-cell subset. The results of this and other studies reviewed herein suggest that these strongly epidermotropic primary cutaneous CD8+ cytotoxic T-cell lymphomas represent a distinct type of CTCL with an aggressive clinical behavior (Berti et al. 1999). Recent studies showing overlap of these cases with primary cutaneous gamma-delta T-cell lymphoma (PCGD-TCL), using paraffin reactive anti-delta, are further discussed in Chap. 10.

Primary Cutaneous Gamma-Delta T-Cell Lymphoma (PCGD-TCL)

PCGD-TCL is a rare lymphoma composed of clonal activated T$\gamma\delta$ cells with a cytotoxic pheno-type. Patients typically present with generalized skin lesions predominantly affecting the extremities. Mucosal lesions are common. There are three major histologic types of cutaneous lesions—epidermotropic, dermal, and subcutaneous (Fig. 6.25). Epidermotropism is associated with patch/plaque lesions. Deep dermal and subcutaneous lesions are associated with necrosis. Subcutaneous cases may show rimming of fat cells but also show dermal and epidermal involvement. Neoplastic cells are

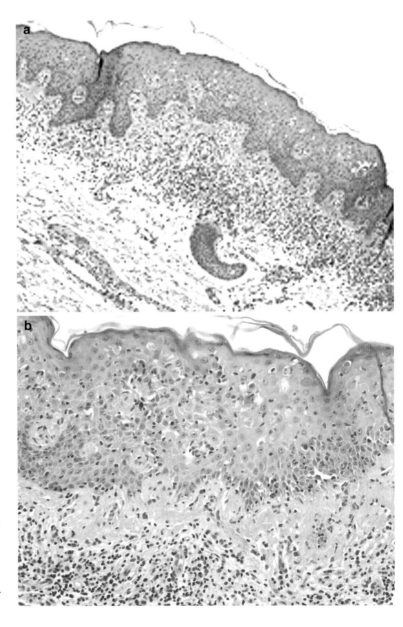

Fig. 6.25 Epidermotropic gamma-delta T-cell lymphoma. (**a**) Band-like infiltrate at DE junction. (**b**) Exocytosis of lymphocytes with keratinocyte necrosis and formation of pink Civatte bodies. (**c**) CD3. (**d**) CD4 (tumor cells unstained). (**e**) Granzyme B

Fig. 6.25 (continued)

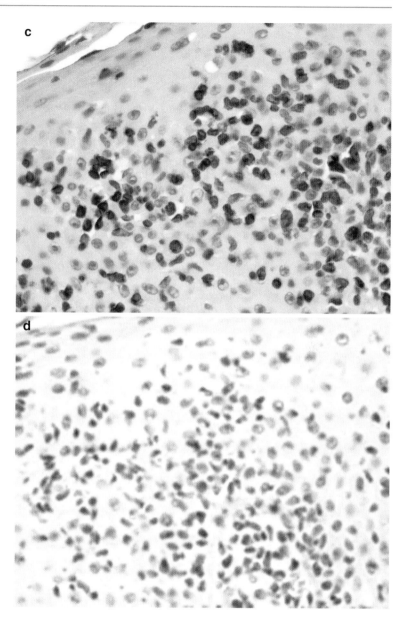

Fig. 6.25 (continued)

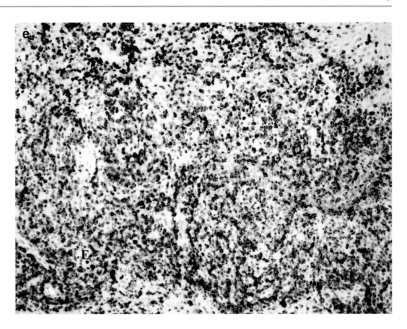

medium- to large-sized with clumped chromatin. Apoptosis and necrosis are common. Neoplastic cells express cytotoxic proteins and are usually negative for both CD4 and CD8 but may be CD8+. Lesions are resistant to radiation and multiagent chemotherapy. Prognosis is poor and patient median survival is 15 months.

Cutaneous Lesions in HTLV-1 Adult T-Cell Lymphoma/Leukemia

Cutaneous lesions occur in more than 50 % of patients with ATLL. Lesions may be erythematous rashes, papules, or nodules. Chronic ATLL is often associated with an exfoliative skin rash. Epidermotropism with Pautrier microabscesses are common and pose a differential diagnosis with MF. Distinction of ATLL from MF is multifactorial. ATLL patients are mostly from Japan or the Caribbean. Serology reveals antibodies against HTLV-1. Peripheral blood shows multilobated "flower cells" (Fig. 6.26). ATLL patients often have hypercalcemia. Opportunistic infections of the skin are frequent as a result of an impaired immune response. This is due to the FoxP3 phenotype of the neoplastic T cells which function as immunosuppressive regulatory T cells. Tumor cells in most cases are CD4+ and CD25+ and in some cases may be CD30+, but negative for cytotoxic proteins and ALK oncoprotein.

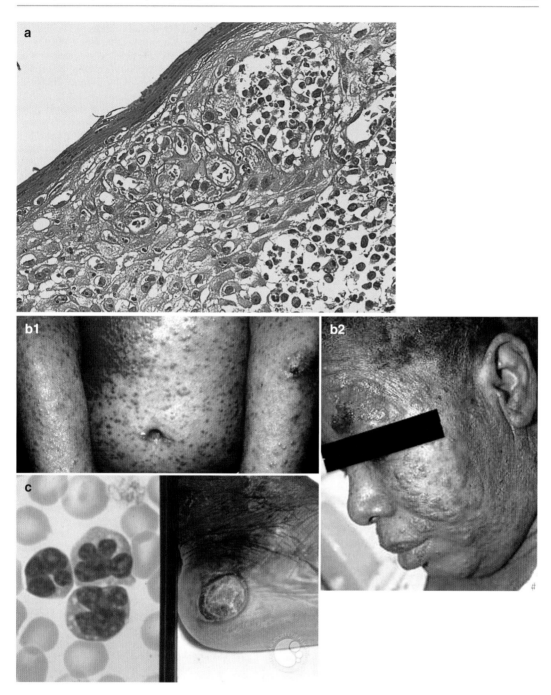

Fig. 6.26 HTLV-1+ adult T-cell leukemia/lymphoma (ATLL). (**a**) Epidermotropic infiltrate of ATLL cells forming Pautrier microabscess that could be confused with mycosis fungoides. (**b1**) Haitian ATLL patient with extensive maculopapular rash on trunk and extremities. (**b2**) Facial nodules of a Caribbean native with ATLL. (**c**) *Left* – Typical "flower cells" of ATLL in peripheral blood. Note that nuclear lobes of ATLL cells are more exaggerated than those of Sézary cells. *Right* – Ulceration of skin on heel of patient from Caribbean region. ATLL is associated with human T-cell leukemia virus type 1 (HTLV-1). It was first described in Japanese patients but later was found to be also endemic in the Caribbean region (This image was originally published in ASH Image Bank. Marshall Kadin. Adult T-cell Leukemia - 1. ASH Image Bank. 2005; 00002084 © the American Society of Hematology)

References

Agar NS, Wedgeworth E, Crichton S, Mitchell TJ, Cox M, Ferreira S, et al. Survival outcomes and prognostic factors in mycosis fungoides/Sezary syndrome: validation of the revised International Society for Cutaneous Lymphomas/European Organisation for Research and Treatment of Cancer staging proposal. J Clin Oncol. 2010;28:4730–9.

Agnarsson BA, Vonderheid EC, Kadin ME. Cutaneous T cell lymphoma with suppressor/cytotoxic (CD8) phenotype: identification of rapidly progressive and chronic subtypes. J Am Acad Dermatol. 1990;22: 569–77.

Bakels V, van Oostveen JW, Gordijn RL, Walboomers JM, Meijer CJ, Willemze R. Diagnostic value of T-cell receptor beta gene rearrangement analysis on peripheral blood lymphocytes of patients with erythroderma. J Invest Dermatol. 1991;97:782–6.

Benharroch D, Meguerian-Bedoyan Z, Lamant L, Amin C, Brugieres L, Terrier-Lacombe MJ, et al. ALK-positive lymphoma: a single disease with a broad spectrum of morphology. Blood 1998;91:2076–84.

Benner MF, Jansen PM, Vermeer MH, Willemze R. Prognostic factors in transformed mycosis fungoides: a retrospective analysis of 100 cases. Blood. 2012; 119:1643–9.

Bernengo MG, Novelli M, Quaglino P, Lisa F, De Matteis A, Savoia P, et al. The relevance of the CD4+ CD26- subset in the identification of circulating Sezary cells. Br J Dermatol. 2001;144:125–35.

Berti E, Tomasini D, Vermeer MH, Meijer CJ, Alessi E, Willemze R. Primary cutaneous CD8-positive epidermotropic cytotoxic T cell lymphomas. A distinct clinicopathological entity with an aggressive clinical behavior. Am J Pathol. 1999;155:483–92.

Borowitz MJ, Weidner A, Olsen EA, Picker LJ. Abnormalities of circulating T-cell subpopulations in patients with cutaneous T-cell lymphoma: cutaneous lymphocyte-associated antigen expression on T cells correlates with extent of disease. Leukemia. 1993; 7:859–63.

Burg G, Dummer R, Haeffner A, Kempf W, Kadin M. From inflammation to neoplasia: mycosis fungoides evolves from reactive inflammatory conditions (lymphoid infiltrates) transforming into neoplastic plaques and tumors. Arch Dermatol. 2001;137:949–52.

Campbell JJ, Clark RA, Watanabe R, Kupper TS. Sezary syndrome and mycosis fungoides arise from distinct T-cell subsets: a biologic rationale for their distinct clinical behaviors. Blood. 2010;116:767–71.

Fink-Puches R, Wolf P, Kerl H, Cerroni L. Lichen aureus: clinicopathologic features, natural history, and relationship to mycosis fungoides. Arch Dermatol. 2008;144:1169–73.

Fraser-Andrews EA, Woolford AJ, Russell-Jones R, Seed PT, Whittaker SJ. Detection of a peripheral blood T cell clone is an independent prognostic marker in mycosis fungoides. J Invest Dermatol. 2000;114:117–21.

Galindo LM, Garcia FU, Hanau CA, Lessin SR, Jhala N, Bigler RD, et al. Fine-needle aspiration biopsy in the evaluation of lymphadenopathy associated with cutaneous T-cell lymphoma (mycosis fungoides/ Sezary syndrome). Am J Clin Pathol. 2000;113: 865–71.

Gelmetti C, Cerri D, Grimalt R. Lichen aureus in childhood. Pediatr Dermatol. 1991;8:280–3.

Guitart J, Peduto M, Caro WA, Roenigk HH. Lichenoid changes in mycosis fungoides. J Am Acad Dermatol. 1997;36:417–22.

Inchara YK, Rajalakshmi T. Early mycosis fungoides vs. inflammatory mimics: how reliable is histology? Indian J Dermatol Venereol Leprol. 2008;74:462–6.

Jackow CM, Cather JC, Hearne V, Asano AT, Musser JM, Duvic M. Association of erythrodermic cutaneous T-cell lymphoma, superantigen-positive Staphylococcus aureus, and oligoclonal T-cell receptor V beta gene expansion. Blood. 1997;89:32–40.

Jones D, Dang NH, Duvic M, Washington LT, Huh YO. Absence of CD26 expression is a useful marker for diagnosis of T-cell lymphoma in peripheral blood. Am J Clin Pathol. 2001;115:885–92.

Kadin ME, Pavlov IY, Delgado JC, Vonderheid EC. High soluble CD30, CD25, and IL-6 may identify patients with worse survival in CD30+ cutaneous lymphomas and early mycosis fungoides. J Invest Dermatol. 2012;132:703–10.

Karai LJ, Kadin ME, Hsi ED, Sluzevich JC, Ketterling RP, Knudson RA, et al. Chromosomal rearrangements of 6p25.3 define a new subtype of lymphomatoid papulosis. Am J Surg Pathol. 2013;37:1173–81.

Karenko L, Sarna S, Kahkonen M, Ranki A. Chromosomal abnormalities in relation to clinical disease in patients with cutaneous T-cell lymphoma: a 5-year follow-up study. Br J Dermatol. 2003;148:55–64.

Kempf W, Ostheeren-Michaelis S, Paulli M, Lucioni M, Wechsler J, Audring H, et al. Granulomatous mycosis fungoides and granulomatous slack skin: a multicenter study of the Cutaneous Lymphoma Histopathology Task Force Group of the European Organization For Research and Treatment of Cancer (EORTC). Arch Dermatol. 2008;144:1609–17.

Kodama K, Fink-Puches R, Massone C, Kerl H, Cerroni L. Papular mycosis fungoides: a new clinical variant of early mycosis fungoides. J Am Acad Dermatol. 2005;52:694–8.

Mao X, Orchard G, Lillington DM, Russell-Jones R, Young BD, Whittaker SJ. Amplification and overexpression of JUNB is associated with primary cutaneous T-cell lymphomas. Blood. 2003;101:1513–9.

Murphy M, Signoretti S, Kadin ME, Loda M. Detection of TCR-gamma gene rearrangements in early mycosis fungoides by non-radioactive PCR-SSCP. J Cutan Pathol. 2000;27:228–34.

Olsen E, Vonderheid E, Pimpinelli N, Willemze R, Kim Y, Knobler R, et al. Revisions to the staging and classification of mycosis fungoides and Sezary syndrome: a proposal of the International Society for Cutaneous

Lymphomas (ISCL) and the cutaneous lymphoma task force of the European Organization of Research and Treatment of Cancer (EORTC). Blood. 2007;110: 1713–22.

Pappa VI, Hussain HK, Reznek RH, Whelan J, Norton AJ, Wilson AM, et al. Role of image-guided core-needle biopsy in the management of patients with lymphoma. J Clin Oncol. 1996;14:2427–30.

Pimpinelli N, Olsen EA, Santucci M, Vonderheid E, Haeffner AC, Stevens S, et al. Defining early mycosis fungoides. J Am Acad Dermatol. 2005;53:1053–63.

Reddy K, Bhawan J. Histologic mimickers of mycosis fungoides: a review. J Cutan Pathol 2007;34:519–26.

Rizzo FA, Vilar EG, Pantaleao L, Fonseca EC, Magrin PF, Henrique-Xavier M, et al. Mycosis fungoides in children and adolescents: a report of six cases with predominantly hypopigmentation, along with a literature review. Dermatol Online J. 2012;18:5.

Santucci M, Biggeri A, Feller AC, Massi D, Burg G. Efficacy of histologic criteria for diagnosing early mycosis fungoides: an EORTC cutaneous lymphoma study group investigation. European Organization for Research and Treatment of Cancer. Am J Surg Pathol. 2000;24:40–50.

Sausville EA, Worsham GF, Matthews MJ, Makuch RW, Fischmann AB, Schechter GP, et al. Histologic assessment of lymph nodes in mycosis fungoides/Sezary syndrome (cutaneous T-cell lymphoma): clinical correlations and prognostic import of a new classification system. Hum Pathol 1985;16:1098–1109.

Sentis HJ, Willemze R, Scheffer E. Histopathologic studies in Sezary syndrome and erythrodermic mycosis fungoides: a comparison with benign forms of erythroderma. J Am Acad Dermatol. 1986;15: 1217–26.

Smoller BR, Bishop K, Glusac E, Kim YH, Hendrickson M. Reassessment of histologic parameters in the diagnosis of mycosis fungoides. Am J Surg Pathol. 1995;19:1423–30.

Sokolowska-Wojdylo M, Wenzel J, Gaffal E, Steitz J, Roszkiewicz J, Bieber T, et al. Absence of CD26 expression on skin-homing CLA+CD4+ T lymphocytes in peripheral blood is a highly sensitive marker for early diagnosis and therapeutic monitoring of patients with Sezary syndrome. Clin Exp Dermatol. 2005;30:702–6.

Vega F, Luthra R, Medeiros LJ, Dunmire V, Lee SJ, Duvic M, et al. Clonal heterogeneity in mycosis fungoides and its relationship to clinical course. Blood. 2002;100:3369–73.

Vergier B, de Muret A, Beylot-Barry M, Vaillant L, Ekouevi D, Chene G, et al. Transformation of mycosis fungoides: clinicopathological and prognostic features of 45 cases. French Study Group of Cutaneous Lymphomas. Blood. 2000;95:2212–8.

Vonderheid EC. On the diagnosis of erythrodermic cutaneous T-cell lymphoma. J Cutan Pathol. 2006;33 Suppl 1:27–42.

Vonderheid EC, Diamond LW, van Vloten WA, Scheffer E, Meijer CJ, Cashell AW, et al. Lymph node classification systems in cutaneous T-cell lymphoma. Evidence for the utility of the working formulation of non-Hodgkin's lymphomas for clinical usage. Cancer. 1994;73:207–18.

Vonderheid EC, Pavlov I, Delgado JC, Martins TB, Telang GH, Hess AD, et al. Prognostic factors and risk stratification early mycosis fungoides. Leuk Lymphoma. 2013;55:44–50.

Vonderheid EC, Pena J, Nowell P. Sezary cell counts in erythrodermic cutaneous T-cell lymphoma: implications for prognosis and staging. Leuk Lymphoma. 2006;47:1841–56.

Vowels BR, Lessin SR, Cassin M, Jaworsky C, Benoit B, Wolfe JT, et al. Th2 cytokine mRNA expression in skin in cutaneous T-cell lymphoma. J Invest Dermatol. 1994;103:669–73.

Wasik MA, Vonderheid EC, Bigler RD, Marti R, Lessin SR, Polansky M, et al. Increased serum concentration of the soluble interleukin-2 receptor in cutaneous T-cell lymphoma. Clinical and prognostic implications. Arch Dermatol. 1996;132:42–7.

Wolfe JT, Chooback L, Finn DT, Jaworsky C, Rook AH, Lessin SR. Large-cell transformation following detection of minimal residual disease in cutaneous T-cell lymphoma: molecular and in situ analysis of a single neoplastic T-cell clone expressing the identical T-cell receptor. J Clin Oncol. 1995;13:1751–7.

Wood GS, Tung RM, Haeffner AC, Crooks CF, Liao S, Orozco R, et al. Detection of clonal T-cell receptor gamma gene rearrangements in early mycosis fungoides/Sezary syndrome by polymerase chain reaction and denaturing gradient gel electrophoresis (PCR/DGGE). J Invest Dermatol. 1994;103:34–41.

Zhang Y, Wang Y, Yu R, Huang Y, Su M, Xiao C, et al. Molecular markers of early-stage mycosis fungoides. J Invest Dermatol. 2012;132:1698–706.

Nodular B-Lymphocyte Reactive Patterns: Reactive Nodular B-Cell Pattern

Phyu P. Aung and Meera Mahalingam

Introduction

Overview of B-Lymphocyte Ontogeny

All B lymphocytes arise in the bone marrow from a stem cell. Once formed, B lymphocytes mature in the following stages: *a pro-B lymphocyte* followed by a pre-B lymphocyte (the earliest cell type to synthesize detectable Ig gene products such as the μ heavy chains), followed by the immature IgM-bearing B lymphocyte, followed by the mature antigen-responsive B lymphocyte which produces both membrane IgM and IgD, and followed by the activated B lymphocyte which proliferates and differentiates to produce immunoglobulin in a secreted form. All, except the last two stages, which are antigen-induced, are antigen-independent cells. Stem cells and pro-/pre-B lymphocytes are only seen in primary hematopoietic tissues (such as bone marrow and fetal liver), while immature as well as mature B lymphocytes are found in the bone marrow, peripheral blood, and secondary lymphoid organs. Activated and antibody-secreting

B lymphocytes are predominantly seen in the peripheral blood and secondary lymphoid organs (Abbas et al. 1991).

Immunophenotypically, surface markers characterize each of these stages. Pro-B cells express the following immunomarkers: TdT, Pax-5, CD10, CD19, CD40, CD34, and MHC class II antigens; pre-B lymphocytes express TdT, CD79a, CD79b, Pax-5, CD10, CD19, CD40, CD34, CD43, and CD22; mature B lymphocytes express CD19, CD20, CD21, CD23, CD40, and MHC class II antigens (but no longer express TdT, CD10, and CD34) and activated B lymphocytes lose expression of sIgD and CD21 but express CD25, CD80, and CD86 (Fig. 7.1) (LeBien and Tedder 2008).

Historical Overview and Clarification of Nomenclature

Conceptually, the definition of pseudolymphoma is somewhat confusing as the term lacks specificity primarily because it does not provide clues about the etiopathogenesis. Confounding issues include the fact that identification of the antigenic stimulus may not be helpful as more often than not the "process" continues long after the initiating event. The term, coined initially to describe a process in the late 1800s, was used to denote an entity that had a banal clinical course but histopathologically mimicked lymphoma. Since its initial description, the process has been identified in several other organ systems such as the breast,

P.P. Aung, MD, PhD
Dermatopathology Section, Department of Dermatology, Boston Medical Center, Boston University School of Medicine, Boston, MA, USA

M. Mahalingam, MD, PhD, FRCPath (✉)
Dermatopathology Section, Department of Dermatology, Boston University School of Medicine, 609 Albany Street, J 401, Boston, MA 02118, USA
e-mail: mmahalin@bu.edu

H.D. Cualing et al. (eds.), *Cutaneous Hematopathology*,
DOI 10.1007/978-1-4939-0950-6_7, © Springer Science+Business Media New York 2014

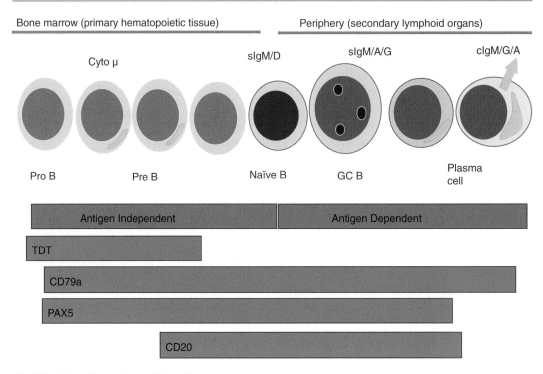

Fig. 7.1 Schematic overview of B-lymphocyte ontogeny

the gastrointestinal tract, the lung, the salivary and lacrimal gland, the skin, the soft tissue, and the thyroid gland. Cutaneous pseudolymphoma was first described as sarcomatosis cutis by Kaposi in 1891 (Bluefarb 1960). A couple of decades later in 1923, the term lymphocytoma cutis was coined by Biberstein (Kerl and Ackerman 1993). In subsequent years, other terms such as lymphadenosis benigna cutis by Bafverstedt in 1943, pseudolymphoma of Spiegler and Fendt introduced by Lever in 1967 (Kerl and Ackerman 1993), cutaneous lymphoid hyperplasia (Caro and Helwig 1969), and cutaneous B-cell pseudolymphomas (CBPL) (Caro and Helwig 1969; Evans et al. 1979) were used to denote an entity with similar if not identical histopathology features.

Prior to the availability of immunophenotyping techniques and immunoglobulin and polymerase chain reaction (PCR) gene rearrangement analyses, the diagnosis of cutaneous pseudolymphoma (CPL) was based primarily on clinicopathologic correlation (Caro and Helwig 1969; Evans et al. 1979). Confirmation of the diagnosis of CPL was based on absence of systemic involvement 5 years

from the date of the original biopsy (Caro and Helwig 1969; Ploysangam et al. 1998; Rijlaarsdam and Willemze 1994).

Histopathologic Overview of Reaction Pattern/s

In a normal lymph node, the cortex is the location of primary and secondary lymphoid follicles. In the absence of immune stimulation, the cortical lymphoid follicles are primary follicles, composed of small B lymphocytes, which may be virgin B lymphocytes or recirculating memory B lymphocytes. There is also a fine meshwork of reticulum cells, usually not visible without special immunolabeling techniques. With antigenic stimulation, antigen recognizing B lymphocytes are stimulated to replicate and differentiate – a process that converts the primary follicle into a secondary follicle or germinal center, surrounded by a mantle zone of transient small lymphocytes, and a central area containing replicating "follicular center cells" and their differentiating progeny (centroblasts and centrocytes). Normal germinal centers are characterized by the presence of tingible body macrophages, a well-formed mantle zone peripherally, normal polarization (darker-staining cells dominating the deeper half of the germinal center), and an increased proliferation index.

Reactive cutaneous lymphoid hyperplasia is characterized by lymphoid follicles with a poorly formed or absent mantle zone. Follicle centers in reactive lymphoid hyperplasia may still maintain polarization and have obvious tingible body macrophages and more centroblasts and immunoblasts than the normal follicle. There are four characteristic histologic patterns of reactive lymphoid hyperplasia (CLH): germinal center (GC) cell clusters forming well-defined lymphoid follicles, GC cell clusters not forming well-defined lymphoid follicles, CLH with a prominent histiocytic component, and CLH with a nonspecific mixed T and B lymphocytes (Bergman et al. 2011).

Classification

Currently, classification of cutaneous pseudolymphoma (CPL) is based on the histopathologic features and results of immunophenotyping and genotyping of the lymphocytes (Rijlaarsdam and Willemze 1994). Cutaneous pseudolymphoma consists of two major subtypes based on the predominant lymphocytes in the infiltrate: (1) cutaneous T-cell pseudolymphomas (CTPL) and (2) cutaneous B-cell pseudolymphomas (CBPL).

Epidemiology

Although it may occur at any age, CBPL characteristically develops in early adult life, with a median age of 34 years (range 1–73 years) (Caro and Helwig 1969). Approximately two-thirds of patients typically present initially below the age of 40 (Ploysangam et al. 1998). The female to male ratio is 3:1 (Brodell and Santa Cruz 1985) with predominance in Caucasians (white to black = 9:1) (Caro and Helwig 1969; Ploysangam et al. 1998). To date, no familial cases have been reported.

While no definite geographic distribution has been identified, CBPL associated with infectious organisms (e.g., *Borrelia burgdorferi*) commonly occurs in endemic regions of the specific infection. The most common sites of involvement include the face (cheek, nose, and ear lobe; 70 %), chest/nipples (36 %), and upper extremities (25 %) (Brodell and Santa Cruz 1985; Caro and Helwig 1969; Kerl and Ackerman 1993; Rijlaarsdam and Willemze 1994).

Etiology

The most common cause of cutaneous nodular reactive B-lymphocyte hyperplasia (cutaneous B-cell pseudolymphoma) is idiopathic. The remaining causes arranged in order of decreasing frequency based on a retrospective literature review of 32 years (1981 to present) include drugs, foreign body reaction, infection (in particular with *Borrelia burgdorferi*, *Treponema pallidum* and herpes simplex virus types 1 and 2, and varicella zoster virus) vaccination, and arthropod assault. Nomenclature based on varied etiopathogenesis includes idiopathic lymphocytoma cutis, persistent nodular arthropod-bite reactions, tattoo-induced lymphocytoma cutis (secondary to a foreign body reaction), lymphocytoma cutis caused by injections/acupuncture (vaccination), lymphomatoid drug-induced pseudo B-cell lymphoma, infectious lymphocytoma cutis (secondary to infection with *Borrelia burgdorferi*, *Treponema pallidum*, herpes simplex virus types 1 and 2, and Varicella zoster virus) and acral pseudolymphomatous angiokeratoma (of unknown etiology) (Crowson and Magro 1995; Kerl and Ackerman 1993; Ploysangam et al. 1998; Rijlaarsdam and Willemze 1994).

Idiopathic Lymphocytoma Cutis

Definition

Idiopathic lymphocytoma cutis, a benign B-cell predominant lymphoproliferative disorder of unknown etiology, is the prototypic example of CBPL.

Clinical Features

Clinically, two distinct forms have been reported: a more common localized form (comprising approximately 72 %) (Brodell and Santa Cruz 1985; Caro and Helwig 1969; Kerl and Ackerman 1993; Rijlaarsdam and Willemze 1994) and a less frequent generalized form (Brodell and Santa Cruz 1985; Gartman 1986; Kerl 1983; Moreno et al. 1991; Self et al. 1969). The former usually presents as a single asymptomatic nodule or tumor of variable consistency, measuring up to 4 cm in diameter. Lesions may be aggregated in small clusters with a few millimeter-sized miliary papules. The color varies from skin-colored to red brown/purple. Scale and ulceration are generally absent (Ploysangam et al. 1998). There is typically no extracutaneous involvement, but local recurrence has been reported (Ploysangam et al. 1998).

Histopathology

Histopathologic features include a dense, superficial, and mid-dermal nodular infiltrate of lymphocytes admixed with a variable number of histiocytes, eosinophils, and plasma cells (Fig. 7.2a). While the infiltrate is typically present predominantly in the papillary dermis ("top-heavy" pattern) (Ackerman 1978; Ackerman et al. 1993; Clark et al. 1974; Connors and Ackerman 1976; Friedmann 1990; Lever et al. 1990; MacKie 1993; Rijlaarsdam et al. 1990; Van Hale and Winkelmann 1985), a few cases of CBPL in which the infiltrate extends into the subcutis and/or in a diffuse pattern have been reported. Two types of nodular infiltrate may be seen: a small-cell variant with a more typical central germinal center that lacks cellular pleomorphism (Fig. 7.2b–d) and a large-cell vari-

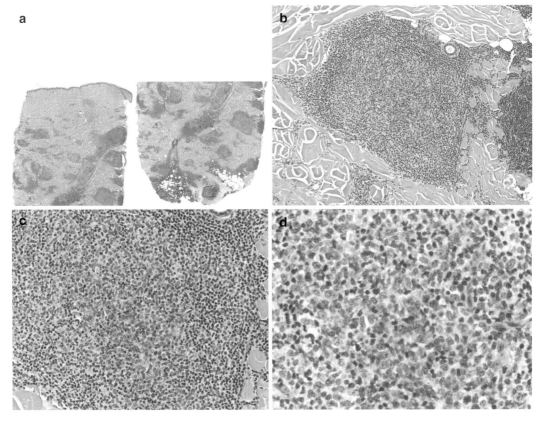

Fig. 7.2 (**a–d**) Prototypic reactive cutaneous B-cell nodular lymphoid hyperplasia (H&E). (**a**) Scanning magnification; (**a1**); upper half, (**a2**); lower half, (**b**) reactive follicle, (**c**) regular germinal center with mantle zone, (**d**) germinal center with polymorphic infiltrate of centrocytes, centroblasts, immunoblasts, and macrophages with tingible bodies

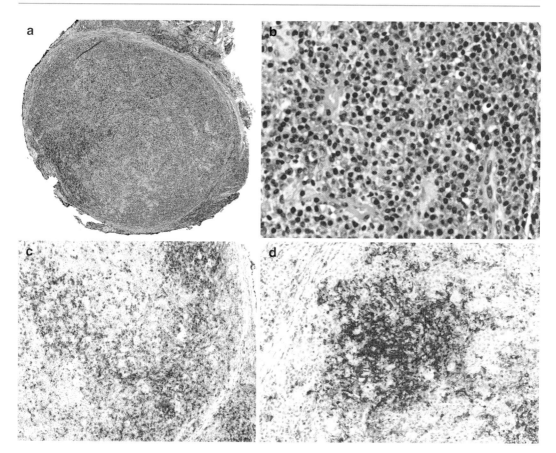

Fig. 7.3 (**a–d**) Plasma cell predominant reactive cutaneous B-cell nodular lymphoid hyperplasia. (**a**) H&E, scanning magnification; (**b**) H&E, plasma cell-rich infiltrate, (**c**) CD3, (**d**) CD20

ant that has large pleomorphic lymphocytes mainly in the central part of the infiltrate. The latter can be difficult to distinguish from lymphoma (Brodell and Santa Cruz 1985). Other cell types that may be found in germinal centers are T-helper lymphocytes, macrophages with tingible bodies, and regular patterned (highlighted by CD21) follicular dendritic cells (Ackerman 1978; Ackerman et al. 1993; Connors and Ackerman 1976; Friedmann 1990; Lever and Schaumburg-Lever 1990; MacKie 1993; Rijlaarsdam et al. 1990; Van Hale and Winkelmann 1985). In rare instances, plasma cells may be the predominant cell type (so-called primary cutaneous plasmacytoma/plasma cell predominant CBPL) (Fig. 7.3a–d) (Brodell and Santa Cruz 1985; Hurt and Santa Cruz 1990; Kerl and Ackerman 1993). A rare histopathology subset of CBPL is "large-cell

lymphocytoma" (Duncan et al. 1980; English et al. 1986; Winkelmann and Dabski 1987) – a variant that can be difficult to differentiate from CBCLs. In the nine cases reported by Duncan et al. (1980; English et al. 1986; Winkelmann and Dabski 1987), seven ended up with a diagnosis of lymphoma. In a similar report of 14 "large-cell lymphocytoma" cases, a diagnosis of lymphoma was made initially, but long-term follow-up showed a benign course (English et al. 1989). These cases, with apparent contradictory clinical courses, were histopathologically described by Winkelmann's group as showing "sharply marginated, dense clusters of small lymphocytes surrounded or infiltrated the large cell component, a juxtaposition that characterizes large cell lymphocytoma" (Winkelmann and Dabski 1987).

Immunophenotype

Immunohistochemical stains reveal a normal phenotype of the germinal center cells (CD20+, CD79a, CD10+, Bcl6+, Bcl2-) (Ploysangam et al. 1998) (Fig. 7.4a–d), normal high proliferation MIB-1/Ki67, with polytypic expression of immunoglobulin light chain. A regular and sharply demarcated network of follicular dendritic cells is highlighted by using CD21 or CD35. A prominent population of reactive CD3+ T lymphocytes is always present admixed with the infiltrate especially at the periphery (Fig. 7.4e).

Cytogenetics and Molecular Findings

In most cases, polyclonality is observed in gene rearrangement of immunoglobulin heavy-chain genes (Leinweber et al. 2004). In addition, there is no light-chain restriction of plasma cells. Of note, several studies have shown clonal gene rearrangement in morphologically reactive lymphoid hyperplasia. These include heavy-chain gene rearrangement detected in 5/14 cases (35 %) in the study by Wood et al., in 2/26 cases (7.7 %) in the study by Hammer et al., in 35/53 cases (66 %) in the study by Bouloc et al., in 27/44 cases (61 %) in the study by Nihal et al., in 1/10 cases (10 %) in the study by Leinweber et al., in 4/30 cases (13 %) in the study by Böer et al. 2008, and more recently in 3/24 cases (13 %) in the study by Bergman et al. 2011. The striking high prevalence of dominant clones in these series may have been the result of a selection bias encountered in a highly specialized referral centers for cutaneous lymphoma. Despite these high numbers, however, only a minority (<10 %) of cases of CBPL with a clonal population of B lymphocytes progressed to cutaneous lymphoma (Nihal et al. 2003).

Clinical Course

Given the fact that the cause is unknown, the clinical course varies considerably, but more often than not tends to be chronic and indolent (Brodell and Santa Cruz 1985; Kerl and Ackerman 1993;

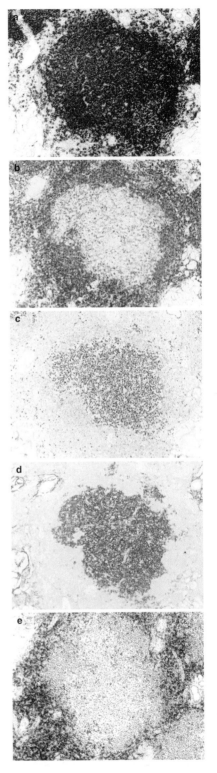

Fig. 7.4 (a–e) Typical immunohistochemical staining pattern of a reactive follicle. (a) CD20, (b) BCL2, (c) BCL6, (d) CD10, (e) CD3

Rijlaarsdam and Willemze 1994). Spontaneous regression may be seen in some lesions after several months or a few years, although local recurrence after prolonged periods has been reported in select cases (Brodell and Santa Cruz 1985; Kerl and Ackerman 1993; Rijlaarsdam and Willemze 1994).

Differential Diagnosis

Differential diagnoses include follicle-center lymphoma, marginal zone B-cell lymphoma, and diffuse large B-cell lymphoma. Helpful features in differentiating a benign from a malignant process include clinical presentation (small, localized lesion in the former vs. large, ulcerated and/or generalized lesions in the latter) (Brodell and Santa Cruz 1985; Kerl and Ackerman 1993; Rijlaarsdam and Willemze 1994), clinical course (spontaneous remission in the former vs. progressive course in the latter) (Brodell and Santa Cruz 1985; Rijlaarsdam and Willemze 1994), light-chain expression (polytypic in the former vs. monotypic in the latter), Bcl2 protein expression within germinal centers (relatively rare in the former vs. expression in 20–58 % of cases in the latter), and immunoglobulin chain gene rearrangements (positive in up to 28 % of cases of the former vs. 75 % of cases the latter) (Ploysangam et al. 1998).

Confounding clinical features include reported cases of primary CBCL without systemic involvement (Berti et al. 1991; Burg et al. 1994; Friedmann et al. 1995; Giannotti and Santucci 1993; Rijlaarsdam et al. 1993; Santucci et al. 1991; van der Putte et al. 1985), primary CBCL with features similar to that of CBPL such as clinical appearance (red- to plum-colored nodules), absence of extracutaneous involvement, response to local treatment, and a favorable prognosis. Thus, differentiating primary CBCL from CBPL on the basis of clinical evaluation alone can sometimes be a problem.

In cases with an atypical diffuse infiltrate, the most helpful differentiating feature is the presence of B lymphocytes with polyclonal light chains in CBPL, in contrast to CBCL in which there is predominance of one light chain

(Halevy and Sandbank 1987; Wantzin et al. 1988). Light-chain restriction is valuable diagnostically only when the kappa to lambda ratios >10:1 or are <0.5:1 (LeBoit et al. 1994). Bcl2 are also useful in distinguishing primary cutaneous follicular lymphomas (follicular CBCL) from CBPL with germinal centers (Chimenti et al. 1996). Of note, positivity with the Bcl2 protein antibody has rarely been found in CBPL within germinal centers (Triscott et al. 1995).

In some subtypes of cutaneous lymphoma, such as the T-lymphocyte-rich CBCL, reactive benign small T lymphocytes can comprise a fairly sizeable population of the infiltrate. This can lead to misdiagnosis on the basis of immunohistochemical studies alone (Cerroni and Kerl 1994). In cases with a discrepancy between the clinical, histologic, and immunohistochemical studies, a search for gene rearrangements in both T and B lymphocytes is useful. Generally, benign or reactive processes are polyclonal, whereas the presence of monoclonality directs a malignant process. However, this distinction is not absolute because monoclonality has been demonstrated in some benign or reactive cutaneous lymphoid hyperplasia (Wechsler et al. 1990; Weinberg et al. 1993).

Lymphomatoid Drug-Induced Pseudo B-Cell Lymphoma

Definition

Lymphomatoid drug-induced pseudo B-cell lymphoma is a subtype of lymphomatoid drug eruptions. The spectrum of drugs reported to induce cutaneous lymphoid infiltrates include anticonvulsants, antipsychotics, antihypertensives (angiotensin-converting enzyme inhibitors, beta-blockers, calcium channel blockers, and diuretics), cytotoxics (cyclosporine, methotrexate, adalimumab, infliximab), antirheumatics (gold, salicylates, phenacetin, D-penicillamine, allopurinol, nonsteroidal antiinflammatory drugs), antibiotics (penicillin, dapsone, nitrofurantoin), antidepressants (fluoxetine, doxepin, desipramine, amitriptyline hydrochloride, lithium), anxiolytics (benzodiazepines), antihistamines (diphenhydramine), H2-antagonists (cimetidine, ranitidine), antiarrhythmics (mexiletine chloride, procainamide), topical agents (menthol, etheric plant oil), sex steroids, lipid-lowering agent (lovastatin), and anti-TNF-α (Imafuku et al. 2012; Kerl and Ackerman 1993; Ploysangam et al. 1998; Rijlaarsdam and Willemze 1994; Sawada et al. 2010; Schmutz and Trechot 2012). Although most cases of lymphomatoid drug eruptions are reportedly of the CTPL type, a few CBPL cases have been reported in association with select drugs that include antihistamines, antidepressants, neuroleptics, and allopurinol (Aguilar et al. 1992; Crowson and Magro 1995; Magro and Crowson 1995; Paley et al. 2006; Torne et al. 1989). A rare type of lymphomatoid drug eruption with numerous CD30+ cells may simulate the CD30+ cutaneous lymphoproliferative disorders (Nathan and Belsito 1998). Of note, the same drug may present with varied skin lesions not only clinically but also with varying histopathology and phenotypic features in different patients.

While the precise etiopathogenesis of lymphomatoid drug eruptions is unknown, possible mechanisms postulated include impaired immunosurveillance by the offending agent which in turn leads to abnormal proliferation of lymphocytes and impairs the ability of cytotoxic/suppressor T lymphocytes to suppress B-lymphocyte differentiation and immunoglobulin production (Behan et al. 1976; Bluming et al. 1976; Brandes et al. 1992; Crowson and Magro 1995; Damle and Gupta 1981; Dosch et al. 1982; Magro and Crowson 1995; McMillen et al. 1985). Precise data concerning the incidence, prevalence, and geographic distribution of a lymphomatoid drug-induced pseudo B-cell lymphoma do not exist; however, anticonvulsant drugs, in particular phenytoin, cause pseudolymphoma syndrome with an increased frequency in African-American patients.

Clinical Features

Clinically, this variant may present as localized or generalized papules, plaques, nodules, or erythroderma (Ploysangam et al. 1998) with accentuation of cutaneous changes in sun-exposed areas. Anticonvulsant drugs, particularly hydantoin,

induce the pseudolymphoma syndrome within the first 2–8 weeks of drug intake, but can occur from 5 days to 5 years after initiation of phenytoin therapy. Clinically, this syndrome is characterized by the triad of fever, lymphadenopathy, and an erythematous eruption (pruritic macules, papules and nodules) in association with eosinophilia, hepatosplenomegaly, leukocytosis, malaise, arthralgia, and severe edema of the face (Choi et al. 2003; Schreiber and McGregor 1968).

Histopathology

Cutaneous lesions usually show the band-like CTPL pattern mimicking MF. However, some cases of lymphomatoid drug eruptions may have the nodular CBPL pattern mimicking non-Hodgkin's lymphoma (Aguilar et al. 1992; Crowson and Magro 1995; Dorfman and Warnke 1974; Kardaun et al. 1988) or lymphocytoma cutis pattern with formation of reactive germinal centers. Eosinophils may or may not be present.

Immunophenotype

The cells in the central portion of the nodular infiltrate express the phenotype of mature lymphocytes (CD20 and CD79a) with a regular follicular dendritic cell pattern highlighted by CD21 and/or CD35. A prominent population of reactive CD3+ T lymphocytes admixed within and/or at the periphery of the B-cell-rich infiltrate is always present.

Cytogenetics and Molecular Findings

There is no immunoglobulin heavy-chain gene rearrangement and no light-chain restriction of plasma cells.

Clinical Course

Characteristically, the lesions disappear after discontinuing of the offending drugs.

Differential Diagnosis

The main differential diagnoses of lymphomatoid drug eruptions include cutaneous T-cell lymphoma, CTCL (mycoses fungoides, Sezary syndrome), CBCL (follicle-center lymphoma or marginal zone B-cell lymphoma) (Aguilar et al. 1992; Crowson and Magro 1995; Magro and Crowson 1995; Paley et al. 2006; Torne et al. 1989), and systemic lymphoma (non-Hodgkin's lymphoma) (Aguilar et al. 1992; Crowson and Magro 1995; Dorfman and Warnke 1974; Kardaun et al. 1988). In addition, in the type of lymphomatoid drug eruption with numerous CD30+ cells, CD30+ cutaneous lymphoproliferative disorders should be considered (Nathan and Belsito 1998). A case of CBCL arising in the fluoxetine-induced CBPL area has been reported in 2006. Therefore, follow-up is essential. Features favoring a reactive process are the same as those mentioned before in the section of differential diagnosis in an idiopathic lymphocytoma cutis.

Cutaneous Lymphoid Hyperplasia Secondary to Foreign Bodies: Reaction to Tattoo

Definition

Cutaneous pseudolymphoma is an unusual immune response that can be caused by various foreign materials such as metals in metal ear piercing and tattoos in particular cinnabar in lesions utilizing a red dye. Cutaneous pseudolymphoma due to tattoo occurs mainly in areas with red pigment (mainly cinnabar), but pseudolymphoma secondary to the blue dye (composed mainly of cobalt salts) and green dye (composed mainly of chrome salts) areas have also been described (Blumental et al. 1982). The precise underlying mechanism in the development of pseudolymphoma in a tattoo is still unclear although a delayed-type inflammatory reaction has been implicated (Lubach and Hinz 1986; Rijlaarsdam et al. 1988; Sanchez-Viera et al. 1992). Despite the popularity of tattooing and its high prevalence rate in adults (8.5 %)

(Kazandjieva and Tsankov 2007), adverse inflammatory reactions to tattoo pigments are relatively infrequent (Stirn et al. 2006). The time of onset ranges from a few months up to 32 years after administration of the tattoo (Kahofer et al. 2003). In one report of two cases, different histologic reactions are reportedly associated with each dye, a lichenoid dermatitis resulting from a reaction to the red pigment, a pseudolymphoma resulting from a reaction to red and lilac pigments, and a photo-induced reaction to a yellow pigment (Cruz et al. 2010).

Clinical Features

Clinically, it typically presents as an asymptomatic red-discolored plaque to nodule limited to areas impregnated with the offending agent. Itching has occasionally been observed in some patients (Blumental et al. 1982; Kahofer et al. 2003; Rijlaarsdam et al. 1988).

Histopathology

Histopathologically, reactions to tattoos are diverse and include spongiotic, lichenoid, granulomatous, and a pseudolymphomatous reaction patterns (Kazandjieva and Tsankov 2007). Of note, granulomatous tattoo reactions, which usually represent hypersensitivity reactions to tattoo pigments, have been reported as a manifestation of systemic sarcoidosis in patients with a known history of the same (i.e sarcoidosis) (Sowden et al. 1992). Granulomatous dermatitis in a tattoo area may also develop in association with other manifestation of sarcoidosis (Sowden et al. 1992).

The pseudolymphomatous reaction pattern comprises a dense, diffuse lymphohistiocytic ("top-heavy" distribution) infiltrate with some eosinophils and occasionally plasma cells interspersed with dark brown, granular, non-refractile foreign body material (more often seen at the bottom of the infiltrate) within the cytoplasm of histiocytes as well as extracellularly between collagen bundles (Fig. 7.5) (Kahofer et al. 2003). The cytomorphology of lesional lymphocytes indicates that they are small. Follicular and nodular structures

Fig. 7.5 Reactive cutaneous B-cell nodular lymphoid hyperplasia secondary to a foreign body (tattoo) H&E, nodular lymphohistiocytic infiltrate with admixed black, granular non-refractile foreign material consistent with tattoo

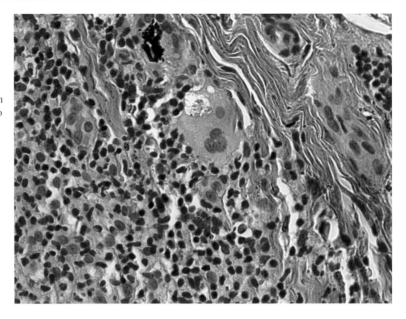

have occasionally been encountered. Rijlaarsdam et al. suggest that there is a follicle-center cell reaction pattern to tattoo pigment with distinct B- and T-lymphocyte compartments, simulating reactive lymph nodes (Rijlaarsdam et al. 1988). Overlying epidermal change in the form of parakeratosis and irregular epidermal hyperplasia with scattered necrotic keratinocytes may be seen.

Immunophenotype

The cells of CBPL express the phenotypes of mature lymphocytes (CD20 and CD79a+) admixed with a prominent population of reactive CD3+ T lymphocytes and polyclonal plasma cells. Antigen-presenting CD1a + Langerhans cells are noted in the T-cell compartment, while CD21+ follicular dendritic cells appear to be confined to the B-cell compartment.

Cytogenetics and Molecular Findings

No heavy-chain gene rearrangement of immunoglobulin heavy-chain genes is present, and there is no light-chain restriction of plasma cells.

Clinical Course

While the lesions generally resolve after nonaggressive treatment, they have been known to persist for months with or without treatment.

Differential Diagnosis

The main differential diagnosis of pseudolymphomatous reactions to tattoo includes follicle-center lymphoma and marginal zone B-cell lymphoma. A case of CBCL arising in a tattoo has been reported. In this report, the patient initially presented with multiple pseudolymphomatous skin lesions, apparently associated with an immune response to the mercury contained in the red tattoo pigment. Over a period of 4 years, his skin lesions evolved from being histopathologically benign (mild-moderate, superficial and deep, predominantly perivascular lymphohistiocytic infiltrate with admixed plasma cells) and immunologically polyclonal pseudolymphoma to histopathologically malignant (dense, superficial and mid, nodular to diffuse infiltrate composed of large atypical lymphoid cells with admixed eosinophils and small lymphocytes) and immunologically monoclonal large B-cell lymphoma indicating that follow-up is essential (Sangueza et al. 1992). In all biopsies, there were common clonal bands of varied intensity relative to the germline bands (reflecting a variability in the proportion of clonal cells) – finding favoring the concept of evolution from an abnormal immune state with multiple B-lymphocyte clones in the pseudolymphoma to a dominant and relatively uncontrollable proliferation of one clonal population in overt lymphoma (Breza et al. 2006).

Pseudo B-Cell Lymphoma Secondary to Infections

These include infections secondary to borreliosis, syphilis, and, albeit less commonly, herpes (as this typically causes CTPL per published reports).

Borreliosis

Definition

Borrelial lymphocytoma cutis is the most common cause of pseudo B-cell lymphoma particularly in endemic areas of Central Europe (Slovenia and Austria), Australia, and the Northeastern part of the United States (Connecticut). Other reported borreliosis cases are from northern Africa (Morocco, Algeria, Egypt, and Tunisia), Asia (Japan, northwest China, Nepal, Thailand, and far eastern Russia), Canada (Ontario), and South America (Brazil). In the United States, according to the CDC 2011 report, 96 % of cases were from the northeast and upper Midwest including Connecticut, Delaware, Maine, Maryland, Massachusetts, Minnesota, New Hampshire, New Jersey, New York, Pennsylvania, Vermont, Virginia, and Wisconsin. This entity is a reactive B-lymphocyte predominant lymphoproliferative disorder caused by a tick bite with *B. burgdorferi*. The diagnosis is made by (1) a history of preceding erythema chronicum migrans or a tick bite, (2) clinical presentation of a blue-red nodule on the earlobe or on the nipple area, (3) histopathology features of lymphocytoma cutis, (4) elevated serum antibody titer to *B. burgdorferi*, and (5) identification of the organism in the tissue by polymerase chain reaction-based techniques (Asbrink and Hovmark 1993).

The prevalence of borrelial lymphocytoma cutis has been reported to be from 0.6 to 1.3 % (Stanek et al. 1985). It most commonly occurs in areas endemic for the Ixodes ricinus tick in Europe, also in North America as mentioned above (Hovmark et al. 1986). It is more common in women than men and may be seen in any age range including children (Colli et al. 2004; Hovmark et al. 1986).

Clinical Features

Clinically, borrelial lymphocytoma cutis often appears at the site of a tick bite or occurs close to the periphery of a large lesion of erythema chronicum migrans (Asbrink and Hovmark 1993). Most patients are aware of having had a tick bite. In comparison with erythema chronicum migrans, borrelial lymphocytoma cutis develops later and lasts longer. The incubation period varies from a few weeks to 10 months (Albrecht et al. 1991; Asbrink and Hovmark 1993; Bratzke et al. 1989; Bucher et al. 1988; Weber et al. 1984). Predilection sites include the earlobe, the nipple and areola, the nose, and the scrotal area (89 % of cases in one series) (Colli et al. 2004), indicating that spirochetes may prefer regions with low skin temperature. Borrelial lymphocytoma cutis usually has an asymptomatic blue-red plaque, papule, or nodule, varying in diameter from 3 mm to 5 cm or more (Wantzin et al. 1982). They may be solitary, grouped or numerous, and widespread (Zackheim et al. 1997).

Histopathology

The histopathologic appearances are varied and there is considerable overlap with primary cutaneous follicle-center cell lymphoma and primary cutaneous marginal zone B-cell lymphoma. There is a variably dense, nodular, mixed-cell infiltrate, which may have a perivascular and periappendageal distribution or be more diffuse (Fig. 7.6a, b). The epidermis is usually spared but some small lymphocytes may be seen traversing the entire epidermis. Although a

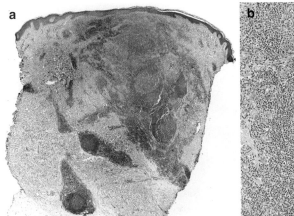
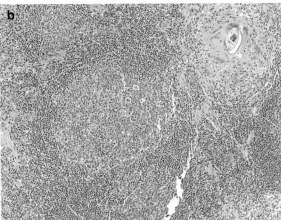

Fig. 7.6 (**a**, **b**) Reactive cutaneous B-cell nodular lymphoid hyperplasia secondary to a tick bite (**a**) H&E, scanning magnification, (**b**) H&E, reactive nodular lymphocytic infiltrate

with germinal center formation (*left*), and a foreign body material reminiscent of part of a tick with an adjacent multinucleate giant cell reaction (*right upper*)

"top-heavy" cellular infiltrate is more typical, the infiltrate may extend into the subcutis. Lymphoid follicles are present in many but not all cases, and well-developed mantle zones are seen in a minority, which may present a difficulty in distinguishing reactive hyperplasia from follicle-center cell lymphoma. Plasma cells and eosinophils are found in almost all cases. However, the composition of follicles is different from that seen in follicle-center cell lymphoma. In CBPL, germinal centers were characterized by predominance of "blastic" cells with features of centroblasts, immunoblasts, and a relatively low number of centrocytes (Colli et al. 2004). Fusion of irregular follicle centers may simulate a pattern of diffuse large B-cell lymphoma (Grange et al. 2002). Presence of an intact or part of a tick argues in favor of a reactive process (Fig. 7.6b).

Immunophenotype
The infiltrate is composed mainly composed of CD10+ and Bcl2− germinal centers and polyclonal plasma cells. Dendritic cells positive for CD1a and S100 are also present in the infiltrate (Bergman et al. 2006).

Cytogenetics and Molecular Findings
Heavy-chain gene rearrangement is typically not seen and there is usually no light-chain restriction of plasma cells.

Clinical Course
If treatment is not given, the lesion may persist for several months with or without regional lymphadenopathy (Asbrink and Hovmark 1993). It has been reported that borrelial lymphocytoma cutis and acrodermatitis chronica atrophicans can be seen in the same patient (Asbrink and Hovmark 1993). Constitutional symptoms or other late manifestations of Lyme disease are found only in a few patients (Asbrink and Hovmark 1993). Serum antibodies to *B. burgdorferi* are elevated in 50 % of cases (Asbrink and Hovmark 1993). *B. burgdorferi* may rarely be the cause of systemic pseudolymphomatous syndrome that recedes after antibiotic treatment (Aigelsreiter et al. 2005).

Differential Diagnosis
The differential diagnoses of pseudolymphomatous reactions caused by *B. burgdorferi* include CBCL (follicle-center lymphoma or marginal zone B-cell lymphoma). Helpful differentiating features are the same as mentioned before under the section of differential diagnosis in an idiopathic lymphocytoma cutis.

Syphilis

Definition
According to the CDC 2010 report, the incidence of syphilis increased from 2001 to 2009 (total

primary and secondary cases, approximately 14,000) but started to decrease in 2010 (by 1.6 %). While the rate of congenital syphilis rate decreased by 15 % since 2008, rates remain high in some urban areas throughout the United States and in select rural areas (in the south). The co-occurrence of syphilis in human immunodeficiency virus (HIV)-positive homosexual men has further contributed to the increased incidence.

Overall, lesions of secondary syphilis characterized by a B-lymphocyte-rich infiltrate and widespread dissemination of spirochetes are still seen (Brown et al. 1999). A reactive B-lymphocyte predominant lymphoproliferative disorder secondary to infection *Treponema pallidum* is typically seen as a manifestation of secondary syphilis, although occasional cases (<25 reported cases in the literature) have been reported as a manifestation of late syphilis (Erfurt et al. 2006; McComb et al. 2003; Moon et al. 2009; ul Bari and Raza 2006).

Clinical Features

Secondary syphilis typically presents 2–6 months after inoculation with the spirochete *Treponema pallidum* (Abell et al. 1975). The classic presentation is that of a generalized papulosquamous/papulonodular eruption involving the skin and mucosa and accompanied by a flu-like prodrome with lymphadenopathy (Sanches 2003). The reddish-purple nodules and plaques, with/without peripheral scaling, are characteristically bilateral, symmetric, more prominent on the upper extremities and, albeit in the early stages, on the palms and soles (Sanches 2003). A case with the clinical presentation of infiltrated, erythematous to violaceous, coalescent plaques on the trunk, limbs, and face, giving an almost leonine facies simulating T- or B-cell lymphoproliferative disease, has been reported (Battistella et al. 2008).

Histopathology

The characteristic histopathology features of secondary syphilis include endarteritis, a superficial and deep, perivascular and perineural, lymphoplasmacytic infiltrate (although plasma cells may be absent or sparse in up to one-third of cases and vascular changes may not be prominent), an inflammatory cell infiltrate obscuring the dermoepidermal junction, and epidermal hyperplasia (lichenoid psoriasiform) with or without exocytosis (Jeerapaet and Ackerman 1974). The composition and depth of the infiltrate can vary from area to area even within a single biopsy. Few cases of secondary syphilis with a dense and diffuse dermal lymphocytic infiltrate have been reported to histologically mimic a lymphoid neoplasm (Cochran et al. 1976; Goffinet et al. 1970; Gollnick et al. 1987; Hodak et al. 1987).

Immunophenotype, Cytogenetics, and Molecular Findings

The plasma cells always reveal a polyclonal pattern of immunoglobulin light-chain expression, and immunohistologic staining for *Treponema pallidum* reveals variable number of microorganisms. Positive serology for syphilis is helpful in confirming the diagnosis.

Differential Diagnosis

The differential diagnoses of benign lymphoid hyperplasia secondary to syphilis are broad given the potential of syphilis to mimic virtually any entity and include lymphoma, reticulohistiocytoma, Hodgkin's disease, lymphomatoid papulosis, and diffuse Kaposi sarcoma (Rashidi et al. 2012) since all of these entities are characterized clinically by a papulosquamous/papulonodular eruption and histopathologically by a dense dermal lymphoplasmacytic infiltrate (Shiino et al. 2012).

Herpes

Definition

Worldwide rates of herpes simplex virus (HSV) infection (herpesviruses; HSV type 1 and HSV type 2) are between 65 and 90 % (Chayavichitsilp et al. 2009). In the United States, the prevalence of HSV-1 was 57.7 % as per a 1999–2004 study (Xu et al. 2006). The data for HSV-2 published in March 2010, based on a National Health and Nutrition Examination Survey study performed between 2005 and 2008 by Centers for Disease Control and Prevention (CDC), revealed about one in six Americans (16.2 %) aged 14–49 is infected with HSV-2. HSV-2 prevalence was nearly twice as high among women (20.9 %)

than men (11.5 %) and was more than three times higher among blacks (39.2 %) than whites (12.3 %) (Xu et al. 2010). HSV-1 especially recurrent disease usually occurs around the lips (herpes labialis). Infection with HSV-2 generally involves the genitalia and surrounding areas and usually sexually transmitted. The usual lesions of herpes simplex consist of a group of clear vesicles. Herpes varicella/zoster virus (VZV) affects 10–20 % of the population with an increased incidence in the elderly and in those who are immunocompromised (Spray and Glaser 2002). An estimated one million cases of herpes zoster occur each year in the United States (Weinberg et al. 1993). It results from reactivation of latent varicella/zoster virus (VZV) infection.

Clinical Features

The characteristic rash has a unilateral dermatomal distribution that most often affects the thoracic and lumbar regions, and sometimes the face although any dermatome can be affected.

Histopathology

The histopathologic appearances of herpes simplex and herpes zoster are very similar and pseudolymphomas caused by both have been reported. Histopathologically, there are epidermal vesicles containing multinucleate ballooning and acantholytic keratinocytes with viral inclusion bodies. In addition there is a dermal inflammatory infiltrate composed of lymphocytes and occasional neutrophils. Atypical large lymphoid cells may be present in the infiltrate. In one study reported by Resnick and Dileonardo, 2010, approximately 70 % of the specimens (32 of 45 cases) showed atypical T lymphocytes. In a study of 65 patients with herpes simplex (HSV-1 and/or 2) and herpes varicella/zoster (VZV), histopathology examination revealed features simulating malignant lymphoma. Briefly these included a dense lymphoid infiltrate, angiotropism, and atypical T lymphocytes (Leinweber et al. 2004). A rapid cytological diagnosis of a vesicular lesion can be made by making a smear from the base of a freshly opened vesicle and staining it with the Giemsa stain (Tzanck test).

Immunophenotype, Cytogenetics, and Molecular Findings

Immunoperoxidase stains and PCR studies with probes specific for HSV-1, HSV-2, and VZV are now available commercially. Immunohistochemistry performed in cases with dense atypical lymphocytes showed a strong preponderance of T lymphocytes with admixed B lymphocytes and scattered CD30+ and CD56+ cells, supporting the T lymphocytes' nature of herpes-induced pseudolymphomas (Leinweber et al. 2004). Heavy-chain gene rearrangement is typically not seen and there is usually no light-chain restriction of plasma cells. Of note, two cases with morphologically pseudolymphomatous appearance histopathologically were found to have a monoclonal population of T lymphocytes by PCR analysis (Leinweber et al. 2004). However, the diagnosis of CPL was confirmed by the presence of histopathology evidence of viral inclusions and PCR analyses.

Differential Diagnosis

The differential diagnosis includes CBCL and CTCL. Helpful differentiating features are the same as those mentioned before under the section of differential diagnosis in an idiopathic lymphocytoma cutis.

Pseudolymphoma at Sites of Vaccination

Definition

This is a relatively rare reaction pattern characterized by a florid lymphocytic inflammatory reaction either immediately or as a delayed hypersensitivity reaction to a vaccine constituent, including aluminum and thimerosal (Chong et al. 2006). There are no precise data concerning the incidence, prevalence, and geographic distribution of this reaction although given the number of reports of this entity in the literature (<15 between 1993 and 2012), it appears to be uncommon. Vaccines associated with this reaction pattern include those to varicella zoster, hepatitis B, early summer meningoencephalitis (Facchetti et al.), tetanus, diphtheria, pertussis, and measles, mumps, and rubella (MMR).

Clinical Features

The clinical presentation is usually that of superficial papules or nodules, at the vaccination site (Cerroni et al. 2007). These may arise immediately or from weeks to months to even, albeit rarely, years after the vaccination.

Histopathology

Histopathologically, about 20 % of the persistent nodules at the vaccination sites showed lymphoid follicles with reactive germinal centers (Fig. 7.7a–c) and a prominent perifollicular infiltrate. Other observed reaction patterns include a lichenoid dermatitis, panniculitis (septal or mixed), and "granuloma annulare-like" (with a palisaded histiocytic infiltrate surrounding foci of necrobiosis) (Chong et al. 2006).

Immunophenotype, Cytogenetics, and Molecular Findings

The demonstration of aluminum by Morin staining and atomic absorption spectrometry on a paraffin-embedded tissue probe can be used to support the diagnosis of vaccination-induced pseudolymphoma. Immunohistochemical analysis reveals a mixed-cell infiltrate containing both CD3-positive T lymphocytes and CD20-positive B lymphocytes. The plasma cells typically show polyclonal expression of immunoglobulin light chains kappa and lambda, and there is no heavy-chain gene rearrangement.

Clinical Course

Lesions may persist for months or years despite intralesional steroid therapy.

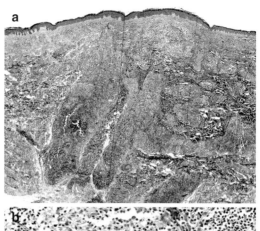
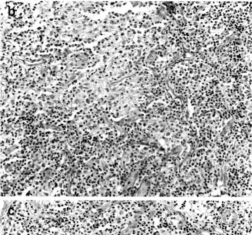
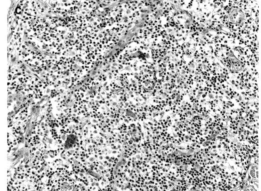

Fig. 7.7 (**a–c**) Reactive cutaneous B-cell nodular lymphoid hyperplasia at hepatitis B vaccine site (H&E). (**a**) Scanning magnification revealing inflammation adjacent scar tract, (**b**) nodular lymphocytic infiltrate with germinal center formation, (**c**) admixed multinucleate giant cells

Differential Diagnosis

The differential diagnosis includes CBCL and CTCL (depending on whether the infiltrate is B or T lymphocyte rich). Helpful differentiating features from CBCL are the same as those mentioned before under the section of differential diagnosis in idiopathic lymphocytoma cutis.

Persistent Nodular Arthropod-Bite Reaction and Nodular Scabies

Definition

This reaction pattern develops most commonly as a result of infestation with the itch mite, Sarcoptes scabiei var. hominis) although it has been known to occur secondary to other arthropod bites. While the cause is not precisely known, it is believed to be a manifestation of a delayed-type hypersensitivity reaction to a component of the mite (Ploysangam et al. 1998).

Scabies is a worldwide disease and a major public health problem in many developing countries, related primarily to poverty and overcrowding. In remote communities in northern Australia, prevalence of up to 50 % among children has been described, despite the availability of effective therapy (Walton and Currie 2007). There are about 300 million cases of scabies in the world each year (Hicks and Elston 2009). An infested person can very easily pass scabies to his or her household members and sexual partners. Scabies in adults frequently is sexually acquired. In the United States and in other developed regions around the world, scabies occurs in epidemics in the institutions such as nursing homes, extended-care facilities, childcare facilities and prisons, and homeless population.

Clinical Features

The clinical presentation is that of multiple, extremely pruritic, firm, round to oval, erythematous to red-brown papules and nodules occurring most commonly between the fingers, wrist, elbows, abdomen, genitalia, nipple, buttocks, shoulder blades, and axillae (Ploysangam et al. 1998). When a person is infested with the scabies mite for the first time, lesions may be asymptomatic for the first 2 months, although an infested person still can spread scabies during this asymptomatic time. If a person has had scabies previously, symptoms appear much sooner (1–4 days) after exposure.

Histopathology

Histopathologically, this reaction pattern is characterized by a dense, superficial and deep, predominantly perivascular lymphohistiocytic infiltrate with eosinophils (Fig. 7.8a–c). Of note, the scabetic mite is seldom identified in a scabetic nodule. Prominent thickened wall vessels lined by reactive endothelial cells and epidermal change (hyperkeratosis and epidermal hyperplasia with mild spongiosis) are frequently seen (Fernandez et al. 1977). Vasculitis can be found in those cases showing tissue eosinophils, an exuberant inflammatory tissue reaction, and many mites. Both the number of circulating eosinophilic granulocytes and serum IgE concentrations correlate with the severity of the skin reaction. In one study, ten of 60 patients (17 %) with scabies had markedly increased numbers of circulating eosinophils during scabies infestation. In most of the patients, however, the number of circulating eosinophils decreased after treatment (Falk and Eide 1981).

Immunophenotype

Immunohistochemical stains indicate a mixed-cell infiltrate containing both T (CD3-positive) and B (CD20-positive) lymphocytes – features arguing in favor of a benign reactive pattern. CD30 may highlight scattered large lymphocytes.

Cytogenetics and Molecular Findings

There is no heavy-chain gene rearrangement and a polyclonal reaction pattern is seen in the immunoglobulin light chains.

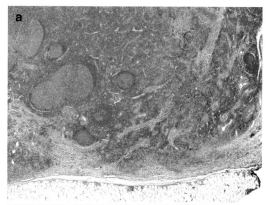

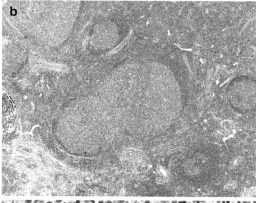

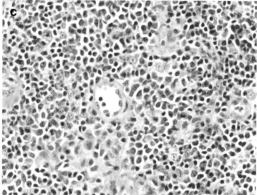

Fig. 7.8 (**a–c**) Reactive nodular lymphoid hyperplasia secondary to an arthropod bite (H&E). (**a**) scanning magnification revealing deep, nodular lymphoid infiltrate, (**b**) reactive follicles, (**c**) admixed eosinophils

Clinical Course

Nodules following infestation with Sarcoptes scabiei var. hominis may persist for many months after adequate anti-scabetic therapy. Spontaneous resolution is seen in all persistent arthropod-bite reactions.

Differential Diagnosis

The differential diagnoses include prurigo nodularis, pseudolymphoma, and lymphoma (CBCL and CTCL). Presence of the scabetic mite, eosinophils, and increased circulating eosinophils and serum IgE are useful clue to the diagnosis. To differentiate from malignant lymphoma, helpful features are as the same as those mentioned earlier (idiopathic lymphocytoma cutis section).

Conclusion

There is no single histopathology criterion to differentiate CBPL from CBCL. Histologic diagnosis of CBPL depends on two considerations: (1) the architecture of the infiltrate and (2) the composition and cytomorphology of cells in the infiltrate. Histopathologic features that favor CBPL over CBCL include (1) acanthosis, (2) a top-heavy infiltrate, (3) a mixed (T- and B-lymphocyte-rich) infiltrate, (4) absence of mitosis outside of the germinal center and/or necrosis, (5) regular appearing germinal centers, (6) presence of tingible bodies in the germinal centers, (7) lack of cohesion of lymphoid cells, (8) infiltrative border (concave), (9) preservation of adnexal structures with the infiltrate respecting adnexal epithelium, and (10) stromal fibrosis (Ploysangam et al. 1998). A useful immunohistochemical feature for distinguishing cutaneous follicle-center cell lymphoma from cutaneous lymphoid hyperplasia is the presence of small clusters of CD10+/Bcl6+ lymphocytes in the interfollicular zones and positive Bcl2 staining in the follicles in the former. Furthermore, there is a low MIB-1 proliferation fraction in lymphoma compared with cutaneous lymphoid hyperplasia.

Mimics

Inflammatory Pseudotumor

Definition

Inflammatory pseudotumor (IPT) also known as inflammatory myofibroblastic tumor (IMT) or plasma cell granuloma (PCG) is a distinct, heterogeneous group of mesenchymal tumors composed of various proportions of myofibroblasts, hyalinized collagenous stroma, and admixed inflammatory cells. It is known to occur in any part of the body and has varied morphology. The one most relevant to this chapter is cutaneous inflammatory myofibroblastic tumor (IMT) or plasma cell granuloma (PCG) – a spectrum of idiopathic benign conditions with pseudolymphomatous pattern, a mixed-cell infiltrate containing numerous plasma cells, prominent germinal centers, and a proliferation of myofibroblasts (Coffin et al. 2007).

Clinical Features

Cutaneous IMT usually presents as a solitary, slowly growing, tender, firm cutaneous, or subcutaneous papule or nodule measuring 1–5 cm in diameter (El Shabrawi-Caelen et al. 2004).

Histopathology

Histopathologically, there is a heavy inflammatory cell infiltrate containing numerous plasma cells with prominent reactive germinal centers dispersed throughout the lesion mimicking CPL or lymphoma (Coffin et al. 1998). Other features include the presence of high endothelial venules, admixed eosinophils and histiocytes, calcification, and large atypical myofibroblasts (CD15–, CD30–, vimentin +) simulating Reed-Sternberg cells (Carlson et al. 2001; El Shabrawi-Caelen et al. 2004; Hurt and Santa Cruz 1990; MacSweeney and Desai 2000; Ramachandra et al. 1995; Yang 1993).

Immunophenotype

CD3 marks small, reactive T lymphocytes, and CD20 detects focal clusters of reactive B lymphocytes (El Shabrawi-Caelen et al. 2004).

Cytogenetics and Molecular Findings

Plasma cells showed a polyclonal reaction pattern with kappa and lambda immunoglobulin light chains. Immunoglobulin heavy-chain gene reveals a polyclonal pattern.

Differential Diagnosis

Main differentiating features from lymphoma especially Hodgkin's lymphoma are the presence of myofibroblasts (CD15–, CD30–, vimentin +) and the density of plasma cells. Differences in the biological behavior (recur locally) and molecular profile (>50 % of cases reveal ALK gene rearrangement) are also of utility in differentiating this entity from ALK-negative IMT lesions with more aggressive clinical course (Coffin et al. 2007).

Lymphocytic Infiltration of the Skin (of Jessner and Kanof)

Definition

Lymphocytic infiltration of the skin (of Jessner and Kanof) or Jessner's lymphocytic infiltrate, a relatively uncommon condition of unknown etiology, was first introduced by Jessner and Kanof in 1953 (Jessner and Kanof 1953). This entity is now regarded as a variant of tumid LE (Remy-Leroux et al. 2008).

Histopathology

Histopathologically, this entity is characterized by a moderately dense, superficial and deep, perivascular and periappendageal infiltrate with occasional involvement of the subcutis. The infiltrate is composed predominantly of small lymphocytes although larger lymphocytes, mimicking CPL, may be present (Cerio et al. 1990; Facchetti et al. 1990; Helm and Muller 1992; Konttinen et al. 1987; Kuo et al. 1994; Willemze et al. 1984).

Immunophenotype

The infiltrate is predominantly T (CD3+) lymphocyte rich with a smaller component of CD20+ B lymphocytes, and negative staining with CD5 and CD43 helps differentiate this entity from cutaneous lesions of CBCL especially CLL.

Cytogenetics and Molecular Findings

The mixed (T and B lymphocytes) and polyclonal nature of the lymphoid infiltrate in Jessner's lymphocytic infiltrate help differentiate this entity from cutaneous lesions of CBCL.

Clinical Course

Lesions often resolve within weeks or months, but recurrences/relapses may occur in the same or different area. The average duration of the disease is 5 years (Toonstra et al. 1989).

Differential Diagnosis
In contrast to CBPL, mucin may be seen between collagen bundles. It has mostly benign, but unpredictable clinical behavior.

Granulomatous Rosacea

Clinical Features
Granulomatous rosacea usually presents as noninflammatory, hard, brown, yellow or red, uniformly sized cutaneous papules or nodules on the cheeks, and periorificial facial skin, although extrafacial lesions have been reported in a minority (15 %) of patients (Helm et al. 1991; Wilkin et al. 2002).

Histopathology
Histopathologically, in granulomatous rosacea, a multinodular, granulomatous, perifollicular, and perivascular lymphohistiocytic infiltrate with varying numbers of multinucleate giant cells is usually seen in the superficial and/or mid-dermis. The infiltrate may be primarily lymphocytic in up to 40 % of patients and primarily histiocytic in up to 34 % of patients. Other features include the presence of damaged follicles, and/or the mite D. folliculorum and marked vascular dilatation (Amichai et al. 1992). The perifollicular granulomas may be noncaseating (epithelioid granulomas in 11 % of patients) or caseating (epithelioid granulomas with caseating necrosis in 11 %) reaction (Helm et al. 1991).

Immunophenotype
Small, reactive T lymphocytes are highlighted by CD3, and CD20 detects focal clusters of reactive B lymphocytes.

Cytogenetics and Molecular Findings
A polyclonal pattern of the immunoglobulin heavy-chain gene is detected by PCR study. No immunoglobulin light-chain restriction is seen.

Differential Diagnosis
Differentiating features from CBPL are the presence of perifollicular lymphocytes and histiocytes with admixed multinucleate giant cells, damage follicles and/or mite D. folliculorum, marked vascular dilatation and the presence of lesion clinically confined to the head and neck area.

Clonality: Significance

In cases with a discrepancy between the clinical, histologic, and immunohistochemical studies, a search for gene rearrangements in both T and B lymphocytes is useful. Generally, benign or reactive processes are polyclonal, whereas the presence of monoclonality directs a malignant process. However, this distinction is not absolute because numerous studies have shown that cutaneous lymphoid hyperplasia, diagnosed both clinically and histologically, harbors a clonal B-lymphocyte population in 4–62 % of cases, as evidenced by monotypic plasma cells or immunoglobulin gene rearrangement (Bergman et al. 2011; Boer et al. 2008; Ceballos et al. 2002; Wechsler et al. 1990; Weinberg et al. 1993). Therefore, the interpretation of clonality result must be done in the context of the clinicopathologic and immunohistochemical features of cutaneous lymphoproliferative processes. Cases of CPL cases with a positive clone should be followed up carefully because a small minority may develop into overt lymphoma (Bergman et al. 2011). Also see differential diagnosis section in cutaneous lymphoid hyperplasia secondary to foreign body's reaction to tattoo.

Clues to Diagnosis: Clinical and Histopathologic

Clinical manifestations of cutaneous pseudolymphoma are variable and usually not helpful for differentiating a benign from a malignant lymphoid process. While benign lesions present most commonly as a solitary nodule, multiple lesions have been reported, albeit rarely. Benign lesions can also present as erythroderma. Benign lesions clinically have a doughy to firm consistency and range from red brown to violaceous in color. Lesions may be pruritic or asymptomatic (Boudova et al. 2005).

Table 7.1 Cutaneous B-cell pseudolymphoma (CBPL) versus cutaneous B-cell lymphoma (CBCL) – helpful differentiating features

	CBPL	CBCL
Clinical features		
Number of lesions	Solitary or multiple	Usually solitary
Extracutaneous involvement	Absent	Possible
Recurrences	Rare	Likely
Histopathologic features		
Acanthosis	Prominent	Minimal or no
Pattern of infiltrate	Nodular (>90 %)	Diffuse or nodular
Structure of infiltrate	Top heavy (75 %)	Bottom heavy (65 %)
Border of the infiltrate	Concave, poorly demarcated	Convex, sharply demarcated
Additional cells (e.g., eosinophils, plasma cells) and epithelioid cell granulomas	Usually present	Less common
Germinal center	More preserved (65 %)	Less preserved (10–20 %)
Mantle zone	Present	Usually absent
Polarity of GC cells	Retained	Loss
Effaced lymphoid follicles	Usually absent	Present
Tingible body macrophages (fragmented basophilic nuclear debris of degenerated lymphoid cells)	Present	Usually absent
Mixed-cell infiltrate with small lymphocytes	Present predominantly in the upper dermis	Less common
Sparing of epithelial and adnexal structures	Present	Usually absent
Immunophenotype		
Immunoglobulin light chain	Polytypic expression (kappa or lambda)	Monotypic expression
B-cell marker expressing cells	<50 % cells (predominantly within the follicles)	>50 % cells
T-cell marker expressing cells	>50 % cells (predominantly outside and between the follicles)	Usually few
CD21-positive dendritic cells	Regular pattern (evenly distributed)	Irregular pattern
MIB-1 immunostain (proliferative rate)	High	Low
Germinal center		
CD10 and Bcl6	Positive	Negative
Bcl2	Negative	Positive
Genotype		
Ig heavy-chain gene rearrangement	Absent in most cases	Present in most cases

Histopathologic clues to the diagnosis of a reactive lymphoid hyperplasia versus one that is malignant include the presence in the former of a mantle zone, polarity of GC cells, absence of effaced lymphoid follicles, tingible body macrophages, mixed-cell infiltrate with small lymphocytes mainly involving the upper dermis, sparing of epithelial and adnexal structures, CD20-positive B lymphocytes predominantly within the follicles, CD3-positive T lymphocytes predominantly outside and between the follicles, evenly distributed CD21 follicular dendritic cells, high proliferative rate as evidence by MIB-1 immunostain, GC cells with positive staining for CD10 and Bcl6, but negative/rare positive staining for Bcl2, the presence of eosinophils, and absence of clonality (Table 7.1). None of the aforementioned criteria, however, is discriminative by itself, and the diagnosis is based on a constellation of several findings (Caro and Helwig 1969).

Acknowledgments The authors would like to acknowledge Amy C Mueller, BA for assistance with formatting and cataloguing of references.

References

Abbas A, Lightman A, Pober J. Maturation of B lymphocytes and expression of immunoglobulin. Philadelphia: W. B. Saunders Company; 1991. 71 p. (Cellular and molecular immunology).

Abell E, Marks R, Jones EW. Secondary syphilis: a clinico-pathological review. Br J Dermatol. 1975; 93(1):53–61.

Ackerman A. Histologic diagnosis of inflammatory skin diseases. Philadelphia: Lea & Febiger; 1978. p. 442–7.

Ackerman A, Briggs P, Bravo F. Differential diagnosis in dermatopathology III. Philadelphia: Lea & Febiger; 1993. p. 46–9.

Aguilar J, Barcelo C, Martin-Urda M, et al. Generalized cutaneous B-cell pseudolymphoma induced by neuroleptics. Arch Dermatol Res. 1992;128:121–3.

Aigelsreiter A, Pump A, Buchhausl W, et al. Successful antibiotic treatment of Borreliosis associated pseudolymphomatous systemic infiltrates. J Infect. 2005; 51(4):e203–6.

Albrecht S, Hofstadter S, Artsob H, et al. Lymphadenosis benigna cutis resulting from Borrelia infection (Borrelia lymphocytoma). J Am Acad Dermatol. 1991;24(4):621–5.

Amichai B, Grunwald MH, Avinoach I, et al. Granulomatous rosacea associated with Demodex folliculorum. Int J Dermatol. 1992;31(10):718–9.

Asbrink E, Hovmark A. Lyme borreliosis. In: Fitzpatrick T, Eisen A, Wolff K, et al., editors. Dermatology in general medicine. 4th ed. New York: McGraw-Hill; 1993. p. 2410–20.

Battistella M, Le Cleach L, Lacert A, et al. Extensive nodular secondary syphilis with prozone phenomenon. Arch Dermatol. 2008;144(8):1078–9.

Behan PO, Behan WM, Zacharias FJ, et al. Immunological abnormalities in patients who had the oculomucocutaneous syndrome associated with practolol therapy. Lancet. 1976;2(7993):984–7.

Bergman R, Khamaysi Z, Sahar D, et al. Cutaneous lymphoid hyperplasia presenting as a solitary facial nodule: clinical, histopathological, immunophenotypical, and molecular studies. Arch Dermatol. 2006;142(12): 1561–6.

Bergman R, Khamaysi K, Khamaysi Z, et al. A study of histologic and immunophenotypical staining patterns in cutaneous lymphoid hyperplasia. J Am Acad Dermatol. 2011;65(1):112–24.

Berti E, Alessi E, Caputo R. Reticulohistiocytoma of the dorsum (Crosti's disease) and other B-cell lymphomas. Semin Diagn Pathol. 1991;8(2):82–90.

Bluefarb S. Lymphocytoma cutis. In: Bluefarb S, editor. Cutaneous manifestations of the benign inflammatory reticuloses. Springfield: Charles C Thomas; 1960. p. 131–99.

Blumental G, Okun MR, Ponitch JA. Pseudolymphomatous reaction to tattoos. Report of three cases. J Am Acad Dermatol. 1982;6(4 Pt 1):485–8.

Bluming A, Homer S, Khiroya R. Selective diphenylhydantoin-induced suppression of lymphocyte reactivity in vitro. J Lab Clin Med. 1976;88(3): 417–22.

Boer A, Tirumalae R, Bresch M, et al. Pseudoclonality in cutaneous pseudolymphomas: a pitfall in interpretation of rearrangement studies. Br J Dermatol. 2008;159(2):394–402.

Boudova L, Kazakov DV, Sima R, et al. Cutaneous lymphoid hyperplasia and other lymphoid infiltrates of the breast nipple: a retrospective clinicopathologic study of fifty-six patients. Am J Dermatopathol. 2005;27(5):375–86.

Brandes LJ, Arron RJ, Bogdanovic RP, et al. Stimulation of malignant growth in rodents by antidepressant drugs at clinically relevant doses. Cancer Res. 1992;52(13):3796–800.

Bratzke B, Stadler R, Gollnick H, et al. Borrelia burgdorferi-induced pseudolymphoma with pathogen cultivation in an HIV-1 positive patient. Hautarzt. 1989;40(8):504–9.

Breza Jr TS, Zheng P, Porcu P, et al. Cutaneous marginal zone B-cell lymphoma in the setting of fluoxetine therapy: a hypothesis regarding pathogenesis based on in vitro suppression of T-cell-proliferative response. J Cutan Pathol. 2006;33(7):522–8.

Brodell RT, Santa Cruz DJ. Cutaneous pseudolymphomas. Dermatol Clin. 1985;3(4):719–34.

Brown TJ, Yen-Moore A, Tyring SK. An overview of sexually transmitted diseases. Part I. J Am Acad Dermatol. 1999;41(4):511–32.

Bucher S, Fluckiger B, Rufli T. Infiltrating lymphadenosis benigna cutis as borreliosis of the skin. Hautarzt. 1988;39:77–81.

Burg G, Schmid MH, Kung E, et al. Semimalignant ("pseudolymphomatous") cutaneous B-cell lymphomas. Dermatol Clin. 1994;12(2):399–407.

Carlson JA, Ackerman AB, Fletcher CD, et al. A cutaneous spindle-cell lesion. Am J Dermatopathol. 2001;23(1):62–6.

Caro WA, Helwig HB. Cutaneous lymphoid hyperplasia. Cancer. 1969;24(3):487–502.

Ceballos KM, Gascoyne RD, Martinka M, et al. Heavy multinodular cutaneous lymphoid infiltrates: clinicopathologic features and B-cell clonality. J Cutan Pathol. 2002;29(3):159–67.

Cerio R, Oliver GF, Jones EW, et al. The heterogeneity of Jessner's lymphocytic infiltration of the skin. Immunohistochemical studies suggesting one form of perivascular lymphocytoma. J Am Acad Dermatol. 1990;23(1):63–7.

Cerroni L, Kerl H. The use of monoclonal antibodies on paraffin sections in the diagnosis of cutaneous lymphoproliferative disorders. Dermatol Clin. 1994;12(2):219–29.

Cerroni L, Borroni RG, Massone C, et al. Cutaneous B-cell pseudolymphoma at the site of vaccination. Am J Dermatopathol. 2007;29(6):538–42.

Chayavichitsilp P, Buckwalter JV, Krakowski AC, et al. Herpes simplex. Pediatr Rev. 2009;30(4):119–29. quiz 30.

Chimenti S, Cerroni L, Zenahlik P, et al. The role of MT2 and anti-bcl-2 protein antibodies in the differentiation of benign from malignant cutaneous infiltrates of B-lymphocytes with germinal center formation. J Cutan Pathol. 1996;23(4):319–22.

Choi TS, Doh KS, Kim SH, et al. Clinicopathological and genotypic aspects of anticonvulsant-induced pseudolymphoma syndrome. Br J Dermatol. 2003;148(4):730–6.

Chong H, Brady K, Metze D, et al. Persistent nodules at injection sites (aluminium granuloma) – clinicopathological study of 14 cases with a diverse range of histological reaction patterns. Histopathology. 2006;48(2):182–8.

Clark WH, Mihm Jr MC, Reed RJ, et al. The lymphocytic infiltrates of the skin. Hum Pathol. 1974;5(1):25–43.

Cochran RE, Thomson J, Fleming KA, et al. Histology simulating reticulosis in secondary syphilis. Br J Dermatol. 1976;95(3):251–4.

Coffin CM, Humphrey PA, Dehner LP. Extrapulmonary inflammatory myofibroblastic tumor: a clinical and pathological survey. Semin Diagn Pathol. 1998; 15(2):85–101.

Coffin CM, Hornick JL, Fletcher CD. Inflammatory myofibroblastic tumor: comparison of clinicopathologic, histologic, and immunohistochemical features including ALK expression in atypical and aggressive cases. Am J Surg Pathol. 2007;31(4):509–20.

Colli C, Leinweber B, Mullegger R, et al. Borrelia burgdorferi-associated lymphocytoma cutis: clinicopathologic, immunophenotypic, and molecular study of 106 cases. J Cutan Pathol. 2004;31(3):232–40.

Connors RC, Ackerman AB. Histologic pseudomalignancies of the skin. Arch Dermatol. 1976;112(12):1767–80.

Crowson AN, Magro CM. Antidepressant therapy. A possible cause of atypical cutaneous lymphoid hyperplasia. Arch Dermatol. 1995;131(8):925–9.

Cruz FA, Lage D, Frigerio RM, et al. Reactions to the different pigments in tattoos: a report of two cases. An Bras Dermatol. 2010;85(5):708–11.

Damle NK, Gupta S. Autologous mixed lymphocyte reaction in man. III. Regulation of autologous MLR by theophylline-resistant and -sensitive human T-lymphocyte subpopulations. Scand J Immunol. 1981;15(5):493–9.

Dorfman RF, Warnke R. Lymphadenopathy simulating the malignant lymphomas. Hum Pathol. 1974;5(5): 519–50.

Dosch HM, Jason J, Gelfand EW. Transient antibody deficiency and abnormal t-suppressor cells induced by phenytoin. N Engl J Med. 1982;306(7):406–9.

Duncan SC, Evans HL, Winkelmann RK. Large cell lymphocytoma. Arch Dermatol. 1980;116(10):1142–6.

El Shabrawi-Caelen L, Kerl K, Cerroni L, et al. Cutaneous inflammatory pseudotumor – a spectrum of various diseases? J Cutan Pathol. 2004;31(9):605–11.

English J, Smith N, Jones WE. Large cell lymphocytoma. J Cutan Pathol. 1986;13:441.

English J, Smith NP, Spaull J, et al. Large cell lymphocytoma – a clinicopathological study. Clin Exp Dermatol. 1989;14(3):181–5.

Erfurt C, Lueftl M, Simon Jr M, et al. Late syphilis mimicking a pseudolymphoma of the skin. Eur J Dermatol. 2006;16(4):431–4.

Evans HL, Winkelmann RK, Banks PM. Differential diagnosis of malignant and benign cutaneous lymphoid infiltrates: a study of 57 cases in which malignant lymphoma had been diagnosed or suspected in the skin. Cancer. 1979;44(2):699–717.

Facchetti F, Boden G, De Wolf-Peeters C, et al. Plasmacytoid monocytes in Jessner's lymphocytic infiltration of the skin. Am J Dermatopathol. 1990;12(4):363–9.

Falk ES, Eide TJ. Histologic and clinical findings in human scabies. Int J Dermatol. 1981;20(9):600–5.

Fernandez N, Torres A, Ackerman AB. Pathologic findings in human scabies. Arch Dermatol. 1977;113(3):320–4.

Friedmann K. Nodular or diffuse infiltrates. In: Farmer E, Hood A, editors. Pathology of the skin. Norwalk: Appleton & Lange; 1990. p. 207–11.

Friedmann D, Wechsler J, Delfau MH, et al. Primary cutaneous pleomorphic small T-cell lymphoma. A review of 11 cases. The French Study Group on Cutaneous Lymphomas. Arch Dermatol. 1995;131(9):1009–15.

Gartman H. Generalisierte pseudolymphoma der haut. Hautarzt. 1986;55:166.

Giannotti B, Santucci M. Skin-associated lymphoid tissue (SALT)-related B-cell lymphoma (primary cutaneous B-cell lymphoma). A concept and a clinicopathologic entity. Arch Dermatol. 1993;129(3):353–5.

Goffinet DR, Hoyt C, Eltringham JR. Secondary syphilis misdiagnosed as a lymphoma. Calif Med. 1970;112(5): 22–3.

Gollnick H, Mayer-da-Silva A, Thies W, et al. Infection with Treponema pallidum and HTLV-1 mimicking cutaneous T-cell lym- phoma. In: Mascaro JM, Orfanos CE editors. Clinical dermatology: the CMD case collection. New York: Schattauer, Stuttgart; 1987. p. 108–10.

Grange F, Wechsler J, Guillaume JC, et al. Borrelia burgdorferi-associated lymphocytoma cutis simulating a primary cutaneous large B-cell lymphoma. J Am Acad Dermatol. 2002;47(4):530–4.

Halevy S, Sandbank M. Transformation of lymphocytoma cutis into a malignant lymphoma in association with the sign of Leser-Trelat. Acta Derm Venereol. 1987;67(2):172–5.

Helm KF, Muller SA. Benign lymphocytic infiltrate of the skin: correlation of clinical and pathologic findings. Mayo Clin Proc. 1992;67(8):748–54.

Helm KF, Menz J, Gibson LE, et al. A clinical and histopathologic study of granulomatous rosacea. J Am Acad Dermatol. 1991;25(6 Pt 1):1038–43.

Hicks MI, Elston DM. Scabies. Dermatol Ther. 2009;22(4):279–92.

Hodak E, David M, Rothem A, et al. Nodular secondary syphilis mimicking cutaneous lymphoreticular process. J Am Acad Dermatol. 1987;17(5 Pt 2):914–7.

Hovmark A, Asbrink E, Olsson I. The spirochetal etiology of lymphadenosis benigna cutis solitaria. Acta Derm Venereol. 1986;66(6):479–84.

Hurt MA, Santa Cruz DJ. Cutaneous inflammatory pseudotumor. Lesions resembling "inflammatory pseudotumors" or "plasma cell granulomas" of extracutaneous sites. Am J Surg Pathol. 1990;14(8):764–73.

Imafuku S, Ito K, Nakayama J. Cutaneous pseudolymphoma induced by adalimumab and reproduced by infliximab in a patient with arthropathic psoriasis. Br J Dermatol. 2012;166(3):675–8.

Jeerapaet P, Ackerman A. Histologic patterns of secondary syphilis. Arch Dermatol Res. 1974;107:373–7.

Jessner M, Kanof N. Lymphocytic infiltration of the skin. Arch Dermatol. 1953;68:447–9.

Kahofer P, El Shabrawi-Caelen L, Horn M, et al. Pseudolymphoma occurring in a tattoo. Eur J Dermatol. 2003;13(2):209–12.

Kardaun SH, Scheffer E, Vermeer BJ. Drug-induced pseudolymphomatous skin reactions. Br J Dermatol. 1988;118(4):545–52.

Kazandjieva J, Tsankov N. Tattoos: dermatological complications. Clin Dermatol. 2007;25(4):375–82.

Kerl H. Cutaneous pseudolymphomas. In: Eisen A; K Wolff K et al. editors. Proceedings of the XVI international congress of dermatology. Tokyo: University of Tokyo Press; 1983. p. 189–95.

Kerl H, Ackerman AB. Inflammatory diseases that simulate lymphomas: cutaneous pseudolymphomas. Dermatology in general medicine. 4th ed. New York: McGraw-Hill; 1993. p. 1315–27.

Konttinen YT, Bergroth V, Johansson E, et al. A long-term clinicopathologic survey of patients with Jessner's lymphocytic infiltration of the skin. J Invest Dermatol. 1987;89(2):205–8.

Kuo TT, Lo SK, Chan HL. Immunohistochemical analysis of dermal mononuclear cell infiltrates in cutaneous lupus erythematosus, polymorphous light eruption, lymphocytic infiltration of Jessner, and cutaneous lymphoid hyperplasia: a comparative differential study. J Cutan Pathol. 1994;21(5):430–6.

LeBien TW, Tedder TF. B lymphocytes: how they develop and function. Blood. 2008;112(5):1570–80.

LeBoit PE, McNutt NS, Reed JA, et al. Primary cutaneous immunocytoma. A B-cell lymphoma that can easily be mistaken for cutaneous lymphoid hyperplasia. Am J Surg Pathol. 1994;18(10):969–78.

Leinweber B, Colli C, Chott A, et al. Differential diagnosis of cutaneous infiltrates of B lymphocytes with follicular growth pattern. Am J Dermatopathol. 2004;26(1):4–13.

Lever W, Schaumburg-Lever G. Lymphocytoma. Odland GF translator. In: Goldsmith LA, editor. Histopathology of the skin. 7 ed. Philadelphia: JB Lippincott; 1990. p. 837–46.

Lubach D, Hinz E. A pseudolymphomatous reaction in tattooing. Hautarzt. 1986;37(10):573–5.

MacKie R. Cutaneous lymphocytic infiltrates and pseudolymphomas. In: Champion R, Burton J, Ebling F, editors. Textbook of dermatology. 5th ed. London: Blackwell Scientific Publications; 1993. p. 2101–5.

MacSweeney F, Desai SA. Inflammatory pseudotumour of the subcutis: a report on the fine needle aspiration findings in a case misdiagnosed cytologically as malignant. Cytopathology. 2000;11(1):57–60.

Magro CM, Crowson AN. Drugs with antihistaminic properties as a cause of atypical cutaneous lymphoid hyperplasia. J Am Acad Dermatol. 1995;32(3):419–28.

McComb ME, Telang GH, Vonderheid EC. Secondary syphilis presenting as pseudolymphoma of the skin. J Am Acad Dermatol. 2003;49(2 Suppl Case Reports):S174–6.

McMillen MA, Lewis T, Jaffe BM, et al. Verapamil inhibition of lymphocyte proliferation and function in vitro. J Surg Res. 1985;39(1):76–80.

Moon HS, Park K, Lee JH, et al. A nodular syphilid presenting as a pseudolymphoma: mimicking a cutaneous marginal zone B-cell lymphoma. Am J Dermatopathol. 2009;31(8):846–8.

Moreno A, Curco N, Serrano T, et al. Disseminated, miliarial type lymphocytoma cutis. A report of two cases. Acta Derm Venereol. 1991;71(4):334–6.

Nathan DL, Belsito DV. Carbamazepine-induced pseudolymphoma with CD-30 positive cells. J Am Acad Dermatol. 1998;38(5 Pt 2):806–9.

Nihal M, Mikkola D, Horvath N, et al. Cutaneous lymphoid hyperplasia: a lymphoproliferative continuum with lymphomatous potential. Hum Pathol. 2003;34(6):617–22.

Paley K, Geskin LJ, Zirwas MJ. Cutaneous B-cell pseudolymphoma due to paraphenylenediamine. Am J Dermatopathol. 2006;28(5):438–41.

Ploysangam T, Breneman DL, Mutasim DF. Cutaneous pseudolymphomas. J Am Acad Dermatol. 1998;38(6 Pt 1):877–95. quiz 96-7.

Ramachandra S, Hollowood K, Bisceglia M, et al. Inflammatory pseudotumour of soft tissues: a clinicopathological and immunohistochemical analysis of 18 cases. Histopathology. 1995;27(4):313–23.

Rashidi A, Dorfler KR, Goodman BM. Diffuse Kaposi's sarcoma. Int J Dermatol. 2012;51(8):964–5.

Remy-Leroux V, Leonard F, Lambert D, et al. Comparison of histopathologic-clinical characteristics of Jessner's lymphocytic infiltration of the skin and lupus erythematosus tumidus: multicenter study of 46 cases. J Am Acad Dermatol. 2008;58(2):217–23.

Rijlaarsdam JU, Bruynzeel DP, Vos W, et al. Immunohistochemical studies of lymphadenosis benigna cutis occurring in a tattoo. Am J Dermatopathol. 1988;10(6):518–23.

Rijlaarsdam JU, Willemze R. Cutaneous pseudolymphomas: classification and differential diagnosis. Semin Dermatol. 1994;13(3):187–96.

Rijlaarsdam J, Meijer C, Willemze R. Differentiation between lymphadenosis benigna cutis and primary cutaneous follicular center cell lymphomas. Cancer Res. 1990;65:2301–6.

Rijlaarsdam JU, van der Putte SC, Berti E, et al. Cutaneous immunocytomas: a clinicopathologic study of 26 cases. Histopathology. 1993;23(2):117–25.

Sanches M. Syphilis. In: Freedberg I, Eisen A, Wolff K, et al., editors. Fitzpatrick's dermatology in general medicine. 6th ed. New York: McGraw Hill; 2003. p. 2163–88. Vol. 2.

Sanchez-Viera M, Hernanz JM, Sampelayo T, et al. Granulomatous rosacea in a child infected with the human immunodeficiency virus. J Am Acad Dermatol. 1992;27(6 Pt 1):1010–1.

Sangueza OP, Yadav S, White Jr CR, et al. Evolution of B-cell lymphoma from pseudolymphoma. A multidisciplinary approach using histology, immunohistochemistry, and Southern blot analysis. Am J Dermatopathol. 1992;14(5):408–13.

Santucci M, Pimpinelli N, Arganini L. Primary cutaneous B-cell lymphoma: a unique type of low-grade lymphoma. Clinicopathologic and immunologic study of 83 cases. Cancer. 1991;67(9):2311–26.

Sawada Y, Yoshiki R, Kawakami C, et al. Valsartan-induced drug eruption followed by CD30+ pseudolymphomatous eruption. Acta Derm Venereol. 2010; 90(5):521–2.

Schmutz JL, Trechot P. Cutaneous pseudolymphoma with two types of anti-TNFalpha: a class effect? Ann Dermatol Venereol. 2012;139(10):695–6.

Schreiber MM, McGregor JG. Pseudolymphoma syndrome. A sensitivity to anticonvulsant drugs. Arch Dermatol. 1968;97(3):297–300.

Self SJ, Carter VH, Noojin RO. Disseminated lymphocytoma cutis. Case reports of miliarial and nodular types. Arch Dermatol. 1969;100(4):459–64.

Shiino S, Kojima M, Arisawa T, et al. Presence of immunoglobulin heavy chain rearrangement in so-called IgG4-related plasma cell granuloma of the eyelid. J Clin Exp Hematop. 2012;52(2):141–3.

Sowden JM, Cartwright PH, Smith AG, et al. Sarcoidosis presenting with a granulomatous reaction confined to red tattoos. Clin Exp Dermatol. 1992;17(6):446–8.

Spray A, Glaser DA. Herpes zoster of the penis: an unusual location for a common eruption. J Am Acad Dermatol. 2002;47(2 Suppl):S177–9.

Stanek G, Wewalka G, Groh V, et al. Differences between Lyme disease and European arthropod-borne Borrelia infections. Lancet. 1985;1(8425):401.

Stirn A, Brahler E, Hinz A. Prevalence, sociodemography, mental health and gender differences of tattooing and body piercing. Psychother Psychosom Med Psychol. 2006;56(11):445–9.

Toonstra J, Wildschut A, Boer J, et al. Jessner's lymphocytic infiltration of the skin. A clinical study of 100 patients. Arch Dermatol. 1989;125(11):1525–30.

Torne R, Roura M, Umbert P. Generalized cutaneous B-cell pseudolymphoma. Report of a case studied by immunohistochemistry. Am J Dermatopathol. 1989; 11(6):544–8.

Triscott JA, Ritter JH, Swanson PE, et al. Immunoreactivity for bcl-2 protein in cutaneous lymphomas and lymphoid hyperplasias. J Cutan Pathol. 1995;22(1):2–10.

ul Bari A, Raza N. Secondary syphilis clinically mimicking pseudolymphoma of the face. Dermatol Online J. 2006;12(3):20.

van der Putte SC, Toonstra J, Schuurman HJ, et al. Immunocytoma of the skin simulating lymphadenosis benigna cutis. Arch Dermatol Res. 1985;277(1): 36–43.

Van Hale HM, Winkelmann RK. Nodular lymphoid disease of the head and neck: lymphocytoma cutis, benign lymphocytic infiltrate of Jessner, and their distinction from malignant lymphoma. J Am Acad Dermatol. 1985;12(3):455–61.

Walton SF, Currie BJ. Problems in diagnosing scabies, a global disease in human and animal populations. Clin Microbiol Rev. 2007;20(2):268–79.

Wantzin GL, Hou-Jensen K, Nielsen M, et al. Cutaneous lymphocytomas: clinical and histological aspects. Acta Derm Venereol. 1982;62(2):119–24.

Wantzin GL, Thomsen K, Ralfkiaer E. Evolution of cutaneous lymphoid hyperplasia to cutaneous T-cell lymphoma. Clin Exp Dermatol. 1988;13(5):309–13.

Weber K, Schierz G, Wilske B, et al. European erythema migrans disease and related disorders. Yale J Biol Med. 1984;57(4):463–71.

Wechsler J, Bagot M, Henni T, et al. Cutaneous pseudolymphomas: immunophenotypical and immunogenotypical studies. Curr Probl Dermatol. 1990; 19:183–8.

Weinberg JM, Rook AH, Lessin SR. Molecular diagnosis of lymphocytic infiltrates of the skin. Arch Dermatol. 1993;129(11):1491–500.

Wilkin J, Dahl M, Detmar M, et al. Standard classification of rosacea: report of the National Rosacea Society Expert Committee on the classification and staging of rosacea. J Am Acad Dermatol. 2002; 46(4):584–7.

Willemze R, Dijkstra A, Meijer CJ. Lymphocytic infiltration of the skin (Jessner): a T-cell lymphoproliferative disease. Br J Dermatol. 1984;110(5):523–9.

Winkelmann RK, Dabski K. Large cell lymphocytoma: follow-up, immunopathology studies, and comparison to cutaneous follicular and Crosti lymphoma. Arch Dermatol Res. 1987;279(Suppl):S81–7.

Xu F, Sternberg MR, Gottlieb SL, et al. Seroprevalence of herpes simplex virus type 2 among persons aged 14–49 years – United States, 2005–2008. Centers for Disease Control and Prevention (CDC). 2010;59(15): 456–9.

Xu F, Sternberg MR, Kottiri BJ, et al. Trends in herpes simplex virus type 1 and type 2 seroprevalence in the United States. JAMA. 2006;296(8):964–73.

Yang M. Cutaneous inflammatory pseudotumor: a case report with immunohistochemical and ultrastructural studies. Pathology. 1993;25(4):405–9.

Zackheim HS, LeBoit PE, Stein KM. Disseminated recurrent papular B-cell pseudolymphoma. Int J Dermatol. 1997;36(8):614–8.

T-Cell Pseudolymphoma Presenting in a Lichenoid and Nodular Pattern

8

Kara M. Trapp, Summer D. Moon, Manojkumar T. Patel, and Michael B. Morgan

Lichenoid Keratosis

Introduction

Lichenoid keratosis (LK), otherwise known as lichen planus-like keratosis and benign lichenoid keratosis, was first described in 1966 by Lumpkin and Helwig as a solitary form of lichen planus (LP) (Lumpkin and Helwig 1966). Ackerman later that year described lesions as lichen planus-like keratosis in distinction with lichen planus (Shapiro and Ackerman 1966). LK is a common cutaneous

K.M. Trapp, BA (✉)
Department of College of Medicine
Georgetown University School of Medicine,
Washington, DC, USA
e-mail: kmt72@georgetown.edu

S.D. Moon, DO
Department of Dermatology, Largo Medical Center,
Nova Southeastern University, Largo, FL, USA

M.T. Patel, MD, FCAP
Department of Dermatopathology, Dermpath
Diagnostics, Bay Area, Tampa, FL, USA

M.B. Morgan, MD
Managing Director Tampa, Pensacola and Atlanta,
Dermpath Diagnostics, Department of Pathology,
University of South Florida College of Medicine,
Tampa, FL, USA

Department of Dermatology, Michigan State
University College of Medicine,
East Lansing, MI, USA

Primary Care Diagnostics Institute, Quest
Diagnostics, Palm Beach Gardens, FL, USA

Tampa, Pensacola and Atlanta Dermpath Diagnostics,
Tampa, FL, USA

entity that is often clinically confused with cutaneous malignancies such as basal cell carcinoma and squamous cell carcinoma. The pathogenesis is thought to involve a chronic inflammatory-mediated involution of a preexisting lentigo.

Clinical Features

Epidemiology

LKs develop between the ages of 36 and 87 years with an average of 59.5 years. The gender distribution in a study of 1,040 cases included 760 females (76 %) and 250 males (24 %) with the majority of lesions occurring in Caucasians (Berger et al. 1984; Morgan et al. 2005).

Clinical Appearance of Lesions

LKs present as solitary pink to red-brown, often scaly, papules ranging from 5 to 20 mm in diameter (Morgan et al. 2005; Prieto et al. 1993). LKs are usually asymptomatic or mildly pruritic and resemble basal or squamous cell carcinoma. Lesions most commonly appear on the trunk and extremities with less frequent occurrences on the head and neck (Bolognia and Jorizzo 2008a; Morgan et al. 2005).

Histopathology

Pattern of Infiltration

LK typically consists of a pronounced band-like lichenoid chronic inflammatory infiltrate nearly indistinguishable from LP (Fig. 8.1a). LK may also

H.D. Cualing et al. (eds.), *Cutaneous Hematopathology*,
DOI 10.1007/978-1-4939-0950-6_8, © Springer Science+Business Media New York 2014

Fig. 8.1 (**a**) Lichenoid
keratosis showing pronounced
band-like (*arrow*) lichenoid
chronic inflammatory infiltrate
with exocytosis. (**b**) Lichenoid
keratosis showing dense
lichenoid and nodular
lymphoid infiltrates

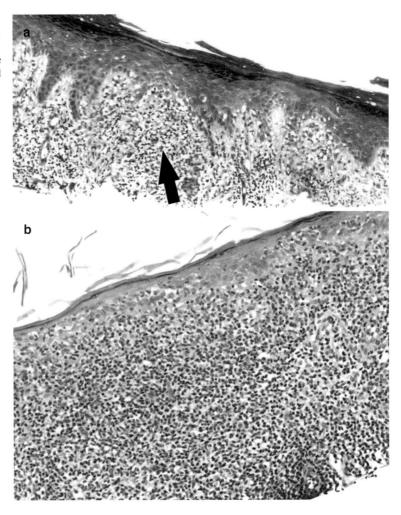

consist of dense lichenoid and nodular lymphoid infiltrates (Fig. 8.1b). As in LP, the epidermis often shows necrotic basilar keratinocytes, epidermal acanthosis, hypergranulosis, and hyperkeratosis (Fig. 8.2). Histological features that differentiate LK from LP include epidermal parakeratosis, an inflammatory infiltrate containing scattered eosinophils and plasma cells, and flanking epidermal foci of lentigo (Fig. 8.3) (Glaun et al. 1996; Jang et al. 2000; Prieto et al. 1993). The lesions of LK are classically divided into one of five histological variants, which include (1) classic form consisting of epidermal acanthosis and hyperkeratosis with an intense lichenoid lymphocyte-predominant inflammatory infiltrate and flanking epidermal foci of lentigo; (2) bullous

form consisting of intra- or subepidermal non-acantholytic bullous cavities with a dense associated lymphocytic infiltrate; (3) an atypical form most readily confused with T-cell lymphoproliferative disorder and consisting of rare (less than 5 %) atypical lymphocytes defined by enlarged, hyperchromatic, and irregularly contoured nuclei that are CD3+ and CD30+ (Fig. 8.4); (4) early or interface form consisting of slightly acanthotic or normal epidermal thickness with lymphocytes aligned along the dermoepidermal junction and adjacent lentigo; (5) and atrophic or senescent form consisting of epidermal atrophy with papillary dermal scarring, patchy lymphocytic infiltrates, and melanin incontinence (Morgan et al. 2005).

Fig. 8.2 Lichenoid keratosis showing necrotic basilar keratinocytes and exocytosis (*arrow*)

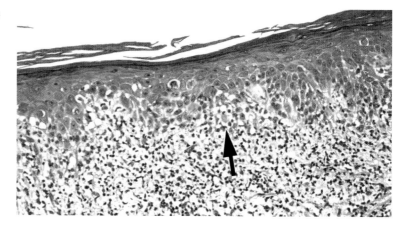

Fig. 8.3 Lichenoid keratosis showing distinguishing characteristics of epidermal parakeratosis, an inflammatory infiltrate containing scattered eosinophils and plasma cells, and flanking epidermal foci of lentigo (*arrow*)

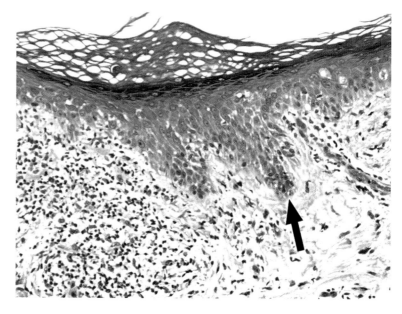

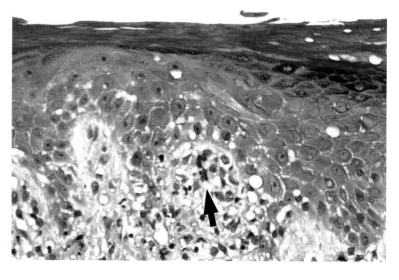

Fig. 8.4 LK showing atypical lymphocytes (*arrow*)

Cytomorphology

In a study of 1,040 cases of BLK, the classic form contained at least one apoptotic or Civatte body in every case (Morgan et al. 2005). The bullous form consists of more conspicuous numbers of apoptotic keratinocytes than the classic form associated with intraepidermal blister formation and subepidermal vesiculation (Morgan et al. 2005). The atypical form contains atypical lymphocytes characterized by enlarged, hyperchromatic, and irregularly contoured nuclei (Morgan et al. 2005).

Immunophenotype

An immunohistochemical study by Jang et al. of 17 patients diagnosed with LK revealed infiltrated epidermal and dermal lymphocytes of mainly CD8+ T cells and partly CD20+ B cells. CD4+ T cells were scarce in LK and cutaneous lymphocyte-associated antigen (CLA) was negative (Jang et al. 2000).

Genetics and Molecular Findings

A polyclonal population of cells was demonstrated by TCR gamma chain rearrangement analysis of 10 cases of benign LK (Smith et al. 2002).

Clinical Course

Clinical examination may not be able to differentiate LK from a solitary malignancy or inflammatory lesion; therefore, a biopsy is recommended. Lesions are usually removed with biopsy. Due to the benign nature of LK, remaining lesions may not require further surgery and may remain stable or undergo spontaneous regression.

Differential Diagnosis

LK can clinically mimic basal or squamous cell carcinoma, actinic keratosis, irritated seborrheic keratosis, melanoma, and nevus. Thus, a biopsy is warranted for accurate diagnosis of LK.

Lichen Aureus

Introduction

Lichen aureus (LA) is a rare variant of chronic pigmented purpuric dermatosis (PPD) first described by Marten in 1958 (Marten 1958). The PPD are a group of skin disorders with overlapping clinical and histopathological features (Graham et al. 1984; Newton and Raimer 1985; Ratnam et al. 1991). The etiologies of PPDs are unknown and the most common variant is Schamberg disease. Cutaneous T-cell lymphoma may begin with clinical lesions that resemble PPDs; thus, clinical and histopathological data is required for diagnosis.

Clinical Features

Epidemiology

Etiology of LA is unknown and lesions commonly occur in young adults and less frequently in children.

Clinical Appearance of Lesions

LA lesions present as one or multiple asymptomatic or mildly pruritic, golden- to rust-colored macules or lichenoid papules. The macules may coalesce into a patch and commonly appear on the lower extremities of young adults. Lesions have also been reported to occur on the trunk, upper extremity, and glans penis (English 1985; Kossard and Shumack 1989; Rudolph 1983). Lesions are frequently unilateral and persist unchanged for years (Graham et al. 1984; Price et al. 1985).

Histopathology

Pattern of Infiltration

LA is characterized by a dense band-like histiocytic and lymphocytic infiltration in the upper dermis; extravasation of erythrocytes and iron pigment in the histiocytes are often noticed. Early LA consists of a lymphocytic capillaritis with extravasated erythrocytes (Fig. 8.5) with mature

Fig. 8.5 Early LA consists of a lymphocytic capillaritis with extravasated erythrocytes (*arrow*)

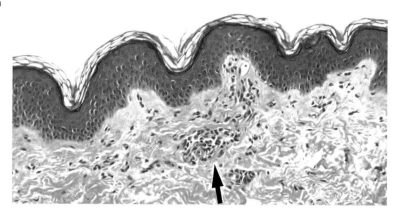

Fig. 8.6 LA mature lesions exhibiting a lichenoid tissue reaction with marked accumulation of hemosiderin-containing macrophages (*arrow*)

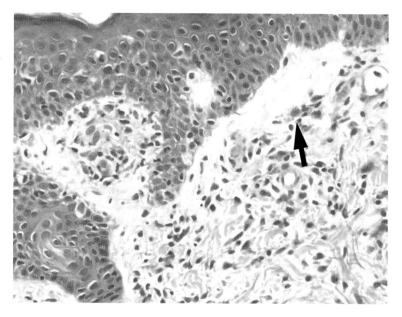

lesions exhibiting a lichenoid tissue reaction with marked accumulation of hemosiderin-containing macrophages (Fig. 8.6) dissimilar to conventional PPD (Price et al. 1985).

Cytomorphology

The infiltrate contains lymphocytes and histiocytes interspersed with extravasated erythrocytes. In one case report of LA, the histiocytes were characterized by convoluted or bean-shaped nuclei and a large amount of eosinophilic cytoplasm (Aoki and Kawana 2002). Additionally, large histiocytic cells consisting of cytoplasmic Birbeck granules were present among the lymphocytes in the upper dermis (Aoki and Kawana 2002). A thinning of the epidermis without evidence of spongiosis or epidermal exocytosis and an increased number of siderophores in the mid-dermis have been observed (Murota and Katayama 2011).

Immunophenotype

The lymphocytic infiltration is predominately composed of T lymphocytes, a majority of which are CD4+, admixed with some reactive CD1a + dendritic cells (Aiba and Tagami 1988; Ghersetich et al. 1994; Smoller and Kamel 1991). Immunofluorescence studies are frequently negative, although one study demonstrated C3 and immunoglobulins present in vessel walls (Iwatsuki et al. 1980).

Genetics and Molecular Findings

T-cell receptor gene rearrangement (TCRGR) is not helpful in the diagnosis of LA. An analysis in 2008 by Fink-Puches et al. of the T-cell receptor gamma gene rearrangement performed in 16 cases of LA revealed an equal number of patients with monoclonal and polyclonal bands (Fink-Puches et al. 2008).

Clinical Course

LA belongs to the expanding spectrum of clonal dermatoses. Possible progression to mycosis fungoides (MF) has been reported in the literature; thus, patients require close follow-up (Brehmer-Andersson 1976; Cather et al. 1998; Guitart and Magro 2007; Martinez et al. 2001; Puddu et al. 1999; Ugajin et al. 2005). LA is difficult to treat and lesions typically remain stable or undergo spontaneous resolution. Anecdotal reports describe some benefit from the use of topical steroids if used for 4–6 weeks. PUVA (psoralen and ultraviolet A), narrow-band UVB, and immunosuppressive therapy have also demonstrated efficacy. If immunosuppression is considered, cutaneous T-cell lymphoma must be excluded (Bolognia and Jorizzo 2008b).

Differential Diagnosis

Angioma serpiginosum, MF, allergic contact dermatitis, non-allergic reactions to topical medica-tions, drug eruptions, and hypergammaglobulinemic purpura of Waldenstrom are included in the differential diagnosis (Bolognia and Jorizzo 2008b). The differentiation between MF and PPDs is frequently challenging because of the overlapping histological and clinical features (Guitart et al. 1997). In the absence of cytological atypia, papillary dermal fibrosis and mild papillary dermal edema favor PPDs. Lymphocytic exocytosis can be seen in both lesions; however, the intraepidermal lymphocytes in MF demonstrate more atypical features than those of PPDs (Boyd and Vnencak-Jones 2003; Crowson et al. 1999; Smoller and Kamel 1991).

Actinic Reticuloid

Introduction

Actinic reticuloid (AR) is a chronic photosensitive dermatosis first described in 1969 by Ive et al. (1969). AR represents the most extreme variant of chronic actinic dermatitis and is characterized by cutaneous lesions simulating cutaneous T-cell lymphoma clinically and histologically. The following criteria must be met in the diagnosis of AR: (1) persistent infiltrated papules and plaques on sun-exposed skin, frequently extending to covered areas or generalized infiltrated erythroderma; (2) photosensitivity to a wide wave length spectrum including UVB, UVA, and some of the visible light spectrum; and (3) a dermal infiltrate with the inclusion of atypical lymphoid cells observed upon histological examination (Toonstra 1991). Cases lacking one or more of the above criteria are denoted with the general term "chronic actinic dermatitis" (Toonstra 1991). Chronic actinic dermatitis encompasses AR, persistent light reaction, photosensitive eczema, and chronic photosensitive dermatitis and is defined by the following criteria: (1) dermatitis of sun-exposed areas, (2) a histological profile resembling eczema or featuring lymphoma-like changes, and (3) a decreased minimal erythema dose (MED) to UVB (mJ/cm^2) and UVA (J/cm^2) (Clark-Loeser 2003; Frain-Bell et al. 1974; Khatri et al. 1994; Oliveira Soares et al. 2002).

The diagnosis and treatment of AR is particularly challenging for physicians as AR may easily be mistaken for the cutaneous T-cell lymphomas, Sézary syndrome (Pacheco et al. 2012; Toonstra et al. 1985), and mycosis fungoides (MF). While it has been demonstrated that a large number of patients with AR do not show an increased susceptibility to malignancy, (Bilsland et al. 1994) De Silva et al. suggest a progression of AR to MF in two patients (De Silva et al. 2000). They hypothesized that the transformation of AR into MF occurred from the chronic immunological stimulation of the skin combined with UV-induced cutaneous immunosuppression (De Silva et al. 2000). Additionally, Thomsen reports on the development of Hodgkin's lymphoma in a patient with AR (Thomsen 1977).

Clinical Features

Epidemiology

AR occurs predominantly in elderly men; however, it has also been shown to occur in young individuals and in women (Guardiola and Sanchez 1980; Healy and Rogers 1995; Kurumaji et al. 1994). AR is considered a rare, idiopathic disease with an incidence of approximately 1 in 6,000 (Ive et al. 1969; Khatri et al. 1994; Toonstra 1991). AR has been demonstrated to occur worldwide, with the greatest frequency in northwestern Europe, most notably, Holland (Healy and Rogers 1995; Toonstra 1991).

Clinical Appearance of Lesions

Erythema and edema on photoexposed areas, including the face, neck, ears, and arms, are common features at initial presentation. At later stages of AR, infiltrated, eczematoid, lichenified patches, plaques, and nodules may arise and extend into nonexposed areas. AR commonly presents in a papular form but has also been demonstrated to present in a nodular or lichenoid form (Evans et al. 2004; Grone et al. 2006; Yap et al. 2003). Patients may demonstrate a history of abnormal photosensitivity. Pruritus and burning are frequently associated with cases of AR. Generalized erythroderma and generalized lymphadenopathy have also been demonstrated to occur (Zak-Prelich and Schwartz 1999). Additional clinical symptoms include lichenoid hyperpigmentation, lichenoid purpuric lesions, palmoplantar hyperkeratosis onycholysis, and alopecia (Toonstra et al. 1989a). Patients with AR may also develop leonine facies, a dermatological condition characterized by deep furrowing of facial skin (Ravic-Nikolic et al. 2012).

Histopathology

Pattern of Infiltration

The histological pattern of AR shares similar features with cutaneous T-cell lymphoma. The infiltrate is present in the upper dermis and may also extend into the middle and lower dermis. Eosinophils, histiocytes, plasma cells, giant cells, IgE + cells with a dendritic morphology, and characteristic multinucleated stellate fibroblasts (Fig. 8.7) are typically present within the infiltrate (Zak-Prelich and Schwartz 1999). Exocytosis of lymphocytes and atypical mononuclear cells infiltrating the epidermis may simulate the Pautrier microabscesses of MF, thus making the diagnosis of AR particularly challenging. However, the atypical lymphocytes of AR are accompanied by conspicuous extracellular epidermal edema (spongiosis) (Fig. 8.8) and, unlike MF, lack pericellular vacuolization. It is also important to note that Pautrier's microabscesses are uncommon in early lesions of MF.

Psoriasiform epidermal hyperplasia may also occur, resulting in the presence of thickened collagen in the papillary dermis. A common histological change seen in AR is the presence of lichen simplex chronicus superimposed upon an inflammatory process; such changes are frequently useful in the differential diagnosis between AR and MF.

Cytomorphology

The infiltrate is perivascular or band-like, is frequently dense, and is composed of atypical mononuclear cells with a cerebriform nucleus (Fig. 8.9) (Clark-Loeser 2003; Ive et al. 1969; Toonstra et al. 1989a).

Fig. 8.7 AR showing characteristic multinucleated stellate fibroblasts (*arrow*)

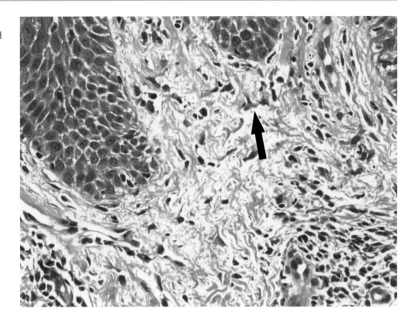

Fig. 8.8 AR showing atypical lymphocytes accompanied by conspicuous extracellular epidermal edema (spongiosis)

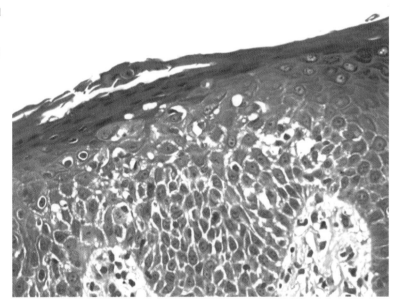

Immunophenotype

Immunohistochemical analysis of the cutaneous infiltrates demonstrates the presence of activated T cells, histiocytes, macrophages, and B cells (Toonstra et al. 1989b). A predominance of CD8+ lymphocytes is most frequently associated with AR, whereas a greater percentage of CD4+ cells is typical in individuals with MF (Toonstra et al. 1989a). An immunohistochemical analysis of 13 patients with AR demonstrated an inverse relationship between dermal infiltrate HLA-DR expression and the number of Leu CD8+ cells, thus indicating a negative correlation between a state of activation and Leu CD8+ cell concentration (Toonstra et al. 1989b). The infiltrate is composed

Fig. 8.9 AR showing psoriasiform epidermal hyperplasia, thickened papillary dermal collagen, and a band-like infiltrate with exocytosis composed of atypical mononuclear cells with a cerebriform nucleus

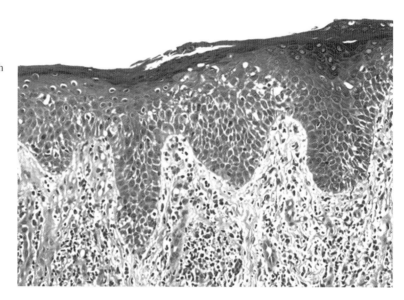

of polyclonal T lymphocytes, Langerhans cells, and HLA-DR + macrophages (Bakels et al. 1998; Toonstra et al. 1989a). The dermal infiltrate will demonstrate a combination of CD8+ cells and CD4+ cells, whereas the epidermal infiltrate will contain predominately CD8 + cells (Heller et al. 1994).

Genetics and Molecular Findings

Genotypic analysis of skin biopsies of patients with AR most frequently demonstrates a lack of T-cell gene receptor rearrangement; however, cases with monoclonal rearrangement have been reported in the literature (Melotti et al. 2008; Pacheco et al. 2012).

Clinical Course

The initial clinical presentation of AR mimics eczema, whereas the chronic stage of AR is characterized by a pseudolymphomatous appearance (Pacheco et al. 2012). Photopatch tests demonstrate one or more positive allergen responses in 75 % of AR cases and are often associated with musk ambrette, sulfanilamide, tetrachlorosalicylanide, lichen acid mix, and P-aminobenzoic acid

(Oliveira Soares et al. 2002; Toonstra et al. 1989a). Increased photosensitivity to UVB, UVA, and part of the visible light spectrum should occur over a duration of at least 1 year for an accurate diagnosis of AR (Zak-Prelich and Schwartz 1999). Laboratory results including serum biochemistry and complete blood count measurements are predominantly normal (Zak-Prelich and Schwartz 1999). Contact allergy recognition and avoidance, photoprotection, photochemotherapy, and systemic immunosuppression may be used in the treatment of chronic AR. Rare cases of AR have demonstrated spontaneous remission (Toonstra 1991).

Differential Diagnosis

The differential diagnosis between AR and cutaneous T-cell lymphomas is significantly challenging for physicians because of the similar clinical and histopathological features between the disorders. Essential features of AR include photosensitivity to a wave length spectrum spanning UVB, UVA, and the inclusion of some of the visible light spectrum. Additionally, AR is characterized by mixed cellular infiltrates and a predominance of CD8+ T cells. Circulating atypical lymphocytes (Sézary-like cells) may occur in both AR and MF; however, fewer numbers and a normal CD4/CD8 ratio are suggestive of AR. Positive patch and photopatch tests are correlated with a high frequency in AR, whereas no association has been shown to occur in MF (De Silva et al. 2000). While clonal T-cell receptor (TCR) gene rearrangement is frequently used in the differential diagnosis between AR and cutaneous T-cell lymphoma, a genetic rearrangement pattern of the beta chain T-cell receptor has been observed in patients with AR (Melotti et al. 2008; Pacheco et al. 2012); therefore, genetic rearrangement should not be used as a definitive marker for malignancy. An accurate diagnosis of AR involves the integrated synthesis of clinical, molecular, immunophenotypical, and morphological data.

Lymphomatoid Contact Dermatitis

Introduction

Lymphomatoid contact dermatitis (LCD) was first described by Orbaneja et al. in 1976 and is characterized as a chronic, persistent variant of allergic contact dermatitis that simulates the cutaneous T-cell lymphoma mycosis fungoides (MF) both clinically and histologically (Orbaneja et al. 1976). The immunological mechanism of LCD is hypothesized to occur from an antigenic stimulus resulting in the production and accumulation of activated lymphocytes that produce clonal selection, proliferate, and transform into blast cells (Evans et al. 2003). LCD is often a challenging disorder to diagnose due to the problematic nature of associating it with a specific allergen (Narganes et al. 2013). The allergens that have been reported to induce LCD include phosphorus, gold, nickel, cobalt, textile dyes, an exotic wood species (teak, *Tectona grandis* L.), benzydamine hydrochloride, para-phenylenediamine, para-tertyl-butyl phenol resin, isopropyl-diphenylenediamine, diaminodiphenylmethane, ethylenediamine dihydrochloride, methylchloroisothiazolinone, quaternium-15, and allergens in an ophthalmological preparation (Alvarez-Garrido et al. 2010; Braun et al. 2000; Calzavara-Pinton et al. 2002; Conde-Taboada

et al. 2007; Danese and Bertazzoni 1995; Evans et al. 2003; Ezzedine et al. 2007; Fleming et al. 1997; Houck et al. 1997; Marliere et al. 1998; Mendese et al. 2010; Narganes et al. 2013; Nigro et al. 1988; Orbaneja et al. 1976; Park et al. 1999; Schena et al. 1995; Wall 1982).

Clinical Features

Epidemiology

LCD is observed in adults of both genders (Wood 2012).

Clinical Appearance of Lesions

LCD is characterized by erythematous, pruritic, scaly plaques and papules that may be discrete or confluent. Exfoliative erythroderma may be present. The lesions grow progressively and may exhibit periods of exacerbation and remission. LCD induced from gold earrings presents clinically as discrete nodules at the sites of contact (Fleming et al. 1997; Park et al. 1999). A nodular clinical presentation has also occurred in a case of LCD caused by an ophthalmological preparation (Braun et al. 2000).

Histopathology

Pattern of Infiltration

T-cell LCD demonstrates a band-like T-cell infiltrate in the upper dermis with prominent epidermotropism (Orbaneja et al. 1976). Superficial dermal (papillary) edema often accompanies the infiltrate permitting distinction with common forms of mycosis fungoides (Fig. 8.10a). Focal extension of the edema and infiltrate to periadnexal and perivascular areas may occur (Calzavara-Pinton et al. 2002). Epidermal spongiosis or spongiotic microvesiculation is typically present (Martinez-Moran et al. 2009) in addition to parakeratosis and acanthosis (Calzavara-Pinton et al. 2002; Ezzedine et al. 2007). Prominent tissue eosinophilia and lymphoid hyperplasia throughout the dermis and subcutaneous tissue were reported in a case of LCD caused by gold earrings (Park et al. 1999).

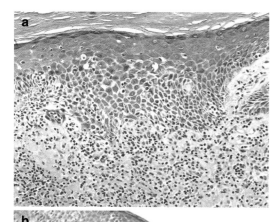

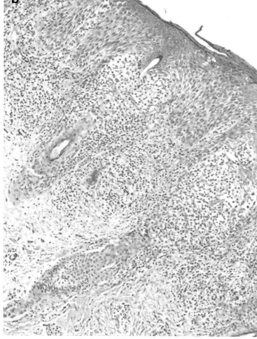

Fig. 8.10 (**a**) LCD showing a band-like T-cell infiltrate in the upper dermis with prominent epidermotropism and superficial dermal edema. (**b**) LCD showing spongiotic microvesiculations with Langerhans cells and few lymphocytes simulating "Pautrier's microabscesses"

Cytomorphology

Hyperchromatic and atypical lymphocytes with focal exocytosis are observed in LCD (Houck et al. 1997). The infiltrate is frequently composed of cells with large, hyperchromatic, convoluted nuclei (Calzavara-Pinton et al. 2002; Martinez-Moran et al. 2009). Multinucleated, giant cells showing birefringent inclusions have also been

demonstrated (Conde-Taboada et al. 2007). The diagnosis of LCD is particularly challenging as the intraepidermal collections of lymphocytes frequently simulate the Pautrier microabscesses of MF (Fig. 8.10b) (Houck et al. 1997; Orbaneja et al. 1976).

Immunophenotype

Immunohistochemical analysis demonstrates a dominant phenotype of CD3+ and CD4+ cells (Evans et al. 2003; Ezzedine et al. 2007; Narganes et al. 2013). A dominance of C8+ cells over CD4+ cells has also been reported (Calzavara-Pinton et al. 2002). The presence of rare CD30+ and CD1a + cells has been observed (Martinez-Moran et al. 2009), in addition to CD2+, CD5+, CD7+, and CD45RO+, cells expressing cutaneous lymphocyte antigen (CLA) (Calzavara-Pinton et al. 2002).

Genetics and Molecular Findings

T-cell receptor gene analysis has demonstrated a lack of a clonal population of T cells (Evans et al. 2003; Ezzedine et al. 2007; Martinez-Moran et al. 2009).

Clinical Course

LCD may present as a localized form, where lesions develop in cutaneous regions in direct contact with the allergen, and as a generalized form, where the lesions are widely dispersed, exhibit an inclination to become erythrodermic and are frequently resistant to treatment (Haynes et al. 1982). Complete resolution of symptoms is most often obtained following removal of the antigenic stimulus. However, a lack of clinical remission despite allergic avoidance and potent topical steroid therapy has been reported (Ezzedine et al. 2007). In such cases, long-term follow-up is necessary as the disorder may evolve into a malignant lymphoma. This was demonstrated by Abraham et al. in their report of the transformation of LCD into T-cell prolymphocytic leukemia (Abraham et al. 2006). However, the premise that these patients had lymphoma from the onset cannot be excluded.

Differential Diagnosis

The differentiation between LCD and mycosis fungoides (MF) remains challenging as the histological presentations of the two disorders may be indistinguishable. An accurate diagnosis of LCD should be made from the clinical and histological data, in combination with immunohistochemical, gene rearrangement, and patch-test analysis. The definitive diagnosis of LCD has been hypothesized to include four criteria: (1) a localized eruption indicating contact dermatitis clinically, (2) histological findings simulating cutaneous T-cell lymphoma, (3) positive patch-test results, and (4) resolution of symptoms following corticosteroid treatment and avoidance of the allergen (Orbaneja et al. 1976).

Lymphomatoid Drug Reactions

Introduction

Lymphomatoid drug reactions are cutaneous drug reactions resulting in atypical lymphoid infiltrates that simulate cutaneous T-cell lymphomas. Additional appellations for this entity include "lymphomatoid drug eruptions," "drug-induced cutaneous pseudolymphoma," and "drug-induced pseudolymphoma syndrome." A large number of drugs have been implicated in the induction of cutaneous atypical lymphoid infiltrates. The lymphomatoid drug reactions are divided into two main categories: (1) anticonvulsant-induced pseudolymphoma syndrome and (2) cutaneous pseudolymphoma induced by drugs other than anticonvulsants. Moreover, externally applied etheric plant oils have also been documented to induce lymphoproliferative reactions simulating malignant lymphomas (Cerroni et al. 2009). The most common anticonvulsant drugs inducing lymphomatoid drug reactions include phenytoin,

primidone, mephenytoin, and trimethadione (Ploysangam et al. 1998). Other classes of drugs associated with lymphocytic eruptions include, but are not limited to, ACE inhibitors, antihistamines, beta blockers, antifungals, antiarrythmics, antirheumatics, and cytotoxics (Gupta et al. 1990; Henderson and Shamy 1990; Kardaun et al. 1988; Magro and Crowson 1995; Ploysangam et al. 1998; Rijlaarsdam and Willemze 1991).

Clinical Features

Epidemiology
Anticonvulsant-induced pseudolymphoma syndrome has been reported to occur more frequently in black patients than in white patients (Ploysangam et al. 1998). Cutaneous pseudolymphoma induced by drugs other than anticonvulsants affects male and females equally (Ploysangam et al. 1998).

Clinical Appearance of Lesions
Anticonvulsant-induced pseudolymphoma syndrome presents as solitary cutaneous plaques, papules, nodules, or macules, and less frequently, as multiple erythematous, pruritic lesions with a widespread distribution (Ploysangam et al. 1998). Cutaneous pseudolymphoma induced by drugs other than anticonvulsants result in localized papules, generalized papulonodular lesions, and single or multiple nodules and plaques (Ploysangam et al. 1998). Erythroderma simulating Sézary syndrome has been reported for both categories of lymphomatoid drug reactions (D'Incan et al. 1992; Souteyrand and d'Incan 1990).

Histopathology

Pattern of Infiltration
Lymphomatoid drug reactions are characterized by an infiltration of lymphocytes into the dermis in a dense band-like or nodular pattern (Rijlaarsdam and Willemze 1991). The band-like lichenoid pattern is the most frequent pattern and it may simulate MF. The nodular pattern may mimic non-Hodgkin's lymphoma (Crowson and

Fig. 8.11 Lymphomatoid drug reaction showing prominent superficial vasculature containing hypertrophied endothelia

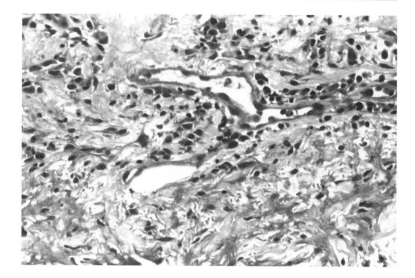

Magro 1995; Dorfman and Warnke 1974; Kardaun et al. 1988; Luelmo Aguilar et al. 1992). A histological presentation compatible with the nodular pattern of pseudo T-cell lymphoma was demonstrated in a patient with pseudolymphoma syndrome due to carbamazepine (Saeki et al. 1999). The infiltrate is frequently composed of atypical nuclei with a cerebriform outline. Nodular lesions are often characterized by significant histiocytes. Eosinophils and plasma cells are typically conspicuous and, along with prominent superficial vasculature containing hypertrophied endothelia (Fig. 8.11), constitute important clues to their distinction with MF (Magro and Crowson 1995). Epidermotropism has also been reported in the literature (Callot et al. 1996).

Cytomorphology

The band and nodular infiltrates are frequently characterized by atypical cells with pleomorphic, hyperchromatic nuclei.

Immunophenotype

Immunohistochemical analysis demonstrates a predominance of T cells in the infiltrate that are CD4+. The predominance of B cells is a rare occurrence and is associated with antihistamines

(Magro and Crowson 1995) and thioridazine (Luelmo Aguilar et al. 1992). Loss of pan-T-cell markers including CD2, CD3, and CD5 antigens has not been observed (Rijlaarsdam et al. 1992). The presence of CD3+, CD30+, and CD20+ atypical dermal lymphocytes was reported in an individual with carbamazepine-induced pseudo-lymphoma (Nathan and Belsito 1998). A polyclonal pattern of immunoglobulin light-chain expression is frequently observed.

Genetics and Molecular Findings

Molecular analysis of TCR genes most frequently demonstrates a polyclonal pattern.

Clinical Course

Patients with anticonvulsant-induced pseudolymphoma syndrome frequently develop symptoms within the first 2–8 weeks following drug intake (Ploysangam et al. 1998). These patients commonly develop generalized or localized lymphadenopathy, hepatosplenomegaly, fever, and erythematous eruptions (Ploysangam et al. 1998). Skin lesions often appear as solitary lesions; however, multiple nodules, papules, and plaques may develop in a widespread distribution (Ploysangam et al. 1998). Circulating Sézary-like cells may be present (Ploysangam et al. 1998). Erythroderma may be present. A digitate dermatitis-like pattern has also been reported (Mutasim 2003). Other clinical symptoms of patients treated with anticonvulsants include arthralgia, leukocytosis, malaise, and severe facial edema. Patients with cutaneous pseudolymphoma induced by drugs other than anticonvulsants develop symptoms within 1–11 months following drug intake (Ploysangam et al. 1998). In most cases, withdrawal of the offending agent results in regression. In rare circumstances, the progression of lymphomatoid drug eruptions into malignant lymphomas may occur, most notably, following a sustained period of anticonvulsant drug therapy (Anthony 1970; Hyman and Sommers 1966; Isobe et al. 1980; Li et al. 1975; Rausing 1978). In such circumstances, withdrawal of the offending agent does not result in clinical remission.

Differential Diagnosis

The differential diagnosis between lymphomatoid drug reactions and cutaneous T-cell lymphomas involves clinicopathological, immunohistochemical, and clonal correlation. In some cases, follow-up data subsequent to the withdrawal of the inciting agent is the only definitive measure used to identify the benign character of the atypical lymphoid infiltrates. The cutaneous T-cell lymphomas involved in the differential diagnosis of lymphomatoid drug reactions include MF and Sézary syndrome.

Solitary T-Cell Pseudolymphoma

Introduction

Solitary T-cell pseudolymphoma was first described in 1986 by van der Putte et al. in their description of three cases of a small, solitary lesion characterized by nonepidermotropic band-like subepidermal infiltrates composed of large T lymphocytes (van der Putte et al. 1986). Since this original description, numerous appellations have been attributed to these solitary lesions composed of T-cell infiltrates, including "solitary lymphomatous papule, nodule, or tumor," "cutaneous lymphoid hyperplasia," "solitary nonepidermotropic T-cell pseudolymphoma," "pseudolymphomatous folliculitis," and "solitary small- to medium-sized pleomorphic T-cell nodules of undetermined significance" (Cerroni 2010). The description of this entity as a lesion of "undetermined significance" was suggested by Leinweber et al. due to inconsistency between the indolent clinical course and histopathological characteristics of the disorder, thus making a definitive diagnosis as precisely benign or malignant challenging (Leinweber et al. 2009).

Clinical Features

Epidemiology
Solitary T-cell pseudolymphoma has been reported to affect individuals of both genders (Leinweber et al. 2009).

Clinical Appearance of Lesions
Solitary T-cell pseudolymphoma presents as slightly elevated, round, erythematous, solitary lesions with a diameter of 1–2 cm (van der Putte et al. 1986). Lesions are commonly located on the head, neck, or trunk (Leinweber et al. 2009). Superficial erosion and ulceration have been observed (Leinweber et al. 2009).

Histopathology

Pattern of Infiltration
The infiltrate may exhibit a band-like subepidermal pattern characterized by large T lymphocytes (van der Putte et al. 1986). A nonepidermotropic, nodular, or diffuse infiltration of small- to medium-sized pleomorphic T lymphocytes was observed in a report of 136 cases of

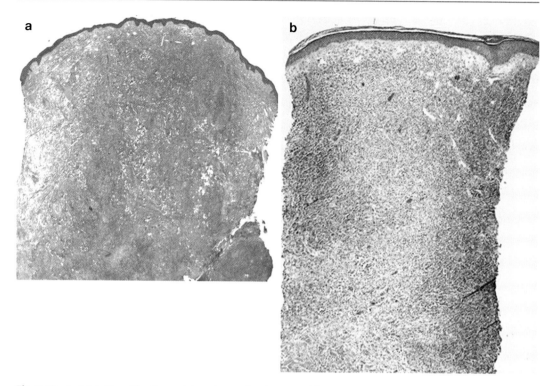

Fig. 8.12 (**a**, **b**) Solitary T-cell pseudolymphoma showing nonepidermotropic nodular or diffuse lymphoid infiltrates located in the entire dermis and with extension into the subcutaneous fat

SMPTCL (Beltraminelli et al. 2009). Dense, nodular, or diffuse lymphoid infiltrates located in the entire dermis and with extension into the subcutaneous fat are typical (Fig. 8.12a, b) (Leinweber et al. 2009). Dermoepidermal alignment or infiltration of the epidermis by lymphocytes is typically absent (Leinweber et al. 2009). Prominent vasculature consisting of hypertrophied or swollen endothelia containing cytoplasmic vacuolization is a helpful diagnostic feature (Fig. 8.13).

Cytomorphology

The lesions are typically composed of dense infiltrates of polymorphic cell population composed of a number of plasma cells, eosinophils, and many small non-atypical lymphocytes without atypia or without cerebriform nuclei (Figs. 8.14 and 8.15). Sheets of plasma cells and eosinophils may also be observed (Fig. 8.16). Adnexal structure effacement and/or angiodestruction, often observed with T-cell

lymphoma, is typically not observed (Leinweber et al. 2009).

Immunophenotype

Immunohistochemical analysis has demonstrated a T-cell phenotype (CD3+) (Fig. 8.17a) and a T-helper phenotype (CD4+) admixed with CD8+/ TIA-1+ cells, with variable proportions of B cells (CD20+) (Fig. 8.17b) (Leinweber et al. 2009). Scattered CD30+ cells representing less than 1 % of the infiltrate has also been observed (Leinweber et al. 2009).

Genetics and Molecular Findings

Although monoclonal rearrangement of the T-cell receptor gamma gene has been reported, these lesions usually are defined by lack of clonality upon T-cell surface receptor gene rearrangement study (Leinweber et al. 2009).

Fig. 8.13 Solitary T-cell
pseudolymphoma showing
prominent vasculature
consisting of hypertrophied or
swollen endothelia (*arrow*)
containing cytoplasmic
vacuolization

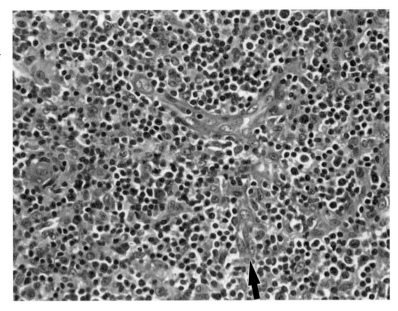

Fig. 8.14 Solitary T-cell
pseudolymphoma showing
sheets of plasma cells and
eosinophils

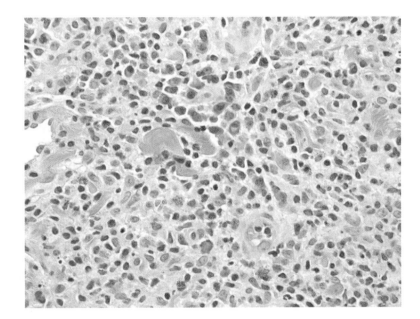

Clinical Course

Patients often present with asymptomatic, solitary, red to purplish plaques or tumors. The lesions often exhibit a tendency to self-regress (van der Putte et al. 1986). Nonaggressive treatment modalities frequently result in an indolent clinical course without extracutaneous manifestations (Leinweber et al. 2009).

Differential Diagnosis

The differential diagnosis of solitary T-cell pseudolymphoma includes "primary cutaneous CD4+ small- to medium-sized pleomorphic T-cell lymphoma (PCSMTCL)." PCSMTCL is characterized by a histopathological profile of dense infiltrates of small- to medium-sized CD4 + pleomorphic T lymphocytes with a small proportion (up to 30 %)

Fig. 8.15 Solitary T-cell pseudolymphoma showing binucleated reactive plasma cells and eosinophils

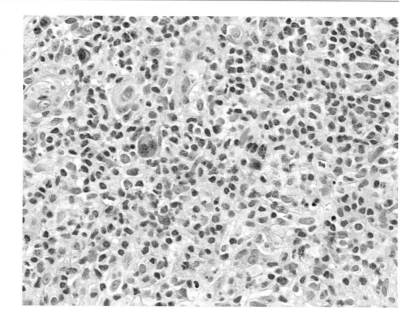

Fig. 8.16 Solitary T-cell pseudolymphoma showing clusters of foamy histiocytes

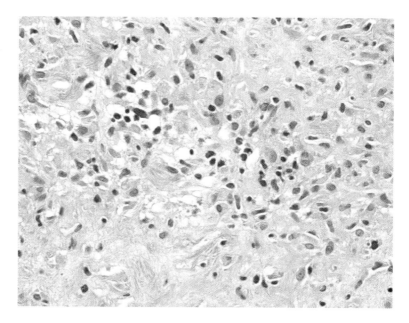

of large pleomorphic cells. The immunohisto-chemical profile of PCSMTCL is a CD3+/CD4+/CD8-/CD30- phenotype; however, CD8+ cases have also been described (Cerroni et al. 2004; Willemze et al. 2005). The difficulty in the diagnosis of PCSMTCL is highlighted by Lienweber et al. in their report on 26 cases that phenotypically and histopathologically met the criteria of PCSMTCL; however, the cases were characterized by excellent prognoses (Leinweber et al. 2009). Additional diagnostic challenges associated with solitary T-cell pseudolymphoma include the frequent predominance of small- to medium-sized pleomorphic T cells in mycosis fungoides (MF) and Sézary syndrome. Thus, the diagnostic criteria for PCSMTCL are limited to cases without

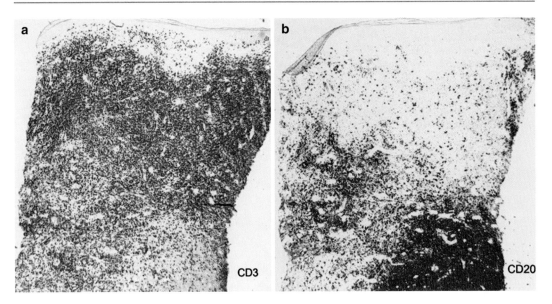

Fig. 8.17 (**a**, **b**) Solitary T-cell pseudolymphoma showing predominantly CD3+ T cells with variable proportions of CD20+ B cells. PCR analysis of TCRGR and IGH genes was negative

a history of MF or Sézary syndrome, without lesions that clinically simulate these disorders, and without distinct epidermotropism (Cerroni et al. 2004; Willemze et al. 2005).

References

Abraham S, Braun RP, Matthes T, Saurat JH. A follow-up: previously reported apparent lymphomatoid contact dermatitis, now followed by T-cell prolymphocytic leukaemia. Br J Dermatol. 2006;155(3):633–4.

Aiba S, Tagami H. Immunohistologic studies in Schamberg's disease. Evidence for cellular immune reaction in lesional skin. Arch Dermatol. 1988;124(7):1058–62.

Alvarez-Garrido H, Sanz-Munoz C, Martinez-Garcia G, Miranda-Romero A. Lymphomatoid photocontact dermatitis to benzydamine hydrochloride. Contact Dermatitis. 2010;62(2):117–9.

Anthony JJ. Malignant lymphoma associated with hydantoin drugs. Arch Neurol. 1970;22(5):450–4.

Aoki M, Kawana S. Lichen aureus. Cutis. 2002;69(2):145–8.

Bakels V, van Oostveen JW, Preesman AH, Meijer CJ, Willemze R. Differentiation between actinic reticuloid and cutaneous T cell lymphoma by T cell receptor gamma gene rearrangement analysis and immunophenotyping. J Clin Pathol. 1998;51(2):154–8.

Beltraminelli H, Leinweber B, Kerl H, Cerroni L. Primary cutaneous CD4+ small-/medium-sized pleomorphic T-cell lymphoma: a cutaneous nodular proliferation of pleomorphic T lymphocytes of undetermined significance? A study of 136 cases. Am J Dermatopathol. 2009;31(4):317–22.

Berger TG, Graham JH, Goette DK. Lichenoid benign keratosis. J Am Acad Dermatol. 1984;11(4 Pt 1):635–8.

Bilsland D, Crombie IK, Ferguson J. The photosensitivity dermatitis and actinic reticuloid syndrome: no association with lymphoreticular malignancy. Br J Dermatol. 1994;131(2):209–14.

Bolognia JL, Jorizzo J. Benign epidermal tumors and proliferations. In: Dermatology. 2nd ed. Philadelphia: Mosby; 2008a.

Bolognia J, Jorizzo J. Purpura and coagulation. In: Dermatology. 2nd ed. Philadelphia: Mosby; 2008b.

Boyd AS, Vnencak-Jones CL. T-cell clonality in lichenoid purpura: a clinical and molecular evaluation of seven patients. Histopathology. 2003;43(3):302–3.

Braun RP, French LE, Feldmann R, Chavaz P, Saurat JH. Cutaneous pseudolymphoma, lymphomatoid contact dermatitis type, as an unusual cause of symmetrical upper eyelid nodules. Br J Dermatol. 2000;143(2):411–4.

Brehmer-Andersson E. Mycosis fungoides and its relation to Sezary's syndrome, lymphomatoid papulosis, and primary cutaneous Hodgkin's disease. A clinical, histopathologic and cytologic study of fourteen cases and a critical review of the literature. Acta Derm Venereol Suppl (Stockh). 1976;56(75):3–142.

Callot V, Roujeau JC, Bagot M, Wechsler J, Chosidow O, Souteyrand P, et al. Drug-induced pseudolymphoma and hypersensitivity syndrome. Two different clinical entities. Arch Dermatol. 1996;132(11):1315–21.

Calzavara-Pinton P, Capezzera R, Zane C, Brezzi A, Pasolini G, Ubiali A, et al. Lymphomatoid allergic contact dermatitis from para-phenylenediamine. Contact Dermatitis. 2002;47(3):173–4.

Cather JC, Farmer A, Jackow C, Manning JT, Shin DM, Duvic M. Unusual presentation of mycosis fungoides as pigmented purpura with malignant thymoma. J Am Acad Dermatol. 1998;39(5 Pt 2):858–63.

Cerroni L, Gatter K, Kerl H. Skin lymphoma: the illustrated guide. London: Wiley-Blackwell; 2009.

Cerroni L, Gatter K, Kerl H. An illustrated guide to skin lymphoma. 2nd ed. Oxford: Blackwell Publishing; 2004.

Cerroni L. Cutaneous lymphoid proliferations: a clinico-pathological continuum. Diagn Histopathol. 2010; 16(9):417–24.

Clark-Loeser L. Chronic actinic dermatitis. Dermatol Online J. 2003;9(4):41.

Conde-Taboada A, Roson E, Fernandez-Redondo V, Garcia-Doval I, De La Torre C, Cruces M. Lymphomatoid contact dermatitis induced by gold earrings. Contact Dermatitis. 2007;56(3):179–81.

Crowson AN, Magro CM. Antidepressant therapy. A possible cause of atypical cutaneous lymphoid hyperplasia. Arch Dermatol. 1995;131(8):925–9.

Crowson AN, Magro CM, Zahorchak R. Atypical pigmentary purpura: a clinical, histopathologic, and genotypic study. Hum Pathol. 1999;30(9):1004–12.

Danese P, Bertazzoni MG. Lymphomatoid contact dermatitis due to nickel. Contact Dermatitis. 1995;33(4):268–9.

De Silva BD, Mclaren K, Kavanagh GM. Photosensitive mycosis fungoides or actinic reticuloid? Br J Dermatol. 2000;142(6):1221–7.

D'Incan M, Souteyrand P, Bignon YJ, Fonck Y, Roger H. Hydantoin-induced cutaneous pseudolymphoma with clinical, pathologic, and immunologic aspects of Sezary syndrome. Arch Dermatol. 1992;128(10):1371–4.

Dorfman RF, Warnke R. Lymphadenopathy simulating the malignant lymphomas. Hum Pathol. 1974;5(5):519–50.

English J. Lichen aureus. J Am Acad Dermatol. 1985;12 (2 Pt 1):377–9.

Evans AV, Banerjee P, McFadden JP, Calonje E. Lymphomatoid contact dermatitis to para-tertyl-butyl phenol resin. Clin Exp Dermatol. 2003;28(3):272–3.

Evans AV, Palmer RA, Hawk JL. Erythrodermic chronic actinic dermatitis responding only to topical tacrolimus. Photodermatol Photoimmunol Photomed. 2004;20(1):59–61.

Ezzedine K, Rafii N, Heenen M. Lymphomatoid contact dermatitis to an exotic wood: a very harmful toilet seat. Contact Dermatitis. 2007;57(2):128–30.

Fink-Puches R, Wolf P, Kerl H, Cerroni L. Lichen aureus: clinicopathologic features, natural history, and relationship to mycosis fungoides. Arch Dermatol. 2008;144(9):1169–73.

Fleming C, Burden D, Fallowfield M, Lever R. Lymphomatoid contact reaction to gold earrings. Contact Dermatitis. 1997;37(6):298–9.

Frain-Bell W, Lakshmipathi T, Rogers J, Willock J. The syndrome of chronic photosensitivity dermatitis and actinic reticuloid. Br J Dermatol. 1974;91(6):617–34.

Ghersetich I, Lotti T, Bacci S. Cell infiltrate in progressive pigmented purpura pigmentosa chronic. J Am Acad Dermatol. 1994;30:193–200.

Glaun RS, Dutta B, Helm KF. A proposed new classification system for lichenoid keratosis. J Am Acad Dermatol. 1996;35(5 Pt 1):772–4.

Graham RM, English JS, Emmerson RW. Lichen aureus – a study of twelve cases. Clin Exp Dermatol. 1984;9(4):393–401.

Grone D, Kunz M, Zimmermann R, Gross G. Successful treatment of nodular actinic reticuloid with tacrolimus ointment. Dermatology. 2006;212(4):377–80.

Guardiola A, Sanchez JL. Actinic reticuloid. Int J Dermatol. 1980;19(3):154–8.

Guitart J, Magro C. Cutaneous T-cell lymphoid dyscrasia: a unifying term for idiopathic chronic dermatoses with persistent T-cell clones. Arch Dermatol. 2007; 143(7):921–32.

Guitart J, Peduto M, Caro WA, Roenigk HH. Lichenoid changes in mycosis fungoides. J Am Acad Dermatol. 1997;36(3 Pt 1):417–22.

Gupta AK, Cooper KD, Ellis CN, Nickoloff BJ, Hanson CA, Brown MD, et al. Lymphocytic infiltrates of the skin in association with cyclosporine therapy. J Am Acad Dermatol. 1990;23(6 Pt 1):1137–41.

Haynes BF, Hensley LL, Jegasothy BV. Phenotypic characterization of skin-infiltrating T cells in cutaneous T-cell lymphoma: comparison with benign cutaneous T-cell infiltrates. Blood. 1982;60(2):463–73.

Healy E, Rogers S. Photosensitivity dermatitis/actinic reticuloid syndrome in an Irish population: a review and some unusual features. Acta Derm Venereol. 1995;75(1):72–4.

Heller P, Wieczorek R, Waldo E, Meola T, Buchness MR, Soter NA, et al. Chronic actinic dermatitis. An immunohistochemical study of its T-cell antigenic profile, with comparison to cutaneous T-cell lymphoma. Am J Dermatopathol. 1994;16(5):510–6.

Henderson CA, Shamy HK. Atenolol-induced pseudolymphoma. Clin Exp Dermatol. 1990;15(2):119–20.

Houck HE, Wirth FA, Kauffman CL. Lymphomatoid contact dermatitis caused by nickel. Am J Contact Dermat. 1997;8(3):175–6.

Hyman GA, Sommers SC. The development of Hodgkin's disease and lymphoma during anticonvulsant therapy. Blood. 1966;28(3):416–27.

Isobe T, Horimatsu T, Fujita T, Miyazaki K, Sugiyama T. Adult T-cell lymphoma following diphenylhydantoin therapy. Nihon Ketsueki Gakkai Zasshi. 1980;43(4):711–4.

Ive FA, Magnus IA, Warin RP, Jones EW. "Actinic reticuloid"; a chronic dermatosis associated with severe photosensitivity and the histological resemblance to lymphoma. Br J Dermatol. 1969;81(7):469–85.

Iwatsuki K, Aoshima T, Tagami H, Ohi M, Yamada M. Immunofluorescence study in purpura pigmentosa chronica. Acta Derm Venereol. 1980;60(4):341–5.

Jang KA, Kim SH, Choi JH, Sung KJ, Moon KC, Koh JK. Lichenoid keratosis: a clinicopathologic study of 17 patients. J Am Acad Dermatol. 2000;43(3):511–6.

Kardaun SH, Scheffer E, Vermeer BJ. Drug-induced pseudolymphomatous skin reactions. Br J Dermatol. 1988;118(4):545–52.

Khatri M, Shafi M, Ben-Ghazeil M. Actinic reticuloid : a study of 12 cases. Indian J Dermatol Venereol Leprol. 1994;60(5):254–7.

Kossard S, Shumack S. Lichen aureus of the glans penis as an expression of Zoon's balanitis. J Am Acad Dermatol. 1989;21(4 Pt 1):804–6.

Kurumaji Y, Kondo S, Fukuro S, Keong CH, Nishioka K. Chronic actinic dermatitis in a young patient with atopic dermatitis. J Am Acad Dermatol. 1994; 31(4):667–9.

Leinweber B, Beltraminelli H, Kerl H, Cerroni L. Solitary small- to medium-sized pleomorphic T-cell nodules of undetermined significance: clinical, histopathological, immunohistochemical and molecular analysis of 26 cases. Dermatology. 2009;219(1):42–7.

Li FP, Willard DR, Goodman R, Vawter G. Malignant lymphoma after diphenylhydantoin (dilantin) therapy. Cancer. 1975;36(4):1359–62.

Luelmo Aguilar J, Mieras Barcelo C, Martin-Urda MT, Castells Rodellas A, Lecha Carralero M, Marti Laborda R. Generalized cutaneous B-cell pseudolymphoma induced by neuroleptics. Arch Dermatol. 1992;128(1):121–3.

Lumpkin LR, Helwig EB. Solitary lichen planus. Arch Dermatol. 1966;93(1):54–5.

Magro CM, Crowson AN. Drugs with antihistaminic properties as a cause of atypical cutaneous lymphoid hyperplasia. J Am Acad Dermatol. 1995;32(3):419–28.

Marliere V, Beylot-Barry M, Doutre MS, Furioli M, Vergier B, Dubus P, et al. Lymphomatoid contact dermatitis caused by isopropyl-diphenylenediamine: two cases. J Allergy Clin Immunol. 1998;102(1):152–3.

Marten R. Case for diagnosis. Trans St Johns Hosp Dermatol Soc. 1958;40(98):2.

Martinez W, del Pozo J, Vazquez J, Yebra-Pimentel MT, Almagro M, Garcia-Silva J, et al. Cutaneous T-cell lymphoma presenting as disseminated, pigmented, purpura-like eruption. Int J Dermatol. 2001;40(2): 140–4.

Martinez-Moran C, Sanz-Munoz C, Morales-Callaghan AM, Garrido-Rios AA, Torrero V, Miranda-Romero A. Lymphomatoid contact dermatitis. Contact Dermatitis. 2009;60(1):53–5.

Melotti F, Mari E, Giorgiana F, Fidanza L, Carlesimo M, Pilozzi E, et al. Actinic reticulosis with clonal TCR (T-cell receptor) gene rearrangement. Eur J Dermatol. 2008;18(5):598–600.

Mendese G, Beckford A, Demierre MF. Lymphomatoid contact dermatitis to baby wipes. Arch Dermatol. 2010;146(8):934–5.

Morgan MB, Stevens GL, Switlyk S. Benign lichenoid keratosis: a clinical and pathologic reappraisal of 1040 cases. Am J Dermatopathol. 2005;27(5):387–92.

Murota H, Katayama I. Lichen aureus responding to topical tacrolimus treatment. J Dermatol. 2011;38(8):823–5.

Mutasim DF. Lymphomatoid drug eruption mimicking digitate dermatosis: cross reactivity between two drugs that suppress angiotensin II function. Am J Dermatopathol. 2003;25(4):331–4.

Narganes LM, Sambucety PS, Gonzalez IR, Rivas MO, Prieto MA. Lymphomatoid dermatitis caused by contact with textile dyes. Contact Dermatitis. 2013; 68(1):62–4.

Nathan DL, Belsito DV. Carbamazepine-induced pseudolymphoma with CD-30 positive cells. J Am Acad Dermatol. 1998;38(5 Pt 2):806–9.

Newton RC, Raimer SS. Pigmented purpuric eruptions. Dermatol Clin. 1985;3(1):165–9.

Nigro A, Patri P, Stradini D. Lymphomatoid contact dermatitis caused by diaminodiphenylmethane. G Ital Dermatol Venereol. 1988;123(7–8):379–82.

Oliveira Soares R, Silva R, Cirne de Castro J. Dermatite actínica crónica, lactonas sesquiterpénicas e líquenes: caso clínico. [Chronic actinic dermatitis, sesquiterpene lactones and lichens: Case report]. Boletim Informativo GPEDC. 2002;9:36–8.

Orbaneja JG, Diez LI, Lozano JL, Salazar LC. Lymphomatoid contact dermatitis: a syndrome produced by epicutaneous hypersensitivity with clinical features and a histopathologic picture similar to that of mycosis fungoides. Contact Dermatitis. 1976;2(3): 139–43.

Pacheco D, Fraga A, Travassos AR, Antunes J, Freitas J, Soares de Almeida L, et al. Actinic reticuloid imitating sezary syndrome. Acta Dermatovenerol Alp Panonica Adriat. 2012;21(3):55–7.

Park YM, Kang H, Kim HO, Cho BK. Lymphomatoid eosinophilic reaction to gold earrings. Contact Dermatitis. 1999;40(4):216–7.

Ploysangam T, Breneman DL, Mutasim DF. Cutaneous pseudolymphomas. J Am Acad Dermatol. 1998; 38(6):877–98.

Price ML, Jones EW, Calnan CD, MacDonald DM. Lichen aureus: a localized persistent form of pigmented purpuric dermatitis. Br J Dermatol. 1985; 112(3):307–14.

Prieto VG, Casal M, McNutt NS. Immunohistochemistry detects differences between lichen planus-like keratosis, lichen planus, and lichenoid actinic keratosis. J Cutan Pathol. 1993;20(2):143–7.

Puddu P, Ferranti G, Frezzolini A, Colonna L, Cianchini G. Pigmented purpura-like eruption as cutaneous sign of mycosis fungoides with autoimmune purpura. J Am Acad Dermatol. 1999;40(2 Pt 2):298–9.

Ratnam KV, Su WP, Peters MS. Purpura simplex (inflammatory purpura without vasculitis): a clinicopathologic study of 174 cases. J Am Acad Dermatol. 1991;25(4):642–7.

Rausing A. Hydantoin-induced lymphadenopathies and lymphomas. Recent Results Cancer Res. 1978;64: 263–4.

Ravic-Nikolic A, Milicic V, Ristic G, Jovovic-Dagovic B, Mitrovic S. Actinic reticuloid presented as facies leonine. Int J Dermatol. 2012;51(2):234–6.

Rijlaarsdam JU, Scheffer E, Meijer CJ, Willemze R. Cutaneous pseudo-T-cell lymphomas. A clinicopathologic study of 20 patients. Cancer. 1992;69(3):717–24.

Rijlaarsdam U, Willemze R. Cutaneous pseudo-T-cell lymphomas. Semin Diagn Pathol. 1991;8(2):102–8.

Rudolph RI. Lichen aureus. J Am Acad Dermatol. 1983;8(5):722–4.

Saeki H, Etoh T, Toda K, Mihm Jr MC. Pseudolymphoma syndrome due to carbamazepine. J Dermatol. 1999;26(5):329–31.

Schena D, Rosina P, Chieregato C, Colombari R. Lymphomatoid-like contact dermatitis from cobalt naphthenate. Contact Dermatitis. 1995;33(3):197–8.

Shapiro L, Ackerman AB. Solitary lichen planus-like keratosis. Dermatologica. 1966;132(5):386–92.

Smith DI, Vnencak-Jones CL, Boyd AS. T-lymphocyte clonality in benign lichenoid keratoses. J Cutan Pathol. 2002;29(10):623–4.

Smoller BR, Kamel OW. Pigmented purpuric eruptions: immunopathologic studies supportive of a common immunophenotype. J Cutan Pathol. 1991;18(6):423–7.

Souteyrand P, D'Incan M. Drug-induced mycosis fungoides-like lesions. Curr Probl Dermatol. 1990;19:176–82.

Thomsen K. The development of Hodgkin's disease in a patient with actinic reticuloid. Clin Exp Dermatol. 1977;2(2):109–13.

Toonstra J. Actinic reticuloid. Semin Diagn Pathol. 1991;8(2):109–16.

Toonstra J, Henquet CJ, van Weelden H, van der Putte SC, van Vloten WA. Actinic reticuloid. A clinical photobiologic, histopathologic, and follow-u study of 16 patients. J Am Acad Dermatol. 1989a;21(2 Pt 1):205–14.

Toonstra J, van der Putte SCJ, van Wichen DF, van Weelden H, Henquet CJM, van Vloten WA. Actinic reticuloid: immunohistochemical analysis of the cutaneous infiltrate in 13 patients. Br J Dermatol. 1989b;120(6):779–86.

Toonstra J, van Weelden H, Gmelig Meyling FH, van der Putte SC, Schiere SI, Baart de la Faille H. Actinic reticuloid simulating Sezary syndrome. Report of two cases. Arch Dermatol Res. 1985;277(3):159–66.

Ugajin T, Satoh T, Yokozeki H, Nishioka K. Mycosis fungoides presenting as pigmented purpuric eruption. Eur J Dermatol. 2005;15(6):489–91.

van der Putte SC, Toonstra J, Felten PC, van Vloten WA. Solitary nonepidermotropic T cell pseudolymphoma of the skin. J Am Acad Dermatol. 1986;14(3):444–53.

Wall LM. Lymphomatoid contact dermatitis due to ethylenediamine dihydrochloride. Contact Dermatitis. 1982;8(1):51–4.

Willemze R, Jaffe ES, Burg G, Cerroni L, Berti E, Swerdlow SH, et al. WHO-EORTC classification for cutaneous lymphomas. Blood. 2005;105(10):3768–85.

Wood GS. Inflammatory diseases that simulate lymphomas: cutaneous pseudolymphomas. 8th ed. New York: McGraw-Hill; 2012. Fitzpatrick's Dermatology in General Medicine.

Yap LM, Foley P, Crouch R, Baker C. Chronic actinic dermatitis: a retrospective analysis of 44 cases referred to an Australian photobiology clinic. Australas J Dermatol. 2003;44(4):256–62.

Zak-Prelich M, Schwartz RA. Actinic reticuloid. Int J Dermatol. 1999;38(5):335–42.

Neoplastic Nodular B-Cell Pattern

9

M. Angelica Selim and Mai P. Hoang

Introduction

Cutaneous B-cell lymphomas (CBCL) encompass a group of B-cell lymphomas that presents in the skin without evidence of extra-cutaneous disease at the time of initial diagnosis (Willemze et al. 1997) (Tables 9.1 and 9.2). Complete laboratory workup and imaging studies are needed to exclude cutaneous involvement by a nodal lymphoma since CBCL have a different biologic course and better prognosis and do not require aggressive treatment in comparison to their nodal counterparts (Kim et al. 2007). The incidence of CBCL was reported to be 20–25 % in several European studies (Willemze et al. 1997; Fink-Puches et al. 2002). From the Surveillance, Epidemiology, and End Results (SEER) registry collected in the United States between 1973 and 2001, the incidence of primary CBCL was 3.9 per million population (Smith et al. 2005).

A new consensus classification for cutaneous lymphoma was introduced by the World Health Organization (WHO) and the European Organization for Research and Treatment of Cancer (EORTC) in 2005 (Willemze et al. 2005;

Burg et al. 2005). It reconciled the differences between the 2001 WHO (histology and molecular parameters) and the 1997 EORTC (histology and skin site) classifications (Jaffe et al. 2001; Willemze et al. 1997). The EORTC categorized these lymphomas in three main groups: cutaneous follicle center lymphomas, cutaneous marginal zone B-cell lymphomas, and cutaneous diffuse large B-cell lymphomas, leg type (Willemze et al. 2005). The new 2008 World Health Organization (WHO) classification of tumors of hematopoietic and lymphoid included cutaneous follicle center lymphomas and cutaneous diffuse large B-cell lymphomas, leg type as separate entities in the classification (Swedlow et al. 2008). Cutaneous marginal zone B-cell lymphomas have been included within the group of extranodal marginal zone lymphomas of mucosa-associated lymphoid tissue (MALT). These classifications are comparable (Table 9.3) and have resulted in improvement in categorization of CBCL and unified criteria for therapeutic trials. In 2007, the International Society for Cutaneous Lymphomas (ISCL) and the Cutaneous Task Force of EORTC proposed a TNM (Tumor Node Metastasis) classification system (Table 9.4) (Kim et al. 2007). Although retrospective studies have been done, large prospective studies are needed to validate this TNM classification (Senff et al. 2007; Senff and Willemze 2007).

B lymphocytes are not normally present in the skin. In response to antigens such as drugs, arthropod bites (e.g., *Borrelia burgdorferi*), and others, B lymphocytes can accumulate resulting

M.A. Selim, MD
Dermatopathology Unit, Department of Pathology,
Duke University Medical Center, Durham, NC, USA

M.P. Hoang, MD (✉)
Department of Pathology, Harvard Medical School,
Massachusetts General Hospital,
55 Fruit Street, Warren 820, Boston, MA 02114, USA
e-mail: mhoang@mgh.harvard.edu

H.D. Cualing et al. (eds.), *Cutaneous Hematopathology*,
DOI 10.1007/978-1-4939-0950-6_9, © Springer Science+Business Media New York 2014

Table 9.1 Clinical features of nodular B-cell lymphomas

	PCFCL	PCMZL	PCLBCL-LT
Median age (years)	58	53	70
M/F ratio	2.1	1.4	0.5
Clinical presentation	Solitary or grouped papules	Solitary or multiple erythematous papules to small nodules	Ulcerated tumors
Sites	Scalp, forehead, trunk	Trunk, upper extremities	One or both lower legs
Therapy	Radiotherapy	Radiotherapy or excision	Solitary: radiotherapy Multiple: combination therapy
5-year overall survival (%)	>95	100	55

M male, *F* female, *PCFCL* primary cutaneous follicle center lymphoma, *PCMZL* primary cutaneous marginal zone lymphoma, *PCLBCL-LT* primary cutaneous large B-cell lymphoma, leg type

Table 9.2 Pathology, cytogenetics, and molecular biology of nodular B-cell lymphomas

Lymphoma type	Histopathology	Immunophenotype	Cytogenetics	Molecular
PCFCL	Proliferation of centrocytes admixed with variable number of centroblasts in a follicular and/or diffuse pattern	CD20+, CD79a+, PAX5+, Bcl6+, CD10+, Bcl2−	Absent t(14;18)	Monoclonal JH gene rearrangement
PCMZL	Nodular or diffuse growth of marginal zone cells with plasma cells at the periphery	CD20+, CD79a+, Bcl2+, Bcl6−, CD10−, CD5−	t(3;14)(p14;q32)	50–60 % monoclonal JH gene rearrangement
PCLBCL-LT	Uniform and large centroblasts and immunoblasts	CD20+, CD79a+, PAX5+, Bcl2+, MUM-1+, IgM+, Bcl6−/+, CD10−		

PCFCL primary cutaneous follicle center lymphoma, *PCMZL* primary cutaneous marginal zone lymphoma, *PCLBCL-LT* primary cutaneous large B-cell lymphoma, leg type, *JH* immunoglobulin heavy chain

Table 9.3 Comparison of the 2008 WHO and 2005 WHO-EORTC classifications for cutaneous B-cell lymphomas (Swedlow et al. 2008; Willemze et al. 2005)

WHO classification 2008	WHO-EORTC classification 2005
Extranodal marginal zone lymphoma of mucosa-associated lymphoid tissue (MALT lymphoma)	Primary cutaneous marginal zone B-cell lymphoma
Primary cutaneous follicle center lymphoma	Primary cutaneous follicle center lymphoma
Primary cutaneous diffuse large B-cell lymphoma, leg type	Primary cutaneous diffuse large B-cell lymphoma, leg type
Intravascular large B-cell lymphoma	Primary cutaneous diffuse large B-cell lymphoma—intravascular large B-cell lymphoma

WHO World Health Organization, *EORTC* European Organization for Research and Treatment of Cancer

in cutaneous lymphoid hyperplasia or pseudo-lymphoma. Studies have suggested that there is a spectrum of cutaneous B-cell lymphoproliferative disorders with a stepwise progression from cutaneous lymphoid hyperplasia to low-grade cutaneous lymphomas (Dummer et al. 2007; Sangueza et al. 1992; Cerroni et al. 1997b). This may partially explain the overlapping clinical and histologic features as well as clonal immunoglobulin gene rearrangement that these two groups shared and the diagnostic difficulty in distinguishing cutaneous lymphoid hyperplasia from low-grade B-cell lymphomas.

Primary Cutaneous Follicle Center Lymphoma

Primary cutaneous follicle center lymphoma (PCFCL) consists of a neoplastic proliferation of germinal center cells confined to the skin (Willemze et al. 2005). In the WHO-EORTC classification, this category includes cases with follicular growth pattern as well as those with diffuse or mixed growth pattern.

Table 9.4 ISCL/EORTC proposal on T classification of cutaneous lymphomas other than mycosis fungoides and Sezary syndrome (Kim et al. 2007)

T1	Solitary	T1a	≤5 cm in diameter
		T1b	≥5 cm in diameter
T2	Multiple	T2a	All encompassing in <15 cm in diameter
		T2b	All encompassing in >15 cm and ≤30 cm in diameter
		T2c	All encompassing in >30 cm in diameter
T3	Generalized	T3a	2 noncontiguous body regions
		T3b	≥3 body regions
N		N0	No clinical or pathologic involvement of lymph node
		N1	Involvement of 1 peripheral lymph node draining current or prior lesion
		N2	Involvement of 2 or more peripheral lymph nodes or involvement of any lymph node that does not drain current or prior lesion
		N3	Involvement of central lymph nodes
M		M0	Absence of extra-cutaneous non-lymph node disease
		M1	Presence of extra-cutaneous non-lymph node disease

ISCL International Society for Cutaneous Lymphomas, *EORTC* European Organization for Research and Treatment of Cancer

Clinical Presentation

PCFCL commonly affects adults of both genders, although rare cases in childhood have been reported (Ghislanzoni et al. 2005). The median age is 58 years (Smith et al. 2005). The male-to-female ratio is 2.1 (Smith et al. 2005). Clinically, it presents with solitary or grouped erythematous papules, plaques, and tumors on the scalp or forehead, trunk, and rarely on the leg (Willemze et al. 2005). If untreated, the tumors grow in size, but spread to extra-cutaneous sites is relatively uncommon. About 11 % show bone marrow spread, and hence a bone marrow examination should be considered (Senff et al. 2008a). Relapse after radiotherapy or excision occurs in 30 %, relapsing almost always in the skin (Senff et al. 2008b). Sporadic cases associated with infections by human herpes virus 8 (HHV-8),

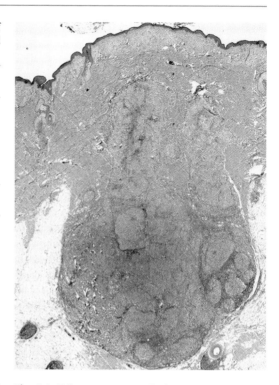

Fig. 9.1 Primary cutaneous follicle cell lymphoma is characterized by a nodular proliferation in the dermis and extending into the subcutaneous tissue

hepatitis C, or *Borrelia burgdorferi* have been identified; however, these infectious agents do not appear to be a significant etiologic factor in these lymphomas (Cerroni et al. 1997b; Viguier et al. 2002). Regardless of the number of lesions, follicular or diffuse growth pattern, or the number of blast cells, PCFCLs have an excellent prognosis, with a 5-year overall survival of greater than 95 % (Willemze et al. 2005). Only tumors present in the leg have a bad prognosis as seen in cutaneous diffuse large B-cell lymphoma, leg type (PCLBCL-LT) (Senff et al. 2008b). Radiotherapy is often the preferred treatment for solitary or few lesions of PCFCLs (Rijlaarsdam et al. 1996).

Histopathology

PCFCLs are tumors located in the dermis with extension to the subcutaneous tissue (Fig. 9.1). As in most cutaneous B-cell lymphomas, the epidermis is spared. They consist of proliferations of

Fig. 9.2 The histologic features of the neoplastic follicles are monomorphism due to the absence of dark and light areas, rarity or absence of tingible body macrophages, and reduction of the mantle zone

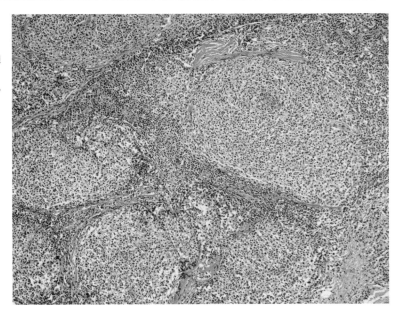

small, medium, and large cleaved cells (centrocytes) admixed with variable number of large and round cells with 1–3 peripheral nucleoli (centroblasts) in a follicular and/or diffuse pattern (Willemze et al. 2005). Immunoblasts are rare. Small reactive T cells are also seen. The histologic features seen in neoplastic follicles are the reduction of the mantle zone, rarity or absence of tingible body macrophages, and monomorphism of follicles due to the absence of dark and light polarized areas (Fig. 9.2). When diffuse and follicular patterns coexist, the neoplastic follicles are localized to the periphery of the tumor. A rare variant formed by spindle cells has been reported and named "spindle cell B-cell lymphoma" (Carbone et al. 2006). Although in the past these cases were classified as large B-cell lymphomas, it is now demonstrated that the spindle cells are centrocytes that show germinal center B-cell origin and therefore they are part of the spectrum of PCFCLs.

Immunophenotype

The neoplastic follicle center cells typically express pan B-cell markers (CD20+, CD79a+, PAX5+) (Fig. 9.3) and are Bcl6+, CD10+, and Bcl2− (Hoefnagel et al. 2003; Cerroni et al. 2000). CD10 is frequently lost in diffuse forms of this

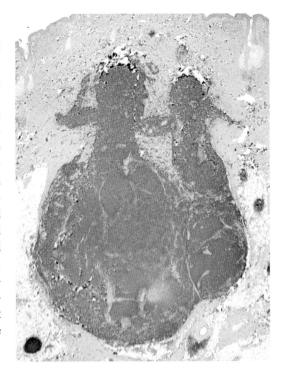

Fig. 9.3 CD20 labels the majority of the neoplastic cells in this case of cutaneous follicle cell lymphoma

lymphoma. CD21, CD23, or CD35 can highlight the distorted follicular dendritic network (Senff et al. 2007). When in doubt if the follicles are reactive or neoplastic in nature, Ki-67 can be used. In reactive follicles around 90 % of the cells react to this marker, while neoplastic follicles have a positivity of less than 50 % (Cerroni et al. 2000). Although Bcl2 is absent in the majority of PCFCLs, in 10–25 % of the cases, Bcl2 and MUM1/IRF4 can be detected (Senff et al. 2007; Lawnicki et al. 2002). PCFCL involving the leg with a diffuse growth pattern has a large component of large cells and can mimic cutaneous diffuse large B-cell lymphoma, leg type. The presence of large cleaved lymphocytes in PCFCLs and the absence of reactivity to Bcl2, IgM, MUM-1, and forkhead box protein (FOX-P1) can differentiate diffuse PCFCL from cutaneous diffuse large B-cell lymphoma, leg type (Koens et al. 2010). As discussed in Chap. 3, a panel of CD20, Bcl2, Bcl6, MUM-1, and IgM is helpful in the distinction of diffuse PCFCL from PCLBCL-LT. Of note, classically the neoplastic follicle center cells are typically positive for the B-cell marker CD20. However, recurrent lymphoma after treatment with anti-CD20 monoclonal antibody (rituximab) may no longer express CD20 (Fink-Puches et al. 2005); therefore, other B-cell-associated markers like CD79a, CD19, and PAX5 should be considered in this clinical scenario.

Cytogenetics and Molecular Findings

The classic translocation (14;18) seen in systemic counterpart of this lymphomas is rarely seen in PCFCLs. For practical purposes, detection of Bcl2 by rearrangements and/or protein expression should raise a concern for a systemic follicular lymphoma with secondary extension to the skin. PCFCLs show a monoclonal rearrangement of the immunoglobulin joining heavy chain (JH) gene by PCR in the majority of cases. Identical clones can be identified in different follicles of the same lymphoma as well as within interfollicular areas (Cerroni et al. 2000).

Primary Cutaneous Marginal Zone B-Cell Lymphoma

Primary cutaneous marginal zone B-cell lymphomas (PCMZLs) include cases previously reported as primary cutaneous immunocytoma and primary cutaneous plasmacytoma (Rijlaarsdam et al. 1993; Torne et al. 1990). The tumor cells are small B cells that are composed of marginal (centrocyte-like) cells, lymphoplasmacytoid cells, and plasma cells.

Clinical Presentation

PCMZLs can present as solitary or multiple erythematous papules to small nodules on the trunk or extremities, especially upper extremities, of young adults with a male predominance (Rijlaarsdam et al. 1993; Cerroni et al. 1997a; Hoefnagel et al. 2005b; Tsuji et al. 2005). The male-to-female ratio is 1.4 (Smith et al. 2005). The median age is 53 years (Smith et al. 2005). Recurrence is common, but systemic or bone marrow (Senff et al. 2008b) involvement is rare (Cerroni et al. 1997a; Tsuji et al. 2005; Hoefnagel et al. 2005b). The recurrences, affecting nearly half of the successfully treated patients, maintain the low-grade features of the primary tumor. The prognosis of PCMZLs is excellent with 5-year survival close to 100 % (Rijlaarsdam et al. 1993; Cerroni et al. 1997a; Tsuji et al. 2005; Hoefnagel et al. 2005b). Although immunocytomas are now considered a variant of PCMZL, they have certain characteristics that differ from the classic PCMZL cases like an increased frequency in older population, involvement of lower extremities, and association with *Borrelia Burgdorferi* infection (Cerroni et al. 1997b). Solitary or few lesions of PCMZL are often treated with radiotherapy or excision (Hoefnagel et al. 2005b). Many patients can be managed with a "watchful waiting" strategy.

Although staging is essential to distinguish PCMZL from secondary cutaneous involvement by a systemic MZL, PCMZL may be seen in younger patients and favors the trunk and extremities, whereas secondary cutaneous involvement is seen in older patients and affects frequently the head and neck (Gerami et al. 2010). It appears that detection of specific cells in the bone marrow does not impact prognosis in PCMZLs; the role of bone marrow biopsy for these patients has been debated (Senff et al. 2008a; Bathelier et al. 2008). Association with *Borrelia burgdorferi* in

Fig. 9.4 Primary cutaneous marginal zone lymphoma affects the dermis in a patchy, nodular, and diffuse pattern and spares the epidermis

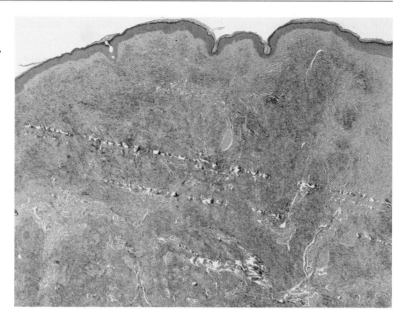

a subset of European cases from endemic and non-endemic areas (Goodlad et al. 2000), tattoo pigment (Sangueza et al. 1992), recurrent herpes simplex virus type 1 infection on the lower lip over 15 years (Zendri et al. 2005), and influenza vaccination (May et al. 2005) has been reported. It has been proven that different samples of cutaneous marginal zone lymphoma recognized similar antigens supporting the hypothesis of an antigen-driven lymphoma parallel to what occurs in gastric MALT lymphoma. On the other hand, the presence of PCMZL in a patient treated with fluoxetine therapy raises the possibility that an inhibitory effect on T-suppressor lymphocytes may originate an excessive antigen-driven B-cell proliferation with PCMZL as end result (Breza et al. 2006).

Histopathology

PCMZL affects the dermis and occasionally the subcutis in a patchy, nodular, or diffuse growth pattern (Rijlaarsdam et al. 1993; Cerroni et al. 1997a). Like most of the B-cell lymphomas, the epidermis is not involved (Fig. 9.4). The most characteristic presentation of PCMZL at low power is the nodular growth pattern with reactive germinal centers (see Fig. 3.2) and peri- and interfollicular proliferation of marginal zone cells (small- to medium-sized cells with indented nuclei and pale cytoplasm) (Fig. 9.5). Commonly, plasma cells aggregate at the periphery of the tumor (Fig. 9.5). In rare cases plasma cells predominate over marginal zone cells, and these cases are classified as PCMZL plasmacytic variant. PCMZL and non-cutaneous MZL cannot be differentiated on histologic ground (Gerami et al. 2010). It should be noted that reactive B and T cells as well as histiocytes and eosinophils are represented in PCMZL creating the challenge of differentiating this lymphoma from reactive processes. It is the expansion of the marginal cell population in association with a clonal population of plasma cells in PCMZL that allows differentiating between lymphoma and reactive process.

Immunophenotype

The marginal zone B cells are typically CD20+, CD79a+, and Bcl2+ (De Leval et al. 2001), and

Fig. 9.5 The neoplastic marginal zone cells are small- to medium-sized cells with indented nuclei and pale cytoplasm. Aggregates of plasma cells are noted

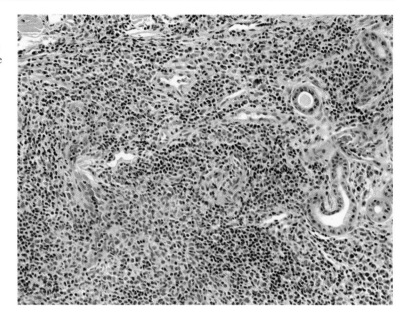

Fig. 9.6 Kappa immunostain demonstrates kappa light chain restriction

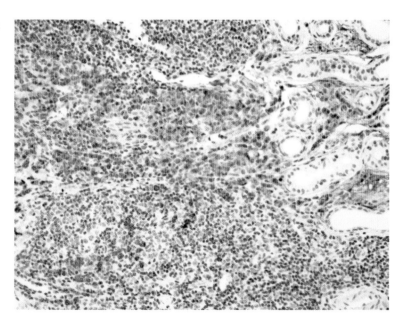

there is monotypic light chain expression by the plasma cells (Figs. 9.6 and 9.7). In contrast to PCFCLs they are CD5−, CD10−, and Bcl6− (Hoefnagel et al. 2005b). Contrary to extranodal marginal zone lymphoma of MALT that expresses IgM, PCMZLs express IgG, IgA, and IgE and lack the chemokine receptor CXCR3 (van Maldegem et al. 2008). As discussed in Chap. 3, a panel of CD3, CD20, Bcl2, Bcl6, CD21, kappa, and lambda in situ hybridization would be helpful in the differential diagnosis of reactive lymphoid hyperplasia versus low-grade B-cell lymphoma.

Fig. 9.7 On the other hand, lambda immunostain is negative

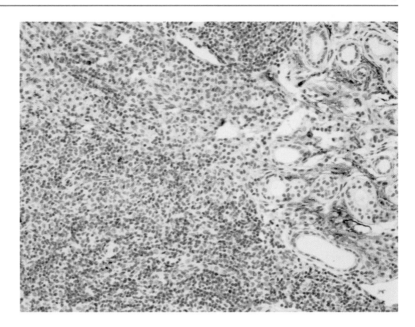

Cytogenetics and Molecular Features

Approximately 50–60 % of the cases possess a monoclonal rearrangement of the immunoglobulin heavy chain (JH) gene (Bahler et al. 2006). A distinct t(14;18)(q32;q21) translocation affecting *IGH* and *MLT* genes has been detected in a subset of PCMZL. The latter has been also identified in other extranodal marginal zone lymphomas involving the liver and ocular, adnexal, and salivary glands highlighting some relationship among a subgroup of PCMZL with extra-cutaneous ones (Streubel et al. 2003). Rare cases of PCMZL may show a conventional t(14;18) involving *IGH* and *BCL2*. A recently described translocation (3;14) (p14;q32) affecting *IGH* and *FOXP1* genes seen in extranodal MALT has been detected in few PCMZL (Streubel et al. 2005). The use of detection of class-switched cases to subclassify PCMZL is still under investigation (Edinger et al. 2010). Aberrant somatic hypermutations could play a role in the pathogenesis of this disease by mutating regulatory and proto-oncogenes such as *PAX5*, *c-MYC*, and *PIM1*, among others (Deutsch et al. 2009). Inactivation of tumor suppressor genes *CDKN2A* and *DAPK* by hypermethylation has frequently been detected in PCMZL.

Cutaneous Plasmacytoma

Primary cutaneous plasmacytoma without bone marrow involvement is an exceedingly rare B-cell lymphoma (Muscardin et al. 2000; Wong et al. 1994; Kazakov et al. 2002). Some have suggested that it is actually marginal zone lymphoma with a prominent plasma cell differentiation (Hussong et al. 1999). It is classified as a peripheral B-cell lymphoma in the REAL and WHO classifications (Harris et al. 1994; Swedlow et al. 2008) and as a provisional entity in the EORTC classification due to limited data (Willemze et al. 1997).

Solitary or clustered, erythematous, reddish-brown or violaceous plaques or nodules are seen on the head and trunk of mostly elderly males. Histopathologically, there is a proliferation of mature and immature plasma cells in the deep dermis and subcutaneous tissue (Fig. 9.8). Amyloid deposition is often seen in the setting of cutaneous involvement by multiple myeloma. The neoplastic plasma cells are CD138+ (Fig. 9.9); CD79a+; light chain restricted, cytoplasmic immunoglobulin + (usually IgA); leukocyte common antigen (LCA)–; and CD20–. They can be positive for EMA and aberrantly for cytokeratins, HMB45, and CD30. A monoclonal rearrangement of the heavy

Fig. 9.8 A diffuse proliferation of plasmacytoid cells is seen in this example of cutaneous plasmacytoma

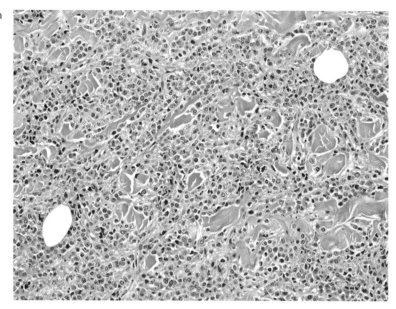

Fig. 9.9 The tumor cells are strongly positive for CD138

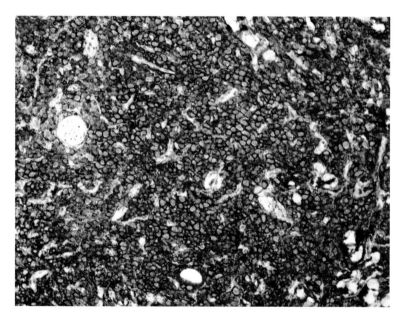

immunoglobulin heavy chain gene is usually detected by molecular analyses. One entity in the differential diagnosis that one must consider is IgG4-related skin disease which is characterized by dense lymphoplasmacytic infiltrates with prominent IgG4+ plasma cells, storiform fibrosis, obliterative phlebitis, and often elevated serum IgG4 level (Deshpande et al. 2012). An IgG4+ to IgG + plasma cell ratio of greater than 40 % is necessary for making the diagnosis (Deshpande et al. 2012).

Primary Cutaneous Large B-Cell Lymphoma, Leg Type

Primary cutaneous large B-cell lymphoma, leg type (PCLBCL), is included as "diffuse large B-cell lymphoma" in the WHO classification (Gatter and Warnke 2001) and as "large B-cell lymphoma of the leg" in the EORTC classification (Willemze et al. 1997).

Clinical Presentation

These lymphomas present as rapidly growing and often ulcerated tumors on one or both lower legs of elderly women (Kodama et al. 2005; Zinzani et al. 2006). The median age is more than 70 years (Smith et al. 2005). The male-to-female ratio is 1:2 (Smith et al. 2005). The skin lesions are present at sites other than the leg in approximately 10–15 % of cases (Kodama et al. 2005; Zinzani et al. 2006). Multiple skin lesions at diagnosis are an adverse risk factor (Grange et al. 2007). Dissemination to extra-cutaneous sites is often seen, and a 5-year survival is approximately 55 % (Vermeer et al. 1996). PCLBCLs are treated as systemic diffuse large B-cell lymphomas with combination therapy (R-CHOP, rituximab, cyclophosphamide, hydroxydaunomycin, Oncovin/vincristine, and prednisone) (Vermeer et al. 1996). Solitary lesions are often treated by radiotherapy.

Histopathology

A diffuse proliferation of uniform and large neoplastic cells, the vast majority (90 % or more) is composed of centroblasts and immunoblasts and is typically seen in the dermis and often in the subcutaneous tissue (Fig. 9.10). A number of unusual histologic variants have been reported including sclerosing pattern, geographic necrosis, anaplastic cell morphology, angioinvasion, starry-sky pattern, spindle cell pattern, histiocytoid morphology, and an epidermotropic pattern (Plaza et al. 2011).

Immunophenotype

The neoplastic B cells are typically CD20+ (Fig. 9.11), CD79a+, Bcl2+, MUM-1/IRF-4+, PAX-5+, Fox-P1+, Bcl6+, monotypic surface immunoglobulin, and CD10– (Hoefnagel et al. 2005a). Ki-67 proliferation index is high. Bcl2 strong expression and higher expression of transcription factors multiple myeloma-1/interferon regulatory factor 4 (*MUM1/IRF4*) (Fig. 9.12) are seen in PCLBCL-LT in comparison to PCFCLs (Hoefnagel et al. 2005a). However, Bcl2 expression can be negative in 10 % of PCLBCL cases. Recently, IgM has been reported as an additional marker in the distinction of PCLBCL-LT from PCFCL (Koens et al. 2010). In the study by Koens and colleagues (2010), IgM expression was seen in all 40 PCLBCL-LT in contrast to only 5 of 53 PCFCL. Bcl6 is expressed in some cases of leg-type large cell lymphoma (Hoefnagel et al. 2005a).

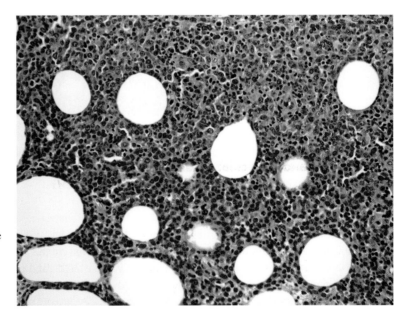

Fig. 9.10 A diffuse infiltrate of atypical lymphoid cells is seen in the subcutaneous tissue in this case of diffuse large B-cell lymphoma, leg type

Fig. 9.11 The neoplastic cells are strongly positive for CD20

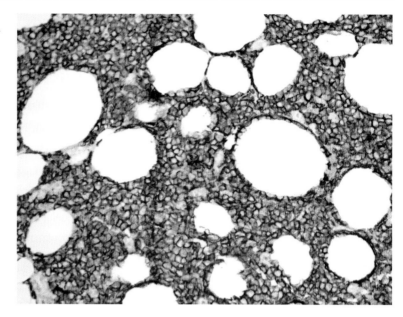

Fig. 9.12 Nuclear MUM1 expression is noted

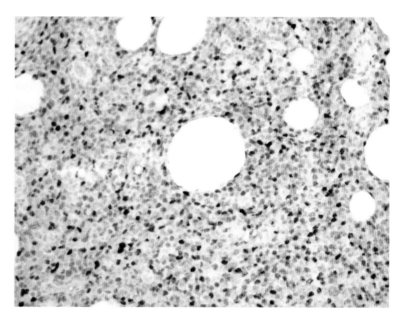

Cytogenetics and Molecular Findings

Although the t(14;18) is absent, amplification of bcl2 gene is present in some cases (Hallermann et al. 2004). Inactivation of p15 and p16 tumor suppressor genes by promotor hypermethylation is noted in 11 % and 14 %, respectively (Child et al. 2002). Chromosomal imbalances, including gains in 18q and 7p and loss of 6q, can be detected in up to 85 % (Mao et al. 2002). Translocations involving *MYC*, *BCL6*, and *IGH* genes were documented in 11 of 14 patients with PCLBCLs (leg type) but not in those with PCFCLs (Hallermann et al. 2004). Deletion of a small region on chromosome 9p21.3 was detected in 67 % of PCLBCLs (leg type), and this feature was associated with worse prognosis (Dijkman et al. 2006a, b).

Other Primary Cutaneous Large B-Cell Lymphomas

Plasmablastic or Anaplastic Lymphoma

Plasmablastic lymphoma (PBL) is a rare subtype of diffuse large B-cell lymphoma that is seen in immunocompromised individuals and also elderly individuals without known immunodeficiency (Heiser et al. 2012; Gilaberte et al. 2005; Jambusaria et al. 2008). PBL is classified by the WHO as a distinct type of non-Hodgkin lymphoma (Gatter and Warnke 2001). It was first reported in human immunodeficiency virus (HIV)-infected individuals (Delecluse et al. 1997; Chetty et al. 2003), but can be seen in patients with organ transplants or receiving chemotherapy (Colomo et al. 2004). PBL preferentially involves the oral cavity, less so in trunk and extremities, and has a poor prognosis with an average survival of 6 months (Delecluse et al. 1997). Cutaneous involvement has rarely been reported in only approximately nine cases documented in the literature (Heiser et al. 2012; Gilaberte et al. 2005; Jambusaria et al. 2008; Chabay et al. 2009; Jordan et al. 2005; Nicol et al. 2003; Liu et al. 2006; Verma et al. 2005; Hernandez et al. 2009).

Clinical Presentation

Cutaneous PBL presents as asymptomatic, solitary or grouped nodules; an erythematous plaque; or ulcerated nodules on either the upper or lower extremities (Jambusaria et al. 2008). The biologic course of cutaneous PBL is indolent with a rare case of spontaneous resolution has been reported (Jordan et al. 2005). Treatment for cutaneous PBL is dependent on the underlying diseases including excision, reduction of immunosuppression drugs in the setting of transplantation, and changing antiretroviral medications to decrease viral load and improve CD4 counts in HIV-positive patients (Jambusaria et al. 2008; Nicol et al. 2003; Gilaberte et al. 2005).

Histopathology

A dense infiltrate of plasmablasts, atypical large neoplastic cells with eccentric nuclei and abundant cytoplasm with a paranuclear hof, is typically seen in the dermis and often the subcutaneous tissue. Numerous mitotic figures and apoptotic bodies are often seen. The differential diagnoses include immunoblastic variant of DLBCL and other aggressive large B-cell and plasma cell neoplasms with plasmablastic morphology.

Immunophenotype

The tumors cells are CD38+, CD138+, CD43+, CD45+, and MUM1+ and show immunoglobulin light chain restriction (Delecluse et al. 1997). They are negative for B-cell (CD20, CD79a, PAX5) and T-cell (CD3, CD4, CD5, CD8) markers, CD10, CD15, Bcl2, Bcl6, CD56, CD57, TIA-1, CD34, and myeloperoxidase (Gilaberte et al. 2005; Liu et al. 2006). In cases associated with HHV-8, immunostain for HHV-8 latency-associated nuclear antigen would be positive (Liu et al. 2006).

Cytogenetics and Molecular Findings

Immunoglobulin heavy chain (FR1 and FR3 regions) gene rearrangement was reported by Liu et al. (2006) in one case. Epstein-Barr virus mRNA and HHV-8 were detected by in situ hybridization and polymerase chain reaction, respectively (Gilaberte et al. 2005). EBV in situ hybridization is positive in approximately 60 % of cases (Gilaberte et al. 2005).

Primary Cutaneous T-Cell/ Histiocyte-Rich B-Cell Lymphoma

This rare variant often presents as solitary lesions on the head, trunk, or extremities. Its biologic course is similar to those of PCFCL and PCMZL (Li et al. 2001). Surgical excision and/or local radiotherapy is often the treatment

(Sander et al. 1996). It is characterized by scattered neoplastic B cells (less than 15 % of the infiltrate) in a background of numerous reactive T cells (Li et al. 2001). The neoplastic B cells are CD20+, CD30−, and often Bcl6+. The reactive T cells are CD3+, CD4+, and CD8+ (Sander et al. 1996). Molecular studies show a monoclonal rearrangement of the immunoglobulin heavy chain gene (Li et al. 2001; Sander et al. 1996; Dunphy and Nahass 1999).

References

Bahler DW, Kim BK, Gao A, Swerdlow SH. Analysis of immunoglobulin V genes suggests cutaneous marginal zone B-cell lymphomas recognise similar antigens. Br J Haematol. 2006;132(5):571–5.

Bathelier E, Thomas L, Balme B, Coiffier B, Salles G, Berger F, et al. Asymptomatic bone marrow involvement in patients presenting with cutaneous marginal zone B-cell lymphoma. Br J Dermatol. 2008;159(2): 498–500. doi:10.1111/j.1365-2133.2008.08659.x.

Breza Jr TS, Zheng P, Porcu P, Magro CM. Cutaneous marginal zone B-cell lymphoma in the setting of fluoxetine therapy: a hypothesis regarding pathogenesis based on in vitro suppression of T-cell-proliferative response. J Cutan Pathol. 2006;33(7):522–8.

Burg G, Kempf W, Cozzio A, Feit J, Willemze R, Jaffe ES, et al. WHO-EORTC classification for cutaneous lymphomas 2005: histological and molecular aspects. J Cutan Pathol. 2005;32(10):647–74.

Carbone A, Gloghini A, Libra M, Gasparotto D, Navolanic PM, Spina M, Tirelli U. A spindle cell variant of diffuse large B-cell lymphoma possesses genotypic and phenotypic markers characteristic of a germinal center B-cell origin. Mod Pathol. 2006; 19(2):299–306.

Cerroni L, Arzberger E, Putz B, Hofler G, Metze D, Sander CR, et al. Primary cutaneous follicular center cell lymphoma with follicular growth pattern. Blood. 2000;95(12):3922–8.

Cerroni L, Signoretti S, Hofler G, Annessi G, Putz B, Lackinger E, et al. Primary cutaneous marginal B-cell lymphoma: a recently described entity of low-grade malignant cutaneous B-cell lymphoma. Am J Surg Pathol. 1997a;21(11):1307–15.

Cerroni L, Zöchling N, Pütz B, Kerl H. Infection by Borrelia burgdorferi and cutaneous B-cell lymphoma. J Cutan Pathol. 1997b;24(8):457–61.

Chabay P, de Matteo E, Lorenzetti M, Gutierrez M, Narbaitz M, Aversa L, Preciado MV. Vulvar plasmablastic lymphoma in a HIV-positive child: a novel extraoral localization. J Clin Pathol. 2009;62(7):644–6. doi:10.1136/jcp.2009.064758.

Chetty R, Hlatswayo N, Muc R, Sabaratnam R, Gatter K. Plasmablastic lymphoma in HIV+ patients: an expanding spectrum. Histopathology. 2003;42(6):605–9.

Child FJ, Scrisbrick JJ, Calonje E, Orchard G, Russell-Jones R, Whittaker SJ. In activation of tumor suppressor genes p15INK4b and p16INK4a in primary cutaneous B cell lymphoma. J Invest Dermatol. 2002;118(6):941–8.

Colomo L, Loong F, Rives S, Pittaluga S, Martinez A, Lopez-Guillermo A, et al. Diffuse large B-cell lymphomas with plasmablastic differentiation represent a heterogeneous group of disease entities. Am J Surg Pathol. 2004;28(6):736–47.

De Leval L, Harris NL, Longtine J, Ferry JA, Duncan LM. Cutaneous B-cell lymphomas of follicular and marginal zone types: use of Bcl-6, CD10, Bcl-2, and CD21 in differential diagnosis and classification. Am J Surg Pathol. 2001;25(6):732–41.

Delecluse HJ, Anagnostopoulos I, Dallenbach F, Hummel M, Marafioti T, Schneider U, et al. Plasmablastic lymphomas of the oral cavity: a new entity associated with the human immunodeficiency virus infection. Blood. 1997;89(4):1413–20.

Deshpande V, Zen Y, Chan JK, Yi EE, Sato Y, Yoshino T, et al. Consensus statement on the pathology of IgG4-related disease. Mod Pathol. 2012;25(9):1181–92. doi:10.1038/modpathol.2012.72.

Deutsch AJ, Frühwirth M, Aigelsreiter A, Cerroni L, Neumeister P. Primary cutaneous marginal zone B-cell lymphomas are targeted by aberrant somatic hypermutation. J Invest Dermatol. 2009;129(2):476–9. doi:10.1038/jid.2008.243.

Dijkman R, Tensen CP, Buettner M, Niedobitek G, Willemze R, Vermeer MH. Primary cutaneous follicle center lymphoma and primary cutaneous large B-cell lymphoma, leg type, are both targeted by aberrant somatic hypermutation but demonstrate differential expression of AID. Blood. 2006a;107(12):4926–9.

Dijkman R, Tensen CP, Jordanova ES, Knijnenburg J, Hoefnagel JJ, Mulder AA, et al. Array-based comparative genomic hybridization analysis reveals recurrent chromosomal alterations and prognostic parameters in primary cutaneous large B-cell lymphoma. J Clin Oncol. 2006b;24(2):296–305.

Dummer R, Asagoe K, Cozzio A, Burg G, Doebbeling U, Golling P, et al. Recent advances in cutaneous lymphomas. J Dermatol Sci. 2007;48(3):157–67.

Dunphy CH, Nahass GT. Primary cutaneous T-cell-rich B-cell lymphomas with flow cytometric immunophenotypic findings: report of 3 cases and review of the literature. Arch Pathol Lab Med. 1999;123(12):1236–40.

Edinger JT, Kant JA, Swerdlow SH. Cutaneous marginal zone lymphomas have distinctive features and include 2 subsets. Am J Surg Pathol. 2010;34(12):1830–41. doi:10.1097/PAS.0b013e3181f72835.

Fink-Puches R, Wolf IH, Zalaudek I, Kerl H, Cerroni L. Treatment of primary cutaneous B-cell lymphoma with rituximab. J Am Acad Dermatol. 2005;52(5): 847–53.

Fink-Puches R, Zenahlik P, Bäck B, Smolle J, Kerl H, Cerroni L. Primary cutaneous lymphomas: applicability of current classification schemes (European Organization for Research and Treatment of Cancer, World Health Organization) based on clinicopathologic features observed in a large group of patients. Blood. 2002;99(3):800–5.

Gatter KC, Warnke RA. Diffuse large B-cell lymphoma. In: Jaffe ES, Harris NL, Stein H, Vardiman JW, editors. World Health Organization classification of tumors: tumors of haematopoietic and lymphoid tissues. Lyon: International Agency for Research on Cancer (IARC) Press; 2001. p. 171–6.

Gerami P, Wickless SC, Querfeld C, Rosen ST, Kuzel TM, Guitart J. Cutaneous involvement with marginal zone lymphoma. J Am Acad Dermatol. 2010;63(1):142–5. doi:10.1016/j.jaad.2009.07.047.

Ghislanzoni M, Gambini D, Perrone T, Alessi E, Berti E. Primary cutaneous follicular center cell lymphoma of the nose with maxillary sinus involvement in a pediatric patient. J Am Acad Dermatol. 2005;52(5 Suppl 1): S73–5.

Gilaberte M, Gallardo F, Bellosillo B, Saballs P, Barranco C, Serrano S, Pujol RM. Recurrent and self-healing cutaneous monoclonal plasmablastic infiltrates in a patient with AIDS and Kaposi sarcoma. Br J Dermatol. 2005;153(4):828–32.

Goodlad JR, Davidson MM, Hollowood K, Ling C, MacKenzie C, Christie I, et al. Primary cutaneous B-cell lymphoma and Borrelia burgdorferi infection in patients from the Highlands of Scotland. Am J Surg Pathol. 2000;24(9):1279–85.

Grange F, Beylot-Barry M, Courville P, Maubec E, Bagot M, Vergier B, et al. Primary cutaneous diffuse large B-cell lymphoma, leg type: clinicopathologic features and prognostic analysis in 60 cases. Arch Dermatol. 2007;143(9):1144–50.

Hallermann C, Kaune KM, Gesk S, Martin-Subero JI, Gunawan B, Griesinger F, et al. Molecular cytogenetic analysis of chromosomal breakpoints in the *IGH*, *MYC*, *BCL6* and *MALT1* gene loci in primary cutaneous B-cell lymphomas. J Invest Dermatol. 2004;123(1):213–9.

Harris NL, Jaffe ES, Stein H, Banks PM, Chan JK, Cleary ML, et al. A revised European-American classification of lymphoid neoplasms: a proposal from the international lymphoma study group. Blood. 1994;84(5): 1361–92.

Heiser D, Muller H, Kempf W, Eisendle K, Zelger B. Primary cutaneous plasmablastic lymphoma of the lower leg in an HIV-negative patient. J Am Acad Dermatol. 2012;67(5):e202–5. doi:10.1016/j.jaad.2012.02.021.

Hernandez C, Cetner AS, Wiley EL. Cutaneous presentation of plasmablastic post-transplant lymphoproliferative disorder in a 14-month-old. Pediatr Dermatol. 2 0 0 9 ; 2 6 (6) : 7 1 3 – 6 . doi:10.1111/j.1525-1470.2009.01019.x.

Hoefnagel JJ, Dijkman R, Basso K, Jansen PM, Hallermann C, Willemze R, et al. Distinct types of primary cutaneous large B-cell lymphoma identified by gene expression profiling. Blood. 2005a;105(9):3671–8.

Hoefnagel JJ, Vermeer MH, Janssen PM, Fleuren GJ, Meijer CJ, Willemze R. Bcl-2, Bcl-6 and CD10 expression in cutaneous B-cell lymphoma: further support for a follicle centre cell origin and differential diagnostic significance. Br J Dermatol. 2003;149(6):1183–91.

Hoefnagel JJ, Vermeer MH, Jansen PM, Heule F, van Voorst Vader PC, Sanders CJ, et al. Primary cutaneous marginal zone B-cell lymphoma: clinical and therapeutic features of 50 patients. Arch Dermatol. 2005b;141(9):1139–45.

Hussong JW, Perkins SL, Schnitzer B, Hargreaves H, Frizzera G. Extramedullary plasmacytoma: a form of marginal zone cell lymphoma? Am J Clin Pathol. 1999;111(1):111–6.

Jaffe E, Harris N, Stein H, et al. Pathology and genetics of tumors of haematopoietic and lymphoid tissues. In: World Health Organization (WHO), editor. Classification of tumors. Lyon: World Health Organization; 2001.

Jambusaria A, Shafer D, Wu H, Al-Saleem T, Perlis C. Cutaneous plasmablastic lymphoma. J Am Acad Dermatol. 2008;58(4):676–8. doi:10.1016/j. jaad.2007.08.009.

Jordan LB, Lessells AM, Goodlad JR. Plasmablastic lymphoma arising at a cutaneous site. Histopathology. 2005;46(1):113–5.

Kazakov DV, Belousova IE, Muller B, Palmedo G, Samtsov AV, Burge G, Kempf W. Primary cutaneous plasmacytoma: a clinicopathologic study of two cases with a long-term follow-up and review of the literature. J Cutan Pathol. 2002;29(4):244–8.

Kim YH, Willemze R, Pimpinelli N, Whittaker S, Olsen EA, Ranki A, Dummer R, Hoppe RT. ISCL and the EORTC. TNM classification system for primary cutaneous lymphomas other than mycosis fungoides and Sezary syndrome: a proposal of the International Society for Cutaneous Lymphomas (ISCL) and the Cutaneous Lymphoma Task Force of the European Organization of Research and Treatment of Cancer (EORTC). Blood. 2007;110(2):479–84.

Kodama K, Massone C, Chott A, Metze D, Kerl H, Cerroni L. Primary cutaneous large B-cell lymphomas: clinicopathologic features, classification, and prognostic factors in a large series of patients. Blood. 2005;106(7):2491–7.

Koens L, Vermeer MH, Willemze R, Jansen PM. IgM expression on paraffin sections distinguishes primary cutaneous large B-cell lymphoma, leg type from primary cutaneous follicle center lymphoma. Am J Surg Pathol. 2010;34(7):1043–8. doi:10.1097/ PAS.0b013e3181e5060a.

Lawnicki LC, Weisenburger DD, Aoun P, Chan WC, Wickert RS, Greiner TC. The t(14;18) and bcl-2 expression are present in a subset of primary cutaneous follicular lymphoma: association with lower grade. Am J Clin Pathol. 2002;118(5):765–72.

Li S, Griffin CA, Mann RB, Borowitz MJ. Primary cutaneous T-cell rich B-cell lymphoma: clinically distinct from its nodal counterpart? Mod Pathol. 2001;14(1): 10–3.

Liu W, Lacouture ME, Jiang J, Kraus M, Dickstein J, Soltani K, Shea CR. KSHV/HHV8-associated primary cutaneous plasmablastic lymphoma in a patient with Castleman's disease and Kaposi's sarcoma. J Cutan Pathol. 2006;33 Suppl 2:46–51.

Mao X, Lillington D, Child F, Russell-Jones R, Young B, Whittaker S. Comparative genomic hybridization analysis of primary cutaneous B-cell lymphomas: identification of common genomic alterations in disease pathogenesis. Genes Chromosomes Cancer. 2002;35(2):144–55.

May SA, Netto G, Domiati-Saad R, Kasper R. Cutaneous lymphoid hyperplasia and marginal zone B-cell lymphoma following vaccination. J Am Acad Dermatol. 2005;53(3):512–6.

Muscardin LM, Pulsoni A, Cerroni L. Primary cutaneous plasmacytoma: report of a case with review of the literature. J Am Acad Dermatol. 2000;43(5 Pt 2):962–5.

Nicol I, Boye T, Carsuzaa F, Feier L, Collet Villette AM, Xerri L, et al. Post-transplant plasmablastic lymphoma of the skin. Br J Dermatol. 2003;149:889–91.

Plaza JA, Kacerovska D, Stockman DL, Buonaccorsi JN, Baillargeon P, Suster S, Kazakov DV. The histomorphologic spectrum of primary cutaneous diffuse large B-cell lymphoma: a study of 79 cases. Am J Dermatopathol. 2011;33(7):649–58. doi:10.1097/DAD.0b013e3181eeb433.

Rijlaarsdam JU, Toonstra J, Meijer OW, Noordijk EM, Willemze R. Treatment of primary cutaneous B-cell lymphomas of follicular center cell origin: a clinical follow-up study of 55 patients treated with radiotherapy or polytherapy. J Clin Oncol. 1996;14(2):549–55.

Rijlaarsdam JU, van der Putte SCJ, Berti E, Kerl H, Rieger E, Toonstra J, et al. Cutaneous immunocytomas: a clinicopathologic study of 26 cases. Histopathology. 1993;23(2):117–25.

Sander CA, Kaudewitz P, Kutzner H, Simon M, Schirren CG, Sioutos N, et al. T-cell rich B-cell lymphoma presenting in the skin: a clinicopathologic analysis of six cases. J Cutan Pathol. 1996;23(2):101–8.

Sangueza OP, Yadav S, White Jr CR, Braziel RM. Evolution of B-cell lymphoma from pseudolymphoma. Am J Dermatopathol. 1992;14(5):408–13.

Senff NJ, Hoefnagel JJ, Jansen PM, Vermeer MH, van Baarlen J, Blokx WA, et al. Reclassification of 300 primary cutaneous B-Cell lymphomas according to the new WHO-EORTC classification for cutaneous lymphomas: comparison with previous classifications and identification of prognostic markers. J Clin Oncol. 2007;25(12):1581–7.

Senff NJ, Kluin-Nelemans HC, Willemze R. Results of bone marrow examination in 275 patients with histological features that suggest an indolent type of cutaneous B-cell lymphoma. Br J Haematol. 2008a;142(1):52–6.

Senff NJ, Noordijk EM, Kim YH, Bagot M, Berti E, Cerroni L, et al. European organization for research and treatment of cancer and international society for cutaneous lymphoma consensus recommendations for the management of cutaneous B-cell lymphomas. Blood. 2008b;112(5):1600–9. doi:10.1182/blood-2008-04-152850.

Senff NJ, Willemze R. The applicability and prognostic value of the new TNM classification system for primary cutaneous lymphomas other than mycosis fungoides and Sézary syndrome: results on a large cohort of primary cutaneous B-cell lymphomas and comparison with the system used by the Dutch Cutaneous Lymphoma Group. Br J Dermatol. 2007;157(6):1205–11.

Smith BD, Smith GL, Cooper DL, Wilson LD. The cutaneous B-cell lymphoma prognostic index: a novel prognostic index derived from a population-based registry. J Clin Oncol. 2005;23(15):3390–5.

Streubel B, Lamprecht A, Dierlamm J, Cerroni L, Stolte M, Ott G, Raderer M, Chott A. T(14;18)(q32;q21) involving IGH and MALT1 is a frequent chromosomal aberration in MALT lymphoma. Blood. 2003;101(6):2335–9.

Streubel B, Vinatzer U, Lamprecht A, Raderer M, Chott A. T(3;14)(p14.1;q32) involving IGH and FOXP1 is a novel recurrent chromosomal aberration in MALT lymphoma. Leukemia. 2005;19(4):652–8.

Swedlow SH, Campo E, Harris NL, Jaffe ES, Pileri SA, Stein H, et al., editors. WHO classification of tumours of haematopoietic and lymphoid tissues. 4th ed. Lyon: IARC Press; 2008.

Torne R, Su WPD, Smolle J, Kerl H. Clinicopathologic study of cutaneous plasmacytoma. Int J Dermatol. 1990;29(8):562–6.

Tsuji K, Suzuki D, Naito Y, Sato Y, Yoshino T, Iwatsuki K. Primary cutaneous marginal zone B-cell lymphoma. Eur J Dermatol. 2005;15(6):480–3.

van Maldegem F, van Dijk R, Wormhoudt TA, Kluin PM, Willemze R, Cerroni L, et al. The majority of cutaneous marginal zone B-cell lymphomas expresses class-switched immunoglobulins and develops in a T-helper type 2 inflammatory environment. Blood. 2008;112(8):3355–61.

Verma S, Nuovo GJ, Porcu P, Baiocchi RA, Crowson AN, Magro CM. Epstein-Barr virus-and human herpesvirus 8-associated primary cutaneous plasmablastic lymphoma in the setting of renal transplantation. J Cutan Pathol. 2005;32(1):35–9.

Vermeer MH, Geelen FAMJ, van Haselen CW, van Voorst Vader PC, Geerts ML, van Vloten WA, Willemze R. Primary cutaneous large B-cell lymphomas of the legs: a distinct type of cutaneous B-cell lymphoma with an intermediate prognosis. Arch Dermatol. 1996;132(11):1304–8.

Viguier M, Rivet J, Agbalika F, Kerviler E, Brice P, Dubertret L, Bachelez H. B-cell lymphomas involving the skin associated with hepatitis C virus infection. Int J Dermatol. 2002;41(9):577–82.

Willemze R, Jaffe ES, Burg G, Cerroni L, Berti E, Swerdlow SH, et al. WHO-EORTC classification for cutaneous lymphomas. Blood. 2005;105(10):3768–85.

Willemze R, Kerl H, Sterry W, Berti E, Cerroni L, Chimenti S, et al. EORTC classification for primary cutaneous lymphoma: a proposal from the cutaneous lymphoma study group of the European organization for research and treatment of cancer. Blood. 1997;90(1):354–71.

Wong KF, Chang JKC, Li LPK, Yau TK, Lee AWM. Primary cutaneous plasmacytoma: report of two cases and review of the literature. Am J Dermatopathol. 1994;16(4):392–7.

Zendri E, Venturi C, Ricci R, Giordano G, De Panfilis G. Primary cutaneous plasmacytoma: a role for a triggering stimulus? Clin Exp Dermatol. 2005;30(3): 229–31.

Zinzani PL, Quaglino P, Pimpinelli N, Berti E, Baliva G, Rupoli S, et al. Prognostic factors in primary cutaneous B-cell lymphoma: the Italian study group for cutaneous lymphomas. J Clin Oncol. 2006;24(9):1376–82.

Neoplastic Nodular T-Cell Pattern: An Approach to Diagnosis of Neoplastic Nodular T-Cell Lymphomas of the Skin

10

Hernani D. Cualing, Michael B. Morgan, and Marshall E. Kadin

Introduction

Primary cutaneous lymphomas have an estimated annual incidence of 1.0–1.5/100,000 and are the second most common group of extranodal lymphomas. Despite their relative rarity, there has been an increasing incidence of cutaneous lymphomas in the United States from 5 to 13 per million person-years over 25 years reported on 2005 (SEER data) (Bradford et al. 2009). Peripheral T-cell lymphomas comprise 12 % of all lymphomas, a minority compared to the more common non-Hodgkin B-cell lymphomas (Swerdlow et al. 2008). Diagnosis of these rare T-cell lymphomas, especially those that arise in the skin, is challeng-

H.D. Cualing, MD (✉)
Department of Hematopathology and Cutaneous Lymphoma, IHCFLOW Diagnostic Laboratory, 18804 Chaville Rd, Lutz, FL 33558, USA
e-mail: ihcflow@verizon.net

M.B. Morgan, MD
Department of Pathology, University of South Florida College of Medicine, Tampa, FL, USA

Department of Dermatology, Michigan State University College of Medicine, East Lansing, MI, USA

Primary Care Diagnostics Institute, Quest Diagnostics, Palm Beach Gardens, FL, USA

Tampa, Pensacola and Atlanta Dermpath Diagnostics, Tampa, FL, USA

M.E. Kadin, MD
Department of Dermatology, Roger Williams Medical Center, Boston University School of Medicine, Providence, RI, USA

ing. Of all peripheral T-cell lymphomas (PTCLs), four out of five are extranodal, and a majority of the peripheral location involves the skin (Groves et al. 2000).

Of the primary cutaneous lymphomas in the United States, primary cutaneous T-cell lymphomas (MF/Sezary syndrome (SS), PTCL-u, CD30 T-cell lymphomas, and the rare types) represent 71 % of all primary cutaneous lymphomas, whereas primary cutaneous B-cell lymphomas account for the remainder of cases (Bradford et al. 2009). Mycosis fungoides (MF) is the most frequent CTCL representing more than half of this group (Bradford et al. 2009). The overall annual age-adjusted incidence of CTCL was 6.4 per million persons. Incidence was higher among blacks (9.0×10^{-6}) than among whites (6.1×10^{-6}) and was higher among men (8.7×10^{-6}) than among women (4.6×10^{-6}). Incidence was correlated with high physician density, high family income, high percentage of population with a bachelor's degree or higher, and high home values. The incidence appears to be increasing both in North America and in Europe (Criscione and Weinstock 2007; Jenni et al. 2011). Although MF is an indolent disease, histologic and clinical progression is seen over time. Transformed MF occurs up to 7 % of early but up to 23 % in advanced cases, especially higher in tumor stage (Lai et al. 2012).

The term primary cutaneous T-cell lymphoma (pCTCL) refers to cases of cutaneous T-cell lymphomas that present in the skin without extracutaneous involvement at the time of diagnosis

(Willemze et al. 2005). For prognostic and therapeutic reasons, this has to be differentiated from the similar other non-MF cutaneous T-cell lymphomas, identical-appearing secondary lymphomas, or even T-cell lymphomas masquerading as sarcoma (Alekshun et al. 2008; Rezania et al. 2007). Secondary lymphomas that involve the skin at presentation derived from systemic loci represent 25 % of all cutaneous lymphomas.

While mycosis fungoides generally presents with a protracted indolent course, the non-MF group of cutaneous PTCLs has a wide range of clinical behaviors. For example, primary cutaneous CD30+ anaplastic large cell lymphoma (c-ALCL) has good prognosis and rarely disseminates, with an estimated 5-year survival greater than 90 % (Bekkenk et al. 2000; Liu et al. 2003; Yu et al 2008), while primary cutaneous peripheral T-cell lymphoma, unspecified (PTCL-u), presents with a more aggressive generalized presentation that frequently spreads systemically and is often resistant to chemotherapy, with an estimated 5-year survival of 15 % (Beljaards et al. 1994; Grange et al. 1999; Bekkenk et al. 2003).

Some of the difference in frequency rates reported among PTCLs may be related to the use of less than precise terminology. For example, the relative frequency between cutaneous PTCLs reported by Bradford et al. differs from the WHO-EORTC data because the former used cutaneous PTCL as a group, while the latter used the more exact PTCL-u for that category. In the Surveillance, Epidemiology, and End Results (SEER) incidence rate data of 3,884 cutaneous lymphomas in the United States from 2001 to 2005, the primary cutaneous peripheral T-cell lymphoma (PTCL) group frequency is 20.8 %, and the CD30 lymphoproliferative group comprise 10.2 %, and the rare PTCLs like gamma-delta, angioimmunoblastic, subcutaneous panniculitic T-cell lymphoma, extranodal NK/T, and adult T-cell lymphoma/leukemia represent about 1 % of all cutaneous lymphomas (Bradford et al. 2009). In this regard, the terminology in the SEER study did not use PTCL, unspecified, but instead called this group " primary cutaneous PTCL" which is a heterogeneous group. In support of this observation is the reported longer overall 5-year survival rate in primary cutaneous PTCL category compared to the generally reported shorter rate in PTCL-u in most literature. In contrast, the frequency data used by WHO-EORTC was based on terminology PTCL-u; hence the CD30 + lymphoproliferative diseases are the second most common lymphoma after MF, instead of PTCL-u (Willemze et al. 2005).

Markers in Transformed MF

Additionally, a subset of these cells show increased expression of activation markers such as CD25 (interleukin 2 receptor family) and CD30 receptors (Zhang et al. 1996; Wasik et al. 1996). Activated B and T cells compose the transformed neoplastic tumor cells. These cells, usually medium or large in size, also express activation antigen CD30, a member of the tumor necrosis family (az-Cascajo 2001; Cepeda et al. 2003; Droc et al. 2007; Eckert et al. 1989; Edinger et al. 2009; Gallardo et al. 2002; Gniadecki and Rossen 2003; Kadin 2006; Kempf et al. 2012; Kikuchi et al. 1992). Similarly, the interleukin-2 family of receptors (Boehncke et al. 1993; Jakob et al. 1996; Kelley and Parker 2010) is noted to be present. Both antigens are seen in certain T- and B-cell lymphomas of the skin. In addition, high levels of Bcl2 proteins are expressed in transformed MF (Benner et al. 2009; Adachi and Horio 2008).

Follicle Helper T Cell as Putative Origin of Nodular T-Cell Lymphomas in the Skin

Germinal or follicle center T cells co-localize in B-cell-dominant germinal centers recognizable as rounded nodules in the dermis or subcutis. This T helper subset expresses follicle helper T-cell markers CD279, CD10, CD4, BCL-6, and CD57. Programmed death-1 (PD1, CD279a)-positive T cells localize in the ridge between germinal centers and the mantle and are an often used marker of follicle helper T cells (Blank and

Mackensen 2007; del Rio et al. 2005; Kantekure et al. 2012; Wang et al. 2007).

Many of the nodular neoplastic T-cell tumors discussed here that arise from helper T cells, the follicle helper T cells, the CD30 + T cells, and the gamma-delta T-cell subset, have putative histogenetic origin from lymph nodes to the skin via homing receptors cutaneous lymphocyte antigen (CLA) and cell chemokine CCR10 as part of the innate or adaptive immune system (Kim et al. 2006; Hudak et al. 2002; Kabelitz and He 2012; Kabelitz et al. 2005; Lanier et al. 1986; Lanier 2005). T-cell lymphomas that present in a nodular or follicular pattern may have this growth pattern presumably owing to their expression of follicle helper phenotype such as CD10 or PD-1. This group, which comprises the tumors forming the neoplastic nodular pattern, is postulated to include angioimmunoblastic T-cell lymphoma (AITCL), CD4 + pleomorphic T-cell lymphoma, the nodular subsets of PTCL-U, or cutaneous ALCL (Battistella et al. 2012; Ferenczi 2009; Gammon and Guitart 2012; Gaulard and de Leval 2011; Hu et al. 2012; Huang et al. 2009). In parallel, the cutaneous gamma-delta T-cell lymphoma is seen to localize following the normal predilections in the subcutaneous, dermis, and follicle epidermis via other idiopathic means.

Pathogenesis: Genotypic and Cellular Signal Pathway Profiles

For the majority of T-cell lymphomas, the pathogenesis is uncertain, although recent DNA profiling studies suggest that immunophenotypic profile and the T helper cytokine profile of the malignant T cells drive the pathogenesis and lead to dysregulation of normal immunity.

Gene expression profiling results show distinct signatures that predispose some types to stay within the skin environment and other genes predispose to dissemination and more aggressive course, as previously noted with MF and Sezary cells, but are also seen in skin-trophic c-ALCL and systemic-trophic cPTCL, also refered to as cPTCL, NOS or cPTCL, u (Ballabio et al. 2010; van Kester et al. 2010, 2011, 2012; Tracey et al.

2002, 2003). Increasing evidence also suggests that genetic and epigenetic profiles are key to clinical and biological behavior. There is evidence for epigenetic instability and promoter methylation in CTCL as well as their aggressive forms (Scarisbrick et al. 2003). *DNA profiling* studies showed inactivation of tumor suppressor genes (Scarisbrick et al. 2002), cell cycle dysregulation, defective DNA repair, disruption of apoptosis signaling, and, in advanced tumor stage MF, promoter hypermethylation of the *p16* gene (Navas et al. 2000). Tumor promotion in MF is postulated to be due to a combination of apoptosis signaling breakdown through increased tumor necrosis factor expression and promotion of apoptosis through inhibition of signal caspases. More practically, increased T-cell proliferation (higher *Ki67* expression) occurs in transformation of patch/plaque stages to advanced IIb tumor stage (Tracey et al. 2003; Wozniak et al. 2009).

Discussion of Individual Entities

Primary Cutaneous Peripheral T-Cell Lymphoma, Unspecified

Definition

All cutaneous peripheral T-cell neoplasms that do not fit the better defined subtypes of PTCLs entities under the WHO-EORTC classification (Willemze et al. 2005) and that could be delineated from the provisional categories of pleomorphic CD4 + T-cell lymphoma, cutaneous gamma-delta, and epidermotropic CD8-positive T-cell lymphoma. Morphologically, PTCL-u comprise at least 30 % large cells and, phenotypically, lack CD30 surface membrane antigen (Bekkenk et al. 2003; Zucca and Zinzani 2005; Fink-Puches et al. 2002).

Epidemiology

PTCL-u affects middle-aged to elderly individuals (median age 68 years, range 20–87 years), with a male to female ratio of 2.5:1 (Bekkenk et al. 2003; Beljaards et al. 1994). In the WHO-EORTC classification, PTCL-u ranks third in incidence, after the CD30+ lymphoproliferative disease, which is the second most common after

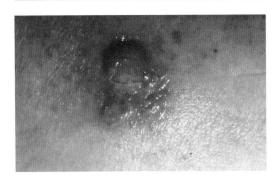

Fig. 10.1 Peripheral T-cell lymphoma, unspecified, showing clustered pustular plaque/nodule with satellite lesions

MF/Sezary syndrome (Willemze et al. 2005). PTCL-u cases have concurrent extranodal disease in 78 % of which skin involvement comprises about a fifth of cases so a diagnosis of PTCL-u in the skin requires a search for disseminated disease elsewhere including bone marrow disease (Savage et al. 2004).

Clinical Appearance of Lesions

Localized but more frequently generalized plaques or nodules are usually present (Fig. 10.1). These cases may be associated with systemic lymphoma, especially upon relapse (Willemze et al. 2005; Bekkenk et al. 2003; Zucca and Zinzani 2005).

Pattern of Infiltration

Diffuse and nodular (82 %) or band-like pattern (18 %) infiltrates occur in the dermis (Fig. 10.2a–c). Epidermotropism (27 %) is generally limited or absent. In less than 10 % of these cases, folliculotropism was present with less than 15 % with angiodestructive pattern (Bekkenk et al. 2003) (Fig. 10.3a–c).

Cytomorphology

For the designation of PTCL, the large cells (the neoplastic cells in which the nuclei are larger than macrophage nuclei or alternatively at least 4× the nuclear diameter of small lymphocytes) (Fig. 10.4a, b) represent at least 30 % of the total tumor cell population. Mitosis is frequent (Beljaards et al. 1994; Zucca and Zinzani 2005; Savage et al. 2004). This characteristic delineates

pleomorphic small- and medium-sized CD4+ T-cell lymphomas (also called primary cutaneous small and medium-sized T-cell lymphoma) which show less than 30 % large cells. There is variable admixture with small lymphocytes and histiocytes and less commonly with sparse eosinophils and plasma cells (Bekkenk et al. 2003) (Fig. 10.5).

Immunophenotype

The neoplastic cells are often CD4 positive and by definition lack CD30, the latter delineating this heterogeneous group from CD30-positive T-cell lymphomas. And in many cases, one or more "mature" T-cell antigens are coexpressed, absent, or diminished (Fig. 10.6) (Savage et al. 2004; Bekkenk et al. 2003). Rare CD56 expression is seen, but a third of the cases express cytotoxic proteins (granzyme B, TIA-1) (Bekkenk et al. 2003). CD8+, double CD4-/CD8-negative, or CD4-/CD8-positive cases account for a minority (Fig. 10.7) (Bekkenk et al. 2003). Admixed B cells (5–10 %) were observed in less than 10 % of biopsies (Bekkenk et al. 2003), and sometimes tumor cells are weakly coexpressing CD20 or CD79a (Fig. 10.8). The prognostic significance of Th1 or Th2 chemokine receptor expression appears to divide PTCL-u into favorable and unfavorable groups. Those with expression of CCR4 (Th2), which correlates with CD25 expression, appear to have poorer clinical outcome than those with a Th1 profile (Tsuchiya et al. 2004; Ishida et al. 2004; Ishida and Ueda 2011).

Cytogenetics and Molecular Findings

TCR genes are clonally rearranged, but no specific karyotypic lesions are found (Bekkenk et al. 2003).

Clinical Behavior

Although primary cutaneous form is seen in practice, this disease presents in a largely systemic fashion with advanced tumor stage, albeit with a high frequency of the extranodal and skin involvement at presentation (Savage et al. 2004). Prognosis is poor, with a 5-year survival rate of less than 20 % (Willemze et al. 2005). No difference has been observed between patients who present with solitary and those who have generalized skin involvement (Bekkenk et al. 2003).

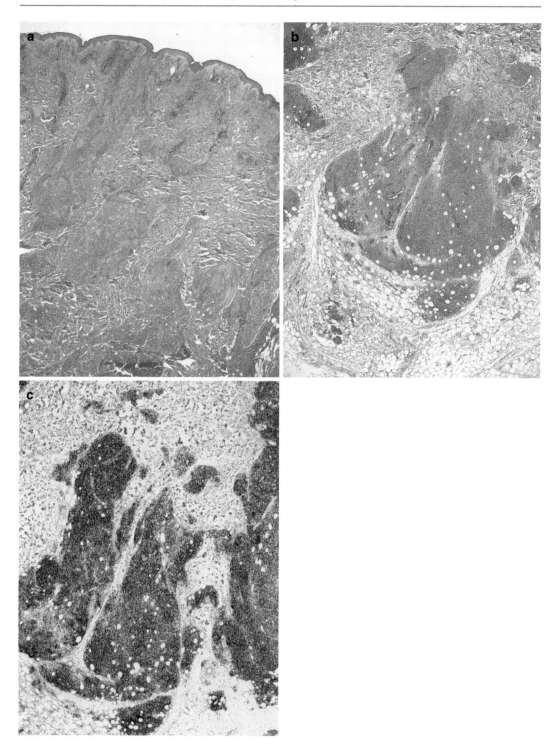

Fig. 10.2 The low-power histologic patterns of lichenoid with dermal (**a**), nodular, and diffuse (**b**) as well as CD3+ T-cell immunostain (**c**) in peripheral T-cell lymphoma, unspecified

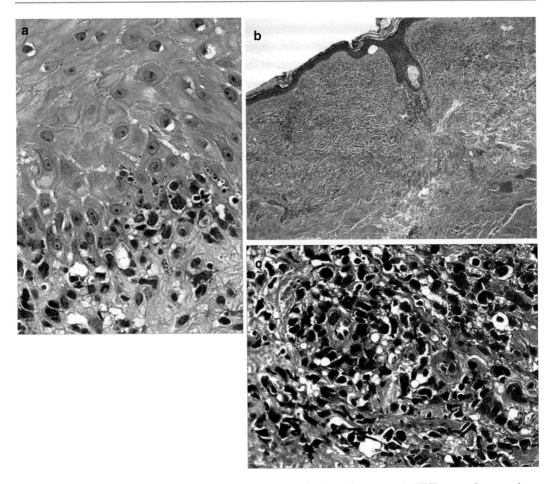

Fig. 10.3 (**a**) Epidermotropism, (**b**) folliculotropism, and (**c**) angiodestructive pattern in PTCL-u are also sometimes seen

Differential Diagnosis

MF transformed type, primary cutaneous small- and medium-sized T-cell lymphoma, or other aggressive cutaneous peripheral T-cell lymphomas (Rezania et al. 2007) (see Tables 10.1 and 10.2) or systemic lymphomas involving the skin are included in the differential diagnosis. Please refer to the discussion of the above entities within this chapter. Systemic PTCL-u has to be considered in the differential, especially considering that this predominantly nodal or viscerotropic lymphoma has predilection for skin involvement (Zucca and Zinzani 2005).

Systemic PTCL-u or Peripheral T-Cell Lymphoma, NOS

This group has an incidence rate of about 6 % of all non-Hodgkin lymphoma (Rudiger et al. 2002) and accounts for about a third of all PTCLs in western countries (Agostinelli et al. 2008; Rizvi et al. 2006). Patients are usually adults with 2:1 male to female ratio and present with nodal or visceral disease as the main clinical picture (Swerdlow et al. 2008). There is heterogeneity in pathology, and about half show morphological and molecular variability that echoes the term

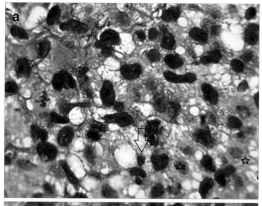

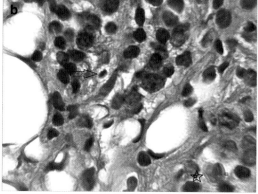

Fig. 10.4 PTCL-u. (**a**) The large neoplastic cell nuclei are larger than macrophage nuclei (*stars*) or (**b**) alternatively at least 4× the nuclear diameter of small lymphocytes (*arrows*) and represent at least 30 % of the cells. Note the atypical mitoses

"not otherwise specified" (Agostinelli et al. 2008; Went et al. 2006). Hence, diagnosis is made when other specific T-cell lymphomas are excluded. Tumor cells are invariably positive for βF1 and variably express CD4+, CD52+, and CD8 +/− immunophenotypes, with frequent antigen loss; double positive or negative CD4/CD8 are seen in more than half and Ki67 in greater than 80 % (Went et al. 2006). CD56 is seen in neoplastic T cells (Went et al. 2006). CD30, CD15, and CD20 are aberrantly seen in less than 10 % suggesting Hodgkin and B-cell non-Hodgkin in the differential (Quintanilla-Martinez et al. 1994, 1999; Yao et al. 2001). There is a high predilection to involve extranodal sites such as the liver, bone marrow, gastrointestinal tract, soft tissue, and skin (Zucca and Zinzani 2005; (Alekshun et al. 2008). The 5-year overall survival is 30–35 %, an intermediate rate, using standard chemotherapy (Savage et al. 2004). Extranodal presentations predict an even poorer prognosis. For example, cases with skin involvement as a primary that have progressed to systemic disease have a poorer prognosis, with a 5-year overall survival rate of less than 20 % (Willemze et al. 2005). No difference has been observed in patients presenting with solitary or generalized skin involvement (Bekkenk et al. 2003).

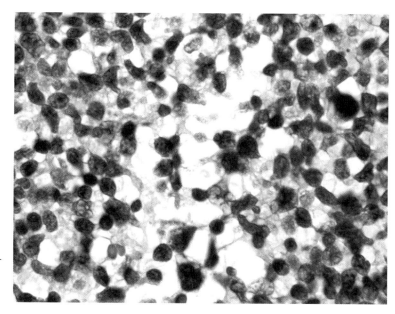

Fig. 10.5 PTCL-u. Variable admixture with small lymphocytes, histiocytes, and less commonly with sparse eosinophils and plasma cells

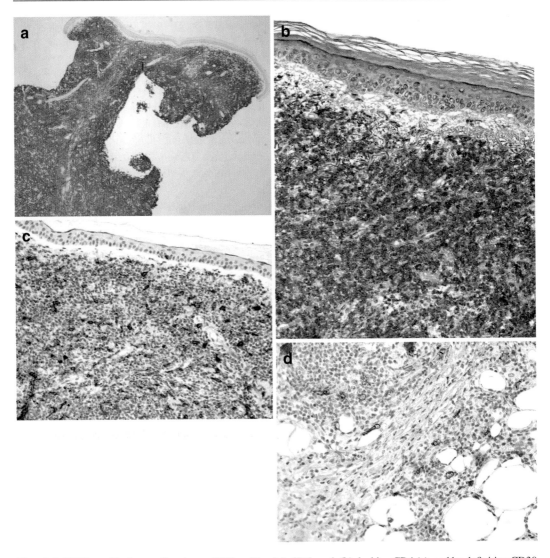

Fig. 10.6 PTCL-u with aberrant T antigens: CD7 positive (**a**), CD5 weak (**b**), lacking CD4 (**c**), and by definition CD30 negative or sparse (**d**)

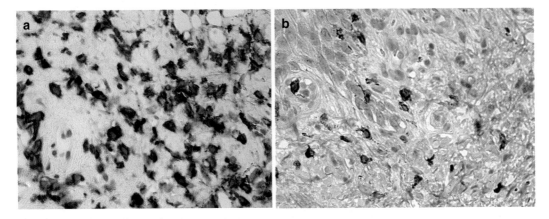

Fig. 10.7 CD8-positive PTCL-u cases are not infrequent (**a**). One or more "mature" T-cell antigens are aberrantly decreased or lost; (**b**) in this case, CD3-positive cells are much decreased

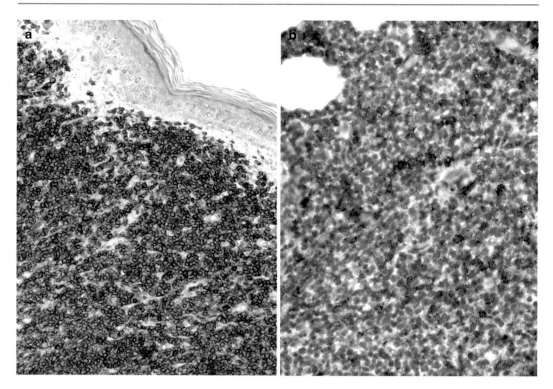

Fig. 10.8 (**a**) CD4-positive PTCL-u with (**b**) coexpression aberrantly of B-cell antigen, CD20

Table 10.1 Pathology, cytogenetics, and molecular biology of rare subtypes of mature T/NK-cell lymphoma

Lymphoma type	Morphology	Immunophenotype	Cytogenetics	Molecular biology	References
Cutaneous γδ T-cell lymphoma	Epidermal, dermal, subcutaneous perivascular cytophagic histiocytes, psoriasiform epidermal hyperplasia	CD3+/CD2+/ CD56+/ cytotoxic proteins+ (TIA-1, granzyme B, and perforin/CD4–/CD8±/ βF1± γ/δ +/CD5–)	Nonspecific	TCR genes are rearranged, EBV absent	Willemze et al. 2005 Toro et al. 2000
Primary cutaneous peripheral T-cell lymphoma, unspecified	Medium- to large-sized pleomorphic or immunoblast-like >30 %	CD4+/CD30–	Nonspecific	TCR genes are rearranged	Willemze et al. 2005 Bekkenk et al. 2003
Primary cutaneous small- to medium-sized T-cell lymphoma	Nodular infiltrates, small to medium lymphocytes <30 % large pleomorphic cells	CD3+/CD4+/CD8–/ or CD8+/CD30–/cytotoxic proteins–(granzyme B, TIA)	Nonspecific	TCR genes are rearranged	Willemze et al. 2005 Bekkenk et al. 2003
Extranodal NK/T-cell lymphoma, nasal type	Angiodestructive necrosis, polymorphous infiltrate admixed with inflammatory cells	CD56+/CD2+/cytoplasmic CD3ε+/cytotoxic granule proteins+(TIA-1, granzyme B, and perforin)/sCD3–/ CD4–/CD8–	del 6(q16–q27), del 13(q14–q34)	TCR genes are gcrm line, EBV+, mutations of k-*ras*	Willemze et al. 2005 Santucci et al. 2003

Table 10.2 Clinical features of rare subtypes of mature T/NK-cell lymphoma

	Cutaneous γδ T-cell lymphoma	Primary cutaneous peripheral T-cell lymphoma, unspecified	Primary cutaneous T-cell lymphoma CD4+ small/medium	Extranodal NK/T-cell lymphoma, nasal type
Median age, years (range)	61 (25–91)	68 (20–87)	53 (3–90)	50
M/F ratio	1.5	2.5	1:1	3.2
Clinical presentation	Disseminated plaques, nodules, tumors with ulceration, necrosis	Solitary or generalized nodules, tumors	Solitary plaques tumors, papules	Localized: destructive tumor of nasal cavity/nasopharynx Disseminated: plaques, tumors ± ulceration
Therapy	Systemic combined CT (chemotherapy)	Anthracycline-based combined CT ± RT	Solitary lesion: excision, RT (radiotherapy) Disseminated: PUVA, IFN-α, cyclophosphamide	Limited stage: RT ± CT Disseminated: CT or CT+RT
5-year disease spec survival rate	0 %	20 %	75 %	17–40 %
Median overall survival (months)	15–31	22	See text	45 (skin only)

Transformed Mycosis Fungoides

Introduction

Transformation of cutaneous T-cell lymphoma was first described by Lukes and Collins (1974). Because of the adverse effect on prognosis, a number of reports have been published since then to better identify and diagnose these cases. The presence of tumor MF clinically is not a sine qua non for a diagnosis of large cell transformation, and tumor MF may not show histologic evidence of transformation (Cerroni et al. 1992). Indeed, large cell transformation could be seen in both early and advanced MF (Lai et al. 2012). Hence, the diagnosis of large cell transformation of mycosis fungoides always requires histologic and cytological confirmation (Salhany et al. 1988; Dmitrovsky et al. 1987).

Tumor MF is one of the three facets of clinical progression; the others include nodal or visceral dissemination. Biopsy may show diffuse to nodular infiltrates with histologic evidence of large cell transformation of small cerebriform cells, which are sometimes referred to as "blastic" cells (Kamarashev et al. 2007), or histology may not contain a significant number of large cells in close to half of cases of tumor MF (Cerroni et al.

1992). Hence, accurate diagnosis of large cell transformation requires the histopathologist to count the number of large cells.

Definition

Large cell transformation is defined as having large cells (nuclei ≥4 times the size of a small lymphocyte) (Vergier et al. 2000), in 25 % or more of the dermal infiltrate or as cohesive nodules composed of large cells. Similar dire prognosis is noted if large cells comprise greater than 25 % or 50 % of cells (Vergier et al. 2000). This distinction from MF is very important since the course of MF is generally protracted except when superimposed with large cell transformation, development of tumors, or dissemination.

Epidemiology

About 8–55 % of MF patients undergo transformation, with 65 years as the average age at transformation (Vergier et al. 2000; Salhany et al. 1988; Greer et al. 1990; Cerroni et al. 1992). The incidence of transformation of mycosis fungoides varies according to the stage, being very rare in early stage MF reported to be from 0.5 to 7 % (Lai et al. 2012) to as much 31 % in stages IIB–IV and as much as 46 % in those with T3 tumors

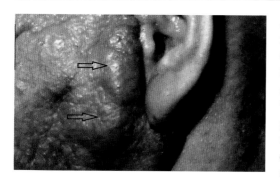

Fig. 10.9 Mycosis fungoides tumor stage (*arrows*) with histologic large cell transformation commonly occurs in the skin, here with antecedent macules, plaques, and papules

(Diamandidou et al. 1998). Tumor stage T3 has the highest incidence of transformation.

The median time to transformation from the time of initial diagnosis was reported to range from about a year to 6.5 years, dependent on varying length of clinical follow-up (Greer et al. 1990; Vergier et al. 2000). About a quarter presented before 2 years from diagnosis. The cumulative probability of transformation is 39 % happening between 1 year and about 12 years (Diamandidou et al. 1998).

A clinically advanced stage higher than tumor stage IIB predict up to 31 % will have large cell transformation versus 14 % in the lower stages. Once transformation occurs, the survival from disease of patch, plaque, and tumor stages was 7.2, 2.3, and 1.8 years, respectively (Kamarashev et al. 2007). The proposed ISCL/EORTC classification revision requires the size of at least one tumor to be at least 1.5 cm in diameter to meet the definition of tumor in T_3 (Olsen et al. 2007). However, biopsy is needed early on as transformed MF may be seen in 13 % of MF patients without clinical evidence of tumor formation (Vergier et al. 2000).

Clinical Appearance of Lesions

The most common location of transformation occurs in the skin (Fig. 10.9), but other uncommon sites like CNS are reported. Transformation often occurs in lymph nodes, where transformation is detected first in 35 % (Salhany et al. 1988; Vergier et al. 2000). In the skin, transformed MF are usually associated with multiple skin lesions and plaques or tumors (Cerroni et al. 1990) or rarely as solitary nodules (Vergier et al. 2000; Greer et al. 1990). Painful: ulcerations that may be reddish, indurated, or elevated, and pruritic; and dry well-demarcated tumors are observed. These tumors are usually located in sun-unexposed areas such as the abdomen, breast, buttocks, trunks, or neck (Berger et al. 2011; Greer et al. 1990). True de novo transformed MF at presentation is reported but probably very rare, considering that 18 % (Vergier et al. 2000) to 36 % (Diamandidou et al. 1998) of cases that presented within months of diagnosis as MF transformation have had a long history of dermatitis that were suggestive of MF.

Extracutaneous disease noted in about 1 % of a large multivariate survival study is associated with clinical evidence of tumors (T3 stage) in 61 %, noted commonly in the lung, oronasopharynx, and central nervous system (Agar et al. 2010).

Pattern of Infiltration

Most of the transformed cases showed a diffuse pattern (Fig. 10.10), sometimes forming micronodules, with lichenoid and patchy pattern in the minority (Diamandidou et al. 1998). Other reports show tumor nodules or large cells located in upper dermal to subcutaneous tissue (Vergier et al. 2000). There is often a decrease in epidermotropism and increased large cells, usually away from hair follicles or epithelia but within the dermis or subcutis (Salhany et al. 1988). The large transformed cells in the dermis often extend from the dermal-epidermal interface into the subcutaneous tissue. A narrow grenz zone, sometimes with reactive fibrosis, frequently separates the epidermis from the dermal tumor in the central portion of the mass. Epidermis may be ulcerated, rarely show Pautrier's microabscesses, and if present usually are comprised of cerebriform cells and large transformed cells (Fig. 10.11) (Salhany et al. 1988).

Cytomorphology

The large cells have round to oval vesicular nuclei, large nucleoli, and moderately abundant amphophilic cytoplasm; sometimes these cells show nuclear irregularity, and along with conspicuous

Fig. 10.10 Transformed tumor stage MF, histologically with a diffuse pattern

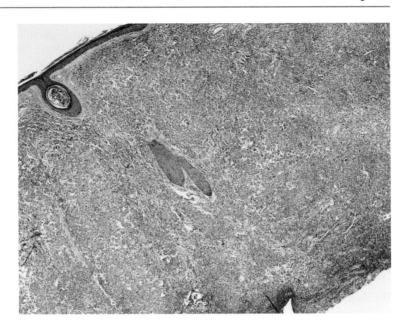

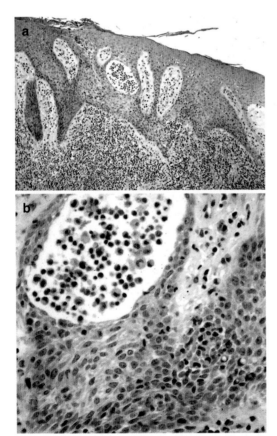

Fig. 10.11 Transformed tumor stage M. (**a**) Pautrier's microabscesses overlying lichenoid pattern. (**b**) Closer view of microabscess with hyperchromatic cerebriform and large transformed cells with lobated nuclei

nucleolus, these cells appear as multinucleated or Reed-Sternberg-like cells although classic Reed-Sternberg cells are rare (Fig. 10.12) (Salhany et al. 1988). The cytopathology of transformed cells appears variously as either medium to large pleomorphic, anaplastic, immunoblastic, or unclassified (Fig. 10.13) (Cerroni et al. 1992). Mitoses are often numerous. Admixed histiocytes along with Langerhans cells are always seen within the dermal infiltrates but must be differentiated from tumor cells. The number of large cells has to be counted, because of similarly bad prognosis of patients with 25–50 % of large cells (Fig. 10.14). Large cells could be defined as above or more precisely greater than 35 μm (Salhany et al. 1988) or more conventionally as greater than the size of macrophage nuclei. Small to large cerebriform or atypical "dysplastic" cells are scattered or easily seen along the periphery of the dermal mass (Salhany et al. 1988), and this salient feature may differentiate transformed MF from similar neoplasm such as ALCL or PTCL-u.

Immunophenotype

Similar to other cutaneous peripheral T-cell lymphomas, transformed MF may lose or gain some T-cell antigens such as CD7, CD5, CD3, or betaF1. Transformed MF often have CD3+ T

Fig. 10.12 MF with large cell transformed lymphoma cells showing lobated irregular nuclei, with conspicuous nucleoli, with occasional Reed-Sternberg-like cells although classic Reed-Sternberg cells are rare

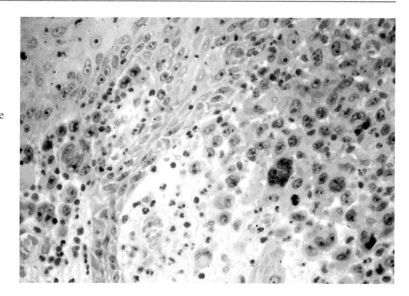

Fig. 10.13 The transformed cells in MF appear variously as either medium to large pleomorphic, anaplastic, immunoblastic, or unclassified, with frequent mitosis, all represented here

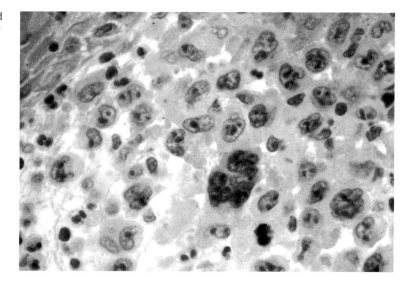

helper phenotype expressing CD4 in 70 % of cases, CD8 in 19 %, and absent CD4 and CD8 in 4 %; and most have partial loss of one or more T antigens and, in 4 %, aberrant expression of B-cell antigens CD20 and CD79 (Benner et al. 2012b).

A decreased intensity or diminution of total number of positive cells may be seen in CD7, CD26, CD45RO, CD5, or CD3 (Jones et al. 2001; Salhany et al. 1988). Absent or diminished pan-T antigens can be observed, while CD30, CD15, or CD75 (LN2) may appear as aberrant additional antigens simulating that seen in Reed-Sternberg cells, each noted in about half of the cases (Salhany et al. 1988). CD25 may be expressed weakly in all of the few cases tested (Diamandidou et al. 1998). Varying expression of CD30 in the large transformed cells (Fig. 10.15) from 31 to

Fig. 10.14 Deep subcutaneous tissue is often involved
as in this case

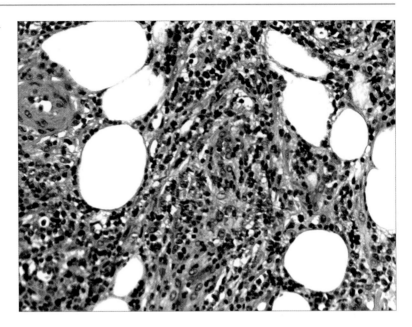

Fig. 10.15 CD30-positive
transformed MF cells with
cytoplasmic and surface
brown staining

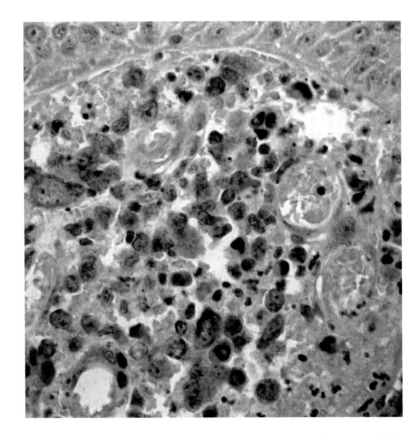

50 % is seen (Olsen et al. 2007; Arulogun et al. 2008; Barberio et al. 2007; Vergier et al. 2000). High expression (greater than 75 % CD30-positive cells) is seen in 15 % (Vergier et al. 2000) to 39 %, while low level (less than 5 %) noted in 45 %, with the remainder of cases (Benner et al. 2012b) showing intermediate expression. Interestingly, Benner et al. reported that CD30 expression in transformed MF is associated with a significantly better survival (Benner et al. 2012b). Their finding raises the question of whether the improved prognosis of those patients was due to inclusion of ALCL masquerading as T-MF.

Immunophenotypes of large cell lymphoma arising from MF are similar to the original MF. The small cerebriform malignant cells gave rise to large cell lymphoma in transformed MF because both cells contain identical T-cell surface v-beta antigens as detected by flow cytometry technique using a set of monoclonal antibodies to T-cell receptor V-beta region families (Wolfe et al. 1995).

Cytogenetics and Molecular Findings

A majority of T-cell gene rearrangement results in MF/SS (84 %) show a clonal T-cell population using PCR or GeneScan capillary electrophoresis (Ponti et al. 2005, 2008). Furthermore, this clone of MF and its large cell transformation are singular. They show identical clones upon V-beta or PCR nucleotide sequences, using molecular genetics of the low grade and its transformed lesion years apart (Wood et al. 1993). Hence, transformation is an evolution instead of an emergence of new malignant clones.

In untransformed MF, an abnormal cytogenetics is found in 66 %, ranging from hypo- to hypertetraploid, with same malignant clones found in the skin, blood, and lymph nodes (Nowell et al. 1982). Losses and gains of chromosome materials are also documented likewise using comparative genomic hybridization with most frequent loss in chromosomes 1p, 17p, 10q, and 19 and gains in chromosomes 4q, 18, and 17q (Mao et al. 2002). FISH analysis documented evidence of chromosome 1 and 17q rearrangements in a third of Sezary syndrome cases.

Similarly, multicolor FISH (SKY) detected structural and recurrent chromosomal abnormality in 47 % with chromosome 10 showing the most frequent abnormality (Batista et al. 2006).

However, conventional cytogenetics data on large cell transformation is surprisingly scant when compared with the molecular genetics and nucleotide profiling analysis data. Using gene profiling analysis, a total of five genes are significantly upregulated in tumor stage compared with patch/plaque stage MF. Tumorigenesis is here associated with upregulation of antiapoptotic and inhibition of proapoptotic pathways leading to growth advantage via TRAF1 and tumor necrosis factor receptors (Tracey et al. 2003). In addition, using microRNA profiling, there are different miRNAs expressed in tumor stage MF that allows differentiation from nontumor MF and ALCL (Benner et al. 2012a; van Kester et al. 2011, 2012; Berger et al. 1988; Karenko et al. 2007). Inflammatory versus MF gene expression profile has also been reported (van Kester et al. 2012). Of targeted therapy significance, genes associated with Th1 immune response and cytotoxicity are downregulated, while CD52 and interleukin seven genes were upregulated in mycosis fungoides/Sezary syndrome (Hahtola et al. 2006).

Clinical Behavior

The 10-year disease-specific survival of MF shows an indolent course with over 80 % surviving, while development of tumor reduces survival to 42 % (Agar et al. 2010; van Doorn et al. 2000) and presence of large cell transformation reduces survival to between 2 and 36 months in most series (Dmitrovsky et al. 1987; Greer et al. 1990; Salhany et al. 1988; Vergier et al. 2000; Barberio et al. 2007; Arulogun et al. 2008; Diamandidou et al. 1998; Benner et al. 2012b) and in a specially large series (Agar et al. 2010) up to 100 months. Similarly, a cohort of patients with tumors in contrast to those with plaques/patches fared poorly (Suzuki et al. 2010b). The presence or absence of large cell transformation in all patients that *already had tumor stage* did not show difference in survival (Vonderheid et al. 1981; Benner et al. 2012b).

Early transformation less than 2 years from diagnosis, advanced stage (IIB–IV vs. I–IIA) (Diamandidou et al. 1998; Berlingeri-Ramos et al. 2007), and extracutaneous dissemination are poor prognostic signs. In patients with disease limited to only skin lesion at transformation, findings of folliculotropic MF, lack of CD30 in large cells, and extracutaneous disease are significantly associated with reduced survival (Benner et al. 2012b). In contrast when studying earlier stages of MF, Edinger found that increasing numbers of CD30+ cells conferred a worse prognosis, as did increased numbers of Ki-67+ cells, although the two markers were independent of each other (Edinger et al. 2009). Increased serum levels of soluble CD30 are also associated with a poorer survival for patients with early (stages 1–IIa) MF (Kadin et al. 2012).

Differential Diagnosis

1. CD30 anaplastic large cell lymphomas: It is important to have an accurate measurement of the CD30-positive cells to differentiate transformed MF from the CD30-positive (ALCL) lymphomas. The diagnosis of T-MF with CD30 + large cells instead of a de novo CD30 + lymphoma is made if clinical evidence of patch and/or plaque skin lesions compatible with MF precedes the transformation, along with a morphology composed of a pleomorphic types from small cerebriform to large cells. This diagnosis is supported if there are less than 75 % CD30-positive large cells among the T cells, but differentiation cannot be made reliably if more than 75 % of large cells are CD30 (Vergier et al. 2000). Beylot-Berry reported that perforin expression by large cells is significantly more frequent in ALCL complicating MF than in T-MF (personal communication 2nd World Congress on Cutaneous Lymphomas, Berlin, Feb 6–10, 2013).

2. Histiocyte-rich or granulomatous MF, histiocytic clusters: Histiocyte-rich or granulomatous MF is characterized by nodules of large histiocytic cells mimicking large lymphoma cells. It is important to separate this type with

large cell transformation of tumor cells composed of T lymphocytes because the clinical course of "histiocyte-rich MF" or "granulomatous MF" parallels MF without transformation (Vergier et al. 2000). In contrast to the latter, histiocytes or granulomatous nodules mark with CD68 (KP1 or PGM1 clones) instead of pan-T antibodies. In one series of transformed MF, upwards of 67 % of these cases show clusters of histiocytes (Vergier et al. 2000). CD68 staining for histiocytes should be performed in suspected transformed MF. This is because if using routine histology only in the assessment of large cells, these cells may not be of T-cell origin but of macrophage lineage. Although the nuclei of macrophage are also large like tumor cells, there are subtle clues to tell them apart. Histiocytic cells are morphologically different from T cells, the former showing scant to very pale and sparse heterochromatin vesicles while the latter tend to have thicker darker chromatin and prominent chromocenters. Macrophages tend to have round to oval thin pinkish nuclear membranes and small nucleolus, while transformed MF may have thick irregular, lobated membranes and prominent nucleolus. However, when clusters of histiocytes are closely admixed with large tumor cells, their differentiation from neoplastic cells may be difficult.

3. Large B-cell lymphoma: The presence of sheets of B cells could be seen in transformed MF and hence may cause confusion with B-cell lymphomas. Clusters of large cells in MF may not be T cells as up to 45 % has been found to be of CD20+ B cells in origin. Hence, CD20 staining for B cells is also an essential panel for working these cases (Vergier et al. 2000). Interpretation is further complicated by the aberrant expression of B-cell antigens, e.g., CD20 by tumor T cells in some T-MF (Merlio communication) (2nd World Congress on Cutaneous Lymphomas, Berlin, Feb. 6–10, 2013).

4. *Tumor d'emblée*: Although the classic Alibert description of MF (Alibert 1806) included

patches, plaques, and progression to ulcerated tumors, a number of literature reports beginning with Vidal-Bronc in 1805 (Habermann and Pittelkow 2007) to the beginning of the twentieth century (Pernet 1912; Pringle 1914) and in the 1950s (Olivier 1951; Pernet 1912; Pringle 1914) described *tumor d' emblée* as an initial presentation of MF. However, current CTCL classification raises concern that *tumor d' emblée* could largely represent a type of nodular cutaneous PTCL, instead of a variant of MF, when seen in a setting that is not accompanied by a longstanding MF. The prevailing view is that when a patient initially presents with only tumor without previous or current patches or plaques, a diagnosis of MF is not likely, but may instead be diagnostic for other T-cell lymphomas infiltrating the skin (Willemze et al. 2005) or perhaps a variant of a systemic peripheral T-cell lymphoma that involves the skin.

Early series of MF tumor stage study include tumor MF detected at presentation (Salhany et al. 1988), but more recent case series excluded "tumor d' emblée" cases. Vergier et al. excluded cases that present without clinical history or histologically confirmed MF if the initial presentation was a large T-cell lymphoma without proven previous clinical and histologic MF (Vergier et al. 2000). In a review of the historical evolution of cutaneous lymphoma classification, Kempf noted that the WHO-EORTC classification (Willemze et al. 2005) excluded *d' emblée* form of MF and in those presenting with tumor should instead consider other T-cell lymphomas such as cutaneous PTCL, unspecified (Kempf and Sander 2010).

5. Non-MF subtypes of CTCL: For patients presenting with tumors, it is important to differentiate tumor stage MF from non-MF subtypes of CTCL such a pleomorphic CD4 small- and medium-sized T-cell lymphoma and PTCL-U (see discussions on each type in this chapter).

Primary Cutaneous Small- to Medium-Sized T-Cell Lymphoma (PCSM-TCL)

Introduction

This provisional entity in the 2008 WHO and 2005 WHO-EORTC classification was called primary cutaneous CD4-positive small/medium T-cell lymphoma (Swerdlow et al. 2008; Willemze et al. 2005). Subsequent case series addressing whether this is a valid entity have indicated that this "entity" may be heterogeneous (Garcia-Herrera et al. 2008; Williams et al. 2011). Hence, phenotypically this group may present as CD8 + tumors, or the CD4 + type may be seen presenting as one of these categories: (1) "solitary… T-cell nodules of undetermined significance" that overlap with reactive pseudolymphomas (Beltraminelli et al. 2009; Leinweber et al. 2009), (2) indolent T-cell lymphoma (Garcia-Herrera et al. 2008; Williams et al. 2011), and (3) a more aggressive subset that may clinically simulate PTCL-u with an adverse course (Garcia-Herrera et al. 2008; Williams et al. 2011).

Because of the nodular T-cell-rich immunohistology and its indolent course, this disease group overlaps with the wide variety of T-cell pseudolymphomas (Beltraminelli et al. 2009; Leinweber et al. 2009) and presents a diagnostic challenge. Accurate diagnosis may require an optimal combination of morphology with accurate large cell identification, immunohistology, clonality, and clinical features for adequate distinction (Williams et al. 2011). A histologic subset of PCSM-TCL with eosinophilia and recurrent skin nodules reported by Campo and the Barcelona group (Garcia-Herrera et al. 2008) may especially mimic allergic/drug-induced T-cell nodular form of pseudolymphoma or cutaneous lymphoid hyperplasia.

Definition

Primary cutaneous small- and medium-sized T-cell lymphoma (PCSM-TCL) presents most commonly as a solitary nodule and histologically as nodules of "pleomorphic" small and medium cells admixed with less than 30 % large or immunoblastic cells (Willemze et al. 2005; Kempf and Sander 2010; Beljaards et al. 1994; Swerdlow et al. 2008). As part of the definition, there should be no clinical evidence of patches and plaque seen in MF. For convenience, we will use the term pleomorphic T-cell lymphoma interchangeably with PCSM-TCL.

A unifying list of criteria for diagnosis may include the following criteria as modified from Cerroni et al. (2009), Garcia-Herrera et al. (2008), and Williams et al. (2011):

1. Absent history or lesions diagnostic of MF or marked epidermotropism.
2. Molecular evidence of monoclonal T lymphocytes.
3. T cells expressing CD3/alpha-beta (either CD4 or CD8), not gamma-delta TCR framework.
4. Absent CD30 (to exclude CD30 lymphomas).
5. Nodular or diffuse infiltrate of neoplastic small- and medium-sized T cells.
6. Admixture of many reactive B, reactive T, histiocytes, eosinophils, and polyclonal plasma cells.
7. Histologic evidence of fewer than 30 % large cells (to exclude PTCL-u).
8. Accurate quantification of proliferative count of Ki67 of less than 25 % and in CD4 tumors with less than 10 % CD8 reactive T cells will exclude the aggressive variant of PCSM-TCL (Garcia-Herrera et al. 2008; Williams et al. 2011) which were clinically recommended to be included with and may behave like a PTCL-u (Garcia-Herrera et al. 2008; Williams et al. 2011).

Epidemiology

A rare disease accounting for 2 % of all CTCLs (Willemze et al. 2005). There is a wide age range of presentation with a median age of 53 years (range 3–90 years), with a male to female ratio of 1:1 (Beltraminelli et al. 2009; Leinweber et al. 2009).

Clinical Appearance of Lesions

The most common locations are in the head and neck, upper trunk, and rarely lower extremities

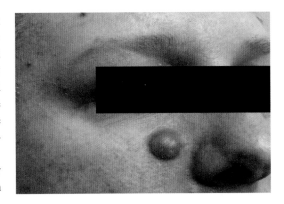

Fig. 10.16 Primary cutaneous small- and medium-sized T-cell lymphoma showing as a solitary reddish nodule on the face

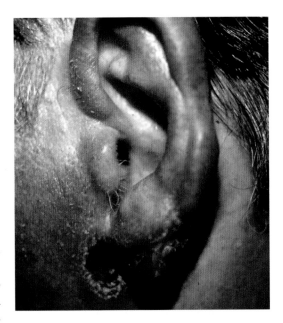

Fig. 10.17 The CD8+ variant of PCSM-TCL has predilection for the ear

(Bekkenk et al. 2003; Garcia-Herrera et al. 2008) (Fig. 10.16).

The CD8+ type has predilection for the ear (Fig. 10.17) as described below. A minority of clinical presentations include multiple nodules or large tumors; otherwise systemic symptoms are usually not present (Beltraminelli et al. 2009; Garcia-Herrera et al. 2008; Leinweber et al. 2009).

Fig. 10.18 Primary cutaneous small- and medium-sized T-cell lymphoma showing a dense nodular involvement throughout the upper and deep dermis close to subcutaneous tissue

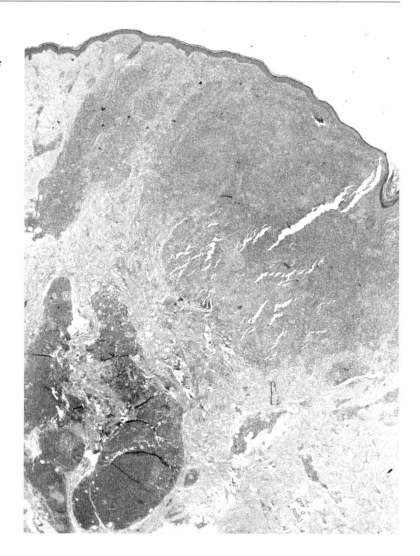

Pattern of Infiltration

Infiltrates are dense, diffuse, or nodular within the dermis (Fig. 10.18), with a tendency to infiltrate the upper portions of the subcutaneous tissue (Fig. 10.19). There is minimal or no epidermotropism (Fig. 10.20). Significant epidermotropism should raise consideration of MF and higher magnification evaluation for typical cerebriform morphology for exclusion of the latter.

Cytomorphology

Cells are pleomorphic composed of majority of small- to medium-sized lymphocytes with scattered or more specifically less than 30 % large cells (Fig. 10.21). Reactive small lymphocytes, many eosinophils, and histiocytes may also be seen (Fig. 10.22) (Bekkenk et al. 2003). A subset with intense eosinophilia has been described as a possible histologic variant of this disease (Garcia-Herrera et al. 2008). The term pleomorphic is

Fig. 10.19 Primary
cutaneous small- and
medium-sized T-cell
lymphoma with focal spread
to the upper portions of the
subcutaneous tissue

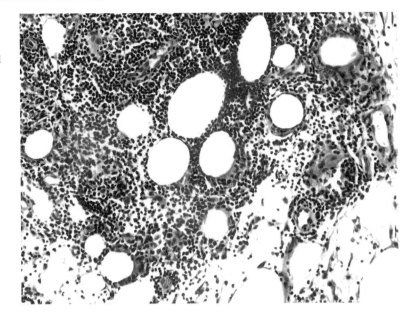

Fig. 10.20 Primary
cutaneous small- and
medium-sized T-cell
lymphoma with minimal to
absent epidermotropism,
unlike that seen in mycosis
fungoides

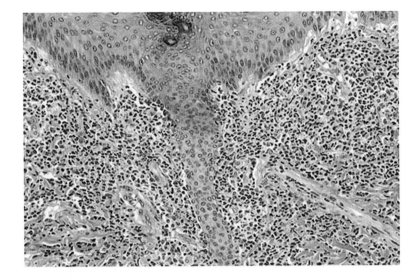

Fig. 10.21 Primary cutaneous small- and medium-sized T-cell lymphoma cells are pleomorphic composed of small- to medium-sized lymphocytes with less than 30 % large cells

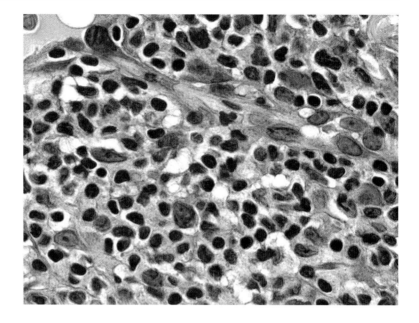

Fig. 10.22 Some primary cutaneous small- and medium-sized T-cell lymphoma cases may show a mixture of small lymphocytes, few plasma cells, many eosinophils, scattered histiocytes, and many capillaries and vessels

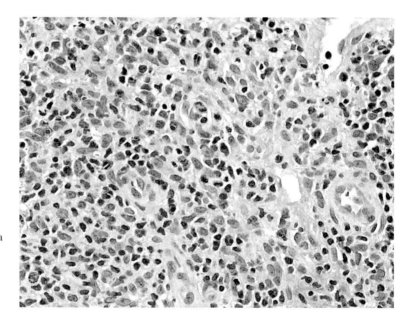

Fig. 10.23 Primary
cutaneous small- and
medium-sized T-cell
lymphoma cells are usually
positive for CD4, in diffuse
and nodular pattern

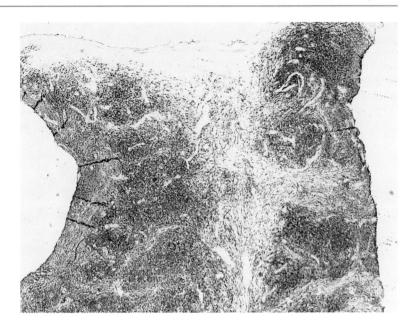

Fig. 10.24 PCSM-TCL may
present as a variant
composed of CD8-positive
tumor cells, particularly
when the nodules are located
in earlobes

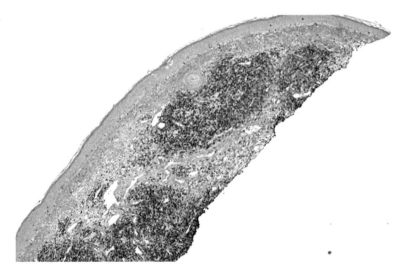

mostly included in the diagnostic terms but have also been substituted by (SM) small- and medium-sized descriptors and the presence of less than 30 % large cells (Beljaards et al. 1994).

Immunophenotype

The neoplastic cells are positive for CD3 and CD4 (Fig. 10.23) in most cases and positive in CD8 in a minor subset, usually localized in the

ear (Fig. 10.24). Cytotoxic proteins (granzyme B, TIA) and Epstein-Barr virus and CD30 and CD56 antigens are not seen in CD4 + tumor cells, and T-cell antigens are aberrantly lost in some cases (Garcia-Herrera et al. 2008; Von Den and Coors 2002).

Originally described as showing only CD4-positive T cells, a collection of recent reports suggest a primary cutaneous small- and medium-sized

T-cell lymphoma may have CD8 immunopheno-type. Almost uniformly, the reports described an indolent, nonepidermotropic, pleomorphic nodular tumor in the ear, with CD8 immunophenotype (Geraud et al. 2011; Beltraminelli et al. 2010; Petrella et al. 2007; Swick et al. 2011; Suchak et al. 2010). Hence, if accepted as part of this group, more recent terminology of PCSM-TCL is notable for absence of the CD4 descriptor. Despite the similar CD8 immunophenotype, this former group is not to be confused with the aggressive and epidermotropic CD8+ T-cell lymphoma, often with ulcerated skin lesions and localized in other skin regions (Berti et al. 1999; Gormley et al. 2010; Nofal et al. 2012).

Along with the dominant neoplastic T cells, admixed reactive CD20 + B cells and polyclonal plasma cells, dotted with eosinophils and histiocytes, are findings that overlap with pseudolymphoma or cutaneous lymphoid hyperplasia (Sterry 1986; Sterry et al. 1992).

Cytogenetics and Molecular Findings

Diagnosis requires molecular genetic analysis and positive TCR gene rearrangement for unequivocal diagnosis of PCSM-T-cell lymphoma versus the similar-looking T-cell pseudolymphoma. TCR genes are rearranged in 60 % (Beltraminelli et al. 2009) to 100 % of reported cases (Grogg et al. 2008; Rodriguez Pinilla et al. 2009). In practice, we tend to consider TCR-negative cases as T-cell pseudolymphoma and positive cases as PCSM-TCL.

Clinical Behavior

The WHO 2008 classification of lymphomas included two provisional categories under PTCL-u. Of these two, only primary cutaneous small- and medium-sized pleomorphic CD4+ T-cell lymphomas have a good prognosis (Swerdlow et al. 2008; Willemze et al. 2005). Localized lesions have a good prognosis with local treatments. A disease-specific 5-year survival rate of up to 75 % and an overall 5-year survival rate of 45 % have been reported (Bekkenk et al. 2003). A large series with long follow-up revealed most were alive without lymphoma after a median follow-up of 63 months (Beltraminelli et al. 2009).

About 200 cases of this provisional entity have been reported, and despite the presence of clonal T cells in many reported cases, the indolent behavior of these lesions perhaps has earned them a recommendation to consider the term "cutaneous nodular proliferation of pleomorphic T cells of undetermined significance" in lieu of small and medium pleomorphic T-cell lymphoma (Von Den and Coors 2002; Bekkenk et al. 2003; Friedmann et al. 1995; Grogg et al. 2008; Beltraminelli et al. 2009; Leinweber et al. 2009; Garcia-Herrera et al. 2008; Sterry et al. 1992; Rodriguez Pinilla et al. 2009; Kim and Vandersteen 2001).

However, a group of five cases with clinical and histologic features of PCSM-TCL was described that followed an aggressive clinical outcome, with a median survival of 23 months, akin to PTCL-u (Garcia-Herrera et al. 2008). Although others believe these cases are different from PCSM-TCL, by using histologic criteria alone, these cases appear to fit that category if one were to exclude one case with an associated nodal Langerhans cell sarcoma (Garcia-Herrera et al. 2008). What sets this group apart from the typical course for PCSM-TCL and may perhaps be useful in practice to exclude these cases from the indolent PCSM-TCL are the following: differences in clinical behavior, high proliferative rate, and different tumor-reactive microenvironments. The markers were scored objectively using commercial image analysis techniques as previously described (Carreras et al. 2006). Hence, this group is characterized by having rapidly growing large tumors (>5 cm) versus less than 3 cm in the indolent group, high mitotic index with median Ki67 % of 22 (15–43) versus 9 % (range 1–20) and low CD8 infiltrating lymphocytes (0.3–8 %) versus 20 % (range 9–47) in indolent, respectively, and, finally, sparse B cells versus nodules of B cells in indolent (Garcia-Herrera et al. 2008).

Because of the clinical difference, a proposal to lump this set in the PTCL-u disease category, instead of as a variant of PCSM-TCL, appears reasonable (Williams et al. 2011). However, to accurately delineate this group, an accurate count of immunomarkers was done by the Barcelona group (Garcia-Herrera et al. 2008). This is

Table 10.3 T-cell lymphoma versus T-cell pseudolymphoma

	Nodular PCSM-TCL	Nodular pseudo-T-cell lymphoma	PTCL, unspecified
Clinical	Solitary, rare multiple	Solitary, rare multiple	Multiple, rare solitary
Course	Indolent	Benign	Aggressive with high mortality
Pattern	Nodular diffuse, nonepidermotropic, dermal to focal subcutaneous tissue	Nodular, also may be band-like or perivascular, usually just dermal	Diffuse and nodular, dermal to subcutaneous tissue
Cytology	Small and medium size, less than 30% large cells	Small and medium size, with immunoblasts and histiocytes	Large cells > 30% of cells
T and B clonality	Monoclonal T	Polyclonal T and B	Monoclonal T
Phenotype	CD4, rare CD8, few or CD30 negative; loss of T-cell antigens; Ki67 increased >25%	CD4,CD8 mixed with CD20 sheets, scattered CD30,ki67 wide range low to less than 40%	CD4, CD8, some CD20 aberrant, loss of T-cell antigens,CD30 negative or few; ki67 increased 60 % of more
Reactive components			
Plasma cells	Few	Few or many sheets	Few
Eosinophils	Few	Few or many sheets	Few
Histiocytes	Few	Many diffuse or granulomas	Few
CD20	Few	Sheets or clusters	Few
CD8, if CD4 tumor	Few	Increased	Few

because by using histologic criteria alone (of less than 30 % large cells) and without using immunomarkers, this aggressive group may inadvertently and unfortunately be assigned to the category of PCSM-TCL. To nullify this heterogeneity and standardize the criteria for diagnosis of PCSM-TCL, clinical and immunomeasurement analysis (immunometric or hematometric analysis) may be used. Those that are aggressive appear to present with a large rapidly growing tumor bigger than 5 cm and decreased CD8 and CD20 cells. A validated 2-D image analysis computerized tools that perform the function of cell population statistic automation applied to fixed tissue immunostains may be helpful in this regard (Nielsen et al. 2012; Baatz et al. 2009; Cualing et al. 2007; Carreras et al. 2006, 2009; Garcia-Herrera et al. 2008).

Differential Diagnosis

T-cell nodular pseudolymphoma – the most important differential diagnosis is from the nodular and diffuse type of T-cell pseudolymphoma. Two major histo-architectural types of T-cell pseudolymphoma include the MF-like band and the nodular T-cell pattern (Smolle et al. 1990;

Wirt et al. 1985). Clinically, a clear-cut etiology from either a recent drug intake, insect bite, or chemical exposure though uncommon may lead to an easy diagnosis. However, since most pseudolymphomas are idiopathic, a thorough correlation for clinical regression on follow-up along with a biopsy for immunohistology, morphology, and molecular genetics may all be useful. See Table 10.3 (Rijlaarsdam et al. 1992; Adams 1981; Albrecht et al. 2007; Arai et al. 1999; Bakels et al. 1997; Barr-Nea et al. 1976; Bendelac et al. 1986; Bergman 2010; Bernstein et al. 1974; Bignon and Souteyrand 1990; Blazejak and Holzle 1990; Blumental et al. 1982; Bocquet et al. 1996; Brodell and Santa Cruz 1985; Cerroni and Goteri 2003; Delaporte et al. 1995; Good and Gascoyne 2009; Griesser et al. 1990; Kulow et al. 2002; Landa et al. 1993; McComb et al. 2003; Rijlaarsdam and Willemze 1994; Smolle et al. 1990; Sterry 1986; Tallon et al. 2010; Van Der Putte et al. 1986; Wirt et al. 1985).

In general, pseudo-T-cell lymphomas may show a nodular pattern (Fig. 10.25) and minimal nuclear atypia of lymphocytes and, by immunostains, show increased number of reactive lymphoid cells in clusters positive for CD8 T cells or

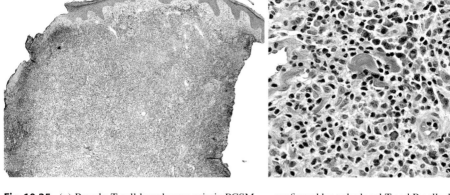

Fig. 10.25 (**a**) Pseudo-T-cell lymphomas mimic PCSM-TCL because they may also often present as a solitary nodule and histologically may likewise show a diffuse to nodular pattern. This biopsy is from a coin-sized nodule on an arm close to an IV drug line, the reactive nature confirmed by polyclonal T and B cells demonstrated with negative TCR and IgG gene rearrangements. (**b**) On high power, there are many capillaries with histiocytes, eosinophils, and clusters of plasma cells

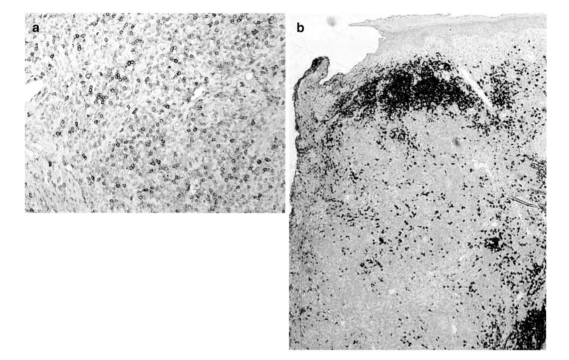

Fig. 10.26 T-cell pseudolymphoma with increased number of reactive cells positive for CD8 T cells (**a**) and CD20 B cells in clusters (**b**)

CD20 B cells (Fig. 10.26), and low Ki67 (Fig. 10.27) as well as increased in eosinophils or plasma cells (Fig. 10.28) and CD68+ histiocytes (Fig. 10.29), sometimes with histiocytic clusters and granulomas (Smolle et al. 1990; Wirt et al. 1985; Rijlaarsdam et al. 1992), and tend to be polyclonal (Bakels et al. 1997). In a comparative series on CD4+ T-cell pseudolymphomas, the CD8+ small T cells ranged between 15 % and 60 % (median, 25 %) compared to between 2 %

Fig. 10.27 T-cell pseudolymphoma with low Ki67

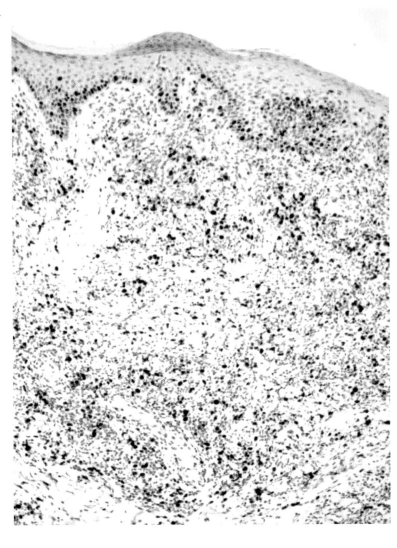

Fig. 10.28 T-cell pseudolymphoma with single and clusters
of CD68+ histiocytes

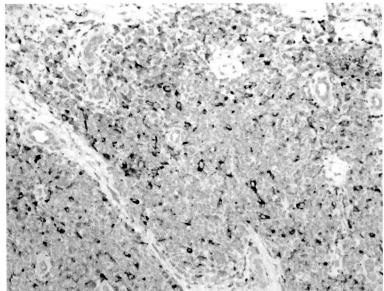

Fig. 10.29 T-cell pseudo-lymphoma with clusters of histiocytes and small granulomas

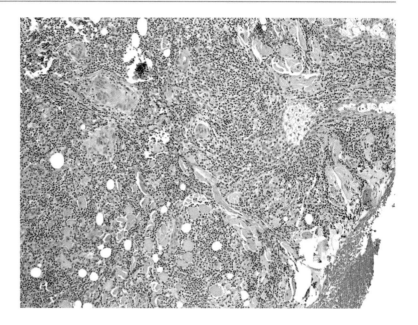

and 15 % (median, 5 %) in transformed MF and between 1 % and 10 % (median, 2 %) in the aggressive PTCL-u. In indolent nodular pleomorphic T-cell lymphoma, however, the CD8 + T cells overlap with the nodular pseudo-T-cell lymphoma (15 and 35 % CD8+). Similar pattern has been observed in the proportion of CD20+ B (Bakels et al. 1997).

Despite utilizing all these tools for diagnosis, distinction may not be possible since it is widely understood that there is a spectrum of clonal benign dermatitis to frank clonal malignant lymphoma (Wood 2001; Kulow et al. 2002; Gniadecki 2004; Gniadecki and Lukowsky 2005; Burg et al. 2005; Guitart and Magro 2007).

PTCL, unspecified, is also a differential diagnosis since some of these cases may rarely present as solitary or few nodules presenting a clinical challenge from PCSM-TCL. The distinction is mainly histopathologic, with the accurate evaluation of the presence of more than 30 % large cells in PTCL-u and less than 30 % in small- and medium-sized T-cell lymphoma. Here the large cells have been variously defined as having nuclei greater than 4×, the size of small lymphocyte nuclei or in those terminologies borrowed from hematopathology lymph node workup as those

cells with nuclei larger than macrophage nuclei. See Table 10.1.

The relation of PCSM-TCL with the few cases described as "primary cutaneous follicle center T cell lymphoma" (Battistella et al. 2012) must be clarified because of the clinical and immunohistologic overlap with PCSM-TCL especially if Bcl6, PD1, and CD10 immunostains are routinely performed. This distinction may not be possible since a number of reports indicated the PCSM-TCL of CD4 type may be of follicle center cell derivation. Hence, the CD4 PCSM-TCL tumors show expression of a subset identified with the follicle helper T cells, typically forming rosettes around B immunoblasts (Rodriguez Pinilla et al. 2009). Follicular T helper cells express PD1 (CD279), Bcl6 (follicle center cell), and CXCL13 (Rodriguez Pinilla et al. 2009). Programmed death-1 (PD1) expression, normally associated with germinal center cells (Fig. 10.30), may be used in workup of these tumors. The PD1 immunoreactivity is decreased or lacking in MF, PTCL-u, CD30 lymphomas, and aggressive CD8 epidermotropic lymphomas but note that PD1 will not separate from the immunophenotypically similar PD1 expression in T-cell pseudolymphomas (Cetinozman et al. 2012).

Fig. 10.30 PD1 expression in germinal center T cells in subepidermal location. Note the weaker staining scattered interfollicular T cells

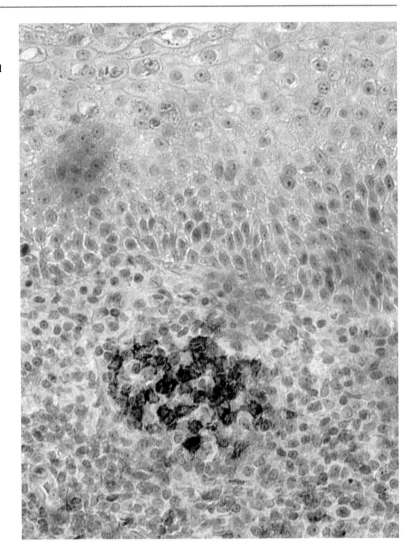

Cutaneous Gamma-Delta T-Cell Lymphoma

Introduction

Primary cutaneous γδ T-cell lymphoma is a rare subset of cutaneous T-cell lymphoma that needs to be delineated from the more common CTCLs and from the similar hepatosplenic lymphoma because of its unique presentation, adverse course, and its hematologic complications (Kadin 2000; Guitart et al. 2012). It has to be noted that both mucosal and cutaneous T γδ lymphomas are different from the hepatosplenic γδ T-cell lymphomas, which are derived from immature γδ T cells and which are positive for TIA-1, but negative for granzyme B and perforin (Toro et al. 2000). Hepatosplenic γδ T-cell lymphomas do not involve the skin. They cause splenomegaly, hepatomegaly, and relatively minimal lymphadenopathy. They usually affect middle-aged men and cause pancytopenia and early death. They are characterized by specific chromosomal abnormalities including isochromosome 7q (Gaulard et al. 2003).

Although primary cutaneous γδ T-cell lymphoma is a provisional entity under the WHO-EORTC (Willemze et al. 2005), it has been included in the WHO 2008 (Swerdlow et al. 2008) under the umbrella of primary cutaneous peripheral T-cell lymphoma, rare subtypes (Gaulard et al. 2008).

It would be useful to review the nosology of this rare cutaneous lymphoma. The T-cell membrane cell surface is specified by a CD3 complex in association with either a T-cell alpha-beta (T αβ) or a T gamma-delta (T γδ) protein subset (Bluestone et al. 1995; Bluestone and Matis 1990). The either/or exclusivity of these markers in normal T cells has been a given for decades, and the presence of TCR βF1 is assumed to identify alpha-beta T cells and exclude T γδ cells, but recent reports suggest a group of cytotoxic T-cell lymphomas may express both. Using an anti-T γδ immunoreactive with human paraffin tissue suggests that TCRT γ expression in primary cutaneous T-cell lymphoma may not be mutually exclusive, and therefore some of these tumors may express both T αβ and T γδ (Rodriguez-Pinilla et al. 2013).

Nevertheless, in human physiology, the majority of mature T cells express T αβ heterodimer framework, but about 5 % of normal T cells express the T-cell γδ framework. The function of the T γδ cells in the skin appears to be protective, has cytotoxic effector properties, and can secrete lymphokines or proliferate (Girardi 2004; Kabelitz 1995; Kabelitz et al. 2000; Kabelitz and Wesch 2003). These cells can be detected by antibodies to T-cell δ1 (TCR delta1) and lack βF1 (antibody to framework beta 1) (Kabelitz 1995). These are mature T cells that express cytotoxic TIA-1 and release granzyme B and perforin causing apoptosis. Most T γδ cells lack both CD4 and CD8 surface markers, but in the human peripheral blood, some are CD8+. This skin and mucosal distribution of disease reflects their role in normal epithelial immune responses, but extracutaneous presentation in lung, nasolaryngeal, and intestinal (Arnulf et al. 1998) as well as splenic and liver sites (Cooke et al. 1996, 1996; Garcia-Herrera et al. 2011; Gaulard et al. 2003) has been well documented.

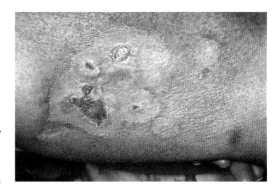

Fig. 10.31 Primary cutaneous T γδ tends to form nodules that ulcerate

Definition

Cutaneous γδ T-cell lymphomas are composed of clonally activated γ/δ T cells with a cytotoxic phenotype, with a dermotrophic and deep subcutaneous pattern of infiltration, and present with ulceronecrotic skin plaques, deep nodules, and aggressive panniculitis-like tumors and hemophagocytic syndrome in less than 10 % of cases (Koch et al. 2009; Toro et al. 2000, 2003; Willemze et al. 2005; Guitart et al. 2012). Whether this is a pure category identified by immunostaining characteristics alone is controversial.

Epidemiology

Young to middle-aged, presenting with skin lesion of a median duration of 1.25 years, and with a median age of 61 years (25–91 range) (Guitart et al. 2012), and a male to female ration of 1.5:1 (Toro et al. 2003).

Clinical Appearance of Cutaneous Lesions

Presentations include most commonly scaly deep plaques resembling panniculitis, or patches resembling MF, as well as nodules or tumors which tend to ulcerate (Fig. 10.31). These are commonly located on the lower and upper extremities, followed by the torso (Guitart et al. 2012). Solitary lesions are seen in 15 % and in those with limited disease; about half are associated with fever, malaise, fatigue, chills, and weight loss (Guitart et al. 2012). Systemic involvement has been reported, but rare with low

Fig. 10.32 Cutaneous T γδ lymphoma shows a mixed epidermal, mid-dermal, periadnexal, and subcutaneous pattern

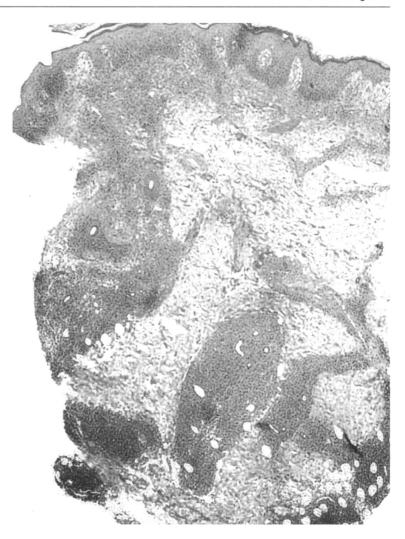

frequency of involvement of the lymph nodes, spleen, or bone marrow. LDH is elevated in more than half of the cases (Kadin 2000; Toro et al. 2003).

Pattern of Infiltration

In the early stages, the pattern is mid-dermal, periadnexal, and perivascular (Fig. 10.32) (Salhany et al. 1998). In later stages, dense lymphocytic infiltrates are located in the mid-dermis, with variable epidermotropism and nodular extensions into subcutaneous fat and ischemic necrosis of overlying skin (Fig. 10.33). Necrosis and psoriasiform epidermal changes are common

(Koch et al. 2009). Pagetoid pattern has been described (Guitart et al. 2012). There are frequently mixed histologic patterns: epidermotropic and subcutaneous panniculitic-like, associated with dense dermal involvement. All cases involved the subcutis with extension upwards into the dermis and epidermis (Fig. 10.34) (Garcia-Herrera et al. 2011; Toro et al. 2000, 2003; Salhany et al. 1998).

Cytomorphology

These tumors have a range of cytomorphology (Rodriguez-Pinilla et al. 2013; Salhany et al. 1998), composed of either small-/medium-sized

Fig. 10.33 Cutaneous T γδ: perivascular and nodular extensions into dermis, hair adnexa, and subcutaneous fat and ischemic necrosis of overlying skin

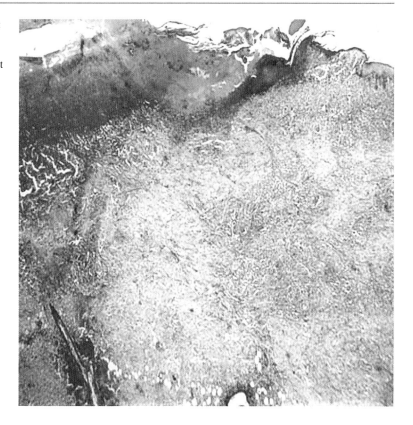

Fig. 10.34 Cutaneous CD8 + T γδ lymphoma involving the epidermis, dermis, and focally subcutis

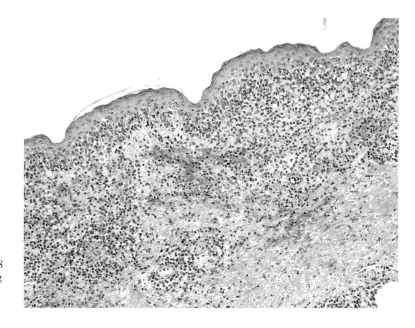

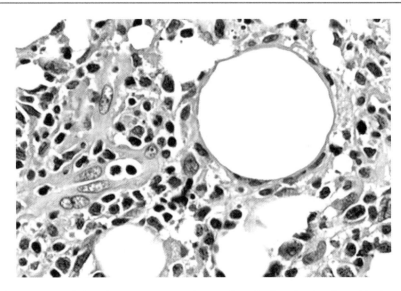

Fig. 10.35 Cutaneous T γδ lymphoma composed of medium-sized or large atypical lymphocytes with irregular hyperchromatic nuclei and coarse chromatin, with small nucleoli and a few large blastic cells which are localized in between fat globules and not rimming the fat cells

atypical lymphocytes (Garcia-Herrera et al. 2011) or medium-sized or large atypical lymphocytes with irregular hyperchromatic nuclei and coarse chromatin, with small nucleoli and a few large blastic cells with vesicular nuclei and conspicuous nucleoli (Toro et al. 2000). Most cases do not show rimming of fat cells as characteristic of subcutaneous panniculitic-like T-cell lymphomas, although rare cases had predominant subcutis infiltrate, some with rimming (Rodriguez-Pinilla et al. 2013) (Fig. 10.35). Cerebriform nuclei are not seen (Toro et al. 2000, 2003; Kadin 2000). Numerous apoptosis are described. In those cases, with cytophagic histiocytes or hemophagocytic syndrome, histiocytes phagocytizing red and white blood cells and platelets may be present in the skin and bone marrow (Craig et al. 1998; Toro et al. 2003; Salhany et al. 1998).

Immunophenotype

Many cutaneous T γδ cases, as originally described, are CD56 + (Fig. 10.36), lacking both CD4 and CD8 and sometimes lose CD5 and variably positive for CD8 and CD7 (Arnulf et al. 1998; Boulland et al. 1997) and negative for CD20, CD79a, and CD30. The γδ expression and the subcutaneous localization of primary cutane-

ous T γδ define adverse prognostic parameters so it is important to be certain (Toro et al. 2003). The lack of betaf1 (βF1) may be due to T antigen loss and cannot be equated with a T γδ lymphoma. T-cell δ1 expression is further defined as positive if more than 80 % of cells have *membrane* expression (Toro et al. 2003).

In a series of eight primary cutaneous T γδ tumors cases (Garcia-Herrera et al. 2011), using paraffin-reactive antibodies to T-cell receptor (TCR) delta (δ) portion of the heterodimer γδ on CD3 T-cell complex (antihuman TCRδ constant region) (Human Pan TCRγδ1, clone 5A6.E9, Thermo Scientific, IL), primary cutaneous T γδ tumors were described to have an activated cytotoxic phenotype, of which six cases were double negative for CD4 and CD8 and two cases expressed CD8. CD56 immunoreacted in three of seven patients. In TCR γδ-positive cases, expression was evaluated by membranous staining for TCRδ chain and additionally for TCRγ chain (using paraffin-reactive monoclonal antibody TCR 1153 clone γ3.20, Thermo Scientific, IL), in which the TCRγ immunoreactivity was previously characterized (Roullet et al. 2009).

Nevertheless, in many previous other studies, these T cells are usually positive for CD3, CD43,

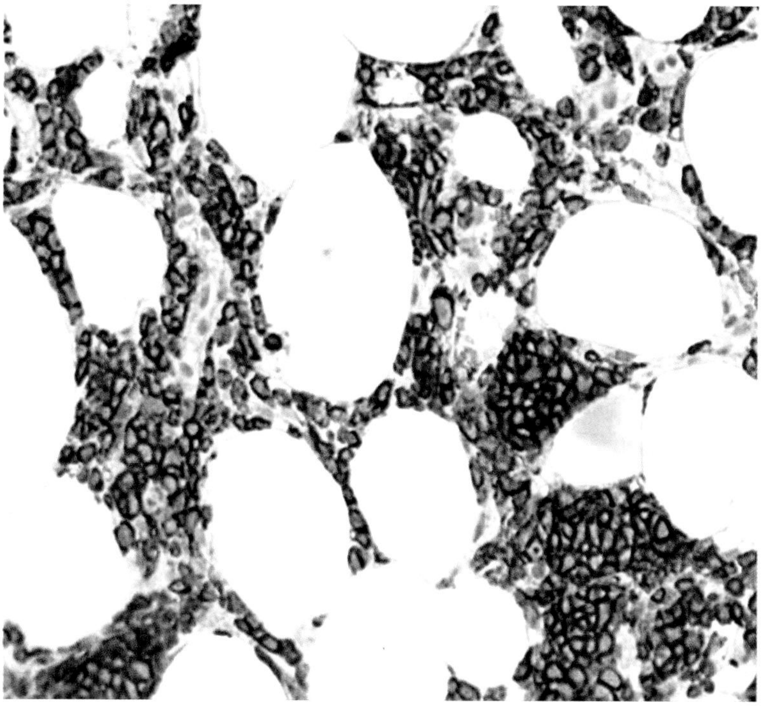

Fig. 10.36 CD3 + CD56 + T cells (*below*) are the typical coexpressed markers

and T-cell δ1, with cytotoxic markers TIA-1 and granzyme B (Salhany et al. 1998; Toro et al. 2003; Go and Wester 2004; Koch et al. 2009). These or similar tumors with overlapping features with primary cutaneous CD8 epidermotropic T-cell lymphoma have been described to be variably positive for βF1, CD4, and CD8 (Guitart et al. 2012). Most reports in which EBER was done showed absence of Epstein-Barr virus (Salhany et al. 1998; Toro et al. 2003; Go and Wester 2004; Rodriguez-Pinilla et al. 2013). High Ki67 expression upwards of 70 % has been reported (Koch et al. 2009).

Cytogenetics and Molecular Findings
TCR (γ/δ) genes are rearranged. There is no specific karyotypic abnormality (Toro et al. 2003. EBV is absent (Salhany et al. 1998; Go and Wester 2004).

Clinical Behavior
Generally characterized as aggressive with progressive clinical course resistant to various chemotherapies (Toro et al. 2000, 2003). The median survival is 15 (Toro et al. 2003) to 31 months (Guitart et al. 2012). If there is hemophagocytic syndrome with resulting pancytopenia, the prognosis is especially poor (Salhany et al. 1998). Patients with subcutaneous fat involvement may fare worse than those with only dermal involvement (Salhany et al. 1998; Toro et al. 2000, 2003).

Differential Diagnosis
The expression of TCRγ may not be confined to primary cutaneous T γδ and include other CTCLs of mycosis fungoides type, lymphomatoid papulosis type D, tumor MF, or MF with large cells, and hence caution is warranted in using one positive parameter alone (Rodriguez-Pinilla et al. 2013). In this report, TCRγ can be found in other CTCLs other than primary cutaneous γδ.

The neoplastic cells show overlapping features with primary cutaneous CD8 epidermotropic T cell (Guitart et al. 2012) and other cytotoxic primary cutaneous lymphoma and had coexpression of TCR αβ with TCR γδ (Rodriguez-Pinilla et al. 2013). Interestingly, Rodriguez-Pinilla et al., using different clones and methodology, showed dual cytoplasmic instead of surface membranous immunostaining pattern, in tumor cells with positivity for both TCR T αβ and TCR γδ. (Paraffin-immunoreactive monoclonal antibodies 8A3 Endogen, Dako autostainer with protease, and Gamma 3.20 Thermo, Dako autostainer, Tris EDTA, both antigen retrieved using said reactants, were used for detecting TCR αβ- and TCR γδ-positive cells, respectively.) (Rodriguez-Pinilla et al. 2013) In 5 of 12 of primary cutaneous γδ cases, coexpression of TCR αβ and TCR γδ markers was noted, which indicated possibly an aberrancy of marker expression in a neoplasm such as cutaneous T-cell lymphomas, in contradistinction with the exclusive expression of these markers in normal cells (Bluestone and Matis 1990; Kabelitz 1995).

Primary cutaneous aggressive CD8+ cytotoxic lymphoma is a challenging differential, if CD8 or CD56 are coexpressed, but one clue may be that cutaneous γδ lymphomas tend to have more subcutaneous involvement. Whether there is a subset of cutaneous γδ which are not distinguishable from primary cutaneous CD8 epidermotropic type is still a standing question given that recent studies indicate an overlap between these groups (Guitart et al. 2012). Although CD8 epidermotropic CTCL can form *nodular patterns*, because of its eponymic label and its current evolving nosology, that particular type is discussed in Chap. 6 (see Fig. 6.24).

Another group to differentiate include lymphomas in the skin with prominent subcutaneous involvement, such as PTCL-u, subcutaneous panniculitic T-cell lymphoma, and nasal-type extranodal NK/T-cell lymphoma and CD30 lymphomas (Koch et al. 2009; Toro et al. 2000, 2003) which all can present with deep subcutaneous tumors. For each of the above categories, an accurate evaluation for the number of large cells, a dominant subcutis tumor infiltrate pattern with no dermal tumor, EBV positivity, and strong CD30 decorated large cells may be useful clues, respectively. CD30 lymphomas are notable differential especially if CD56 and cytotoxic markers are strongly

expressed as is known to be so for this group (Chang et al. 2000; Bekkenk et al. 2001).

The subcutaneous panniculitic T-cell lymphoma expressing T αβ appears to have a predominant subcutaneous distribution, rimming of fat by tumor cells, and prominent apoptosis, whereas the cutaneous T γδ shows pandistributed epidermic, dermic, and subcutaneous infiltration (Kumar et al. 1998; Salhany et al. 1998). Because of the involvement of the subcutaneous fat on histology alone, benign conditions mainly that of lupus erythematosus profundus and other reactive panniculitis are in large part the benign differential diagnosis. In this regard, an absence of clonal T cells or clinical features may distinguish reactive processes from T-cell lymphomas with fat involvement (Aguilera et al. 2007).

Finally, when there is intense epidermotropic component, MF has to be ruled out since MF has been described to also present with a CD56+ (Wain et al. 2005), CD4-negative, and CD8-negative phenotype and may involve the subcutaneous tissue as well, especially on progression.

Cutaneous Angioimmunoblastic T-Cell Lymphoma (cAITL)

Skin involvement is often not primary and often occurs in patients with generalized disease. Primary cAITL has been described in about 10 % of cases (Martel et al. 2000) and documented in many case reports and few series (Smithberger et al. 2010; Batinac et al. 2003; Bayerl et al. 2010; Bernstein et al. 1979; Brown et al. 2001; Ferran et al. 2006; Huang and Chuang 2004; Martel et al. 2000; Suarez-Vilela and Izquierdo-Garcia 2003).

Four main histologic patterns, in the order of frequency, are seen in cutaneous involvement of AITL (Martel et al. 2000), and the findings may be similar to that of primary cAITL:
1. Vascular hyperplasia, with "high" endothelial vessels (HEVs) associated with sparse superficial perivascular atypical lymphoid infiltrates. Endothelial cells are plump and protrude into the lumina. Atypical lymphocytes are pleomorphic with large RS-like cells (Fig. 10.37a, b).

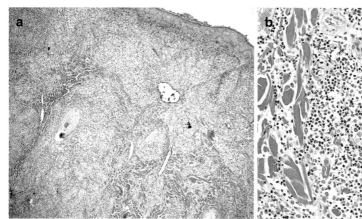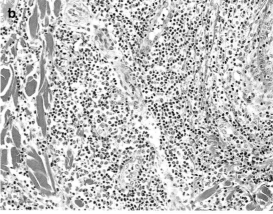

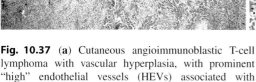

Fig. 10.37 (**a**) Cutaneous angioimmunoblastic T-cell lymphoma with vascular hyperplasia, with prominent "high" endothelial vessels (HEVs) associated with perivascular atypical lymphoid infiltrates. (**b**) High-power view of venules with many endothelial cells which are plump and protrude into the lumina

2. Vascular hyperplasia with dense pleomorphic atypical lymphoid infiltrate in superficial and deep dermis.
3. Vasculitis with no pleomorphic atypical lymphocytes.
4. Capillary hyperplasia, mild perivascular infiltrate in superficial dermis of non-atypical lymphocytes associated with eosinophils (Fig. 10.38a–c).

Systemic *Angioimmunoblastic T-Cell Lymphoma* (*AITL*): This lymphoma primarily presents in lymph nodes but often at a disseminated stage with involvement of the liver and spleen and clinically associated with hypergammaglobulinemia and B symptoms such as fever and malaise (Frizzera et al. 1975; Sallah and Gagnon 1998; Attygalle et al. 2004, 2007; Dogan et al. 2003). Originally included in the atypical lymphoproliferative disorders, this entity is now firmly included in the WHO monograph under the PTCLs based on typical clonal molecular and karyotypic findings (Swerdlow et al. 2008).

The pathologic distinction from cPTCL-u can be difficult, but salient morphological and phenotypic features may be useful (Agostinelli et al. 2008). The main findings in favor of AITL, primary or cutaneous, include prominent or arborizing vascularization, expansile CD21+ dendritic cell networks, and coexpression of CD10 (a precursor and follicular lymphoma-associated antigen) and other follicle center helper T-cell markers by the neoplastic T cells (Grogg et al. 2005; Attygalle et al. 2004, 2007; Dogan et al. 2003). Immunoblasts of varying size along with clear medium-sized cells are present (Swerdlow et al. 2008). EBV association has been described with secondary oligoclonal or monoclonal EBV + B-cell lymphomas in some patients (Attygalle et al. 2004, 2007; Dogan et al. 2003).

The neoplastic cells are often CD4 positive with variable loss of T-cell antigens and expression of follicular T helper cells which show immunoreactivity to CD10, BCL6, CXCL13, and PD1 (de Leval and Gaulard 2011; Gaulard and de Leval 2011; Attygalle et al. 2004, 2007; Dogan et al. 2003). Clonal T-cell gene rearrangements with strong, distinct bands with oligoclonal pattern favor AITL over reactive angioimmunoblastic proliferation (Attygalle et al. 2004, 2007; Dogan et al. 2003).

AITL is found mostly in the elderly and has an aggressive clinical course. The 5-year overall survival rate, as well as the 3-year median survival rate, is about 30 % (Savage et al. 2004).

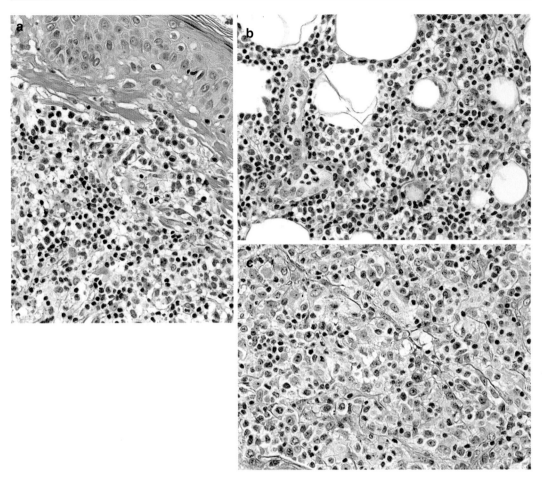

Fig. 10.38 Cutaneous angioimmunoblastic T-cell lymphoma with (**a**) capillary hyperplasia, mild perivascular infiltrate in superficial dermis, (**b**) lymphocytes associated with eosinophils, and (**c**) high-power view with atypical pleomorphic lymphocytes with mitosis, some with scattered large nucleolated mononuclear cells. Note the "clear-" appearing cytoplasm of cells

"Extanasal (Cutaneous)" Subtype of Extranodal NK/T-Cell Lymphoma, Nasal Type

Definition

This is an extranodal lymphoid neoplasm of NK cells or, less commonly, from cytotoxic T cells (Chan et al. 1997; Mraz-Gernhard et al. 2001). Skin involvement may be a primary or secondary manifestation of the disease, but the "extranasal" type is often associated with skin lesions (Gniadecki et al. 2004). Nasal cases and extranasal cases are two major types of extranodal NK/T-cell lymphomas designated as "nasal type" (Swerdlow et al. 2008; Willemze et al. 2005).

Extranodal NK/T-cell lymphoma, nasal type, has also been synonymous with past cases described as "lethal midline reticulosis, polymorphic reticulosis." For our purposes here, we will focus on the extranasal (cutaneous) NK/T-cell lymphomas with skin involvement instead of the extranodal NK/T-cell lymphoma, nasal type (with frequent upper aerodigestive tract involvement).

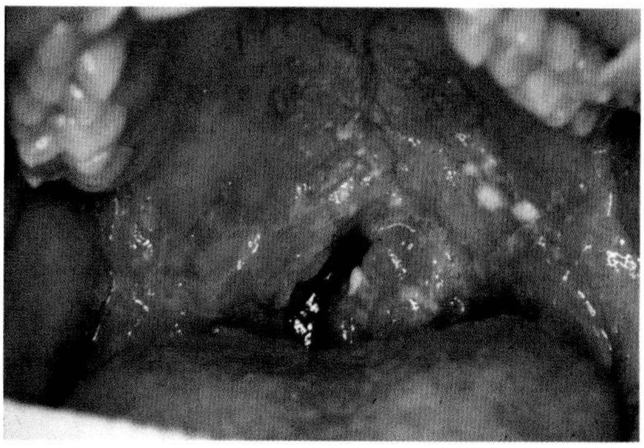

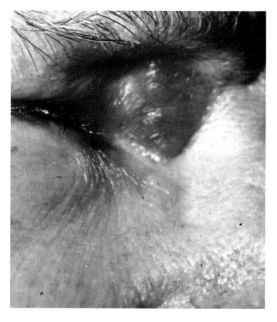

Fig. 10.39 Extranodal NK/T-cell lymphoma, nasal type, oropharyngeal lesions with pustular deformed uvular ulcerated mucosa

Fig. 10.40 Skin involvement of extranodal NK/T-cell lymphoma, nasal type, adjacent to the nose

Epidemiology

The whole spectrum of diseases that include extranodal NK/T-cell lymphoma (nasal and extranasal) and aggressive NK-cell leukemia is rare. The "nasal" type comprised 4 % of the peripheral T-cell lymphomas in Europe (Gallamini et al. 2004). Mostly adults of middle age to elderly (median age 50 years), with a male to female ratio of 3:2, are described (Mraz-Gernhard et al. 2001; Savage et al. 2012). Rare

pediatric cases with cutaneous involvement have been reported (Pol-Rodriguez et al. 2006).

Race Predilection

The nasal and extranasal types were originally described in Oriental/Asian patients, but patients of Mexican and South American descent (Chan et al. 1997; Cheung et al. 2003), as well as European Caucasians (Assaf et al. 2007; Bekkenk et al. 2003, 2004; Bekkenk and Willemze 2001), have also been reported as well as individual reports of patients from North America (Aladily et al. 2012; Summers et al. 2011; Wood et al. 2011).

Clinical Appearance of Lesions

Oropharyngeal lesions (Fig. 10.39), may present without skin lesions or be concurrently associated with cutaneous lesions (Fig. 10.40). Skin lesions appear in about a third of the cases (Chan et al. 1997) and, although rare, are increasingly recognized (Mraz-Gernhard et al. 2001; Natkunam et al. 1999; Savoia et al. 1997; Ansai et al. 1997). Clinical features include confluent or multiple reddish plaques, tumors, or nodules that may ulcerate, but flat lesions have been described. Lesions may be located on the extremities, trunk, and, less frequently, head and neck (Chan et al. 1997). Rare cases with bruise-like skin lesions have been reported (Dummer et al. 1996). Systemic symptoms such as weight loss, malaise, and fever may be present, and cytopenia due to hemophagocytic syndrome has been reported in some cases (Brodkin et al. 2008; Takahashi et al. 2001).

Pattern of Infiltration

Nodules and ulcerated skin along with dermal and subcutaneous angiocentric lymphoid infiltrate are seen (Fig. 10.41). Epidermotropism may be present (Fig. 10.42). A dense infiltrate in the dermis may be seen extending to the subcutaneous tissue, with associated angiodestructive growth pattern and occlusion of the blood vessel lumens by lymphoid cells, which are both common but not evident in all cases (Fig. 10.43). Vascular occlusion can cause ischemic necrosis of both tumor cells and normal tissue (Fig. 10.44).

Fig. 10.41 Extranodal NK/T-cell lymphoma, nasal type. A dense infiltrate of perivascular atypical lymphocytes which extends from the ulcerated epidermis to the dermis and into the subcutaneous tissue is seen

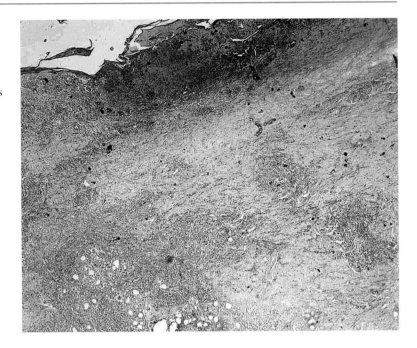

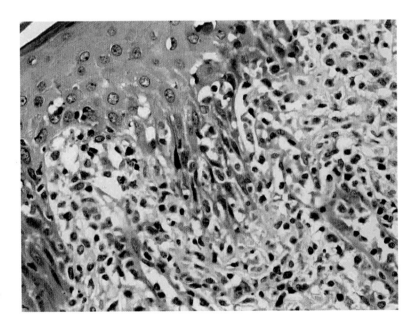

Fig. 10.42 Extranodal NK/T-cell lymphoma, nasal type. Epidermotropism may be present

Fig. 10.43 Extranodal
NK/T-cell lymphoma, nasal
type. Angiodestructive
growth pattern and occlusion
of the blood vessel lumens
by lymphoid cells are
common but not evident in
all cases

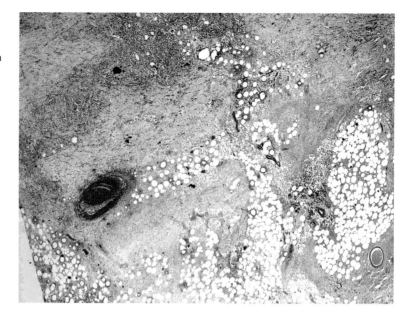

Fig. 10.44 Extranodal
NK/T-cell lymphoma, nasal
type. Vascular occlusion can
cause ischemic necrosis of
both tumor cells and normal
tissue

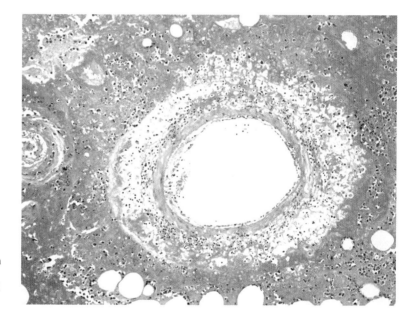

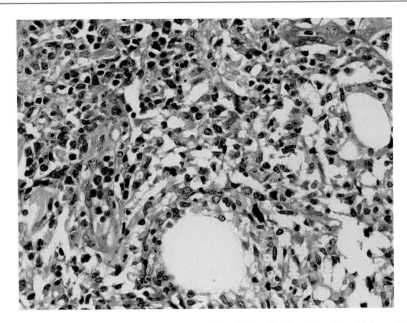

Fig. 10.45 Polymorphous infiltrate admixed with inflammatory cells, with the malignant cells composed of a mixture of normal-appearing small lymphocytes and atypical lymphoid cells of varying size with irregular nuclei, moderately dense granular chromatin, and pale to clear to finely granular cytoplasm with high mitotic activity

Cytomorphology

These cases feature polymorphous infiltrate admixed with inflammatory cells, with the malignant cells composed of a mixture of normal-appearing small lymphocytes and atypical lymphoid cells of varying size with irregular nuclei, moderately dense granular chromatin, and pale to clear to finely granular cytoplasm with high mitotic activity (Fig. 10.45) (Chan et al. 1989, 1997). The cytological spectrum of extranodal NK/T-cell lymphoma "nasal type" is very broad ranging from bland cytology (Fig. 10.46) to large atypical cells with necrosis (Fig. 10.47). In most cases, the lymphoma is composed of medium-sized cells with irregular nuclei, granular cytoplasm, and frequent mitosis (Pagano et al. 2006).

Immunophenotype

The neoplastic cells are usually positive for CD2, CD7, CD45RO, CD43, cytoplasmic CD3ε (cd3 epsilon cytoplasmic portion), CD56, and cytotoxic granule proteins (TIA-1, granzyme B, and perforin) (Chan et al. 1989, 1997; Pagano et al. 2006). They are usually negative for surface CD3, CD4, and CD8, but some that may lack CD56 antigens may still be classified as extranodal NK/T cells, nasal-type lymphoma, if they also express cytotoxic markers and EBV (Chan et al. 1989, 1997; Swerdlow et al. 2008; Pagano et al. 2006). CD4+ and CD7+ immunophenotypes have also been described (Chan et al. 1989, 1997; Pagano et al. 2006; Bekkenk et al. 2004). EBV is almost always (94 %) positive (Chan et al. 1989, 1997; Pagano et al. 2006; Bekkenk et al. 2004; Cheung et al. 1998, 2003). EBV positivity is helpful since it is rare in other cutaneous lymphomas and similar-looking extranasal or nasal-type CD3+ CD56 – lymphomas lacking EBV may be a type of PTCL-u or other neoplasms. EBER in situ hybridization is the most consistent test for the presence of EBV. CD30+ expression has been suggested to be of good prognostic parameter via p21 expression and increased apoptosis (Hubinger et al. 2001; Mraz-Gernhard et al. 2001).

Expression of killer cell inhibitor receptors via KIR immunophenotype or molecular RT-PCR techniques have been used to determine clonality

Fig. 10.46 Extranodal
NK/T-cell lymphoma, nasal
type. The cytological
spectrum of extranodal
NK/T-cell lymphoma "nasal
type" is very broad ranging
from bland cytology below

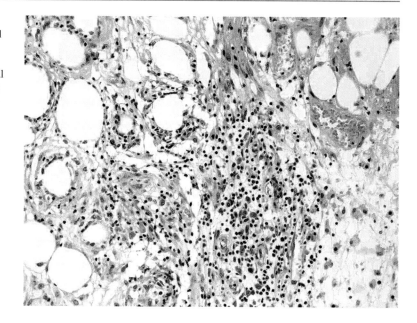

Fig. 10.47 Extranodal
NK/T-cell lymphoma, nasal
type, also showing medium-
large atypical cells

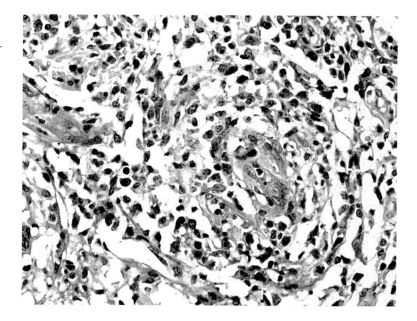

or oligoclonality of true NK-cell lymphomas and
other cytotoxic cell lymphomas (Dukers et al.
2001; Kamarashev et al. 2001; Lin et al. 2001;
Urosevic et al. 2004).

Cytogenetics and Molecular Findings

TCR genes are germ line since NK cells do not
have rearrangement of TCR genes (Chan et al.
1989, 1997; Bekkenk et al. 2004; Siu et al. 1999).

Table 10.4 Summary of NK/T-cell lymphoma, nasal type, extranasal (cutaneous) NKTL, and aggressive NK/T-cell leukemia/lymphoma

	Nasal (aerodigestive) NK/T	Extranasal (cutaneous) NKTL	NK/T-cell leukemia/lymphoma
Epidemiology	Asia, Central America, South America, and Mexico; men are affected more than women; occurs most often in the fifth decade of life	Similar to EN-NK/T-NT	Asia; men and women affected equally; median age of onset of 42 years
Sites frequently involved	Aerodigestive tract can disseminate to the skin, soft tissue, gastrointestinal tract, testes, and rarely bone marrow	Skin torso but also extremities, salivary gland, and viscera and has overlap with aggressive NK when BM is involved	Bone marrow, blood, liver, spleen, skin rarely involved
Immunophenotype	EBV+, CD16−, CD56+−, cytoplasmic CD3; CD7−, surface CD3−; CD4, CD8, CD57, and TCR βF1 or δγ are usually negative; cytotoxic proteins are positive; no clonal TCR gene rearrangement	EBV+, CD16− cytotoxic phenotype similar to nasal-type TCR βF1 or δγ are usually negative; cytotoxic proteins are positive; no clonal TCR gene rearrangement	EBV+,CD16+ ;no clonal TCR gene rearrangement
Prognosis	Median survival of advanced disease 12 months (40 % alive 5 years)	Most die within 6 months of diagnosis (17 % alive 5 years)	Most die within a few weeks of diagnosis

Deletions of chromosomes 6 (q16–q27) and 13 (q14–q34) are common karyotypic findings (Siu et al. 1999). Mutations of k-*ras* have been described, and p53 is overexpressed in many patients (Hongyo et al. 2005; Hoshida et al. 2003; Kurniawan et al. 2006). In both cutaneous and non-cutaneous cases, both disease-free and overall survival have been poor, perhaps related to the presence of multidrug resistance genes (Suzuki et al. 2010a).

Clinical Behavior

The single most important prognostic factor in cutaneous form of extranodal NK/T-cell lymphoma, nasal type, is extracutaneous involvement to the lymph node, viscera, or bone marrow. Those patients with extracutaneous disease had a median survival of 7.6 months compared with 44.9 months for those with disease limited to the skin (Mraz-Gernhard et al. 2001).

In a more encompassing review of these cases, the 5-year overall survival ranged from 17 to 40 % (meta-analysis of European, Asian, South American reported cases) (Pagano et al. 2006), and at this juncture, the prognosis appears better when compared with the original reported skin and extra-skin series of Asian patients who had median survival of 3.5 months (Chan et al. 1997) and a small series of three cases of primary cuta-

neous NK-cell lymphoma with a reported 0 % 5-year survival (Fink-Puches et al. 2002). Nonetheless, patients with tumors associated with aggressive NK-cell leukemia have the worst outcome, with a median survival of 6 weeks (Chan et al. 1997).

Differential Diagnosis

In the previous classifications, these cases were classified among cutaneous CD56+ neoplasm, blastic NK, or PTCL-u or CD30-negative cutaneous large T-cell lymphoma, so these cases present a differential matrix, especially when these tumors express CD56. Lack of EBV and a nongerm line T-cell receptor gene rearrangement result appear to be the crucial commonality in the above cases.

When confronted with an EBV + lymphoma, however, with immunohistologic features of NK/T-cell type, it is helpful to differentiate between the different clinical variants of extranodal NK/T-cell lymphoma, nasal type, such (primary cutaneous) as extranasal NK/T-cell lymphoma or the aggressive natural killer (NK) cell leukemia. See Table 10.4.

Although not absolute, skin involvement favors extranasal NK/T-cell lymphoma, while bone marrow, blood, and disseminated visceral disease favor aggressive natural killer (NK) cell

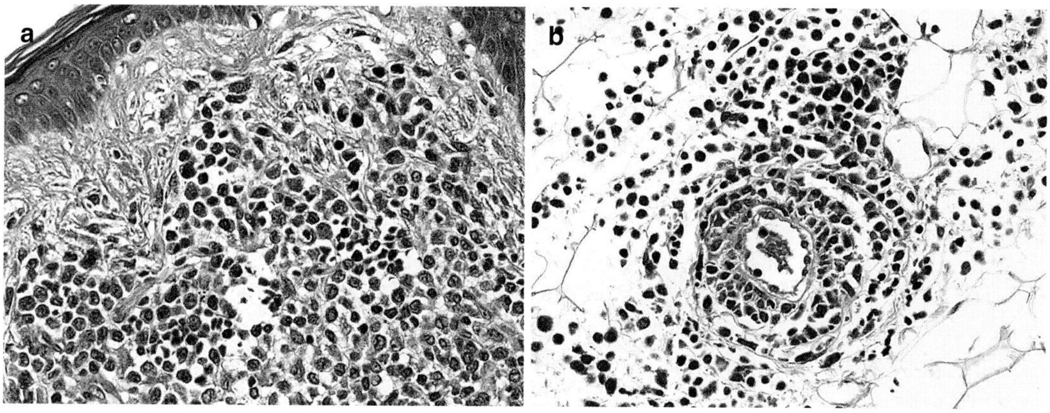

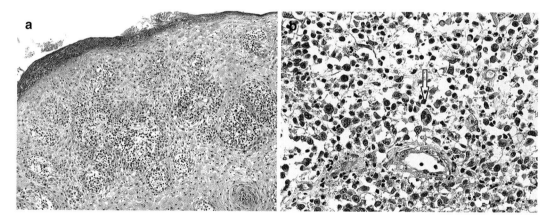

Fig. 10.48 Plasmacytoid dendritic cell neoplasm is derived from marrow precursor dendritic cells and not a true natural killer cell blast. (**a**) Blastic cells with fine nuclear chromatin. (**b**) Angiotropic blasts in single file targetoid pattern, a common arrangement of blasts in leukemia involving the skin

Fig. 10.49 Cutaneous adult T-cell leukemia/lymphoma (cATLL) showing epidermotropism. Tumor cells are medium to large size with nuclear pleomorphism and Reed-Sternberg-like narrow

leukemia. All of these cases may involve the aerodigestive tracts and therefore belong to the umbrella of extranodal NK/T-cell lymphoma, nasal type.

These above diseases are currently separated from the previous category of extranodal "blastic-NK" cell types which are not lymphoid in origin but derived from precursor plasmacytoid dendritic cells (also called "hematodermic neoplasm" because of common involvement of skin and marrow). The skin involvement of blast is recognized by the immature cells with blastic finely dispersed chromatin and the single file pattern often seen in leukemic skin involvement (Fig. 10.48a, b) (please see Chap. 16 for discussion of plasmacytoid dendritic cell neoplasm).

Cutaneous Adult T-Cell Leukemia/ Lymphoma

This entity will be discussed in more detail in Chap. 6 since occasional cases may present in a tumor nodular pattern, but cases are largely epidermotropic. A short description is provided here.

The tumor cells may show occasional deep dermal atypical cerebriform to large pleomorphic/immunoblastic cells, especially in cases with deep dermal tumor nodules (Fig. 10.49). The tumor cells have a T regulatory phenotype – FoxP3+, CD4+, and CD25+ (Fig. 10.50). This explains their ability to suppress local immunity and the propensity of ATLL patients to be

Fig. 10.50 CD25+ T helper cells in most cells are typical of cATLL

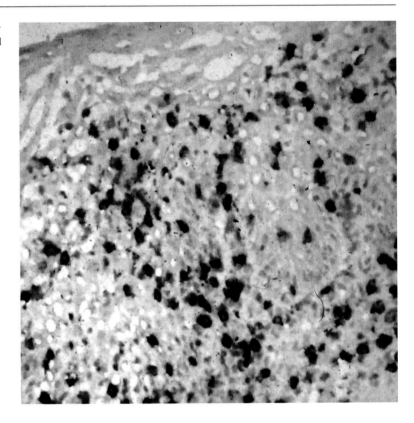

extraordinarily susceptible to opportunistic infection. Serum levels of IL-10 and TGF-beta1 are increased (Tokura, oral abstract #40, 2nd World Congress of Cutaneous Lymphomas, Feb 6–10, 2014).

Differential Diagnosis

MF is the principal differential diagnosis.

References

Adachi Y, Horio T. Chronic actinic dermatitis in a patient with adult T-cell leukemia. Photodermatol Photoimmunol Photomed. 2008;24(3):147–9.

Adams JD. Localized cutaneous pseudolymphoma associated with phenytoin therapy: a case report. Australas J Dermatol. 1981;22(1):28–9.

Agar NS, Wedgeworth E, Crichton S, Mitchell TJ, Cox M, Ferreira S, Robson A, Calonje E, Stefanato CM, Wain EM, Wilkins B, Fields PA, Dean A, Webb K, Scarisbrick J, Morris S, Whittaker SJ. Survival outcomes and prognostic factors in mycosis fungoides/Sezary syndrome: validation of the revised International Society for Cutaneous Lymphomas/European Organisation for Research and Treatment of Cancer staging proposal. J Clin Oncol. 2010;28(31): 4730–9.

Agostinelli C, Piccaluga PP, Went P, Rossi M, Gazzola A, Righi S, Sista T, Campidelli C, Zinzani PL, Falini B, Pileri SA. Peripheral T cell lymphoma, not otherwise specified: the stuff of genes, dreams and therapies. J Clin Pathol. 2008;61(11):1160–7.

Aguilera P, Mascaro Jr JM, Martinez A, Esteve J, Puig S, Campo E, Estrach T. Cutaneous gamma/delta T-cell lymphoma: a histopathologic mimicker of lupus erythematosus profundus (lupus panniculitis). J Am Acad Dermatol. 2007;56(4):643–7.

Aladily TN, Nathwani BN, Miranda RN, Kansal R, Yin CC, Protzel R, Takowsky GS, Medeiros LJ. Extranodal NK/T-cell lymphoma, nasal type, arising in association with saline breast implant: expanding the spectrum of breast implant-associated lymphomas. Am J Surg Pathol. 2012;36(11):1729–34.

Albrecht J, Fine LA, Piette W. Drug-associated lymphoma and pseudolymphoma: recognition and management. Dermatol Clin. 2007;25(2):233–44, vii.

Alekshun TJ, Rezania D, Ayala E, Cualing H, Sokol L. Skeletal muscle peripheral T-cell lymphoma. J Clin Oncol. 2008;26(3):501–3.

Alibert JLM. Tableau de plan fongoide: description des mala- dies de la peau observee a l'hopital St. Louis, et exposition des meilleures methods suivies pour leur traitement. Paris: Bar rior l'Aine et Files; 1806.

Ansai S, Maeda K, Yamakawa M, Matsuda M, Saitoh S, Suwa S, Saitoh H, Ohtsuka M, Iwatsuki K. CD56-positive (nasal-type T/NK cell) lymphoma arising on the skin. Report of two cases and review of the literature. J Cutan Pathol. 1997;24(8):468–76.

Arai E, Okubo H, Tsuchida T, Kitamura K, Katayama I. Pseudolymphomatous folliculitis: a clinicopathologic study of 15 cases of cutaneous pseudolymphoma with follicular invasion. Am J Surg Pathol. 1999;23(11): 1313–9.

Arnulf B, Copie-Bergman C, fau-Larue MH, Lavergne-Slove A, Bosq J, Wechsler J, Wassef M, Matuchansky C, Epardeau B, Stern M, Bagot M, Reyes F, Gaulard P. Nonhepatosplenic gammadelta T-cell lymphoma: a subset of cytotoxic lymphomas with mucosal or skin localization. Blood. 1998;91(5):1723–31.

Arulogun SO, Prince HM, Ng J, Lade S, Ryan GF, Blewitt O, McCormack C. Long-term outcomes of patients with advanced-stage cutaneous T-cell lymphoma and large cell transformation. Blood. 2008;112(8):3082–7.

Assaf C, Gellrich S, Whittaker S, Robson A, Cerroni L, Massone C, Kerl H, Rose C, Chott A, Chimenti S, Hallermann C, Petrella T, Wechsler J, Bagot M, Hummel M, Bullani-Kerl K, Bekkenk MW, Kempf W, Meijer CJ, Willemze R, Sterry W. CD56-positive haematological neoplasms of the skin: a multicentre study of the Cutaneous Lymphoma Project Group of the European Organisation for Research and Treatment of Cancer. J Clin Pathol. 2007;60(9):981–9.

Attygalle AD, Chuang SS, Diss TC, Du MQ, Isaacson PG, Dogan A. Distinguishing angioimmunoblastic T-cell lymphoma from peripheral T-cell lymphoma, unspecified, using morphology, immunophenotype and molecular genetics. Histopathology. 2007;50(4): 498–508.

Attygalle AD, Diss TC, Munson P, Isaacson PG, Du MQ, Dogan A. CD10 expression in extranodal dissemination of angioimmunoblastic T-cell lymphoma. Am J Surg Pathol. 2004;28(1):54–61.

az-Cascajo C. Strong immunoexpression of the monoclonal antibody CD-30 in lymphocytic infiltrates of the skin not by itself evidence for diagnosing malignant lymphoma. Am J Dermatopathol. 2001;23(1):79–80.

Baatz M, Zimmermann J, Blackmore CG. Automated analysis and detailed quantification of biomedical images using definiens cognition network technology. Comb Chem High Throughput Screen. 2009;12(9): 908–16.

Bakels V, van Oostveen JW, Van Der Putte SC, Meijer CJ, Willemze R. Immunophenotyping and gene rearrangement analysis provide additional criteria to differentiate between cutaneous T-cell lymphomas and pseudo-T-cell lymphomas. Am J Pathol. 1997;150(6): 1941–9.

Ballabio E, Mitchell T, van Kester MS, Taylor S, Dunlop HM, Chi J, Tosi I, Vermeer MH, Tramonti D, Saunders NJ, Boultwood J, Wainscoat JS, Pezzella F, Whittaker SJ, Tensen CP, Hatton CS, Lawrie CH. MicroRNA expression in Sezary syndrome: identification, function, and diagnostic potential. Blood. 2010;116(7): 1105–13.

Barberio E, Thomas L, Skowron F, Balme B, Dalle S. Transformed mycosis fungoides: clinicopathological features and outcome. Br J Dermatol. 2007;157(2): 284–9.

Barr-Nea L, Sandbank M, Ishay J. Pseudolymphoma of skin induced by oriental hornet (Vespa orientalis) venom. Experientia. 1976;32(12):1564–5.

Batinac T, Zamolo G, Jonjic N, Gruber F, Nacinovic A, Seili-Bekafigo I, Coklo M. Angioimmunoblastic lymphadenopathy with dysproteinemia following doxycycline administration. Tumori. 2003;89(1): 91–5.

Batista DA, Vonderheid EC, Hawkins A, Morsberger L, Long P, Murphy KM, Griffin CA. Multicolor fluorescence in situ hybridization (SKY) in mycosis fungoides and Sezary syndrome: search for recurrent chromosome abnormalities. Genes Chromosom Cancer. 2006;45(4):383–91.

Battistella M, Beylot-Barry M, Bachelez H, Rivet J, Vergier B, Bagot M. Primary cutaneous follicular helper T-cell lymphoma: a new subtype of cutaneous T-cell lymphoma reported in a series of 5 cases. Arch Dermatol. 2012;148(7):832–9.

Bayerl MG, Hennessy J, Ehmann WC, Bagg A, Rosamilia L, Clarke LE. Multiple cutaneous monoclonal B-cell proliferations as harbingers of systemic angioimmunoblastic T-cell lymphoma. J Cutan Pathol. 2010;37(7):777–86.

Bekkenk MW, Geelen FA, van Voorst Vader PC, Heule F, Geerts ML, van Vloten WA, Meijer CJ, Willemze R. Primary and secondary cutaneous CD30(+) lymphoproliferative disorders: a report from the Dutch Cutaneous Lymphoma Group on the long-term follow-up data of 219 patients and guidelines for diagnosis and treatment. Blood. 2000;95(12):3653–61.

Bekkenk MW, Jansen PM, Meijer CJ, Willemze R. CD56+ hematological neoplasms presenting in the skin: a retrospective analysis of 23 new cases and 130 cases from the literature. Ann Oncol. 2004;15(7):1097–108.

Bekkenk MW, Kluin PM, Jansen PM, Meijer CJ, Willemze R. Lymphomatoid papulosis with a natural killer-cell phenotype. Br J Dermatol. 2001;145(2): 318–22.

Bekkenk MW, Vermeer MH, Jansen PM, van Marion AM, Canninga-van Dijk MR, Kluin PM, Geerts ML, Meijer CJ, Willemze R. Peripheral T-cell lymphomas unspecified presenting in the skin: analysis of prognostic factors in a group of 82 patients. Blood. 2003;102(6): 2213–9.

Bekkenk MW, Willemze R. CD56-positive 'natural killer'/T-cell lymphoma. Ned Tijdschr Geneeskd. 2001;145(31):1524–5.

Beljaards RC, Meijer CJ, Van Der Putte SC, Hollema H, Geerts ML, Bezemer PD, Willemze R. Primary cutaneous T-cell lymphoma: clinicopathological features and prognostic parameters of 35 cases other than mycosis fungoides and CD30-positive large cell lymphoma. J Pathol. 1994;172(1):53–60.

Beltraminelli H, Leinweber B, Kerl H, Cerroni L. Primary cutaneous CD4+ small-/medium-sized pleomorphic T-cell lymphoma: a cutaneous nodular proliferation of pleomorphic T lymphocytes of undetermined significance? A study of 136 cases. Am J Dermatopathol. 2009;31(4):317–22.

Beltraminelli H, Mullegger R, Cerroni L. Indolent CD8+ lymphoid proliferation of the ear: a phenotypic variant of the small-medium pleomorphic cutaneous T-cell lymphoma? J Cutan Pathol. 2010;37(1):81–4.

Bendelac A, Lesavre P, Boitard C, O'Connor NT, Laure F, Laroche L, Teillac D, de Prost Y, Bach JF. Cutaneous pheomorphic T cell lymphoma. Immunologic, virologic, and T-cell receptor gene rearrangement studies in one European case with initial pseudolymphoma presentation. J Am Acad Dermatol. 1986;15(4 Pt 1):657–64.

Benner MF, Ballabio E, van Kester MS, Saunders NJ, Vermeer MH, Willemze R, Lawrie CH, Tensen CP. Primary cutaneous anaplastic large cell lymphoma shows a distinct miRNA expression profile and reveals differences from tumor-stage mycosis fungoides. Exp Dermatol. 2012a;21(8):632–4.

Benner MF, Jansen PM, Meijer CJ, Willemze R. Diagnostic and prognostic evaluation of phenotypic markers TRAF1, MUM1, BCL2 and CD15 in cutaneous CD30-positive lymphoproliferative disorders. Br J Dermatol. 2009;161(1):121–7.

Benner MF, Jansen PM, Vermeer MH, Willemze R. Prognostic factors in transformed mycosis fungoides: a retrospective analysis of 100 cases. Blood. 2012b;119(7):1643–9.

Berger E, Altiner A, Chu J, Patel R, Sanders S, Latkowski JA. Mycosis fungoides stage IB progressing to cutaneous tumors. Dermatol Online J. 2011;17(10):5.

Berger R, Baranger L, Bernheim A, Valensi F, Flandrin G. Cytogenetics of T-cell malignant lymphoma. Report of 17 cases and review of the chromosomal breakpoints. Cancer Genet Cytogenet. 1988;36(1):123–30.

Bergman R. Pseudolymphoma and cutaneous lymphoma: facts and controversies. Clin Dermatol. 2010;28(5):568–74.

Berlingeri-Ramos AC, De JG, Sanchez JL, Gonzalez JR. Disease evolution of patients with mycosis fungoides–a report of 30 cases. P R Health Sci J. 2007;26(2):151–4.

Bernstein H, Shupack J, Ackerman B. Cutaneous pseudolymphoma resulting from antigen injections. Arch Dermatol. 1974;110(5):756–7.

Bernstein JE, Soltani K, Lorincz AL. Cutaneous manifestations of angioimmunoblastic lymphadenopathy. J Am Acad Dermatol. 1979;1(3):227–32.

Berti E, Tomasini D, Vermeer MH, Meijer CJ, Alessi E, Willemze R. Primary cutaneous CD8-positive epidermotropic cytotoxic T cell lymphomas. A distinct clinicopathological entity with an aggressive clinical behavior. Am J Pathol. 1999;155(2):483–92.

Bignon YJ, Souteyrand P. Genotyping of cutaneous T-cell lymphomas and pseudolymphomas. Curr Probl Dermatol. 1990;19:114–23.

Blank C, Mackensen A. Contribution of the PD-L1/PD-1 pathway to T-cell exhaustion: an update on implications for chronic infections and tumor evasion. Cancer Immunol Immunother. 2007;56(5):739–45.

Blazejak T, Holzle E. Phenothiazine-induced pseudolymphoma. Hautarzt. 1990;41(3):161–3.

Bluestone JA, Khattri R, Sciammas R, Sperling AI. TCR gamma delta cells: a specialized T-cell subset in the immune system. Annu Rev Cell Dev Biol. 1995;11:307–53.

Bluestone JA, Matis LA. Are TCR alpha beta cells and TCR gamma delta cells that different? Res Immunol. 1990;141(7):606–10.

Blumental G, Okun MR, Ponitch JA. Pseudolymphomatous reaction to tattoos. Report of three cases. J Am Acad Dermatol. 1982;6(4 Pt 1):485–8.

Bocquet H, Bagot M, Roujeau JC. Drug-induced pseudolymphoma and drug hypersensitivity syndrome (Drug Rash with Eosinophilia and Systemic Symptoms: DRESS). Semin Cutan Med Surg. 1996;15(4):250–7.

Boehncke WH, Gerdes J, Wiese M, Kaltoft K, Sterry W. A majority of proliferating T cells in cutaneous malignant T cell lymphomas may lack the high affinity IL-2 receptor (CD25). Arch Dermatol Res. 1993;285(3):127–30.

Boulland ML, Kanavaros P, Wechsler J, Casiraghi O, Gaulard P. Cytotoxic protein expression in natural killer cell lymphomas and in alpha beta and gamma delta peripheral T-cell lymphomas. J Pathol. 1997;183(4):432–9.

Bradford PT, Devesa SS, Anderson WF, Toro JR. Cutaneous lymphoma incidence patterns in the United States: a population-based study of 3884 cases. Blood. 2009;113(21):5064–73.

Brodell RT, Santa Cruz DJ. Cutaneous pseudolymphomas. Dermatol Clin. 1985;3(4):719–34.

Brodkin DE, Hobohm DW, Nigam R. Nasal-type NK/T-cell lymphoma presenting as hemophagocytic syndrome in an 11-year-old Mexican boy. J Pediatr Hematol Oncol. 2008;30(12):938–40.

Brown HA, Macon WR, Kurtin PJ, Gibson LE. Cutaneous involvement by angioimmunoblastic T-cell lymphoma with remarkable heterogeneous Epstein-Barr virus expression. J Cutan Pathol. 2001;28(8):432–8.

Burg G, Dummer R, Kempf W. Dyscrasias with "undetermined significance". Arch Dermatol. 2005;141(3):382–4.

Carreras J, Lopez-Guillermo A, Fox BC, Colomo L, Martinez A, Roncador G, Montserrat E, Campo E, Banham AH. High numbers of tumor-infiltrating FOXP3-positive regulatory T cells are associated with improved overall survival in follicular lymphoma. Blood. 2006;108(9):2957–64.

Carreras J, Lopez-Guillermo A, Roncador G, Villamor N, Colomo L, Martinez A, Hamoudi R, Howat WJ, Montserrat E, Campo E. High numbers of tumor-infiltrating programmed cell death 1-positive regulatory lymphocytes are associated with improved overall survival in follicular lymphoma. J Clin Oncol. 2009;27(9):1470–6.

Cepeda LT, Pieretti M, Chapman SF, Horenstein MG. CD30-positive atypical lymphoid cells in common non-neoplastic cutaneous infiltrates rich in neutrophils and eosinophils. Am J Surg Pathol. 2003;27(7):912–8.

Cerroni L, Gatter K, Kerl H. Skin lymphoma: the illustrated guide. 3rd ed. Hoiboken, NJ: Wiley-Blackwell; 2009.

Cerroni L, Goteri G. Differential diagnosis between cutaneous lymphoma and pseudolymphoma. Anal Quant Cytol Histol. 2003;25(4):191–8.

Cerroni L, Peris K, Torlone G, Chimenti S. Immunophenotype of lymphocytic infiltrate in mycosis fungoides at the plaque stage and at the tumor stage. A comparative study. G Ital Dermatol Venereol. 1990;125(7–8):313–7.

Cerroni L, Rieger E, Hodl S, Kerl H. Clinicopathologic and immunologic features associated with transformation of mycosis fungoides to large-cell lymphoma. Am J Surg Pathol. 1992;16(6):543–52.

Cetinozman F, Jansen PM, Willemze R. Expression of programmed death-1 in primary cutaneous CD4-positive small/medium-sized pleomorphic T-cell lymphoma, cutaneous pseudo-T-cell lymphoma, and other types of cutaneous T-cell lymphoma. Am J Surg Pathol. 2012;36(1):109–16.

Chan JK, Sin VC, Ng CS, Lau WH. Cutaneous relapse of nasal T-cell lymphoma clinically mimicking erythema multiforme. Pathology. 1989;21(3):164–8.

Chan JK, Sin VC, Wong KF, Ng CS, Tsang WY, Chan CH, Cheung MM, Lau WH. Nonnasal lymphoma expressing the natural killer cell marker CD56: a clinicopathologic study of 49 cases of an uncommon aggressive neoplasm. Blood. 1997;89(12):4501–13.

Chang SE, Park IJ, Huh J, Choi JH, Sung KJ, Moon KC, Koh JK. CD56 expression in a case of primary cutaneous CD30+ anaplastic large cell lymphoma. Br J Dermatol. 2000;142(4):766–70.

Cheung MM, Chan JK, Lau WH, Foo W, Chan PT, Ng CS, Ngan RK. Primary non-Hodgkin's lymphoma of the nose and nasopharynx: clinical features, tumor immunophenotype, and treatment outcome in 113 patients. J Clin Oncol. 1998;16(1):70–7.

Cheung MM, Chan JK, Wong KF. Natural killer cell neoplasms: a distinctive group of highly aggressive lymphomas/leukemias. Semin Hematol. 2003;40(3):221–32.

Cooke CB, Krenacs L, Stetler-Stevenson M, Greiner TC, Raffeld M, Kingma DW, Abruzzo L, Frantz C, Kaviani M, Jaffe ES. Hepatosplenic T-cell lymphoma: a distinct clinicopathologic entity of cytotoxic gamma delta T-cell origin. Blood. 1996;88(11):4265–74.

Craig AJ, Cualing H, Thomas G, Lamerson C, Smith R. Cytophagic histiocytic panniculitis – a syndrome associated with benign and malignant panniculitis: case

comparison and review of the literature. J Am Acad Dermatol. 1998;39(5 Pt 1):721–36.

Criscione VD, Weinstock MA. Incidence of cutaneous T-cell lymphoma in the United States, 1973–2002. Arch Dermatol. 2007;143(7):854–9.

Cualing HD, Zhong E, Moscinski L. "Virtual flow cytometry" of immunostained lymphocytes on microscopic tissue slides: iHCFlow tissue cytometry. Cytometry B Clin Cytom. 2007;72(1):63–76.

de Leval L, Gaulard P. Pathology and biology of peripheral T-cell lymphomas. Histopathology. 2011;58(1):49–68.

del Rio ML, Penuelas-Rivas G, Dominguez-Perles R, Ramirez P, Parrilla P, Rodriguez-Barbosa JI. Antibody-mediated signaling through PD-1 costimulates T cells and enhances CD28-dependent proliferation. Eur J Immunol. 2005;35(12):3545–60.

Delaporte E, Catteau B, Cardon T, Flipo RM, Lecomte-Houcke M, Piette F, Delcambre B, Bergoend H. Cutaneous pseudolymphoma during treatment of rheumatoid polyarthritis with low-dose methotrexate. Ann Dermatol Venereol. 1995;122(8):521–5.

Diamandidou E, Colome-Grimmer M, Fayad L, Duvic M, Kurzrock R. Transformation of mycosis fungoides/Sezary syndrome: clinical characteristics and prognosis. Blood. 1998;92(4):1150–9.

Dmitrovsky E, Matthews MJ, Bunn PA, Schechter GP, Makuch RW, Winkler CF, Eddy J, Sausville EA, Ihde DC. Cytologic transformation in cutaneous T cell lymphoma: a clinicopathologic entity associated with poor prognosis. J Clin Oncol. 1987;5(2):208–15.

Dogan A, Attygalle AD, Kyriakou C. Angioimmunoblastic T-cell lymphoma. Br J Haematol. 2003;121(5):681–91.

Droc C, Cualing HD, Kadin ME. Need for an improved molecular/genetic classification for CD30+ lymphomas involving the skin. Cancer Control. 2007;14(2):124–32.

Dukers DF, Vermeer MH, Jaspars LH, Sander CA, Flaig MJ, Vos W, Willemze R, Meijer CJ. Expression of killer cell inhibitory receptors is restricted to true NK cell lymphomas and a subset of intestinal enteropathy-type T cell lymphomas with a cytotoxic phenotype. J Clin Pathol. 2001;54(3):224–8.

Dummer R, Potoczna N, Haffner AC, Zimmermann DR, Gilardi S, Burg G. A primary cutaneous non-T, non-B CD4+, CD56+ lymphoma. Arch Dermatol. 1996;132(5):550–3.

Eckert F, Schmid U, Kaudewitz P, Burg G, Braun-Falco O. Follicular lymphoid hyperplasia of the skin with high content of Ki-1 positive lymphocytes. Am J Dermatopathol. 1989;11(4):345–52.

Edinger JT, Clark BZ, Pucevich BE, Geskin LJ, Swerdlow SH. CD30 expression and proliferative fraction in nontransformed mycosis fungoides. Am J Surg Pathol. 2009;33(12):1860–8.

Ferenczi K. Could follicular helper T-cells play a role in primary cutaneous CD4+ small/medium-sized pleomorphic T-cell lymphomas? J Cutan Pathol. 2009;36(6):717–8.

Ferran M, Gallardo F, Baena V, Ferrer A, Florensa L, Pujol RM. The 'deck chair sign' in specific cutaneous involvement by angioimmunoblastic T cell lymphoma. Dermatology. 2006;213(1):50–2.

Fink-Puches R, Zenahlik P, Back B, Smolle J, Kerl H, Cerroni L. Primary cutaneous lymphomas: applicability of current classification schemes (European Organization for Research and Treatment of Cancer, World Health Organization) based on clinicopathologic features observed in a large group of patients. Blood. 2002;99(3):800–5.

Friedmann D, Wechsler J, Delfau MH, Esteve E, Farcet JP, de Muret A, Parneix-Spake A, Vaillant L, Revuz J, Bagot M. Primary cutaneous pleomorphic small T-cell lymphoma. A review of 11 cases. The French Study Group on Cutaneous Lymphomas. Arch Dermatol. 1995;131(9):1009–15.

Frizzera G, Moran EM, Rappaport H. Angioimmunoblastic lymphadenopathy. Diagnosis and clinical course. Am J Med. 1975;59(6):803–18.

Gallamini A, Stelitano C, Calvi R, Bellei M, Mattei D, Vitolo U, Morabito F, Martelli M, Brusamolino E, Iannitto E, Zaja F, Cortelazzo S, Rigacci L, Devizzi L, Todeschini G, Santini G, Brugiatelli M, Federico M. Peripheral T-cell lymphoma unspecified (PTCL-U): a new prognostic model from a retrospective multicentric clinical study. Blood. 2004;103(7):2474–9.

Gallardo F, Barranco C, Toll A, Pujol RM. CD30 antigen expression in cutaneous inflammatory infiltrates of scabies: a dynamic immunophenotypic pattern that should be distinguished from lymphomatoid papulosis. J Cutan Pathol. 2002;29(6):368–73.

Gammon B, Guitart J. Intertriginous mycosis fungoides: a distinct presentation of cutaneous T-cell lymphoma that may be caused by malignant follicular helper T cells. Arch Dermatol. 2012;148(9):1040–4.

Garcia-Herrera A, Colomo L, Camos M, Carreras J, Balague O, Martinez A, Lopez-Guillermo A, Estrach T, Campo E. Primary cutaneous small/medium CD4+ T-cell lymphomas: a heterogeneous group of tumors with different clinicopathologic features and outcome. J Clin Oncol. 2008;26(20):3364–71.

Garcia-Herrera A, Song JY, Chuang SS, Villamor N, Colomo L, Pittaluga S, Alvaro T, Rozman M, de Anda GJ, Arrunategui AM, Fernandez E, Gonzalvo E, Estrach T, Colomer D, Raffeld M, Gaulard P, Campo E, Jaffe ES, Martinez A. Nonhepatosplenic gammadelta T-cell lymphomas represent a spectrum of aggressive cytotoxic T-cell lymphomas with a mainly extranodal presentation. Am J Surg Pathol. 2011;35(8):1214–25.

Gaulard P, Belhadj K, Reyes F. Gammadelta T-cell lymphomas. Semin Hematol. 2003;40(3):233–43.

Gaulard P, Berti E, Willemze R, Jaffe ES. Primary cutaneous peripheral T-cell lymphoma, rare subtypes. In: Swerdlow SH, Campo E, Harris NL, Jaffe ES, Pileri SA, Stein H, editors. WHO classification of tumors of hematopoietic and lymphoid tissues. 4th ed. Lyon: IARC; 2008:302–5.

Gaulard P, de Leval L. Follicular helper T cells: implications in neoplastic hematopathology. Semin Diagn Pathol. 2011;28(3):202–13.

Geraud C, Goerdt S, Klemke CD. Primary cutaneous CD8+ small/medium-sized pleomorphic T-cell lymphoma, eartype: a unique cutaneous T-cell lymphoma with a favourable prognosis. Br J Dermatol. 2011;164(2):456–8.

Girardi M. Cutaneous biology of gammadelta T cells. Adv Dermatol. 2004;20:203–15.

Gniadecki R. Neoplastic stem cells in cutaneous lymphomas: evidence and clinical implications. Arch Dermatol. 2004;140(9):1156–60.

Gniadecki R, Lukowsky A. Monoclonal T-cell dyscrasia of undetermined significance associated with recalcitrant erythroderma. Arch Dermatol. 2005;141(3):361–7.

Gniadecki R, Rossen K. Expression of T-cell activation marker CD134 (OX40) in lymphomatoid papulosis. Br J Dermatol. 2003;148(5):885–91.

Gniadecki R, Rossen K, Ralfkier E, Thomsen K, Skovgaard GL, Jonsson V. CD56+ lymphoma with skin involvement: clinicopathologic features and classification. Arch Dermatol. 2004;140(4):427–36.

Go RS, Wester SM. Immunophenotypic and molecular features, clinical outcomes, treatments, and prognostic factors associated with subcutaneous panniculitis-like T-cell lymphoma: a systematic analysis of 156 patients reported in the literature. Cancer. 2004;101(6):1404–13.

Good DJ, Gascoyne RD. Atypical lymphoid hyperplasia mimicking lymphoma. Hematol Oncol Clin North Am. 2009;23(4):729–45.

Gormley RH, Hess SD, Anand D, Junkins-Hopkins J, Rook AH, Kim EJ. Primary cutaneous aggressive epidermotropic CD8+ T-cell lymphoma. J Am Acad Dermatol. 2010;62(2):300–7.

Grange F, Hedelin G, Joly P, Beylot-Barry M, D'Incan M, Delaunay M, Vaillant L, Avril MF, Bosq J, Wechsler J, Dalac S, Grosieux C, Franck N, Esteve E, Michel C, Bodemer C, Vergier B, Laroche L, Bagot M. Prognostic factors in primary cutaneous lymphomas other than mycosis fungoides and the Sezary syndrome. The French Study Group on Cutaneous Lymphomas. Blood. 1999;93(11):3637–42.

Greer JP, Salhany KE, Cousar JB, Fields JP, King LE, Graber SE, Flexner JM, Stein RS, Collins RD. Clinical features associated with transformation of cerebriform T-cell lymphoma to a large cell process. Hematol Oncol. 1990;8(4):215–27.

Griesser H, Feller AC, Sterry W. T-cell receptor and immunoglobulin gene rearrangements in cutaneous T-cell-rich pseudolymphomas. J Invest Dermatol. 1990;95(3):292–5.

Grogg KL, Attygalle AD, Macon WR, Remstein ED, Kurtin PJ, Dogan A. Angioimmunoblastic T-cell lymphoma: a neoplasm of germinal-center T-helper cells? Blood. 2005;106(4):1501–2.

Grogg KL, Jung S, Erickson LA, McClure RF, Dogan A. Primary cutaneous CD4-positive small/medium-sized pleomorphic T-cell lymphoma: a clonal T-cell lymphoproliferative disorder with indolent behavior. Mod Pathol. 2008;21(6):708–15.

Groves FD, Linet MS, Travis LB, Devesa SS. Cancer surveillance series: non-Hodgkin's lymphoma incidence by histologic subtype in the United States from 1978 through 1995. J Natl Cancer Inst. 2000;92(15):1240–51.

Guitart J, Magro C. Cutaneous T-cell lymphoid dyscrasia: a unifying term for idiopathic chronic dermatoses with persistent T-cell clones. Arch Dermatol. 2007;143(7): 921–32.

Guitart J, Weisenburger DD, Subtil A, Kim E, Wood G, Duvic M, Olsen E, Junkins-Hopkins J, Rosen S, Sundram U, Ivan D, Selim MA, Pincus L, Deonizio JM, Kwasny M, Kim YH. Cutaneous gammadelta T-cell lymphomas: a spectrum of presentations with overlap with other cytotoxic lymphomas. Am J Surg Pathol. 2012;36(11):1656–65.

Habermann TM, Pittelkow MR. Cutaneous T-cell lymphoma and cutaneous B-cell lymphoma. In: Abeloff MD, Armitage JO, Niederhuber JE, Kastan MB, McKenna WG, editors. Clinical Oncology. 3rd ed. New York, NY: Churchill Livingstone; 2004: 3077–108.

Hahtola S, Tuomela S, Elo L, Hakkinen T, Karenko L, Nedoszytko B, Heikkila H, Saarialho-Kere U, Roszkiewicz J, Aittokallio T, Lahesmaa R, Ranki A. Th1 response and cytotoxicity genes are downregulated in cutaneous T-cell lymphoma. Clin Cancer Res. 2006;12(16):4812–21.

Hongyo T, Hoshida Y, Nakatsuka S, Syaifudin M, Kojya S, Yang WI, Min YH, Chan H, Kim CH, Harabuchi Y, Himi T, Inuyama M, Aozasa K, Nomura T. p53, K-ras, c-kit and beta-catenin gene mutations in sinonasal NK/T-cell lymphoma in Korea and Japan. Oncol Rep. 2005;13(2):265–71.

Hoshida Y, Hongyo T, Jia X, He Y, Hasui K, Dong Z, Luo WJ, Ham MF, Nomura T, Aozasa K. Analysis of p53, K-ras, c-kit, and beta-catenin gene mutations in sinonasal NK/T cell lymphoma in northeast district of China. Cancer Sci. 2003;94(3):297–301.

Hu S, Young KH, Konoplev SN, Medeiros LJ. Follicular T-cell lymphoma: a member of an emerging family of follicular helper T-cell derived T-cell lymphomas. Hum Pathol. 2012;43(11):1789–98.

Huang CT, Chuang SS. Angioimmunoblastic T-cell lymphoma with cutaneous involvement: a case report with subtle histologic changes and clonal T-cell proliferation. Arch Pathol Lab Med. 2004;128(10):e122–4.

Huang Y, Moreau A, Dupuis J, Streubel B, Petit B, Le Gouill S, Martin-Garcia N, Copie-Bergman C, Gaillard F, Qubaja M, Fabiani B, Roncador G, Haioun C, fau-Larue MH, Marafioti T, Chott A, Gaulard P. Peripheral T-cell lymphomas with a follicular growth pattern are derived from follicular helper T cells (TFH) and may show overlapping features with angioimmunoblastic T-cell lymphomas. Am J Surg Pathol. 2009;33(5):682–90.

Hubinger G, Muller E, Scheffrahn I, Schneider C, Hildt E, Singer BB, Sigg I, Graf J, Bergmann L. CD30-mediated cell cycle arrest associated with induced expression of p21(CIP1/WAF1) in the anaplastic large cell lymphoma cell line Karpas 299. Oncogene. 2001;20(5):590–8.

Hudak S, Hagen M, Liu Y, Catron D, Oldham E, McEvoy LM, Bowman EP. Immune surveillance and effector functions of CCR10(+) skin homing T cells. J Immunol. 2002;169(3):1189–96.

Ishida T, Inagaki H, Utsunomiya A, Takatsuka Y, Komatsu H, Iida S, Takeuchi G, Eimoto T, Nakamura S, Ueda R. CXC chemokine receptor 3 and CC chemokine receptor 4 expression in T-cell and NK-cell lymphomas with special reference to clinicopathological significance for peripheral T-cell lymphoma, unspecified. Clin Cancer Res. 2004;10(16):5494–500.

Ishida T, Ueda R. Immunopathogenesis of lymphoma: focus on CCR4. Cancer Sci. 2011;102(1):44–50.

Jakob T, Neuber K, Altenhoff J, Kowalzick L, Ring J. Stage-dependent expression of CD7, CD45RO, CD45RA and CD25 on CD4-positive peripheral blood T-lymphocytes in cutaneous T-cell lymphoma. Acta Derm Venereol. 1996;76(1):34–6.

Jenni D, Karpova MB, Seifert B, Golling P, Cozzio A, Kempf W, French LE, Dummer R. Primary cutaneous lymphoma: two-decade comparison in a population of 263 cases from a Swiss tertiary referral centre. Br J Dermatol. 2011;164(5):1071–7.

Jones D, Dang NH, Duvic M, Washington LT, Huh YO. Absence of CD26 expression is a useful marker for diagnosis of T-cell lymphoma in peripheral blood. Am J Clin Pathol. 2001;115(6):885–92.

Kabelitz D. Analysis of the human T-cell receptor V gamma gene usage by flow cytometry. Ann N Y Acad Sci. 1995;756:103–5.

Kabelitz D, Glatzel A, Wesch D. Antigen recognition by human gammadelta T lymphocytes. Int Arch Allergy Immunol. 2000;122(1):1–7.

Kabelitz D, He W. The multifunctionality of human Vgamma9Vdelta2 gammadelta T cells: clonal plasticity or distinct subsets?Scand. J Immunol. 2012;76(3): 213–22.

Kabelitz D, Marischen L, Oberg HH, Holtmeier W, Wesch D. Epithelial defence by gamma delta T cells. Int Arch Allergy Immunol. 2005;137(1):73–81.

Kabelitz D, Wesch D. Features and functions of gamma delta T lymphocytes: focus on chemokines and their receptors. Crit Rev Immunol. 2003;23(5–6):339–70.

Kadin ME. Cutaneous gamma delta T-cell lymphomas – how and why should they be recognized? Arch Dermatol. 2000;136(8):1052–4.

Kadin ME. Pathobiology of CD30+ cutaneous T-cell lymphomas. J Cutan Pathol. 2006;33 Suppl 1:10–7.

Kadin ME, Pavlov IY, Delgado JC, Vonderheid EC. High soluble CD30, CD25, and IL-6 may identify patients with worse survival in CD30+ cutaneous lymphomas and early mycosis fungoides. J Invest Dermatol. 2012;132(3 Pt 1):703–10.

Kamarashev J, Burg G, Mingari MC, Kempf W, Hofbauer G, Dummer R. Differential expression of cytotoxic molecules and killer cell inhibitory receptors in CD8+ and CD56+ cutaneous lymphomas. Am J Pathol. 2001;158(5):1593–8.

Kamarashev J, Theler B, Dummer R, Burg G. Mycosis fungoides–analysis of the duration of disease stages in patients who progress and the time point of high-grade transformation. Int J Dermatol. 2007;46(9):930–5.

Kantekure K, Yang Y, Raghunath P, Schaffer A, Woetmann A, Zhang Q, Odum N, Wasik M. Expression patterns of the immunosuppressive proteins PD-1/CD279 and PD-L1/CD274 at different stages of cutaneous T-cell lymphoma/mycosis fungoides. Am J Dermatopathol. 2012;34(1):126–8.

Karenko L, Hahtola S, Ranki A. Molecular cytogenetics in the study of cutaneous T-cell lymphomas (CTCL). Cytogenet Genome Res. 2007;118(2–4):353–61.

Kelley TW, Parker CJ. CD4 (+)CD25 (+)Foxp3 (+) regulatory T cells and hematologic malignancies. Front Biosci (Sch Ed). 2010;2:980–92.

Kempf W, Kazakov DV, Palmedo G, Fraitag S, Schaerer L, Kutzner H. Pityriasis lichenoides et varioliformis acuta with numerous CD30(+) cells: a variant mimicking lymphomatoid papulosis and other cutaneous lymphomas. A clinicopathologic, immunohistochemical, and molecular biological study of 13 cases. Am J Surg Pathol. 2012;36(7):1021–9.

Kempf W, Sander CA. Classification of cutaneous lymphomas – an update. Histopathology. 2010;56(1):57–70.

Kikuchi A, Sakuraoka K, Kurihara S, Akiyama M, Shimizu H, Nishikawa T. CD8+ cutaneous anaplastic large-cell lymphoma: report of two cases with immunophenotyping, T-cell-receptor gene rearrangement and electron microscopic studies. Br J Dermatol. 1992;126(4):404–8.

Kim EJ, Lin J, Junkins-Hopkins JM, Vittorio CC, Rook AH. Mycosis fungoides and sezary syndrome: an update. Curr Oncol Rep. 2006;8(5):376–86.

Kim YC, Vandersteen DP. Primary cutaneous pleomorphic small/medium-sized T-cell lymphoma in a young man. Br J Dermatol. 2001;144(4):903–5.

Koch R, Jaffe ES, Mensing C, Zeis M, Schmitz N, Sander CA. Cutaneous gamma/delta T-cell lymphoma. J Dtsch Dermatol Ges. 2009;7(12):1065–7.

Kulow BF, Cualing H, Steele P, VanHorn J, Breneman JC, Mutasim DF, Breneman DL. Progression of cutaneous B-cell pseudolymphoma to cutaneous B-cell lymphoma. J Cutan Med Surg. 2002;6(6):519–28.

Kumar S, Krenacs L, Medeiros J, Elenitoba-Johnson KS, Greiner TC, Sorbara L, Kingma DW, Raffeld M, Jaffe ES. Subcutaneous panniculitic T-cell lymphoma is a tumor of cytotoxic T lymphocytes. Hum Pathol. 1998;29(4):397–403.

Kurniawan AN, Hongyo T, Hardjolukito ES, Ham MF, Takakuwa T, Kodariah R, Hoshida Y, Nomura T, Aozasa K. Gene mutation analysis of sinonasal lymphomas in Indonesia. Oncol Rep. 2006;15(5):1257–63.

Lai P, Hsiao Y, Hsu J, Wey SJ. Early stage mycosis fungoides with focal CD30-positive large cell transformation. Dermatol Sin. 2013;31(2):73–7. doi:http://dx.doi.org/10.1016/j.dsi.2012.06.006

Landa NG, Zelickson BD, Peters MS, Muller SA, Pittelkow MR. Lymphoma versus pseudolymphoma of the skin: gene rearrangement study of 21 cases with clinicopathologic correlation. J Am Acad Dermatol. 1993;29(6):945–53.

Lanier LL. NK cell recognition. Annu Rev Immunol. 2005;23:225–74.

Lanier LL, Cwirla S, Federspiel N, Phillips JH. Human natural killer cells isolated from peripheral blood do not rearrange T cell antigen receptor beta chain genes. J Exp Med. 1986;163(1):209–14.

Leinweber B, Beltraminelli H, Kerl H, Cerroni L. Solitary small- to medium-sized pleomorphic T-cell nodules of undetermined significance: clinical, histopathological, immunohistochemical and molecular analysis of 26 cases. Dermatology. 2009;219(1):42–7.

Lin CW, Lee WH, Chang CL, Yang JY, Hsu SM. Restricted killer cell immunoglobulin-like receptor repertoire without T-cell receptor gamma rearrangement supports a true natural killer-cell lineage in a subset of sinonasal lymphomas. Am J Pathol. 2001;159(5):1671–9.

Liu HL, Hoppe RT, Kohler S, Harvell JD, Reddy S, Kim YH. CD30+ cutaneous lymphoproliferative disorders: the Stanford experience in lymphomatoid papulosis and primary cutaneous anaplastic large cell lymphoma. J Am Acad Dermatol. 2003;49(6):1049–58.

Lukes RJ, Collins RD. Immunologic characteristics of human malignant lymphomas. Cancer. 1974;34:1488.

Mao X, Lillington D, Scarisbrick JJ, Mitchell T, Czepulkowski B, Russell-Jones R, Young B, Whittaker SJ. Molecular cytogenetic analysis of cutaneous T-cell lymphomas: identification of common genetic alterations in Sezary syndrome and mycosis fungoides. Br J Dermatol. 2002;147(3):464–75.

Martel P, Laroche L, Courville P, Larroche C, Wechsler J, Lenormand B, Delfau MH, Bodemer C, Bagot M, Joly P. Cutaneous involvement in patients with angioimmunoblastic lymphadenopathy with dysproteinemia: a clinical, immunohistological, and molecular analysis. Arch Dermatol. 2000;136(7):881–6.

McComb ME, Telang GH, Vonderheid EC. Secondary syphilis presenting as pseudolymphoma of the skin. J Am Acad Dermatol. 2003;49(2 Suppl Case Reports): S174–6.

Mraz-Gernhard S, Natkunam Y, Hoppe RT, LeBoit P, Kohler S, Kim YH. Natural killer/natural killer-like T-cell lymphoma, CD56+, presenting in the skin: an increasingly recognized entity with an aggressive course. J Clin Oncol. 2001;19(8):2179–88.

Natkunam Y, Smoller BR, Zehnder JL, Dorfman RF, Warnke RA. Aggressive cutaneous NK and NK-like T-cell lymphomas: clinicopathologic, immunohistochemical, and molecular analyses of 12 cases. Am J Surg Pathol. 1999;23(5):571–81.

Navas IC, Ortiz-Romero PL, Villuendas R, Martinez P, Garcia C, Gomez E, Rodriguez JL, Garcia D, Vanaclocha F, Iglesias L, Piris MA, Algara P. p16(INK4a) gene alterations are frequent in lesions of mycosis fungoides. Am J Pathol. 2000;156(5): 1565–72.

Nielsen PS, Riber-Hansen R, Raundahl J, Steiniche T. Automated quantification of MART1-verified Ki67 indices by digital image analysis in melanocytic lesions. Arch Pathol Lab Med. 2012;136(6):627–34.

Nofal A, bdel-Mawla MY, Assaf M, Salah E. Primary cutaneous aggressive epidermotropic CD8(+) T-cell lymphoma: proposed diagnostic criteria and therapeutic evaluation. J Am Acad Dermatol. 2012;67(4): 748–59.

Nowell PC, Finan JB, Vonderheid EC. Clonal characteristics of cutaneous T cell lymphomas: cytogenetic evidence from blood, lymph nodes, and skin. J Invest Dermatol. 1982;78(1):69–75.

OLIVIER J. Mycosis fungoides a tumeurs d'emblee; remission during 3 1/2 years. Arch Belg Dermatol Syphiligr. 1951;7(3):131–2.

Olsen E, Vonderheid E, Pimpinelli N, Willemze R, Kim Y, Knobler R, Zackheim H, Duvic M, Estrach T, Lamberg S, Wood G, Dummer R, Ranki A, Burg G, Heald P, Pittelkow M, Bernengo MG, Sterry W, Laroche L, Trautinger F, Whittaker S. Revisions to the staging and classification of mycosis fungoides and Sezary syndrome: a proposal of the International Society for Cutaneous Lymphomas (ISCL) and the cutaneous lymphoma task force of the European Organization of Research and Treatment of Cancer (EORTC). Blood. 2007;110(6):1713–22.

Pagano L, Gallamini A, Trape G, Fianchi L, Mattei D, Todeschini G, Spadca A, Cinieri S, Iannitto E, Martelli M, Nosari A, Bona ED, Tosti ME, Petti MC, Falcucci P, Montanaro M, Pulsoni A, Larocca LM, Leone G. NK/T-cell lymphomas 'nasal type': an Italian multicentric retrospective survey. Ann Oncol. 2006;17(5): 794–800.

Pernet G. Drawing and photograph of a case of mycosis fungoides d'emblee. Proc R Soc Med. 1912;5(Dermatol Sect):207–8.

Petrella T, Maubec E, Cornillet-Lefebvre P, Willemze R, Pluot M, Durlach A, Marinho E, Benhamou JL, Jansen P, Robson A, Grange F. Indolent CD8-positive lymphoid proliferation of the ear: a distinct primary cutaneous T-cell lymphoma? Am J Surg Pathol. 2007;31(12):1887–92.

Pol-Rodriguez MM, Fox LP, Sulis ML, Miller IJ, Garzon MC. Extranodal nasal-type natural killer T-cell lymphoma in an adolescent from Bangladesh. J Am Acad Dermatol. 2006;54(5 Suppl):S192–7.

Ponti R, Fierro MT, Quaglino P, Lisa B, Paola FC, Michela O, Paolo F, Comessatti A, Novelli M, Bernengo MG. TCRgamma-chain gene rearrangement by PCR-based GeneScan: diagnostic accuracy improvement and clonal heterogeneity analysis in multiple cutaneous T-cell lymphoma samples. J Invest Dermatol. 2008;128(4):1030–8.

Ponti R, Quaglino P, Novelli M, Fierro MT, Comessatti A, Peroni A, Bonello L, Bernengo MG. T-cell receptor gamma gene rearrangement by multiplex polymerase chain reaction/heteroduplex analysis in patients with cutaneous T-cell lymphoma (mycosis fungoides/

Sezary syndrome) and benign inflammatory disease: correlation with clinical, histological and immunophenotypical findings. Br J Dermatol. 2005; 153(3):565–73.

Pringle JJ. Mycosis Fungoides a Tumeurs d'Emblee. Proc R Soc Med. 1914;7(Dermatol Sect):155–8.

Quintanilla-Martinez L, Fend F, Moguel LR, Spilove L, Beaty MW, Kingma DW, Raffeld M, Jaffe ES. Peripheral T-cell lymphoma with Reed-Sternberg-like cells of B-cell phenotype and genotype associated with Epstein-Barr virus infection. Am J Surg Pathol. 1999;23(10):1233–40.

Quintanilla-Martinez L, Preffer F, Rubin D, Ferry JA, Harris NL. CD20+ T-cell lymphoma. Neoplastic transformation of a normal T-cell subset. Am J Clin Pathol. 1994;102(4):483–9.

Rezania D, Sokol L, Cualing HD. Classification and treatment of rare and aggressive types of peripheral T-cell/natural killer-cell lymphomas of the skin. Cancer Control. 2007;14(2):112–23.

Rijlaarsdam JU, Scheffer E, Meijer CJ, Willemze R. Cutaneous pseudo-T-cell lymphomas. A clinicopathologic study of 20 patients. Cancer. 1992;69(3):717–24.

Rijlaarsdam JU, Willemze R. Cutaneous pseudolymphomas: classification and differential diagnosis. Semin Dermatol. 1994;13(3):187–96.

Rizvi MA, Evens AM, Tallman MS, Nelson BP, Rosen ST. T-cell non-Hodgkin lymphoma. Blood. 2006;107(4):1255–64.

Rodriguez Pinilla SM, Roncador G, Rodriguez-Peralto JL, Mollejo M, Garcia JF, Montes-Moreno S, Camacho FI, Ortiz P, Limeres-Gonzalez MA, Torres A, Campo E, Navarro-Conde P, Piris MA. Primary cutaneous CD4+ small/medium-sized pleomorphic T-cell lymphoma expresses follicular T-cell markers. Am J Surg Pathol. 2009;33(1):81–90.

Rodriguez-Pinilla SM, Ortiz-Romero PL, Monsalvez V, Tomas IE, Almagro M, Sevilla A, Camacho G, Longo MI, Pulpillo A, Az-Perez JA, Montes-Moreno S, Castro Y, Echevarria B, Trebol I, Gonzalez C, Sanchez L, Otin AP, Requena L, Rodriguez-Peralto JL, Cerroni L, Piris MA. TCR-gamma expression in primary cutaneous T-cell Lymphomas. Am J Surg Pathol. 2013;37(3):375–84.

Roullet M, Gheith SM, Mauger J, Junkins-Hopkins JM, Choi JK. Percentage of {gamma}{delta} T cells in panniculitis by paraffin immunohistochemical analysis. Am J Clin Pathol. 2009;131(6):820–6.

Rudiger T, Weisenburger DD, Anderson JR, Armitage JO, Diebold J, Maclennan KA, Nathwani BN, Ullrich F, Muller-Hermelink HK. Peripheral T-cell lymphoma (excluding anaplastic large-cell lymphoma): results from the Non-Hodgkin's Lymphoma Classification Project. Ann Oncol. 2002;13(1):140–9.

Salhany KE, Cousar JB, Greer JP, Casey TT, Fields JP, Collins RD. Transformation of cutaneous T cell lymphoma to large cell lymphoma. A clinicopathologic and immunologic study. Am J Pathol. 1988; 132(2):265–77.

Salhany KE, Macon WR, Choi JK, Elenitsas R, Lessin SR, Felgar RE, Wilson DM, Przybylski GK, Lister J, Wasik MA, Swerdlow SH. Subcutaneous panniculitis-like T-cell lymphoma: clinicopathologic, immunophenotypic, and genotypic analysis of alpha/beta and gamma/delta subtypes. Am J Surg Pathol. 1998; 22(7):881–93.

Sallah S, Gagnon GA. Angioimmunoblastic lymphadenopathy with dysproteinemia: emphasis on pathogenesis and treatment. Acta Haematol. 1998;99(2): 57–64.

Santucci M, Pimpinelli N, Massi D, et al. Cytotoxic/natural killer cell cutaneous lymphomas. Report of EORTC Cutaneous Lymphoma Task Force Workshop. Cancer 2003;97:610–27.

Savage KJ, Chhanabhai M, Gascoyne RD, Connors JM. Characterization of peripheral T-cell lymphomas in a single North American institution by the WHO classification. Ann Oncol. 2004;15(10):1467–75.

Savage NM, Johnson RC, Natkunam Y. The spectrum of lymphoblastic, nodal and extranodal T-cell lymphomas: characteristic features and diagnostic dilemmas. Hum Pathol. 2012;44(4):451–71.

Savoia P, Fierro MT, Novelli M, Quaglino P, Verrone A, Geuna M, Bernengo MG. CD56-positive cutaneous lymphoma: a poorly recognized entity in the spectrum of primary cutaneous disease. Br J Dermatol. 1997;137(6):966–71.

Scarisbrick JJ, Mitchell TJ, Calonje E, Orchard G, Russell-Jones R, Whittaker SJ. Microsatellite instability is associated with hypermethylation of the hMLH1 gene and reduced gene expression in mycosis fungoides. J Invest Dermatol. 2003;121(4):894–901.

Scarisbrick JJ, Woolford AJ, Calonje E, Photiou A, Ferreira S, Orchard G, Russell-Jones R, Whittaker SJ. Frequent abnormalities of the p15 and p16 genes in mycosis fungoides and sezary syndrome. J Invest Dermatol. 2002;118(3):493–9.

Siu LL, Wong KF, Chan JK, Kwong YL. Comparative genomic hybridization analysis of natural killer cell lymphoma/leukemia. Recognition of consistent patterns of genetic alterations. Am J Pathol. 1999;155(5):1419–25.

Smithberger ES, Rezania D, Chavan RN, Lien MH, Cualing HD, Messina JL. Primary cutaneous angioimmunoblastic T-cell lymphoma histologically mimicking an inflammatory dermatosis. J Drugs Dermatol. 2010;9(7):851–5.

Smolle J, Torne R, Soyer HP, Kerl H. Immunohistochemical classification of cutaneous pseudolymphomas: delineation of distinct patterns. J Cutan Pathol. 1990;17(3):149–59.

Sterry W. Criteria for the differentiation of pseudolymphomas and malignant lymphomas of the skin. Z Hautkr. 1986;61(10):705–8.

Sterry W, Siebel A, Mielke V. HTLV-1-negative pleomorphic T-cell lymphoma of the skin: the clinicopathological correlations and natural history of 15 patients. Br J Dermatol. 1992;126(5):456–62.

Suarez-Vilela D, Izquierdo-Garcia FM. Angioimmunoblastic lymphadenopathy-like T-cell lymphoma: cutaneous clinical onset with prominent granulomatous reaction. Am J Surg Pathol. 2003;27(5): 699–700.

Suchak R, O'Connor S, McNamara C, Robson A. Indolent CD8-positive lymphoid proliferation on the face: part of the spectrum of primary cutaneous small-/medium-sized pleomorphic T-cell lymphoma or a distinct entity? J Cutan Pathol. 2010;37(9):977–81.

Summers E, Samadashwily G, Florell SR. A unique presentation of an Epstein-Barr virus-associated natural killer/T-cell lymphoproliferative disorder in a white male adolescent. Arch Dermatol. 2011;147(2):216–20.

Suzuki R, Suzumiya J, Yamaguchi M, Nakamura S, Kameoka J, Kojima H, Abe M, Kinoshita T, Yoshino T, Iwatsuki K, Kagami Y, Tsuzuki T, Kurokawa M, Ito K, Kawa K, Oshimi K. Prognostic factors for mature natural killer (NK) cell neoplasms: aggressive NK cell leukemia and extranodal NK cell lymphoma, nasal type. Ann Oncol. 2010a;21(5):1032–40.

Suzuki SY, Ito K, Ito M, Kawai K. Prognosis of 100 Japanese patients with mycosis fungoides and Sezary syndrome. J Dermatol Sci. 2010b;57(1):37–43.

Swerdlow SJ, Campo E, Harris NL, Jaffe ES, Pileri S, Stein H, Thiele J, Vardiman JW, editors. WHO classification of tumors of haematopoieitic and lymphoid tissues, 4th ed. Lyon: IARC press; 2008.

Swick BL, Baum CL, Venkat AP, Liu V. Indolent CD8+ lymphoid proliferation of the ear: report of two cases and review of the literature. J Cutan Pathol. 2011;38(2):209–15.

Takahashi N, Miura I, Chubachi A, Miura AB, Nakamura S. A clinicopathological study of 20 patients with T/natural killer (NK)-cell lymphoma-associated hemophagocytic syndrome with special reference to nasal and nasal-type NK/T-cell lymphoma. Int J Hematol. 2001;74(3):303–8.

Tallon B, Kaddu S, Cerroni L, Kerl H, Aberer E. Pseudolymphomatous tumid lupus erythematosus of the oral mucosa. Am J Dermatopathol. 2010;32(7):704–7.

Toro JR, Beaty M, Sorbara L, Turner ML, White J, Kingma DW, Raffeld M, Jaffe ES. gamma delta T-cell lymphoma of the skin: a clinical, microscopic, and molecular study. Arch Dermatol. 2000;136(8):1024–32.

Toro JR, Liewehr DJ, Pabby N, Sorbara L, Raffeld M, Steinberg SM, Jaffe ES. Gamma-delta T-cell phenotype is associated with significantly decreased survival in cutaneous T-cell lymphoma. Blood. 2003;101(9):3407–12.

Tracey L, Villuendas R, Dotor AM, Spiteri I, Ortiz P, Garcia JF, Peralto JL, Lawler M, Piris MA. Mycosis fungoides shows concurrent deregulation of multiple genes involved in the TNF signaling pathway: an expression profile study. Blood. 2003;102(3):1042–50.

Tracey L, Villuendas R, Ortiz P, Dopazo A, Spiteri I, Lombardia L, Rodriguez-Peralto JL, Fernandez-Herrera J, Hernandez A, Fraga J, Dominguez O, Herrero J, Alonso MA, Dopazo J, Piris MA. Identification of genes involved in resistance to interferon-alpha in cutaneous T-cell lymphoma. Am J Pathol. 2002;161(5):1825–37.

Tsuchiya T, Ohshima K, Karube K, Yamaguchi T, Suefuji H, Hamasaki M, Kawasaki C, Suzumiya J, Tomonaga M, Kikuchi M. Th1, Th2, and activated T-cell marker and clinical prognosis in peripheral T-cell lymphoma, unspecified: comparison with AILD, ALCL, lymphoblastic lymphoma, and ATLL. Blood. 2004;103(1):236–41.

Urosevic M, Kamarashev J, Burg G, Dummer R. Primary cutaneous CD8+ and CD56+ T-cell lymphomas express HLA-G and killer-cell inhibitory ligand, ILT2. Blood. 2004;103(5):1796–8.

Van Der Putte SC, Toonstra J, Felten PC, van Vloten WA. Solitary nonepidermotropic T cell pseudolymphoma of the skin. J Am Acad Dermatol. 1986;14(3):444–53.

van Kester MS, Ballabio E, Benner MF, Chen XH, Saunders NJ, van der Fits L, van Doorn R, Vermeer MH, Willemze R, Tensen CP, Lawrie CH. miRNA expression profiling of mycosis fungoides. Mol Oncol. 2011;5(3):273–80.

van Kester MS, Borg MK, Zoutman WH, Out-Luiting JJ, Jansen PM, Dreef EJ, Vermeer MH, van Doorn R, Willemze R, Tensen CP. A meta-analysis of gene expression data identifies a molecular signature characteristic for tumor-stage mycosis fungoides. J Invest Dermatol. 2012;132(8):2050–9.

van Kester MS, Tensen CP, Vermeer MH, Dijkman R, Mulder AA, Szuhai K, Willemze R, van Doorn R. Cutaneous anaplastic large cell lymphoma and peripheral T-cell lymphoma NOS show distinct chromosomal alterations and differential expression of chemokine receptors and apoptosis regulators. J Invest Dermatol. 2010;130(2):563–75.

van Doorn R, Van Haselen CW, van Voorst V, Geerts ML, Heule F, de Rie M, Steijlen PM, Dekker SK, van Vloten WA, Willemze R. Mycosis fungoides: disease evolution and prognosis of 309 Dutch patients. Arch Dermatol. 2000;136(4):504–10.

Vergier B, de Muret A, Beylot-Barry M, Vaillant L, Ekouevi D, Chene G, Carlotti A, Franck N, Dechelotte P, Souteyrand P, Courville P, Joly P, Delaunay M, Bagot M, Grange F, Fraitag S, Bosq J, Petrella T, Durlach A, de Mascarel A, Merlio JP, Wechsler J. Transformation of mycosis fungoides: clinicopathological and prognostic features of 45 cases. French Study Group of Cutaneious Lymphomas. Blood. 2000;95(7):2212–8.

Von Den DP, Coors EA. Localized cutaneous small to medium-sized pleomorphic T-cell lymphoma: a report of 3 cases stable for years. J Am Acad Dermatol. 2002;46(4):531–5.

Vonderheid EC, Tam DW, Johnson WC, Van Scott EJ, Wallner PE. Prognostic significance of cytomorphology in the cutaneous T-cell lymphomas. Cancer. 1981;47(1):119–25.

Wain EM, Orchard GE, Mayou S, Atherton DJ, Misch KJ, Russell-Jones R. Mycosis fungoides with a CD56+ immunophenotype. J Am Acad Dermatol. 2005;53(1):158–63.

Wang L, Han R, Hancock WW. Programmed cell death 1 (PD-1) and its ligand PD-L1 are required for allograft tolerance. Eur J Immunol. 2007;37(10):2983–90.

Wasik MA, Vonderheid EC, Bigler RD, Marti R, Lessin SR, Polansky M, Kadin ME. Increased serum concentration of the soluble interleukin-2 receptor in cutaneous T-cell lymphoma. Clinical and prognostic implications. Arch Dermatol. 1996;132(1):42–7.

Went P, Agostinelli C, Gallamini A, Piccaluga PP, Ascani S, Sabattini E, Bacci F, Falini B, Motta T, Paulli M, Artusi T, Piccioli M, Zinzani PL, Pileri SA. Marker expression in peripheral T-cell lymphoma: a proposed clinical-pathologic prognostic score. J Clin Oncol. 2006;24(16):2472–9.

Willemze R, Jaffe ES, Burg G, Cerroni L, Berti E, Swerdlow SH, Ralfkiaer E, Chimenti S, az-Perez JL, Duncan LM, Grange F, Harris NL, Kempf W, Kerl H, Kurrer M, Knobler R, Pimpinelli N, Sander C, Santucci M, Sterry W, Vermeer MH, Wechsler J, Whittaker S, Meijer CJ. WHO-EORTC classification for cutaneous lymphomas. Blood. 2005;105(10):3768–85.

Williams VL, Torres-Cabala CA, Duvic M. Primary cutaneous small- to medium-sized CD4+ pleomorphic T-cell lymphoma: a retrospective case series and review of the provisional cutaneous lymphoma category. Am J Clin Dermatol. 2011;12(6):389–401.

Wirt DP, Grogan TM, Jolley CS, Rangel CS, Payne CM, Hansen RC, Lynch PJ, Schuchardt M. The immunoarchitecture of cutaneous pseudolymphoma. Hum Pathol. 1985;16(5):492–510.

Wolfe JT, Chooback L, Finn DT, Jaworsky C, Rook AH, Lessin SR. Large-cell transformation following detection of minimal residual disease in cutaneous T-cell lymphoma: molecular and in situ analysis of a single neoplastic T-cell clone expressing the identical T-cell receptor. J Clin Oncol. 1995;13(7):1751–7.

Wood GS. Analysis of clonality in cutaneous T cell lymphoma and associated diseases. Ann N Y Acad Sci. 2001;941:26–30.

Wood GS, Bahler DW, Hoppe RT, Warnke RA, Sklar JL, Levy R. Transformation of mycosis fungoides: T-cell receptor beta gene analysis demonstrates a common clonal origin for plaque-type mycosis fungoides and CD30+ large-cell lymphoma. J Invest Dermatol. 1993;101(3):296–300.

Wood PB, Parikh SR, Krause JR. Extranodal NK/T-cell lymphoma, nasal type. Proc (Bayl Univ Med Cent). 2011;24(3):251–4.

Wozniak MB, Tracey L, Ortiz-Romero PL, Montes S, Alvarez M, Fraga J, Fernandez HJ, Vidal S, Rodriguez-Peralto JL, Piris MA, Villuendas DR. Psoralen plus ultraviolet A +/− interferon-alpha treatment resistance in mycosis fungoides: the role of tumour microenvironment, nuclear transcription factor-kappaB and T-cell receptor pathways. Br J Dermatol. 2009;160(1): 92–102.

Yao X, Teruya-Feldstein J, Raffeld M, Sorbara L, Jaffe ES. Peripheral T-cell lymphoma with aberrant expression of CD79a and CD20: a diagnostic pitfall. Mod Pathol. 2001;14(2):105–10.

Yu JB, Blitzblau RC, Decker RH, Housman DM, Wilson LD. Analysis of primary CD30+ cutaneous lymphoproliferative disease and survival from the surveillance, epidemiology, and end results database. J Clin Oncol. 2008;26(9):1483–8.

Zhang Q, Nowak I, Vonderheid EC, Rook AH, Kadin ME, Nowell PC, Shaw LM, Wasik MA. Activation of Jak/ STAT proteins involved in signal transduction pathway mediated by receptor for interleukin 2 in malignant T lymphocytes derived from cutaneous anaplastic large T-cell lymphoma and Sezary syndrome. Proc Natl Acad Sci U S A. 1996;93(17):9148–53.

Zucca E, Zinzani PL. Understanding the group of peripheral T-cell lymphomas, unspecified. Curr Hematol Rep. 2005;4(1):23–30.

Subcutaneous Pattern: Subcutaneous Lymphoproliferative Disorders

Marshall E. Kadin and Hernani D. Cualing

Malignant Disorders

Subcutaneous Panniculitis-Like T-Cell Lymphoma (SPTCL), Alpha-Beta Type

Epidemiology

Most patients are adults. Pediatric patients comprise 20 % of cases and can be as young as 5 months of age (Huppmann et al. 2013). Females exceed males. A unique feature is the high frequency of autoimmune disease, especially systemic lupus erythematosus.

Clinical Features

Most patients have multiple skin lesions which appear as nodules ranging from 0.5 to several centimeters in diameter (Fig. 11.1). Extremities and trunk are most common sites. Lymphadenopathy is uncommon. Systemic B symptoms occur in 50 % of patients. Most common laboratory abnormalities include abnormal liver function tests and cytopenias which can result from hemophagocytic

syndrome in up to 35 % of patients (Fig. 11.2) (Gonzalez et al. 1991). SPTCL patients without hemophagocytic syndrome have better survival than patients with the syndrome (5-year OS: 91 % vs. 46 %; $P < 0.001$) (Willemze et al. 2008).

Autoimmune diseases, particularly systemic lupus erythematosus, are common among SPTCL patients. The distinction between SPTCL and lupus erythematosus profundus is not always clear, and some cases appear to show progression of lupus profundus to SPTCL. Magro suggested there may be a spectrum of subcutaneous T-cell dyscrasias including lupus profundus and SPTCL (Magro et al. 2001).

In a multicenter study of the French Cutaneous Lymphoma Group (GFELC), 27 patients with SPTCL diagnosed since 2000 had a median age of 31.1 year; F/M ratio was 22:5 (Michonneau et al. 2013). Five cases occurred in children of whom three were under age 3. Almost half of patients (47 %) had an autoimmune disease, and 24 % were diagnosed with another panniculitis. Three cases occurred after pregnancy and in three young children after infectious events. Hemophagocytic syndrome was present in 35 % of cases. Serum beta2-microglobulin was elevated in 83 % of cases (4.51+/−2 mg/L). Median follow-up was 20.5 months. Complete remission was reached in 74 % of cases. 69.5 % were treated with immunosuppressive agents (group 1), and 30.5 % received chemotherapy (group 2). In both groups, complete remission was 77.7 % and 37.5 % ($P = 0.07$), respectively, and progression was only observed with chemotherapy (37.5 %, $P = 0.02$). The study

M.E. Kadin, MD (✉)
Department of Dermatology, Roger Williams
Medical Center, Boston University School
of Medicine, 50 Maude Street, Elmhurst Bldg.,
Providence, RI 02908, USA
e-mail: mkadin@chartercare.org

H.D. Cualing, MD
Department of Hematopathology and Cutaneous
Lymphoma, IHCFLOW Diagnostic Laboratory,
Lutz, FL, USA
e-mail: ihcflow@verizon.net

H.D. Cualing et al. (eds.), *Cutaneous Hematopathology*,
DOI 10.1007/978-1-4939-0950-6_11, © Springer Science+Business Media New York 2014

indicated that SPTCL in this group of French patients was often associated with autoimmunity or infections, and a good treatment response with low toxicity was encountered with immunosuppressive treatments.

Histology

The pattern is distinctive and evokes an instant sight diagnosis. At low magnification, one sees a dense lymphocytic infiltration of the subcutaneous tissue and usual sparing of the dermis and epidermis (Fig. 11.3). High magnification reveals atypical lymphocytes with irregular nuclei rimming individual fat cells. Reactive histiocytes are common in areas of fat infiltration. Plasma cells which are common in lupus panniculitis are typically absent. Lymphocytes that surround individual fat cells with frequent apoptotic bodies (karyorrhexis) are seen (Fig. 11.4). Fat necrosis occurs in most cases.

Immunophenotype

Tumor cells have a mature T αβ phenotype, expressing TCRβf1. They are usually CD3+, CD8+, CD4−, CD56−, and CD30− and strongly express cytotoxic molecules (granzyme B, perforin, TIA-1) (Fig. 11.5).

Genetics

Comparative genomic hybridization studies on single cell laser-microdissected cells performed by Hahtola et al. revealed large numbers of DNA copy number changes, the most common of

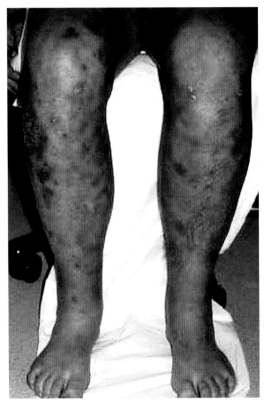

Fig. 11.1 SPTCL – multiple discrete nodular lesions of lower extremities

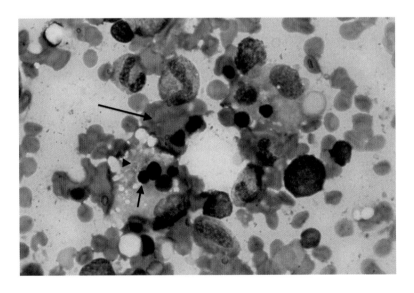

Fig. 11.2 Hemophagocytic syndrome in SPTCL – bone marrow aspirate showing histiocyte phagocytosis of nucleated erythrocytes (*arrows*)

Fig. 11.3 SPTCL – dense lymphocytic infiltrate permeating subcutaneous fat

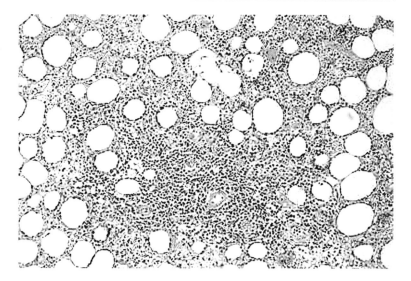

Fig. 11.4 SPTCL – lymphocytic surrounding individual fat cells. Atypical lymphocytes with irregular-shaped nuclei rim fat cells. Apoptotic bodies (karyorrhexis) are seen (*arrows*)

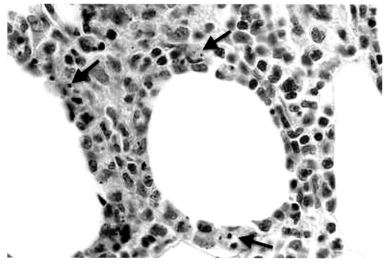

Fig. 11.5 SPTCL – tumor cells strongly express cytotoxic molecules (granzyme B, perforin, TIA-1)

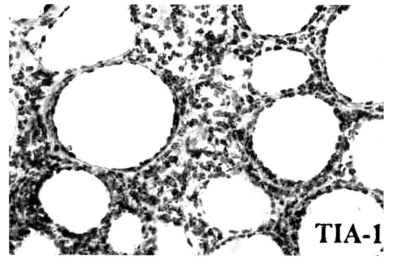

which were losses of chromosomes 1 pter, 2 pter, 10 qter, 11 qter, 12 qter, 16, 19, 20, and 22 and gains of chromosomes 2q and 4q. Some of the DNA copy number aberrations in SPTCL, such as loss of 10q, 17p, and chromosome 19, overlap with those characteristic of mycosis fungoides and Sezary syndrome, whereas 5q and 10q gains are more specific for SPTCL (Hahtola et al. 2008). Analysis of tumors shows clonal rearrangement of TCR genes in most cases. No clonal TCR gene rearrangement was detected in 4 of 17 pediatric cases (Huppmann et al. 2013). Epstein-Barr viral sequences have not been detected.

Differential Diagnosis

Any other condition with a predominant lymphocytic infiltration of subcutaneous tissues can lead to a mistaken diagnosis of SPTCL. Principal differential diagnostic features are summarized in Table 11.1. The prototypic benign condition mimicking SPTCL is lupus profundus. Some cases of cytophagic histiocytic panniculitis (CHP) overlap with SPTCL and could be indistinguishable (see Chap. 4 for discussion). There may be a continuum between the non-clonal indolent CHP and fatal clonal SPTCL (Marzano et al. 2000). The most significant malignant condition that can mimic SPTCL is primary cutaneous gamma-delta T-cell lymphoma (PCGD-TCL). These differential diagnoses are discussed in the following sections.

The deep infiltrating component of CD30+ cALCL can surround individual fat cells in the manner of SPTCL (Fig. 11.6). In contrast to SPTCL, cALCL has large anaplastic CD30+ cells, and the main tumor cell infiltrate is within the dermis.

Primary Cutaneous Gamma-Delta T-Cell Lymphoma (PCGD-TCL)

Clinical Features

Most cases occur in adults. In one series of 53 patients, the median age at presentation was 61 years (range 26–91) (Guitart et al. 2012). There is no gender predilection. The most common presentation is deep plaques, followed by patches resembling psoriasis or mycosis fungoides. Lesions frequently ulcerate (Fig. 11.7). Lesions most often involve the extremities, but the trunk is also frequently affected. Lymphadenopathy has been reported in 3/42 cases and bone marrow involvement in 5/28 cases (Guitart et al. 2012). A mucosal form of gamma-delta T-cell lymphoma occurs and a mucocutaneous form of the disease has been suggested (de Wolf-Peeters and Achten 2000). Approximately one-half of patients report systemic symptoms. Progression of disease is associated with extensive ulcerating lesions and hemophagocytic syndrome (Guitart et al. 2012). PCGD-TCL is resistant to radiation and multi-agent chemotherapy. Median survival in one large patient series is 15 months (Willemze et al. 2008) and in another is 31 months (Guitart et al. 2012).

Histology

Unlike SPTCL, primary cutaneous gamma-delta T-cell lymphomas involve the dermis and epidermis as well as subcutaneous tissue (Fig. 11.8). This is the principal histopathologic difference and explains the clinical manifestation of ulcerating lesions. Most cases have a dense lymphocytic infiltrate with partial involvement of epidermal, dermal, and subcutaneous compartments. Interface changes with exocytosis of erythrocytes and necrotic keratinocytes are common (Fig. 11.9). Although extensive epidermal infiltration with pagetoid features is seen, Pautrier microabscesses do not occur. Cytologically, primary cutaneous gamma-delta T-cell lymphomas reveal medium-sized lymphocytes, some with nuclear pleomorphism with Reed-Sternberg-like appearance (Fig. 11.10).

Immunophenotype

The main feature is the expression of the γδ T-cell phenotype now disclosed with a commercially available antibody that recognizes the TCR-δ subunit of the TCR in paraffin-embedded material (Fig. 11.11) (Rodriguez-Pinilla et al. 2013). It should be noted that tumor cells in some cases of PCGD-TCL also express TCR-βf1 (Rodriguez-Pinilla et al. 2013). All cases of PCGD-TCL express CD3. One-half of cases are double nega-

Table 11.1 Principle features distinguishing subcutaneous panniculitis-like T-cell lymphoma from other entities infiltrating the subcutis

	Demographics	Clinical features	Histology	Cytology	Immunophenotype	TCR clonality	Prognosis
SPTCL	20 % children/F > M	Plaques, tumors, extremities, and trunk	Subcutaneous rimming of fat cells	Minimal pleomorphism, karyorrhexis	TCRβf1+, CD8+, cytotoxic proteins+	+	Fair to good, death associated with hemophagocytic syndrome
PCGD-TCL	Adults, M > F	Ulcerated plaques, nodules, tumors	Epidermal with interface changes, dermal; subcutaneous involvement variable	Pleomorphism of tumor cells, karyorrhexis	TCRγδ+, βf1−/+, CD3+, CD4−, CD56+/−, EBER−/+	+	Poor
NKTCL	Adults, M > F	Nodules, tumors	Angiocentric, necrosis	Variable cell size	EBER+/, CD56+	−	Poor
LP	History of lupus erythematosus (LE)	Cutaneous atrophy	Subcutaneous, germinal centers, plasma cells mucin, hyperkeratotic follicular plugging	Minimal lymphocytic atypia, clusters of plasmacytoid dendritic cells	Human myxovirus resistance protein 1	−/+	No deaths attributed to panniculitis
ILLP	No hx of LE, young male	Painless nodules in extremities	Subcutaneous panniculitis with eccrinotropism	Nuclear atypia, focal necrosis	TCRβf1+, mixed CD4/CD8 with decreased ratio	+	Persistence without progression, constitutional symptoms ominous
EN	Young women; delayed hypersensitivity to bacterial infection or drugs	Painful nodules in extremities	Predominantly septal inflammation between fat lobules	Variable numbers of neutrophils, lymphocytes, and histiocytes as well as variable numbers of necrotic adipocytes, Langhans giant cells	TCRβf1+, mixed lymphohistiocytic infiltrate	−	Etiology varied, commonly infectious, i.e., Mycobacterium TB

LP lupus profundus, *ILLP* indeterminate lymphocytic lobular panniculitis, *EN* erythema nodosum

Fig. 11.6 CD30+ tumor cells in cALCL surrounding fat cells simulating SPTCL

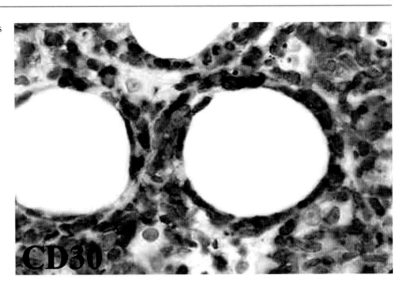

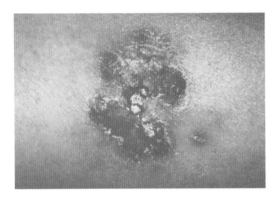

Fig. 11.7 Ulcerating lesions of primary cutaneous gamma-delta T-cell lymphoma

tive for CD4 and CD8 (Guitart et al. 2012). Cytotoxic proteins are expressed in >80 % of cases (Fig. 11.12). EBER by FISH is detected in approximately 10 %. The PCGD-TCL shows the expression of CD56 in about half the cases. The CD56 expression is similar to those of NK cells, which are effector cells together with gamma-delta T cells as part of the immediate immune response to foreign or microbial antigens (Toro et al. 2000; Garcia-Rodriguez et al. 2008; Garcia-Herrera et al. 2011).

Genetics

TCR clonality was detected in skin lesions in 96 % of cases in one large series and also in blood (9/12) and bone marrow (2/4) cases (Guitart et al. 2012).

Differential Diagnosis

The most significant differential diagnosis is SPTCL because some PCGD-TCL can have a predominantly panniculitic pattern (Guitart et al. 2012). Epidermal and dermal infiltrates support the diagnosis of PCGD-TCL. Tumor cell expression of TCR-γ is confirmatory.

The differential diagnosis of PCGD-TCL and extranodal NK/T TCL is often difficult to make (Rodriguez-Pinilla et al. 2013). Both tumors commonly express cytoplasmic CD3, CD2, and cytotoxic proteins, with variable expression of CD7 and CD56. However, most extranodal NK/T TCL are derived from NK cells and lack TCR gene rearrangements which are not characteristic of PCGD-TCL. Also extranodal NK/T TCL do not express TCR-γ. The nasal type of extranodal NK/T is EBV positive by EBER in situ hybridization.

Reactive Panniculitis Disorders

Lupus Profundus

Magro described two main groups of lymphocytic lobular panniculitis having overlapping features with SPTCL: (1) lupus erythematosus profundus (LEP) (Fig. 11.13) and (2) indeterminate lymphocytic lobular panniculitis (ILLP)

Fig. 11.8 Primary cutaneous gamma-delta T-cell lymphoma. Epidermal and dermal involvement with extravasation of erythrocytes distinguish this entity from SPTCL

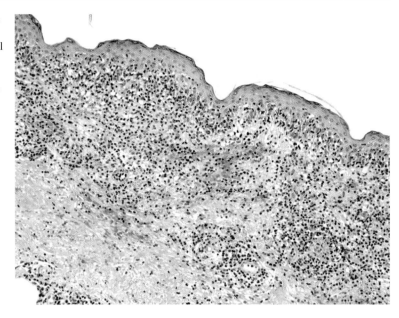

Fig. 11.9 Primary cutaneous gamma-delta T-cell lymphoma. Interface changes shown here occur in approximately one-half of cases

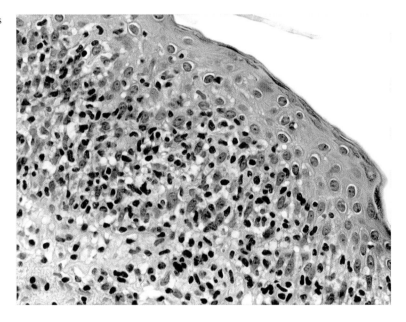

which is not associated with cutaneous or systemic LE (Magro et al. 2001). LEP showed histological similarities to SPTCL including dense lobular lymphocytic infiltration, but with the absence of lymphoid atypia (Fig. 11.14), histiocytes with ingested debris, eosinophilic necrosis of the fat lobule, and thrombosis. The infiltrate in ILLP had a similar cytomorphology and distribution with variable angioinvasion which was of lesser intensity and not associated with significant fat necrosis or vasculitis. Germinal centers, dermal/subcuticular mucin deposition, and an atrophy causing interface dermatitis with hyperkeratosis and follicular plugging were largely confined to the LEP group. The absence of T-cell monoclonality by gene rearrangement analysis

Fig. 11.10 Nuclear pleomorphism in primary cutaneous gamma-delta T-cell lymphoma

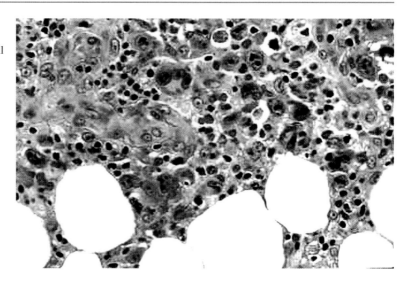

Fig. 11.11 Primary cutaneous gamma-delta T-cell lymphoma. Staining of tumor cells for TCRδ

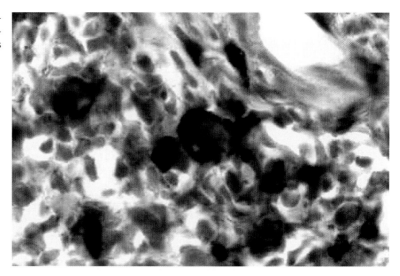

strongly favors LEP (Magro et al. 2001). However, detection of T-cell clonality, whether oligoclonal or stable persistent clone, is also characteristic of ILLP, and therefore ILLP is within the spectrum of lesions in continuity with SPTCL (Magro et al. 2008).

Differential Diagnosis

Recently, Wang and Magro demonstrated the usefulness of IHC staining of human myxovirus resistance protein 1 (MxA) in the differential diagnosis of LEP from SPTCL and PCGD-TCL (Wang and Magro 2012). In SPTCL and GDTCL, MxA was primarily seen in macrophages and generally did not exceed 20 % of the infiltrate. In contrast, a significant portion of the subcutaneous infiltrate was positive for MxA in LEP, with 50 % of the infiltrate staining on average. A greater number of macrophages and lymphocytes stained with a greater intensity as well ($P < 0.001$). Moreover, endothelial cell staining was uniquely identified in LEP but not in lymphoma. Although

Fig. 11.12 Primary cutaneous gamma-delta T-cell lymphoma. Staining of tumor cells for cytotoxic proteins like granzyme B shown here is seen in nearly all cases

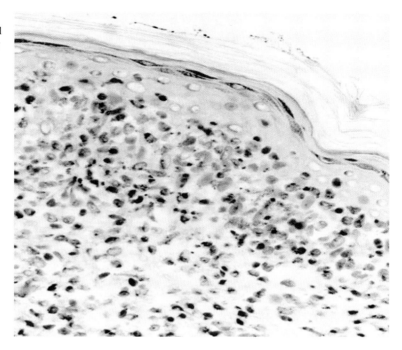

Fig. 11.13 Lupus profundus. Nodular lymphocytic infiltrates of subcutaneous fat. Rimming of fat cells by lymphocytes is not seen in this example

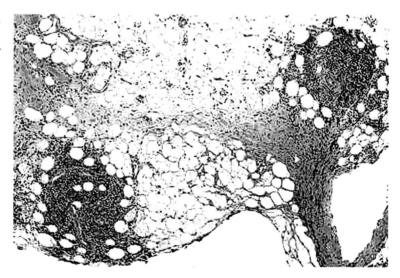

specificity was not 100 %, minimal staining of MxA was a predictor for SPTCL or GDTCL. Conversely, extensive staining for MxA both qualitatively and quantitatively was a feature of LEP. Endothelial staining also appeared to be specific for LEP.

Liau et al. found that the presence of clusters of plasmacytoid dendritic cells is a helpful feature for differentiating lupus panniculitis from subcutaneous panniculitis-like T-cell lymphoma. They also found that the presence of lymphoid follicles, dermal mucin deposition,

Fig. 11.14 Lupus profundus. Dense lymphocytic infiltrate without atypia

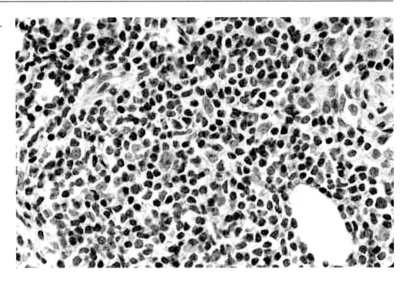

and lack of moderate to marked nuclear atypia or adipocyte rimming were more suggestive of LEP (Liau et al. 2013).

Infectious Panniculitis

Infection is the most frequent cause of panniculitis in developing countries: secondary to acute bacterial etiology such as *Staphylococcus/Streptococcus* infections, followed by cutaneous tuberculosis (Mert et al. 2007). Erythema nodosum (EN) is an inflammatory disease of the skin and subcutaneous tissue that presents with bilateral painful nodules in the extremities, histologically seen in the septa between the subcutaneous fat lobules (Fig. 11.15a–c). The hallmark lesions are tender, reddish nodules that present symmetrically on the extensor surfaces of the lower extremities. Erythema nodosum is considered an immunologic response to a wide variety of antigens or even associated with lymphomas (Fox and Schwartz 1992).

EN is most commonly associated with cutaneous tuberculid disease instead of an active cutaneous tuberculosis (Garcia-Rodriguez et al. 2008). EN is also described in association with nodular vasculitis (erythema induratum) as it is one of the many manifestations of cutaneous tuberculosis (Losada-Lopez et al. 2012). Hence, the diagnosis of an infectious-disease-associated panniculitis vis-a-vis tumor panniculitis is more frequent in the developing world than in developed countries (Mechai et al. 2011). Detection of TB-associated EN is additionally facilitated by molecular PCR methods in cutaneous lesions (Chen et al. 2013).

Although most EN are secondary to infections, including tuberculosis (Bohn et al. 1997), EN is associated with a wide range of disorders, some (Pileckyte and Griniute 2003) systemic diseases such as sarcoidosis (Pileckyte and Griniute 2003), Behcet disease, or inflammatory bowel diseases but also secondary to some drugs, mainly estrogen-progestins, salicylic acid, minocycline, and sulfamidic acid.

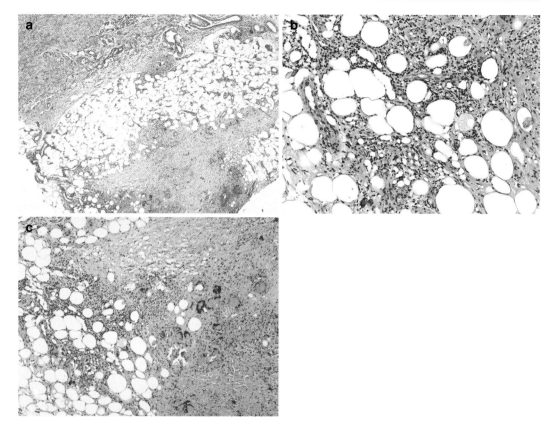

Fig. 11.15 Erythema nodosum. (**a**) Septal lobular panniculitis with fibrosis and Langhans giant cells in fibrotic areas. (**b**) Panniculitis with increased vessels and histiocytes. (**c**) Panniculitis with poorly formed granuloma on the right side with multinucleated Langhans-type giant cells typical of *Mycobacteria*

References

Bohn S, Buchner S, Itin P. Erythema nodosum: 112 cases. Epidemiology, clinical aspects and histopathology. Schweiz Med Wochenschr. 1997;127(27–28): 1168–76.

Chen S, Chen J, Chen L, Zhang Q, Luo X, Zhang W. Mycobacterium tuberculosis infection is associated with the development of erythema nodosum and nodular vasculitis. PLoS One. 2013;8:e62653.

de Wolf-Peeters C, Achten R. Gammadelta T-cell lymphomas: a homogeneous entity? Histopathology. 2000;36:294–305.

Fox MD, Schwartz RA. Erythema nodosum. Am Fam Physician. 1992;46:818–22.

Garcia-Rodriguez JF, Monteagudo-Sanchez B, Marino-Callejo A. Cutaneous tuberculosis: a 15-year descriptive study. Enferm Infecc Microbiol Clin. 2008;26: 205–11.

Gonzalez CL, Medeiros LJ, Braziel RM, Jaffe ES. T-cell lymphoma involving subcutaneous tissue. A clinicopathologic entity commonly associated with hemophagocytic syndrome. Am J Surg Pathol. 1991;15:17–27.

Guitart J, Weisenburger DD, Subtil A, Kim E, Wood G, Duvic M, et al. Cutaneous gammadelta T-cell lymphomas: a spectrum of presentations with overlap with other cytotoxic lymphomas. Am J Surg Pathol. 2012; 36:1656–65.

Hahtola S, Burghart E, Jeskanen L, Karenko L, Abdel-Rahman WM, Polzer B, et al. Clinicopathological characterization and genomic aberrations in subcutaneous panniculitis-like T-cell lymphoma. J Invest Dermatol. 2008;128:2304–9.

Huppmann AR, Xi L, Raffeld M, Pittaluga S, Jaffe ES. Subcutaneous panniculitis-like T-cell lymphoma in the pediatric age group: a lymphoma of low malignant potential. Pediatr Blood Cancer. 2013;60:1165–70.

Liau JY, Chuang SS, Chu CY, Ku WH, Tsai JH, Shih TF. The presence of clusters of plasmacytoid dendritic cells is a helpful feature for differentiating lupus panniculitis from subcutaneous panniculitis-like T-cell lymphoma. Histopathology. 2013;62: 1057–66.

Losada-Lopez I, Garcia-Gasalla M, Taberner R, Cifuentes-Luna C, Arquinio L, Terrasa F, et al. Cutaneous tuberculosis in an area of Mallorca (2003–2011). Rev Clin Esp. 2012;212:179–83.

Magro CM, Crowson AN, Kovatich AJ, Burns F. Lupus profundus, indeterminate lymphocytic lobular panniculitis and subcutaneous T-cell lymphoma: a spectrum of subcuticular T-cell lymphoid dyscrasia. J Cutan Pathol. 2001;28:235–47.

Magro CM, Schaefer JT, Morrison C, Porcu P. Atypical lymphocytic lobular panniculitis: a clonal subcutaneous T-cell dyscrasia. J Cutan Pathol. 2008;35:947–54.

Marzano AV, Berti E, Paulli M, Caputo R. Cytophagic histiocytic panniculitis and subcutaneous panniculitis-like T-cell lymphoma: report of 7 cases. Arch Dermatol. 2000;136:889–96.

Mechai F, Soler C, Aoun O, Fabre M, Merens A, Imbert P, et al. Primary mycobacterium bovis infection revealed by erythema nodosum. Int J Tuberc Lung Dis. 2011;15:1131–2.

Mert A, Kumbasar H, Ozaras R, Erten S, Tasli L, Tabak F, et al. Erythema nodosum: an evaluation of 100 cases. Clin Exp Rheumatol. 2007;25:563–70.

Michonneau D, Bruneau J, Boccara O, Hermine O, Maynade M, Petrall T, et al. Subcutaneous panniculitis-like T-cell lymphoma: a multicentric clinical and pathologic report of the French Cutaneous Lymphoma Group (GFLEC) experience. In 2nd World Congress of Cutaneous Lymphomas. International Program Committee and Local Organizing Committee (Editors), Berlin, Germany; Feb. 609, 2013.

Pileckyte M, Griniute R. Erythema nodosum association with malignant lymphoma. Medicina (Kaunas). 2003;39:438–42.

Rodriguez-Pinilla SM, Ortiz-Romero PL, Monsalvez V, Tomas IE, Almagro M, Sevilla A, et al. TCR-gamma expression in primary cutaneous T-cell lymphomas. Am J Surg Pathol. 2013;37:375–84.

Toro JR, Beaty M, Sorbara L, Turner ML, White J, Kingma DW, et al. gamma delta T-cell lymphoma of the skin: a clinical, microscopic, and molecular study. Arch Dermatol. 2000;136:1024–32.

Wang X, Magro CM. Human myxovirus resistance protein 1 (MxA) as a useful marker in the differential diagnosis of subcutaneous lymphoma vs. lupus erythematosus profundus. Eur J Dermatol. 2012;22:629–33.

Willemze R, Jansen PM, Cerroni L, Berti E, Santucci M, Assaf C, et al. Subcutaneous panniculitis-like T-cell lymphoma: definition, classification, and prognostic factors: an EORTC Cutaneous Lymphoma Group Study of 83 cases. Blood. 2008;111:838–45.

Part III

Specific Patterns Including Granulomas and Infections

CD30+ Cutaneous Lymphoproliferative Disorders and Pseudolymphomas

12

Marshall E. Kadin

Lymphomatoid Papulosis

Definition

Lymphomatoid papulosis (LyP) is a self-healing or spontaneously regressing cutaneous lymphoproliferative disorder (LPD) which histologically resembles a malignant lymphoma (Macaulay 1968).

Epidemiology

LyP is a rare skin disorder. The overall prevalence rate of lymphomatoid papulosis is estimated at 1.2–1.9 cases per 1,000,000 population. The peak incidence of LyP is in women in the fifth decade. We described 35 patients with childhood-onset LyP (19 boys and 16 girls). The age distribution was significantly different, with boys having an earlier onset of LyP ($P=0.03$). Compared with the general population, patients with childhood-onset LyP have a significantly increased risk of developing non-Hodgkin lymphoma (relative risk, 226.2; 95 % confidence interval, 73.4–697.0). More than two-thirds of the patients reported being atopic, which is significantly more than the expected prevalence of atopy (relative risk, 3.1; 95 % confidence interval, 2.2–4.3) (Nijsten et al. 2004). In contrast, all 11 LyP patients initially described with the 6p25.3 rearrangement were elderly; ages of the 11 patients ranged from 67 to 88 years at presentation (mean, 75 years). There was a strong male predominance (9M:2F).

Clinical Features

LyP presents as a waxing and waning intermittent or continuous eruption of reddish papules which may have a central necrotic area. Individual lesions form, while others undergo regression (Fig. 12.1). Upon healing, there may be a scar or change in pigmentation. Lesions are commonly found on the extremities, trunk, or buttock but may also occur on the face, genitalia, and hands. Only rare cases of mucosal, e.g., oral, involvement have been reported (Kato et al. 1998). The prognosis is excellent with >90 % 10-year survival (Bekkenk et al. 2000).

Association of LyP with Lymphoid and Nonlymphoid Malignancies

A higher than expected occurrence of malignant lymphomas in LyP patients is well established (Bekkenk et al. 2000; Beljaards and Willemze 1992; Cabanillas et al. 1995; el-Azhary et al. 1994; Nijsten et al. 2004; Volkenandt et al. 1993;

M.E. Kadin, MD
Department of Dermatology, Roger Williams
Medical Center, Boston University School of Medicine,
50 Maude Street, Elmhurst Bldg,
Providence, RI 02908, USA
e-mail: mkadin@chartercare.org

H.D. Cualing et al. (eds.), *Cutaneous Hematopathology*,
DOI 10.1007/978-1-4939-0950-6_12, © Springer Science+Business Media New York 2014

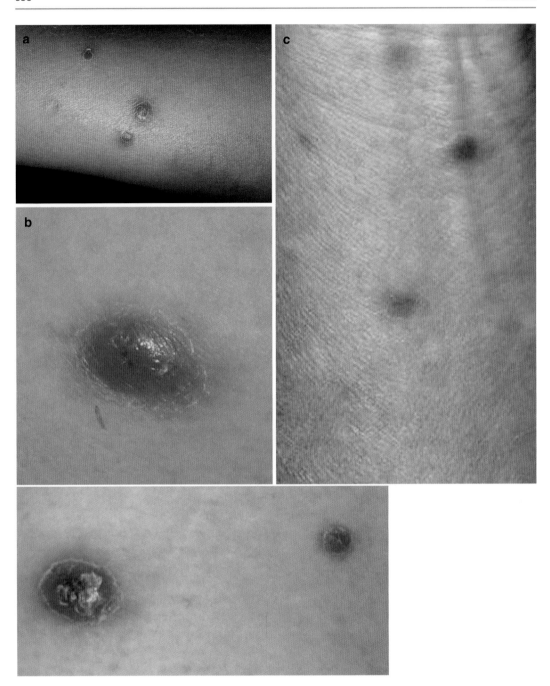

Fig. 12.1 Clinical appearance of LyP lesions. (**a**) Four lesions including developing and healed lesions appearing simultaneously. (**b**) LyP lesions at different stages of development. Single mature lesion *top*. Two lesions undergoing spontaneous regression, *bottom*. (**c**) LyP lesions of type B histology without central necrosis—LyP lesions generally heal more slowly than type A lesions

Wang et al. 1992, 1999; Wood et al. 1995). Moreover, one prognostic study revealed an increased risk of LyP patients to develop *nonlymphoid* cancers (Wang et al. 1999). Associated lymphomas may occur before, after, or concurrent with LyP skin lesions. The most

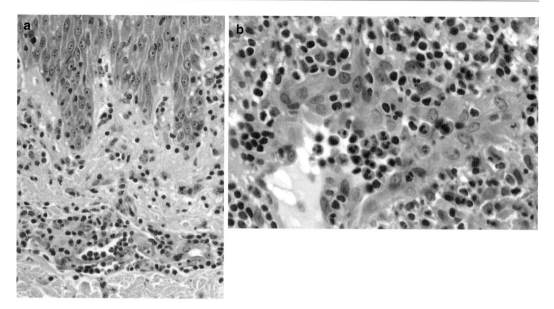

Fig. 12.2 Histology of an early LyP lesion. (**a**) Scan lymphoid infiltrate surrounding dermal capillary with marginating neutrophils. (**b**) Neutrophils egressing through activated endothelial cells

common lymphomas associated with LyP are mycosis fungoides, ALCL, and Hodgkin lymphoma, although other non-Hodgkin lymphomas also occur (Wang et al. 1992). The frequency of LyP-associated lymphomas derived from the literature is between 5 % and 20 %. However, higher numbers have been reported, particularly from referral centers where large numbers of cancer patients are seen, and this may reflect referral bias (Cabanillas et al. 1995). Cabanillas evaluated 21 LyP patients at MD Anderson Cancer Hospital. Five of 21 (24 %) developed lymphoma; the cumulative risk for transformation after 15 years was 80 %. *LyP patients should be monitored for development of an associated lymphoma annually or when a notable change in clinical status or symptoms suggestive of lymphoma occurs.* This will require close cooperation of the patient, their dermatologist, and oncologist when indicated.

Histology

The histology is variable and depends on the state of evolution of the lesion. Early lesions show a perivascular distribution of atypical lymphocytes.

Vascular lumina frequently contain marginated neutrophils (Fig. 12.2) (Kadin 2009). Lymphocytes eventually involve larger portions of the dermis, and mature lesions form a wedge shape which may extend to the deepest portion of the dermis. Neutrophils are numerous and migrate into the epidermis, forming pustules. The superficial epidermis becomes ulcerated, but individual keratinocyte necrosis does not occur (Fig. 12.3). Varying numbers of eosinophils are found. Vascular necrosis occurs in the rare type E described below (Fig. 12.4). Plasma cells are found in clusters in some cases. Macrophages are inconspicuous without special stains. Granulomas are rarely found. The epidermis and adnexal epithelium are sparingly involved by lymphocytes except in type B and the 6p25.3 type to be described below. The different histologic types of LyP are summarized in Table 12.1 and described in greater detail below.

LyP type A is the most common type. It resembles Hodgkin lymphoma in appearance.

It is characterized by large atypical cells surrounded by inflammatory cells, mainly neutrophils and eosinophils (Fig. 12.5). Neutrophils frequently are found in the epidermis and may

Fig. 12.3 Mature LyP lesion
with many atypical, large,
often multinucleated cells.
The epidermis contains many
neutrophils and is undergoing
ulceration

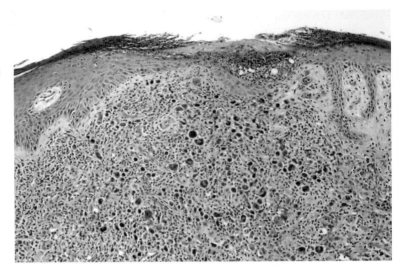

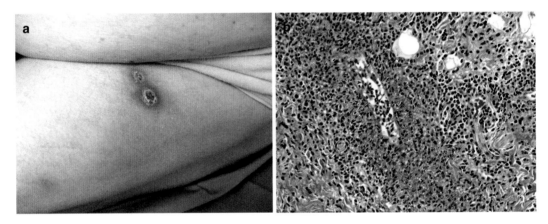

Fig. 12.4 LyP type E lesions. (**a**) Clinical appearance of eschars. (**b**) Vascular necrosis associated with atypical lymphocytic infiltrate

be associated with ulceration. The large atypical cells resemble immunoblasts with basophilic cytoplasm and often prominent nucleoli. Reed-Sternberg-like cells may be seen (Fig. 12.6). Mitoses, sometimes atypical, and apoptotic debris are commonly present. Epidermotropism of atypical cells is infrequent.

LyP type B resembles patch stage mycosis fungoides with cerebriform atypical lymphocytes infiltrating the epidermis, but not forming Pautrier microabscesses (Fig. 12.7). Few or no atypical lymphocytes express CD30, but most express CD4. There is not an interface pattern,

and individual keratinocyte necrosis is usually absent. Extravasation of erythrocytes is uncommon. Neutrophils and eosinophils are generally absent.

LyP type C resembles large cell lymphoma. It contains sheets of CD30+ large atypical cells which also form clusters (Fig. 12.8). Neutrophils and eosinophils are less conspicuous than in type A. Type C has the highest risk of progression to ALCL.

Mixed features of types A, B, and/or C are common. Individual patients may have lesions of more than one histologic type (Chott et al. 1996; El Shabrawi-Caelen et al. 2004).

Table 12.1 Major distinguishing features of CD30+ cutaneous lymphoproliferative disorders

	LyP	ALCL	Borderline
Clinical	Crops of papules/nodules with central necrosis; spontaneous regression occurs in 4–6 weeks	One to several ulcerating nodules or tumors; regression occurs in 25–40 % Extracutaneous spread in 10 %	Intermediate-sized nodules (1–2 cm), slow regression
Histology	Early lesions have upper dermal perivascular lymphocytes. Neutrophils in blood vessels	Deep dermal infiltrate, often sparing the epidermis	Clusters of large atypical cells largely confined to the dermis
	Scattered large atypical cells surrounded by reactive/inflammatory cells	Extensive tumor cell infiltration of the dermis and subcutis	Variable numbers of inflammatory cells
	"Mature" lesions are wedge shaped	Reactive small lymphocytes largely confined to periphery Neutrophil-rich variant with rare tumor cells	Spectrum of cerebriform mononuclear cells to large RS-like cells may be found
Immunophenotype, genetics	CD30+, CD4+, LCA+, TIA-1/granzyme B+ Diploid to aneuploid Poly-, oligo-, or monoclonal TCR gene rearrangement (60 %). 6p25.3 rearrangement in a subset of cases with distinctive pathology	CD30+, CD4+, LCA+, TIA1/granzyme B+ Absence of t(2;5) except in rare cases IRF4 translocation in 25 % Aneuploidy, clonal TCR (>90 %). 6p25.3 rearrangement in 25 % of cases	CD30+, CD4+, LCA+, TIA-1+ No data on cytogenetics Clonal by TCR gene analysis

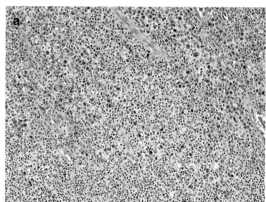
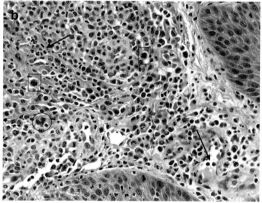

Fig. 12.5 LyP type A. (**a**) Low magnification showing scattered immunoblasts surrounded by many inflammatory cells. (**b**) *Top* portion shows large immunoblasts with basophilic cytoplasm and prominent nucleoli. *Rectangles* contain mitotic figures. *Circle* contains cell with multilobed nuclei. *Arrows* designate neutrophils within and outside blood vessels

LyP type D is an infrequent type with a prominent epidermotropic component which resembles pagetoid reticulosis (Fig. 12.9). This type is CD8+ and coexpresses CD30 (Saggini et al. 2010).

LyP type E is recognized clinically by eschars and histologically by vascular necrosis (Kempf et al. 2013) (Fig. 12.4). It is characterized by oligolesional papules that rapidly ulcerate and evolve into large necrotic eschar-like lesions

Fig. 12.6 LyP. Reed-Sternberg-like cells with multilobed nuclei and prominent eosinophilic nucleoli are seen within *rectangle*

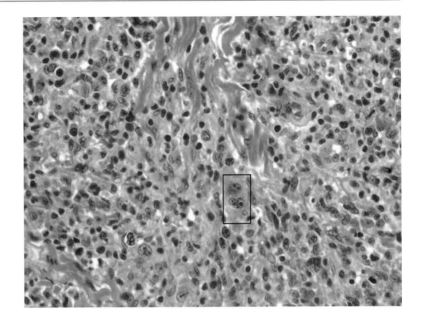

with a diameter of 1–4 cm and an angiocentric and angiodestructive infiltrate of small- to medium-sized atypical lymphocytes expressing CD30 and frequently CD8. Recurrences are common, but the prognosis is excellent with no extracutaneous spread or disease-related deaths reported. Complete remission occurred in 9 of 16 patients (56 %). LyP type E must be distinguished from aggressive forms of angiocentric and angiodestructive and cytotoxic T-cell lymphomas.

LyP with 6p25.3 rearrangement has a biphasic histology noticeable at low magnification (Fig. 12.10). A reproducible finding is the presence of an extensive atypical lymphoid infiltrate in the epidermis simulating lesions of pagetoid reticulosis. The intraepidermal infiltrate appears largely confined to an area overlying a dermal nodule which contains intermediate- to large-sized cells usually lacking typical anaplastic features. Marked periadnexal involvement by small- to medium-sized lymphocytes with markedly irregular nuclei expanding the folliculo-sebaceous units and/or eccrine glands is noted. Mitotic figures and apoptotic bodies are frequent in the dermal infiltrate. Neutrophils and eosinophils are infrequent or absent. Classical cytogenetic studies are not feasible for most cutaneous CD30+ lymphoproliferative disorders. FISH is recommended for cases of LyP which are suspected of harboring the 6p25.3 rearrangement, especially in the presence of a biphasic pattern of CD30+ epidermotropic cerebriform cells and a dense dermal infiltrate of larger CD30+ cells. The prognostic significance of this translocation is not known because of the small number of cases so far reported.

Immunophenotype

The large atypical cells have a phenotype of activated helper T cells expressing Hodgkin lymphoma-associated antigens CD30, CD25, CD71, HLA-DR, and sometimes CD15 (Kadin et al. 1985) and usually CD4+ but may be CD8+ (Kadin et al. 1985; Magro et al. 2006) (Plaza et al. 2013; Ralfkiaer et al. 1987) (Fig. 12.11). The atypical cells contain cytotoxic proteins (TIA-1, granzyme B, and/or perforin in one-half of cases (Kummer et al. 1997) (Fig. 12.12). The atypical cells express cutaneous lymphocyte antigen (CLA).

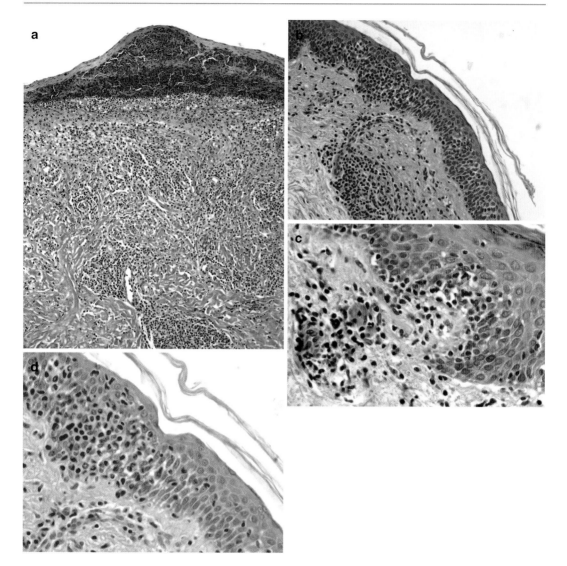

Fig. 12.7 LyP type B. (**a**) Crusted lesion. (**b**) Epidermotropic lymphocytes. (**c**) Epidermotropic cerebriform lymphocytes. (**d**) High magnification of epidermotropic lymphocytes with irregular nuclei

Genetics

We reported cytogenetic findings in an adult female patient with LyP type A. Karyotyping of the CD30+ atypical lymphoid cells revealed numerical and structural aberrations. Trisomy 7, a common finding in hematologic disorders such as adult T-cell leukemia and non-Hodgkin lymphomas, was detected. Additionally, a breakpoint was found at 10q24 in the region of the TCL3 oncogene and tumor suppressor gene PTEN.

These results contrast with cells of a young female patient (age 3) with a type A LyP, which showed a normal karyotype as well as cells of a male adult with type B LyP. None of the cases showed the t(2;5)p(23;q35). Together the results suggest different steps in the development of LyP and distinct forms of this one disease (Peters et al. 1995).

Chromosomal rearrangements of 6p25.3 define a newly recognized type of LyP (Karai et al. 2013). The rearrangement or less frequent

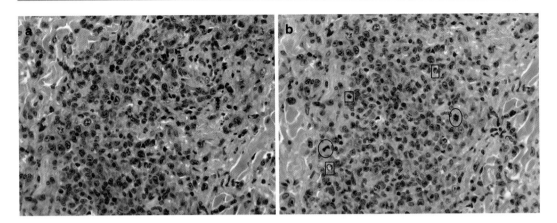

Fig. 12.8 LyP type C. (**a**) Sheets of atypical large cells with no inflammatory cells. (**b**) Mitotic figures in *circles*. Apoptotic bodies in *rectangles*

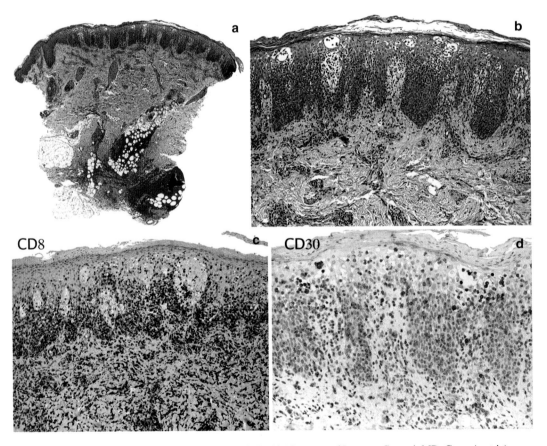

Fig. 12.9 LyP type D. (**a**, **b**) H&E stains. (**c**) CD8. (**d**) CD30 (Courtesy of Lorenzo Cerroni, MD, Graz, Austria)

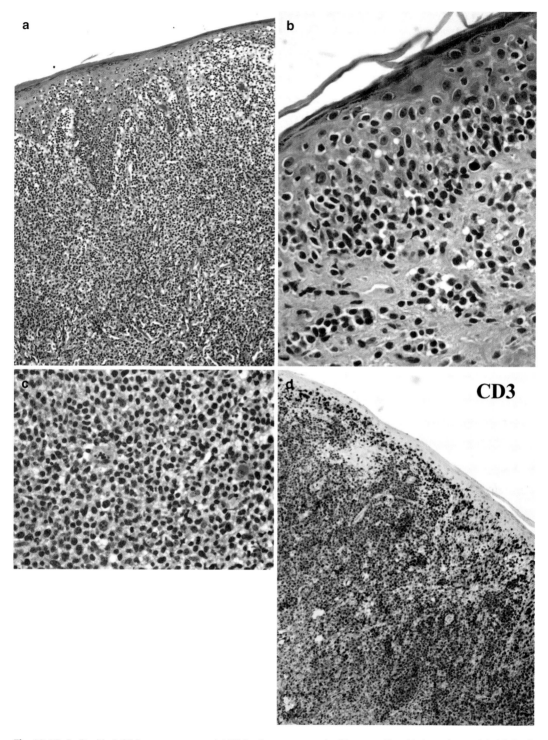

Fig. 12.10 LyP with 6p25.3 rearrangement. (**a**) Biphasic pattern involving the epidermis and dermis. (**b**) Epidermotropic small cells. (**c**) Dermal infiltrate composed of larger cells with irregular nuclei. (**d**) Both dermal and epidermal components stain for CD3

Fig. 12.11 Large atypical cells in LyP type A stain for CD30 antigen

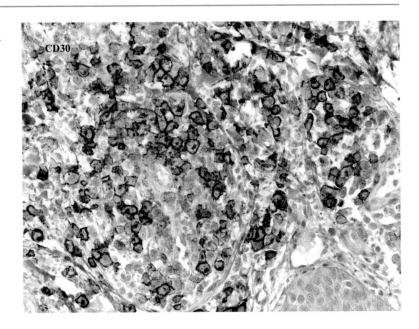

Fig. 12.12 Large atypical cells in LyP type A stain for TIA-1 representing cytotoxic proteins

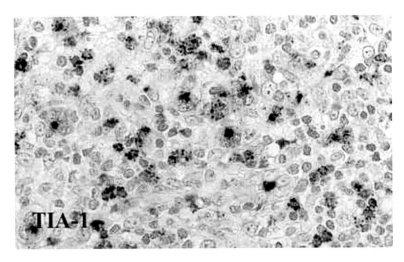

inversion inactivates one DUSP22 allele, while the other is inactivated by constitutive methylation (Cappelin et al. 2013). Inactivation may also occur by biallelic rearrangements (Csikesz et al. 2013). DUSP22 is a dual-action phosphatase which promotes growth and cell migration and appears to act as a tumor suppressor gene.

We studied the clonality of LyP lesions and their clonal relationship to T-cell lymphomas which develop in some LyP patients (Chott et al. 1996). Punch biopsies of skin of 11 adult patients with LyP were analyzed for morphologic subtype of LyP, surface antigens, and clonal T-cell receptor

(TCR) gene rearrangements. Clonal rearrangements were identified by semiquantitative polymerase chain reaction amplification and sequencing of TCR-beta chain genes in nine patients and TCR-gamma chain genes in two patients. A single dominant clone was detected in multiple separate LyP lesions, often of different histologies, in nine patients. The same clone was detected in LyP lesions and the anaplastic large cell lymphoma (ALCL) of two patients and the mycosis fungoides (MF) of two other patients. No dominant clone could be detected in one patient with LyP uncomplicated by lymphoma or in a second patient with LyP and MF. A T-cell lineage was evident for RS-like cells in cell culture and in type A lesions. These results show that multiple regressing skin lesions and associated T-cell lymphomas (MF and ALCL) are clonally related in most LyP patients, which suggests that the disease in these patients was initiated by a nonrandom genetic event as we hypothesized in an earlier study (Davis et al. 1992). Basarab studied 15 patients with LyP associated with MF. LyP either preceded ($n=4$), followed ($n=5$), or occurred concurrently with the MF lesions ($n=6$). They identified a T-cell clone in six of 16 LyP lesions and nine of 16 MF lesions. In the three patients who had clones in both types of skin lesions, the clones were identical (Basarab et al. 1998). Gallardo studied 12 patients who presented with LyP and MF. T-cell clonality was identified in 7 of 12 LyP lesions and six skin biopsies of MF plaque stage. In each individual case where T-cell clonality was established, both MF and LyP specimens were derived from the same clone. Each patient with LyP and MF had an indolent course consistent with prior observations of Beljaards and Williemze (1992).

The nature of the clonal cell in LyP has been controversial. One study of four patients using microdissection and PCR amplification of T-cell receptor genes indicated that the clonal cells are CD3+, CD30 negative (Gellrich et al. 2004). In contrast, Steinhoff showed that the isolated CD30+ cells from individual and separate lesions of LyP patients were clonally related (Steinhoff et al. 2002). They analyzed the T-cell receptor-gamma rearrangements of single CD30+ as well as of single CD30- cells isolated from 14 LyP lesions of 11 patients. By using this approach, they demonstrated that the CD30+ cells represent members of a single T-cell clone in all LyP cases. Moreover, in three patients, the same CD30+ cell clone was found in anatomically and temporally separate lesions. In contrast, with only a few exceptions, the CD30- cells were polyclonal in all instances and unrelated to the CD30+ cell clone. Their results demonstrate that LyP unequivocally represents a monoclonal T-cell disorder of CD30+ cells in all instances. This observation was recently confirmed by Riboni

(2013). TCR clonality assessment revealed a 92 % of monoclonal rearrangement in microdissected CD30+ cells versus 42 % in whole tissue sections. Sequencing of PCR products showed a high degree of matching rearrangements, suggesting clonal identity. No clonal rearrangements were found in a pool of microdissected cells from CD30-negative areas. The high rate of TCR clonality in microdissected cases supports the neoplastic nature of LyP. These findings are consistent with our development of aneuploid CD30+ T-cell lines derived from LyP patients that are clonally related to prior LyP lesions (Davis et al. 1992; Schiemann et al. 1999).

The recurrence of clonally related lesions after many eruptions over years raises questions as to the reservoir of clonal cells. Humme studied peripheral blood as a possible source of these clonal cells (Humme et al. 2009). They demonstrated dominance of nonmalignant T-cell clones and distortion of the TCR repertoire in the peripheral blood of patients with cutaneous CD30+ lymphoproliferative disorders. They investigated genomic DNA of 126 samples of lesional skin and peripheral blood from 31 patients with CLPD, obtained during both active disease and clinical remission. They performed molecular genetic analysis by combining T-cell receptor (TCR)-gamma PCR with the GeneScan technique and assessed the TCR repertoire in selected blood samples by beta-variable complementarity-determining region 3 (CDR3) spectratyping qualitatively and quantitatively. They were able to detect a clonal T-cell population in 36/43 (84 %) skin samples and in 35/83 (42 %) blood samples. Comparison of the compartments in each patient demonstrated different T-cell clones in skin and blood, suggesting a reactive nature of the clonal T cells in the blood. Moreover, CDR3 spectratyping revealed a restricted T-cell repertoire in the blood, suggesting T-cell stimulation by an unknown antigen.

Differential Diagnosis

When LyP tissues are pathologically examined, they are frequently confused with lymphoma,

Table 12.2 CD30+ pseudolymphomatous infiltrates that can be mistaken for LyP and ALCL

Condition	Histology	
Lymphomatoid drug eruption	Spongiotic dermatitis, lichenoid infiltrates, and interface dermatitis with large atypical lymphocytes	Pulitzer et al. (2013)
Milker's nodule		Werner et al. (2008)
Herpes simplex infection	Interface dermatitis and viral inclusions	Werner et al. (2008)
Molluscum contagiosum		Werner et al. (2008)
Nodular scabies	CD30+ large cells, inflammatory cells, presence of mite	Werner et al. (2008)
Leishmaniasis		Werner et al. (2008)
Syphilis		Werner et al. (2008)
Pernio		Werner et al. (2008)
Tsutsugamushi disease	Leukocytoclastic vasculitis and basal vacuolar changes	Lee et al. (2009)

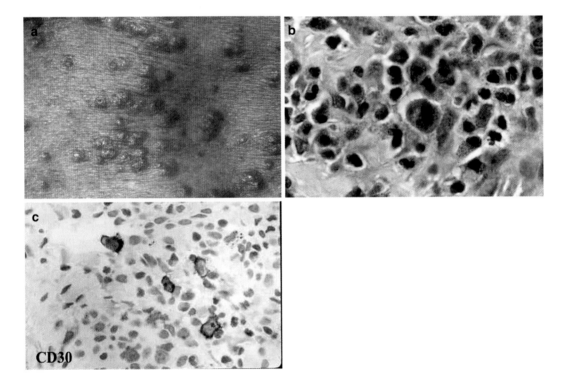

Fig. 12.13 Scabies, an infectious disease that can mimic LyP clinically and immunophenotypically staining scattered large cells for CD30. (**a**) Papular lesions of scabies. (**b**) Higher magnification showing pleomorphism of lymphoid cells. (**c**) CD30 stain

melanoma, or carcinoma. The diagnosis of metastatic melanoma can be complicated by absent characteristic cytology, melanin, or antigen expression in a suspect tumor. Because LyP lesions are characterized by the presence of scattered CD30+ large cells, a variety of other conditions affecting the skin and containing large CD30+ cells can be confused with LyP (Table 12.2). Viral exanthema and drug reactions

are the most common causes of large CD30-positive cells in cutaneous pseudolymphomatous infiltrates. LyP is often mistaken for insect bite, scabies, and pityriasis lichenoides, all of which can have positive staining for CD30 antigen (Fig. 12.13 and Table 12.3). Melanoma may infrequently express CD30 antigen (Polski and Janney 1999). However, the combination of other markers for melanoma, e.g., MART-1, Melan-A,

Table 12.3 Comparison of different LyP histologic types

LyP type	A	B	C	D	E	6p25.3 rearrangement
Pattern	Perivascular and wedge shaped	Epidermotropic	Extensive dermal infiltration	Remarkably pagetoid and perivascular	Angio-invasive	Biphasic epidermotropic and dermal nodule
						Folliculo- and eccrinotropic
Cytology	Immunoblasts, large anaplastic cells, RS-like cells, apoptotic bodies	Cerebriform cells (CMC)	Immunoblasts; sometimes a spectrum of CMC and immunoblasts	Intraepidermal midsized atypical pleomorphic lymphocytes	Small to medium to large atypical pleomorphic lymphocytes	Small to medium size with irregular nuclei in the epidermis
						Medium to large size in the dermis
Inflammatory cells	Numerous	Few	Few to moderate	Few	Focal collections of eosinophils and neutrophils	Few
Mitoses	Frequent	Infrequent	Frequent	Not described	Not described	In dermal component
Immunophenotype	CD30+, CD4+	CD30−/+, CD4+	CD30+, CD4+	CD30+, CD8+	CD30+, CD8+	CD30+, double negative
Regression	4–6 weeks	8–12 weeks	Slow and incomplete	Complete	Recurrences common	Complete

and tyrosinase, will resolve the problem (Shidham et al. 2003).

Pityriasis lichenoides et varioliformis acuta (PLEVA) resembles LyP clinically (Fig. 12.13). It is more often seen in children. Skin lesions in PLEVA appear hemorrhagic and lack the central white core comprised on inflammatory cells often seen in LyP. Importantly, PLEVA usually has a limited clinical course, and the association with malignant lymphomas is controversial (Gelmetti et al. 1990; Magro et al. 2007; Boccara et al. 2012). PLEVA can evolve to pityriasis lichenoides chronica (PLC). An interface dermatitis pattern with basal vacuolation of the epidermis, individual necrotic keratinocytes with Civatte (cytoid) bodies, and extravasation of erythrocytes in the papillary dermis are far more common in PLEVA than in LyP (Fig. 12.14). These features are also present but less frequent in pityriasis lichenoides chronica (PLC) (Fig. 12.15).

Neutrophils and eosinophils which are often numerous in LyP are generally lacking in PLEVA and PLC. Whereas the atypical cells in LyP are CD30+, usually CD4+, the predominant T-cell infiltrate in PLEVA is CD8+ and CD30-. Keratinocytes in PLEVA express HLA-DR. The immunohistochemical distinction between LyP and PLC is more difficult because CD4+ lymphocytes are more common than CD8+ cells in PLC (Kim et al. 2011).

Kempf recently described a variant of PLEVA with numerous CD30+ cells (Kempf et al. 2012). The patient cohort included ten female and three male patients whose ages at diagnosis ranged from 7 to 89 years (mean 41 y; median 39 y). The clinical manifestation was that of PLEVA, with small erythematous macules quickly evolving into necrotic papules. No waxing and waning was seen on follow-up in any of the cases. Histopathologically, typical features

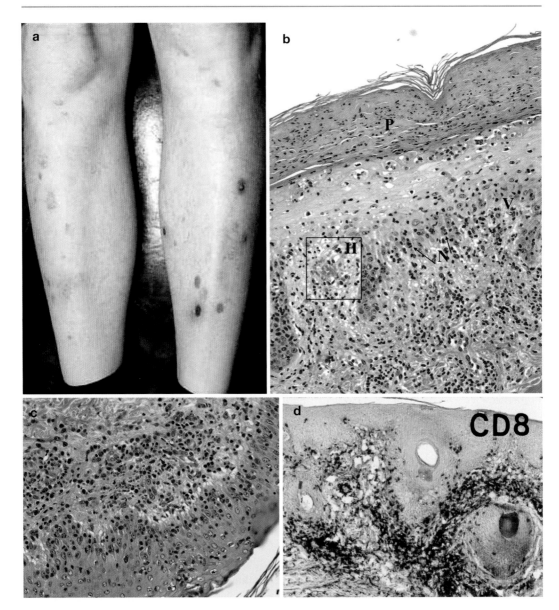

Fig. 12.14 Pityriasis lichenoides et varioliformis acuta (PLEVA). (**a**) Clinical photograph showing multiple hemorrhagic necrotic lesions (Permission pending from Elsevier). (**b**) Parakeratosis (*P*), hemorrhage (*H*), necrotic keratinocytes (*N*), and vacuolar change (*V*). (**c**) Necrotic keratinocytes (*circles*), vacuolar change, and extravasated erythrocytes. (**d**) CD8 stains most interface lymphocytes

of PLEVA were present, but an unusual finding was occurrence of a considerable number of CD30 small lymphocytes as detected immuno-histochemically. Over half of the cases also displayed a large number of CD8 cells and showed coexpression of CD8 and CD30 in the intraepidermal and dermal component of the infiltrate. Of the 11 cases of PLEVA studied for T-cell receptor gene rearrangement, six evidenced a monoclonal T-cell population, and five were polyclonal. Parvovirus B19 (PVB19) DNA was identified in four of ten cases investigated, and positive serology was observed for PVB19 in two patients, altogether suggesting that PVB19 is pathogenetically linked to PLEVA at least in a subset of cases. The main significance of this

PLEVA variant is, however, its potential confusion with LyP or some cytotoxic lymphomas.

Plaza recently reported cutaneous CD30-positive lymphoproliferative disorders with CD8 expression (Plaza et al. 2013). CD8+ cases of LyP were predominated by small lymphocytes exhibiting a prominent epidermotropic pattern consistent with either type B or type D LyP. Four

cases showed coexpression of CD56. The ALCL cases included myxoid features, pseudoepitheliomatous change, and an intravascular component. In all cases that were primary in the skin, an indolent clinical course was seen while one patient with systemic myxoid ALCL is in remission following systemic multiagent chemotherapy. The paucity of neutrophils and eosinophils and

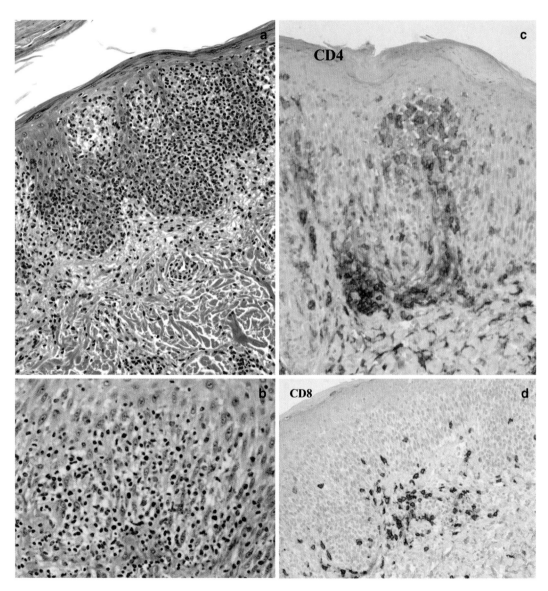

Fig. 12.15 Pityriasis lichenoides chronica (PLC). (**a**) Numerous intraepidermal lymphocytes. (**b**) Interface pattern with vacuolar change. (**c**) Most intraepidermal lymphocytes are CD4+. (**d**) Minor population of CD8+ lymphocytes within the epidermis and adjacent papillary dermis. (**e**) Numerous pink Civatte (cytoid) bodies are seen

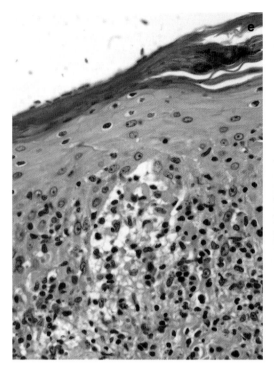

Fig. 12.15 (continued)

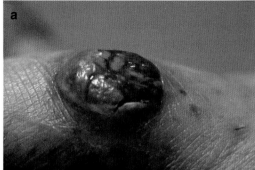

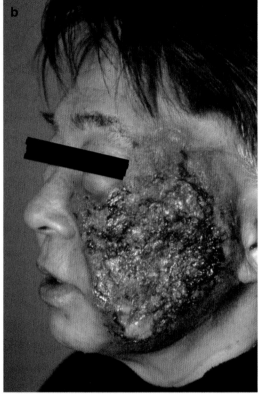

concomitant granulomatous inflammation were distinctive features in cases of type B and type D LyP. CD30 and CD45R0 positivity and a clinical course typical of LyP were useful in differentiating features from an aggressive cytotoxic CD8+ T-cell lymphoma. In all cases that were primary in the skin, an indolent clinical course was observed. CD45 R0 positivity and a clinical course typical of LyP were useful in preventing a misdiagnosis of an aggressive cytotoxic CD8+ T-cell lymphoma.

The border between LyP and C-ALCL is sometimes difficult to discern. Such lesions have been referred to as borderline lesions. MUM1 expression does not differentiate LyP and C-ALCL (Hernandez-Machin et al. 2009). Most borderline lesions would be classified as either LyP type C or pcALCL, both of which probably carry a higher risk of spread to regional lymph nodes. Fortunately, patients with one draining lymph node site have a good prognosis similar to those who have c-ALCL without concurrent lymph node involvement (Bekkenk et al. 2000).

Fig. 12.16 Clinical appearance of primary cutaneous anaplastic large cell lymphoma. (**a**) An ulcerated lesion on the arm. (**b**) Large ulcerated facial tumor

Primary Cutaneous ALCL

Clinical Features

Primary cutaneous ALCL comprises one or more tumor nodules exceeding 2 cm in diameter (Fig. 12.16). While often individual, multiple

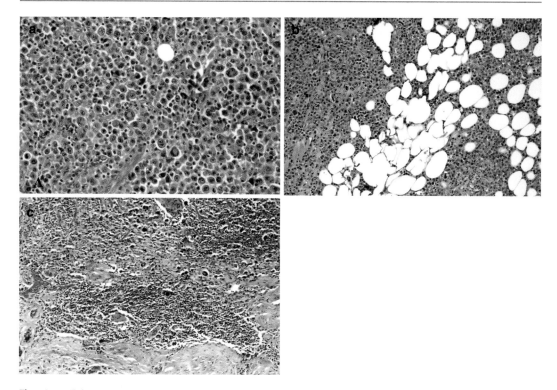

Fig. 12.17 Primary cutaneous anaplastic large cell lymphoma. (**a**) Sheets of anaplastic cells with prominent nucleoli. (**b**) Anaplastic cells infiltrating subcutis. (**c**) Small "reactive" lymphocytes surround large anaplastic cells near edge of tumor

nodules can occur and up to 25 % may show some degree of spontaneous regression. Tumor nodules are often purplish red and frequently become ulcerated. Most common sites are trunk and extremities, but facial lesions occur. Unlike systemic CD30-positive ALCL or tumor stage mycosis fungoides (T-MF), the prognosis of cutaneous ALCL (C-ALCL) is excellent, with a 10-year survival of over 90 % (Diez-Martin et al. 2009). Extracutaneous spread of C-ALCL occurs in only 10 % of cases, and when limited to the draining regional lymph node, such progression does not alter prognosis (Bekkenk et al. 2000).

Histology

The dermis is occupied by sheets of large anaplastic/pleomorphic cells with prominent nucleoli and basophilic cytoplasm (Fig. 12.17). The infiltrate typically extends into the subcutis, a distinguishing feature from LyP type C or borderline lesions. Small reactive lymphocytes are usually confined to the lateral and deep borders of the infiltrate, in contrast to LyP where they surround the large atypical cells. Mitoses and apoptotic bodies are frequent. Inflammatory cells vary but may be numerous as in neutrophil-rich or eosinophil-rich ALCL (Burg et al. 2003) (Fig. 12.18). The epidermis is often spared with a so-called Grenz zone (Fig. 12.19). Adnexa may be heavily infiltrated or replaced by the infiltrate.

Immunophenotype

Tumor cells are CD30+, usually CD4+, but may be CD8+. There is often loss of CD3, CD2, and/or CD5. Cytotoxic proteins (TIA-1, granzyme B, and perforin) are usually present. ALK is usually absent but when present is generally cytoplasmic

Fig. 12.18 Neutrophil-rich anaplastic large cell lymphoma. Numerous neutrophils appear to "attack" tumor cells and cause apoptosis (highlighted in *rectangles*)

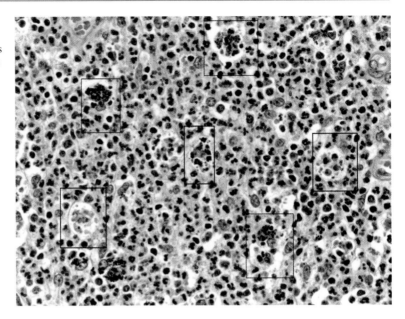

Genetics

Usual Absence of t(2;5)(p23;q35): We studied 43 cases of cutaneous and nodal CD30+ LPDs using reverse transcriptase-polymerase chain reaction (RT-PCR) and/or immunohistochemistry. We found no evidence for the t(2; 5) translocation in 14 cases of primary cutaneous CD30+ LPDs, which included ten cases of LyP, three cases of primary cutaneous CD30+ ALCL, and one borderline case. These findings were in marked contrast to CD30+ ALCL of nodal origin, in which 19 of 29 (66 %) cases were positive for t(2;5), including all five cases with secondary skin involvement (DeCoteau et al. 1996).

The t(2;5) generates a chimeric NPM-ALK transcript encoded by the nucleophosmin (NPM) gene fused to the anaplastic lymphoma kinase gene (ALK). Using an RT-PCR assay, Beylot-Barry detected NPM-ALK transcripts within a minority of CD30+ primary cutaneous T-cell lymphomas. The t(2;5) was identified in 4 out of 9 CD30+ ALCL and in 1 out of 4 CD30+ pleomorphic lymphomas. Moreover, the t(2;5) was detected in 3 of 10 LyPs. All NPM-ALK-positive lymphomas and 1 NPM-ALK-positive LyP exhibited a clonal rearrangement of the TCR-gamma chain gene. The t(2;5) was detected in two cases of LyP without other evidence for a

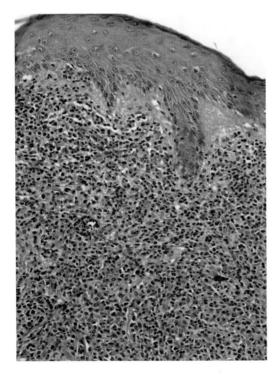

Fig. 12.19 Primary cutaneous anaplastic large cell lymphoma—sparing of the epidermis with uninvolved Grenz zone above dermal component

only (Kadin et al. 2008) (Fig. 12.20). EMA is usually absent in contrast to systemic ALCL. CLA is usually present (de Bruin et al. 1993).

Fig. 12.20 Primary cutaneous anaplastic large cell lymphoma—cytoplasmic staining of ALK

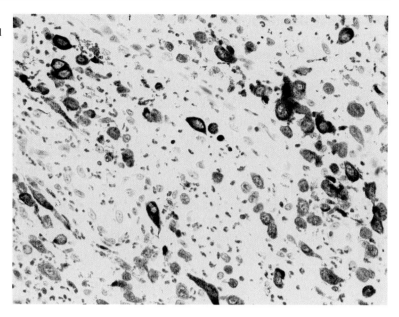

clonal lymphoid population. To identify cells carrying the t(2;5) translocation, they used immunohistochemistry to detect the ALK-encoded p80 protein and in situ hybridization for the specific detection of NPM-ALK transcripts. Both p80 protein and NPM-ALK transcripts were expressed by anaplastic or large CD30+ lymphoma cells with positive NPM-ALK amplification. The presence of t(2;5) in a subset of CD30+ cutaneous lymphomas and LyP may indicate a common pathogenesis with a subset of anaplastic nodal lymphoma (Beylot-Barry et al. 1996).

Approximately 25 % of primary cutaneous ALCL carry a 6p25.3 rearrangement involving DUSP22. Feldman et al. reported IRF4 (interferon regulatory factor-4) translocations in cutaneous ALCL (Feldman et al. 2009). In an expanded study, they investigated the clinical utility of detecting IRF4 translocations in skin biopsies. They performed fluorescence in situ hybridization (FISH) for IRF4 in 204 biopsies involved by T-cell lymphoproliferative disorders from 182 patients at three institutions. In all, 9 of 45 (20 %) cutaneous ALCL and 1 of 32 (3 %) cases of LyP with informative results demonstrated an IRF4 translocation. The one LyP case was the first encountered of the LyP series with 6p23.5 rearrangements described above.

Remaining informative cases were negative for a translocation (7 systemic anaplastic large cell lymphomas; 44 cases of mycosis fungoides/Sezary syndrome (13 transformed); 24 peripheral T-cell lymphomas, not otherwise specified; 12 CD4-positive small/medium-sized pleomorphic T-cell lymphomas; 5 extranodal NK/T-cell lymphomas, nasal type; 4 gamma-delta T-cell lymphomas; and 5 other uncommon T-cell lymphoproliferative disorders). Among all cutaneous T-cell lymphoproliferative disorders, FISH for IRF4 had a specificity and positive predictive value for cutaneous ALCL of 99 and 90 %, respectively ($P=0.00002$, Fisher's exact test). Among anaplastic large cell lymphomas, lymphomatoid papulosis, and transformed mycosis fungoides, specificity and positive predictive value were 98 and 90 %, respectively ($P=0.005$).

Transcription factor JUNB is overexpressed in primary cutaneous ALCL. Using genomic microarray, Mao reported amplification of JUNB in seven of ten cases of primary cutaneous CD30(+) anaplastic large cell lymphoma (Mao et al. 2003). We found that JunB is induced by constitutive CD30-extracellular signal-regulated kinase 1/2 mitogen-activated protein kinase signaling and activates the CD30 promoter in anaplastic large cell lymphoma (Watanabe et al. 2005).

Differential Diagnosis

Secondary Skin Lesions of Systemic ALCL

A most important distinction is that of primary cutaneous ALCL from secondary skin lesions in systemic ALCL. Histologically, there is little difference. Expression of EMA and little or no expression of CLA on tumor cells favors systemic ALCL. The lack of ALK and cytogenetic or molecular evidence of t(2;5)(p23;q35) or NPM-ALK, respectively, supports a diagnosis of primary cutaneous ALCL. However, it should be noted as above that some primary cutaneous ALCL stain for cytoplasmic ALK activity (Kadin et al. 2008).

Large Cell Transformation of MF

One of the most difficult differential diagnoses of primary cutaneous ALCL is large cell transformation of MF which carries a worse prognosis (Benner et al. 2012) (Fig. 12.21). The large MF cells occur in sheets and are usually CD30+, both features shared with C-ALCL. The diagnosis of large cell transformation of MF is generally made clinically when there are accompanying patches and plaques typical of MF. MF tumors with large cell transformation often contain a spectrum of lymphocytes with convoluted nuclei generally lacking in primary cutaneous ALCL. Epidermotropism of CD30+ cells favors large cell transformation MF over primary cutaneous ALCL.

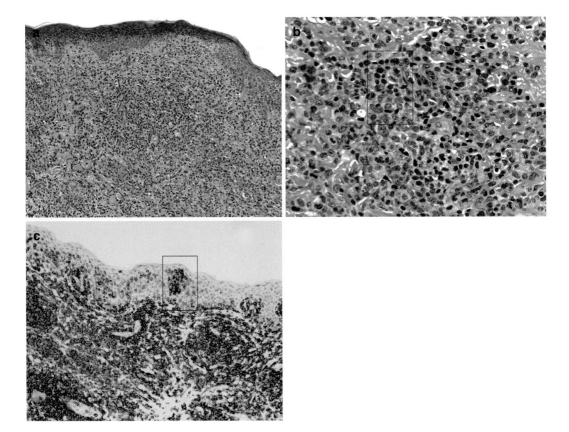

Fig. 12.21 Large cell transformation of mycosis fungoides (LCT-MF). (**a**) More than 25 % of cells are large cells. (**b**) There is a spectrum of cell types (*rectangle*) ranging from small cells with dark staining convoluted nuclei to large cells with open chromatin and convoluted nuclei. These features distinguish LCT-MF from ALCL occurring in MF. (**c**) CD30 stain shows CD30+ cells within the epidermis (*rectangle*)

Neutrophil-Rich ALCL

Neutrophil-rich ALCL can be mistaken for an infectious or other inflammatory process. Tumor cells are obscured by the numerous granulocytes (Fig. 12.18). In such instances, tumor cells may be revealed by staining for CD30 (Kato et al. 2003). In two cases, a strong correlation between tumor growth and interleukin (IL)-8 cytokine pattern as well as the production of IL-8 by tumor cells was demonstrated. The diagnosis of neutrophil-rich ALCL is challenging clinically and histologically as the tumor cell compartment is masked by an extensive inflammatory infiltrate of neutrophils and other reactive cells such as histiocytes which may be mainly due to release of IL-8 by tumor cells (Burg et al. 2003).

LyPs with 6p25.3 rearrangement are easily mistaken for C-ALCL by histology due to the extensive large cell dermal infiltrate, frequent mitoses, and apoptosis. However, LyPs with 6p25.3 have a distinctive epitheliotropism of smaller sometimes cerebriform lymphocytes and often pagetoid appearance. Clinically, the patients with 6p25.3 rearrangements tend to be elderly (over age 50) and have smaller self-healing lesions.

References

Basarab T, Fraser-Andrews EA, Orchard G, Whittaker S, Russel-Jones R. Lymphomatoid papulosis in association with mycosis fungoides: a study of 15 cases. Br J Dermatol. 1998;139:630–8.

Bekkenk MW, Geelen FA, van Voorst Vader PC, Heule F, Geerts ML, van Vloten WA, et al. Primary and secondary cutaneous CD30(+) lymphoproliferative disorders: a report from the Dutch Cutaneous Lymphoma Group on the long-term follow-up data of 219 patients and guidelines for diagnosis and treatment. Blood. 2000;95:3653–61.

Beljaards RC, Willemze R. The prognosis of patients with lymphomatoid papulosis associated with malignant lymphomas. Br J Dermatol. 1992;126:596–602.

Benner MF, Jansen PM, Vermeer MH, Willemze R. Prognostic factors in transformed mycosis fungoides: a retrospective analysis of 100 cases. Blood. 2012;119:1643–9.

Beylot-Barry M, Lamant L, Vergier B, de Muret A, Fraitag S, Delord B, et al. Detection of t(2;5)(p23;q35) translocation by reverse transcriptase polymerase chain reaction and in situ hybridization in CD30-positive primary cutaneous lymphoma and lymphomatoid papulosis. Am J Pathol. 1996;149:483–92.

Boccara O, Blanche S, de Prost Y, Brousse N, Bodemer C, Fraitag S. Cutaneous hematologic disorders in children. Pediatr Blood Cancer. 2012;58:226–32.

Burg G, Kempf W, Kazakov DV, Dummer R, Frosch PJ, Lange-Ionescu S, et al. Pyogenic lymphoma of the skin: a peculiar variant of primary cutaneous neutrophil-rich CD30+ anaplastic large-cell lymphoma. Clinicopathological study of four cases and review of the literature. Br J Dermatol. 2003;148:580–6.

Cabanillas F, Armitage J, Pugh WC, Weisenburger D, Duvic M. Lymphomatoid papulosis: a T-cell dyscrasia with a propensity to transform into malignant lymphoma. Ann Intern Med. 1995;122:210–7.

Cappelin D, Idrissi Y, Prochazkova-Carlotti M, Lahranne E, De Sousa Goes AC, et al. Chromosomal rearrangements at 6p25.3 in cutaneous T-cell lymphomas highlight the role of the DUSP22-phosphatase in oncogenesis. In: The International Program Committee and Local Organizing Committee, editors. Proceedings of 2nd world congress of cutaneous lymphomas; 2013; Berlin.

Chott A, Vonderheid EC, Olbricht S, Miao NN, Balk SP, Kadin ME. The dominant T cell clone is present in multiple regressing skin lesions and associated T cell lymphomas of patients with lymphomatoid papulosis. J Invest Dermatol. 1996;106:696–700.

Csikesz CR, Knudson RA, Greipp PT, Feldman AL, Kadin M. Primary cutaneous CD30-positive T-cell lymphoproliferative disorders with biallelic rearrangements of DUSP22. J Invest Dermatol. 2013;133:1680–2.

Davis TH, Morton CC, Miller-Cassman R, Balk SP, Kadin ME. Hodgkin's disease, lymphomatoid papulosis, and cutaneous T-cell lymphoma derived from a common T-cell clone. N Engl J Med. 1992;326:1115–22.

de Bruin PC, Beljaards RC, van Heerde P, Van Der Valk P, Noorduyn LA, Van Krieken JH, et al. Differences in clinical behaviour and immunophenotype between primary cutaneous and primary nodal anaplastic large cell lymphoma of T-cell or null cell phenotype. Histopathology. 1993;23:127–35.

DeCoteau JF, Butmarc JR, Kinney MC, Kadin ME. The t(2;5) chromosomal translocation is not a common feature of primary cutaneous CD30+ lymphoproliferative disorders: comparison with anaplastic large-cell lymphoma of nodal origin. Blood. 1996;87:3437–41.

Diez-Martin JL, Balsalobre P, Re A, Michieli M, Ribera JM, Canals C, et al. Comparable survival between HIV+ and HIV- non-Hodgkin and Hodgkin lymphoma patients undergoing autologous peripheral blood stem cell transplantation. Blood. 2009;113:6011–4.

El Shabrawi-Caelen L, Kerl H, Cerroni L. Lymphomatoid papulosis: reappraisal of clinicopathologic presentation and classification into subtypes A, B, and C. Arch Dermatol. 2004;140:441–7.

el-Azhary RA, Gibson LE, Kurtin PJ, Pittelkow MR, Muller SA. Lymphomatoid papulosis: a clinical and histopathologic review of 53 cases with leukocyte immunophenotyping, DNA flow cytometry, and T-cell receptor gene rearrangement studies. J Am Acad Dermatol. 1994;30:210–8.

Feldman AL, Law M, Remstein ED, Macon WR, Erickson LA, Grogg KL, et al. Recurrent translocations involving the IRF4 oncogene locus in peripheral T-cell lymphomas. Leukemia. 2009;23:574–80.

Gellrich S, Wernicke M, Wilks A, Lukowsky A, Muche JM, Jasch KC, et al. The cell infiltrate in lymphomatoid papulosis comprises a mixture of polyclonal large atypical cells (CD30-positive) and smaller monoclonal T cells (CD30-negative). J Invest Dermatol. 2004;122:859–61.

Gelmetti C, Rigoni C, Alessi E, Ermacora E, Berti E, Caputo R. Pityriasis lichenoides in children: a long-term follow-up of eighty-nine cases. J Am Acad Dermatol. 1990;23:473–8.

Hernandez-Machin B, de Misa RF, Montenegro T, Rivero JC, Bastida J, Febles C, et al. MUM1 expression does not differentiate primary cutaneous anaplastic large-cell lymphoma and lymphomatoid papulosis. Br J Dermatol. 2009;160:713.

Humme D, Lukowsky A, Steinhoff M, Beyer M, Walden P, Sterry W, et al. Dominance of nonmalignant T-cell clones and distortion of the TCR repertoire in the peripheral blood of patients with cutaneous CD30+ lymphoproliferative disorders. J Invest Dermatol. 2009;129:89–98.

Kadin ME. Current management of primary cutaneous CD30+ T-cell lymphoproliferative disorders. Oncology (Williston Park). 2009;23:1158–64.

Kadin M, Nasu K, Sako D, Said J, Vonderheid E. Lymphomatoid papulosis. A cutaneous proliferation of activated helper T cells expressing Hodgkin's disease-associated antigens. Am J Pathol. 1985;119:315–25.

Kadin ME, Pinkus JL, Pinkus GS, Duran IH, Fuller CE, Onciu M, et al. Primary cutaneous ALCL with phosphorylated/activated cytoplasmic ALK and novel phenotype: EMA/MUC1+, cutaneous lymphocyte antigen negative. Am J Surg Pathol. 2008;32:1421–6.

Karai LJ, Kadin ME, Hsi ED, Sluzevich JC, Ketterling RP, Knudson RA, et al. Chromosomal rearrangements of 6p25.3 define a new subtype of lymphomatoid papulosis. Am J Surg Pathol. 2013;37:1173–81.

Kato N, Tomita Y, Yoshida K, Hisai H. Involvement of the tongue by lymphomatoid papulosis. Am J Dermatopathol. 1998;20:522–6.

Kato N, Mizuno O, Ito K, Kimura K, Shibata M. Neutrophil-rich anaplastic large cell lymphoma presenting in the skin. Am J Dermatopathol. 2003;25:142–7.

Kempf W, Kazakov DV, Palmedo G, Fraitag S, Schaerer L, Kutzner H. Pityriasis lichenoides et varioliformis acuta with numerous CD30(+) cells: a variant mimicking lymphomatoid papulosis and other cutaneous lymphomas. A clinicopathologic, immunohistochemical, and molecular biological study of 13 cases. Am J Surg Pathol. 2012;36:1021–9.

Kempf W, Kazakov DV, Scharer L, Rutten A, Mentzel T, Paredes BE, et al. Angioinvasive lymphomatoid papulosis: a new variant simulating aggressive lymphomas. Am J Surg Pathol. 2013;37:1–13.

Kim JE, Yun WJ, Mun SK, Yoon GS, Huh J, Choi JH, et al. Pityriasis lichenoides et varioliformis acuta and pityriasis lichenoides chronica: comparison of lesional T-cell subsets and investigation of viral associations. J Cutan Pathol. 2011;38:649–56.

Kummer JA, Vermeer MH, Dukers D, Meijer CJ, Willemze R. Most primary cutaneous CD30-positive lymphoproliferative disorders have a CD4-positive cytotoxic T-cell phenotype. J Invest Dermatol. 1997;109:636–40.

Lee JS, Park MY, Kim YJ, Kil HI, Choi YH, Kim YC. Histopathological features in both the eschar and erythematous lesions of Tsutsugamushi Disease: identification of CD30+ cell infiltration in Tsutsugamushi disease. The American Journal of dermatopathology 2009;31:551–6.

Macaulay WL. Lymphomatoid papulosis. A continuing self-healing eruption, clinically benign–histologically malignant. Arch Dermatol. 1968;97:23–30.

Magro CM, Crowson AN, Morrison C, Merati K, Porcu P, Wright ED. CD8+ lymphomatoid papulosis and its differential diagnosis. Am J Clin Pathol. 2006;125:490–501.

Magro CM, Crowson AN, Morrison C, Li J. Pityriasis lichenoides chronica: stratification by molecular and phenotypic profile. Hum Pathol. 2007;38:479–90.

Mao X, Orchard G, Lillington DM, Russell-Jones R, Young BD, Whittaker SJ. Amplification and overexpression of JUNB is associated with primary cutaneous T-cell lymphomas. Blood. 2003;101:1513–9.

Nijsten T, Curiel-Lewandrowski C, Kadin ME. Lymphomatoid papulosis in children: a retrospective cohort study of 35 cases. Arch Dermatol. 2004;140:306–12.

Peters K, Knoll JH, Kadin ME. Cytogenetic findings in regressing skin lesions of lymphomatoid papulosis. Cancer Genet Cytogenet. 1995;80:13–6.

Plaza JA, Feldman AL, Magro C. Cutaneous CD30-positive lymphoproliferative disorders with CD8 expression: a clinicopathologic study of 21 cases. J Cutan Pathol. 2013;40:236–47.

Polski JM, Janney CG. Ber-H2 (CD30) immunohistochemical staining in malignant melanoma. Mod Pathol. 1999;12:903–6.

Pulitzer MP, Nolan KA, Oshman RG, Phelps RG. CD30+ Lymphomatoid Drug Reactions. Am J Dermatopathol 2013;35:343–50.

Ralfkiaer E, Bosq J, Gatter KC, Schwarting R, Gerdes J, Stein H, et al. Expression of a Hodgkin and Reed-Sternberg cell associated antigen (Ki-1) in cutaneous lymphoid infiltrates. Arch Dermatol Res. 1987;279:285–92.

Riboni R, Lucioni M, Araini L, Marta N, Maffie A, Dallera E, et al. High rate of TCR gamma gene rearrangement with clonal identity of microdissected CD30+ cells from lymphomatoid papulosis (LyP). In: The international program committee and Local Organizing Committee, editors. Proceedings of 2nd world congress of cutaneous lymphomas; 2013; Berlin.

Saggini A, Gulia A, Argenyi Z, Fink-Puches R, Lissia A, Magana M, et al. A variant of lymphomatoid papulosis simulating primary cutaneous aggressive epidermotropic CD8+ cytotoxic T-cell lymphoma. Description of 9 cases. Am J Surg Pathol. 2010;34:1168–75.

Schiemann WP, Pfeifer WM, Levi E, Kadin ME, Lodish HF. A deletion in the gene for transforming growth factor beta type I receptor abolishes growth regulation by transforming growth factor beta in a cutaneous T-cell lymphoma. Blood. 1999;94:2854–61.

Shidham VB, Qi D, Rao RN, Acker SM, Chang CC, Kampalath B, et al. Improved immunohistochemical evaluation of micrometastases in sentinel lymph nodes of cutaneous melanoma with 'MCW melanoma cocktail'–a mixture of monoclonal antibodies to MART-1, Melan-A, and tyrosinase. BMC Cancer. 2003;3:15.

Steinhoff M, Hummel M, Anagnostopoulos I, Kaudewitz P, Seitz V, Assaf C, et al. Single-cell analysis of CD30+ cells in lymphomatoid papulosis demonstrates a common clonal T-cell origin. Blood. 2002;100:578–84.

Volkenandt M, Bertino JR, Shenoy BV, Koch OM, Kadin ME. Molecular evidence for a clonal relationship between lymphomatoid papulosis and Ki-1 positive large cell anaplastic lymphoma. J Dermatol Sci. 1993;6:121–6.

Wang HH, Lach L, Kadin ME. Epidemiology of lymphomatoid papulosis. Cancer. 1992;70:2951–7.

Wang HH, Myers T, Lach LJ, Hsieh CC, Kadin ME. Increased risk of lymphoid and nonlymphoid malignancies in patients with lymphomatoid papulosis. Cancer. 1999;86:1240–5.

Watanabe M, Sasaki M, Itoh K, Higashihara M, Umezawa K, Kadin ME, et al. JunB induced by constitutive CD30-extracellular signal-regulated kinase 1/2 mitogen-activated protein kinase signaling activates the CD30 promoter in anaplastic large cell lymphoma and reed-sternberg cells of Hodgkin lymphoma. Cancer Res. 2005;65:7628–34.

Werner B, Massone C, Kerl H, Cerroni L. Large CD30-positive cells in benign, atypical lymphoid infiltrates of the skin. J Cutan Pathol 2008;35:1100–7.

Wood GS, Crooks CF, Uluer AZ. Lymphomatoid papulosis and associated cutaneous lymphoproliferative disorders exhibit a common clonal origin. J Invest Dermatol. 1995;105:51–5.

Lymphohistiocytic and Granulomatous Dermatitis

13

May P. Chan

Kikuchi-Fujimoto Lymphohistiocytic Skin Lesion

Introduction

Kikuchi-Fujimoto disease (KFD) is a self-limited histiocytic necrotizing lymphadenitis of unknown etiology. Many potential causative agents have been proposed, including Epstein-Barr virus (EBV) (Yen et al. 1997), human herpesvirus-6 (HHV-6) (Sumiyoshi et al. 1993), and parvovirus B19 (Zhang et al. 2007), but subsequent confirmatory studies failed to validate direct causality (Hollingsworth et al. 1994; George et al. 2003; Kim et al. 2010).

Diagnosis of KFD requires histologic demonstration of nodal or extranodal tissue necrosis showing abundant histiocytes with karyorrhectic debris but distinctly lacking neutrophilic response (Fujimoto et al. 1972; Kikuchi 1972). Up to 40 % of patients with KFD develop skin eruption, which is the focus of this discussion.

Clinical Features

Kikuchi-Fujimoto disease most often affects young Asians under 40 years of age, with a slight

female predilection (Kim et al. 2010). The clinical hallmarks of KFD are fever and cervical lymphadenopathy, although infrequently other lymph nodes may also be involved (Fujimoto et al. 1972; Kikuchi 1972). The skin is the most common extranodal site of involvement. Clinically, the cutaneous eruptions are relatively nonspecific but most commonly described as "rash," erythematous macules, patches, papules, or plaques (Atwater et al. 2008). The upper body including the face is typically affected (Spies et al. 1999; Kim et al. 2010). The skin lesions may precede, follow, or develop simultaneously with the lymphadenopathy (Kim et al. 2010).

Kikuchi-Fujimoto disease usually affects otherwise healthy individuals. Association with other diseases is relatively rare and, if found, largely those of autoimmune disorders (Sopeña et al. 2012). Aside from systemic lupus erythematosus, which is a close mimic and may be a related disorder of KFD, other autoimmune conditions such as antiphospholipid syndrome, autoimmune thyroiditis, Sjögren's syndrome, and autoimmune hepatitis have also been reported in patients with KFD (Papaioannou et al. 2002; Santana et al. 2005; Paradela et al. 2008; Shusang et al. 2008; Cheng et al. 2010; Vassilakopoulos et al. 2010; Go et al. 2012).

Histopathology

The most common finding in the skin lesions of KFD is a lymphohistiocytic infiltrate associated

M.P. Chan, MD
Departments of Pathology and Dermatology,
University of Michigan Health System,
1301 Catherine Street, Medical Science I, M3261,
Ann Arbor, MI 48109, USA
e-mail: mpchan@med.umich.edu

with non-neutrophilic karyorrhectic debris. The infiltrate involves the superficial and deep dermis and may extend into the subcutis (Atwater et al. 2008; Kim et al. 2010), often with accentuation around blood vessels and adnexal structures (Aqel et al. 1997) (Fig. 13.1). In addition to the predominance of phagocytic histiocytes, the infiltrate is also composed of crescentic macrophages and plasmacytoid monocytes similar to those described in nodal KFD (Spies et al. 1999). Crescentic macrophages are characterized by pale cytoplasm and eccentric U-shaped to crenelated nuclei pushed against the cell membrane (Fig. 13.2 and periphery of Fig. 13.3), whereas plasmacytoid monocytes are usually smaller and ovoid, with purplish cytoplasm and round basophilic nuclei (Fig. 13.3 and periphery of Fig. 13.2). The lymphocytes range from small to medium in size and may appear slightly atypical. The karyorrhectic debris is composed of nuclear dusts in the absence of neutrophils (Fig. 13.4). Another common finding is vacuolar interface change with necrotic keratinocytes (Fig. 13.5). Other histologic changes reported in over 10 % of cases include parakeratosis, papillary dermal edema, mucin deposition, and panniculitis. Plasma cells and eosinophils have been observed only in a small number of cases. The diagnostic criteria for cutaneous KFD as proposed by Kim et al. are listed in Table 13.1 (Kim et al. 2010).

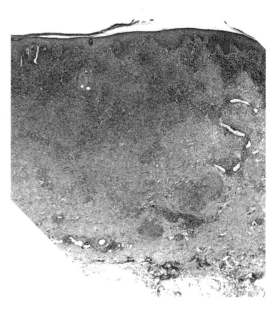

Fig. 13.1 Cutaneous lesion of Kikuchi-Fujimoto disease (KFD). Low magnification shows a brisk lymphoid infiltrate involving the superficial to deep dermis, with accentuation around blood vessels and adnexal structures (Courtesy of Dr. Hernani Cualing)

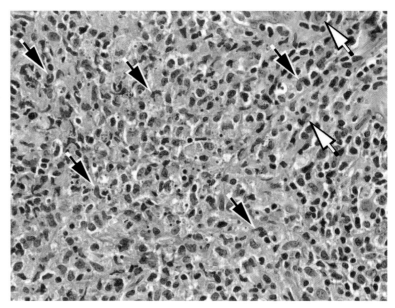

Fig. 13.2 Cutaneous lesion of KFD. The infiltrate in KFD consists of many crescentic macrophages containing pale cytoplasm and eccentric nuclei compressed into a U-shaped crescent against the cell membrane (*black arrows*). There are scattered karyorrhectic debris, but neutrophils are notably absent. Few plasmacytoid monocytes are also present at the periphery of this photomicrograph (*white arrows*) (Courtesy of Dr. Hernani Cualing)

Fig. 13.3 Cutaneous lesion of KFD. Several plasmacytoid monocytes are present in the perivascular infiltrate. Plasmacytoid monocytes contain scant cytoplasm and relatively small, round, and dark nuclei resembling plasma cells (*black arrows*). Few crescentic macrophages are also present at the periphery of this photomicrograph (*white arrows*) (Courtesy of Dr. Hernani Cualing)

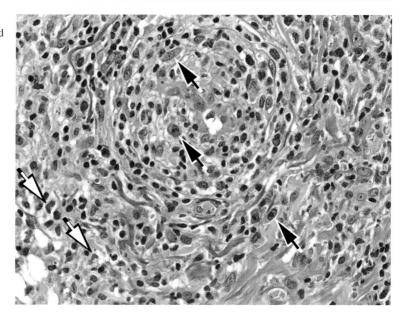

Fig. 13.4 Cutaneous lesion of KFD. A small necrotic focus is present amidst the lymphohistiocytic infiltrate. There is prominent karyorrhexis in the absence of neutrophils (Courtesy of Dr. Hernani Cualing)

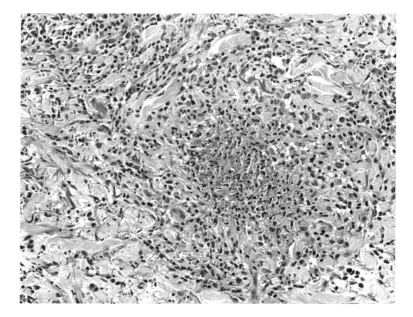

Immunophenotype

The lymphocytes in the skin lesions of KFD are CD3-positive T cells. In most cases, there are slightly more CD8-positive cytotoxic T cells than CD4-positive helper T cells (Kim et al. 2010). Only rare cells express CD30 and TIA-1 (Spies et al. 1999). The histiocytes are positive for CD68 (Fig. 13.6), CD163, and myeloperoxidase (MPO) (Pileri et al. 2001; Fernandez-Flores et al. 2008). In particular, the plasmacytoid monocytes also express CD123 but are negative for fascin, suggesting an immature dendritic cell phenotype (Pilichowska et al. 2009). Occasional cases may demonstrate EBV, HHV-6, parvovirus B19, and other viral

Fig. 13.5 Cutaneous lesion of KFD. The epidermis demonstrates basal vacuolar degeneration consistent with vacuolar interface dermatitis (Courtesy of Dr. Hernani Cualing)

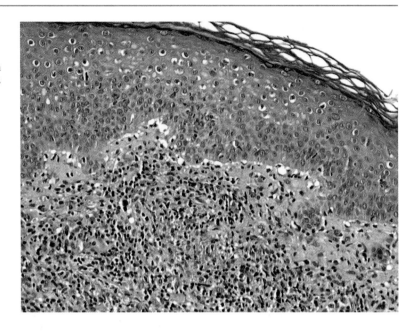

Table 13.1 Diagnostic criteria for the cutaneous lesions of Kikuchi-Fujimoto disease

Major criteria	Minor criteria
1. Presence of karyorrhexis	1. Presence of interface dermatitis
2. Absence of neutrophils	2. Presence of inflammatory cell infiltrate in the reticular dermis or subcutaneous fat
	3. The histiocytes are predominant cells of the inflammatory cells
	4. The CD8-positive cytotoxic T lymphocytes are predominant lymphocytes

Diagnosis requires fulfillment of two major criteria and at least two minor criteria
Reprinted from Kim et al. (2010). With permission from Elsevier

antigens in the atypical lymphocytes by immunohistochemistry, in situ hybridization, or polymerase chain reaction studies (Sumiyoshi et al. 1993; Yen et al. 1997; Zhang et al. 2007).

Genetics and Molecular Findings

A T-cell receptor gene rearrangement study has shown the vast majority of KFD cases to be polyclonal. Although some cases demonstrated oligoclonality at the beta and/or gamma loci, spontaneous resolution of all cases within 6 months supports a benign immune reaction (Lin et al. 2002). A Japanese study examined the HLA class II genes (HLA-DR, HLA-DQ, and HLA-DP) and found significantly higher allele frequencies of DPA1*01 and DPB1*0202 in patients with KFD compared to normal controls (Tanaka et al. 1999). These findings may explain the higher incidence of KFD in Asians as the DPB1*0202 allele is extremely rare in Caucasians and Negroids but relatively frequent in Asians (Imanishi et al. 1992). Another study reported familial occurrence of KFD in two non-twin sisters with identical HLA phenotypes, further suggesting genetic predisposition to the disease (Amir et al. 2002).

Prognosis or Course

Most cases of KFD resolve without intervention within 2–6 months (Spies et al. 1999; Lin et al. 2002). Recurrence is observed in about 15–20 % of patients and is associated with a higher incidence of autoimmune diseases and positive antinuclear antibodies (ANA) (Song et al. 2009; Cheng et al. 2010). While skin involvement alone

Fig. 13.6 Cutaneous lesion of KFD. CD68 highlights many histiocytes in the infiltrate (Courtesy of Dr. Hernani Cualing)

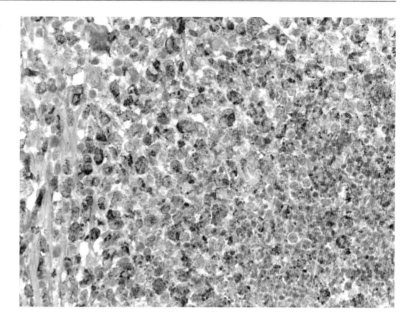

does not seem to be associated with recurrence or development of autoimmune diseases, interface dermatitis was found to be a consistent finding in cases that evolved into systemic lupus erythematosus (Paradela et al. 2008). Long-term follow-up of patients with skin involvement and/or positive ANA is therefore recommended (Cheng et al. 2010).

Differential Diagnosis

The distinction between the skin lesions of KFD and cutaneous lupus erythematosus (LE) can be extremely challenging due to significant histologic overlap, namely, interface dermatitis, dermal mucin deposition, perivascular lymphocytic infiltrate, and panniculitis. The presence of prominent non-neutrophilic karyorrhexis, however, is not a feature of LE. Plasma cells are often present in LE but usually absent or sparse in KFD. Direct immunofluorescence study is useful in confirming LE and excluding KFD when a characteristic "lupus band" (granular immune deposits) is present at the dermoepidermal junction (Kim et al. 2010).

The infiltrate in the cutaneous lesions of KFD may be brisk and, in conjunction with the presence of atypical lymphocytes and larger monocytes, may raise concern for lymphoma. In particular, cases demonstrating subcutaneous involvement by histiocytes, CD8-positive lymphocytes, and karyorrhectic debris may bear close resemblance to subcutaneous panniculitis-like T-cell lymphoma (SPLTCL). However, the absence of rimming of adipocytes by atypical lymphocytes and the significant dermal (and sometimes epidermal) involvement in KFD would help in its distinction from SPLTCL. An immunoprofile showing CD8 predominance and minimal CD56 and TIA-1 staining also helps to exclude other types of T-cell lymphomas. Molecular analysis for T-cell receptor gene rearrangement may be employed to rule out a clonal process in challenging cases.

A comparison of the histologic findings in KFD, LE, and SPLTCL is summarized in Table 13.2.

Rosai-Dorfman Skin Lesion

Introduction

Rosai-Dorfman disease (RDD), also known as sinus histiocytosis with massive lymphadenopathy, is a rare histiocytosis of unclear etiology. An infectious cause has long been suspected but

Table 13.2 Comparison of the skin lesions of Kikuchi-Fujimoto disease (KFD), lupus erythematosus (LE), and subcutaneous panniculitis-like T-cell lymphoma (SPLTCL)

Histologic features	KFD	LE	SPLTCL
Interface dermatitis with necrotic keratinocytes	+	+	–
Dermal infiltrate	+ (may be brisk)	+ (mild)	–
Subcutaneous infiltrate	+/–	+ in lupus panniculitis	+
Rimming of adipocytes by atypical lymphocytes	–	–	+
CD8-predominant T cells	+	+	+
Crescentic macrophages	+	–	+/–
Plasmacytoid monocytes	+	+	–
Non-neutrophilic karyorrhexis	+	–/rare	+
Mucin	+/–	+	–
T-cell receptor gene rearrangement	Polyclonal	Polyclonal	Monoclonal

+, present; –, absent

has not been confirmed. While the condition primarily affects the lymph nodes, up to 43 % of cases also demonstrate extranodal involvement. Skin involvement is present in 10 % of cases and is the most common extranodal manifestation (Rosai and Dorfman 1972). Over the past decades, a rare, pure cutaneous form of RDD (C-RDD) has been increasingly reported and recognized as a distinct clinical entity. Regardless of site, RDD is characterized by the presence of Rosai-Dorfman cells ("RD cells") which engulf intact inflammatory cells in a process known as emperipolesis. This discussion focuses on the skin lesions of RDD.

Clinical Features

Systemic RDD has the highest incidence among African and Caucasian young adults. The disease classically manifests as bilateral, massive, but painless cervical lymphadenopathy, accompanied by fever, leukocytosis, and polyclonal hypergammaglobulinemia (Rosai and Dorfman 1969, 1972). Skin lesions in systemic RDD are usually multiple (Thawerani et al. 1978). In contrast, pure C-RDD mainly affects Asians with a median age of over 40 years (Brenn et al. 2002; Lu et al. 2004; Wang et al. 2006; Kong et al. 2007). Three types of skin lesions have been described, including papulonodular, indurated plaque, and tumor types (Kong et al. 2007). The most common papulonodular type refers to clusters of papules and/or nodules measuring up to 1.5 cm in diameter. The lesions may be erythematous, violaceous, or brown in color. The indurated plaque type refers to flat-topped hyperpigmented plaques with a palpable infiltrated border. Scattered papules may also be found within or surrounding the plaques. The tumor type is the rarest form which presents as exophytic large masses with or without central ulceration.

A case registry study has shown that approximately 10 % of patients with systemic RDD exhibit signs of immune dysfunction (Foucar et al. 1984). Interestingly, a link between systemic RDD and autoimmune lymphoproliferative syndrome (ALPS) has been proposed due to the overlapping clinical features (lymphadenopathy and hypergammaglobulinemia) and the finding of nodal RD cells in over 40 % of patients with ALPS type Ia (Maric et al. 2005). These associations, however, have not been demonstrated in pure C-RDD. Other individual case reports have described the occurrence of RDD in patients with lymphoma, carcinoma, melanoma, sickle cell disease, and morphea; however, no clear association has been established (Ratzinger et al. 2003; Stebbing et al. 2007; Moore et al. 2008; Chappell et al. 2009).

Histopathology

The cutaneous lesions of RDD are composed of a nodular or diffuse infiltrate which may be purely dermal, dermal and subcutaneous, or purely

Fig. 13.7 Cutaneous lesion of Rosai-Dorfman disease (RDD). A dense lymphoid infiltrate is present in the dermis

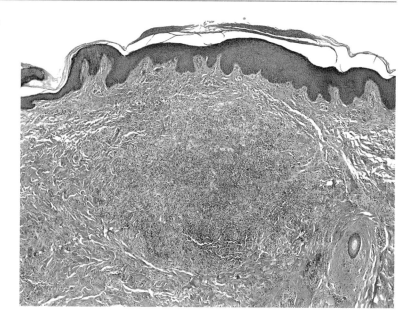

Fig. 13.8 Cutaneous lesion of RDD. This example shows extensive involvement of the subcutaneous fat

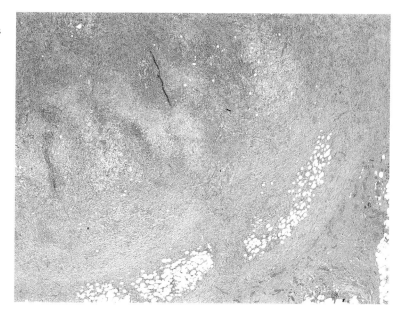

subcutaneous (Figs. 13.7 and 13.8). The overlying epidermis is uninvolved but may be attenuated. Amidst the infiltrate are a variable number of RD cells, which are large polygonal histiocytes containing intact lymphocytes, plasma cells, and/or neutrophils within their pale cytoplasm (Figs. 13.9, 13.10, and 13.11). This process is referred to as "emperipolesis" and is the diagnostic hallmark of this disease. RD cells may sometimes be found within dilated lymphatics (Chu and LeBoit 1992). The rest of the infiltrate consists of lymphocytes, plasma cells, non-RD histiocytes, and neutrophils. Germinal centers and microabscesses may be present (Lu et al. 2004; Kong et al. 2007). A xanthomatous component has been described in a subset of cases (Thawerani et al. 1978; Quaglino et al. 1998), as well as coexisting foci of Langerhans cell histiocytosis

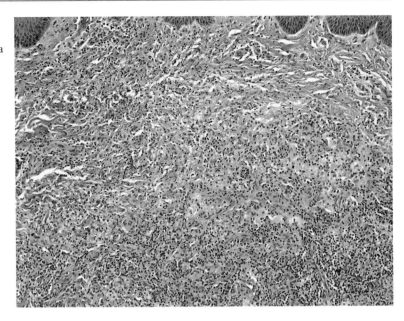

Fig. 13.9 Cutaneous lesion of RDD. Scattered large pale histiocytes are admixed with a dense lymphocytic infiltrate

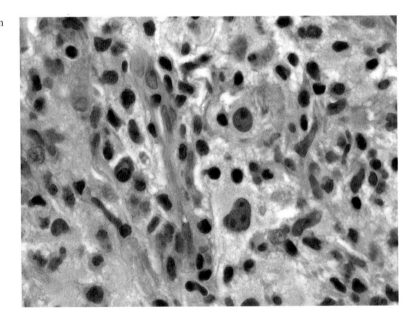

Fig. 13.10 Emperipolesis in cutaneous RDD. Intact lymphocytes are present within the abundant pale cytoplasm of several large Rosai-Dorfman (RD) cells (Courtesy of Dr. David P. Arps, Department of Pathology, University of Michigan)

(LCH) (Wang et al. 2002, 2006; Kong et al. 2007). Eosinophils are rare except in the foci of LCH (Cangelosi et al. 2011). Many cases show various degrees of stromal fibrosis with or without a storiform pattern (Kong et al. 2007; Kuo et al. 2009). When the subcutis is involved, a panniculitis-like pattern with secondary vasculitis may be observed (Kong et al. 2007).

No reliable histologic feature is helpful in distinguishing C-RDD from the cutaneous lesions of systemic RDD. A small series has found pseudoepitheliomatous hyperplasia and eosinophils to be present only in one case of C-RDD but not in systemic RDD; however, the small number of cases precludes any definitive conclusion (Chu and LeBoit 1992). Human herpesvirus-6 has

Fig. 13.11 Emperipolesis in cutaneous RDD. Frequent plasma cells are present, some of which are present within the cytoplasm of RD cells along with lymphocytes and few neutrophils

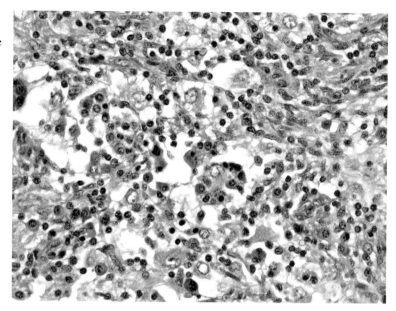

Fig. 13.12 Emperipolesis in cutaneous RDD. S100 immunostain highlights the nuclei and the cytoplasm of RD cells, while the engulfed lymphocytes are negative

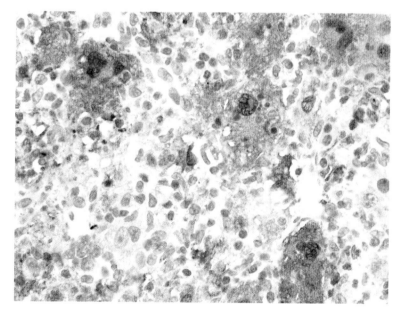

been detected in some cases of systemic RDD (Levine et al. 1992; Luppi et al. 1998) but not in C-RDD (Ortonne et al. 2002). Other rarely detected viruses include parvovirus B19, EBV, and polyomavirus (Levine et al. 1992; Mehraein et al. 2006; Al-Daraji et al. 2010). However, the causal role of these agents has not been confirmed due to the limited number of cases.

Immunophenotype

The RD cells are positive for S100 (Bonetti et al. 1987) (Fig. 13.12), CD68, and lysozyme (Kong et al. 2007). Immunoreactivity for fascin and factor XIIIa has also been reported (Perrin et al. 1993; Jaffe et al. 1998). Unlike Langerhans cells, RD cells lack Birbeck granules and are negative

Table 13.3 Comparison of cutaneous Rosai-Dorfman disease (RDD) with Langerhans cell histiocytosis (LCH) and xanthogranuloma (XG)

	RDD	LCH	XG
Characteristic histiocytes	"RD cells" with abundant pale cytoplasm showing emperipolesis of lymphocytes, plasma cells, and/or neutrophils	Langerhans cells with moderate amount of eosinophilic cytoplasm and reniform/folded nuclei	Xanthomatous cells with foamy cytoplasm
Other common inflammatory cells	Lymphocytes, plasma cells	Eosinophils	Variable
Immunophenotype	RD cells (+) S100, CD68, lysozyme (−) CD1a, langerin	Langerhans cells (+) S100, CD1a, langerin (−) CD68, lysozyme	Xanthomatous cells (+) CD68, lysozyme (+/−) S100 (−) CD1a, langerin

for CD1a and langerin (Rosai and Dorfman 1972; O'Malley et al. 2010). The lymphocytes in RDD are a mixture of T and B cells with T-cell predominance (Yu et al. 2007). The plasma cells are polytypic (Motta et al. 2005). Interestingly, the vast majority of plasma cells in both nodal and extranodal RDD are positive for IgG. There is also an increased proportion of IgG4 positive cells, with a mean IgG4/IgG ratio of over 30 % (Kuo et al. 2009; Zhang et al. 2013). Taken together with the frequent finding of stromal fibrosis, a possible relationship between RDD and IgG4-related sclerosing disease has been suggested and deserves further investigation.

Genetics and Molecular Findings

Polyclonality has been demonstrated in two cases of RDD (Paulli et al. 1995). Despite the possible relationship between ALPS and RDD, no mutation in the Fas-encoding gene has been illustrated in the few RDD cases studied (Maric et al. 2005).

Prognosis or Course

RDD typically runs a benign and indolent course. Spontaneous remission of C-RDD occurs in a subset of patients, while the remainder of cases may be treated effectively by surgical excision (Lu et al. 2004; Kong et al. 2007). Other treatment modalities include high-dose thalidomide

and radiation therapy for extensive or persistent diseases in the skin or soft tissue (Lu et al. 2004; Al-Daraji et al. 2010).

Differential Diagnosis

RDD needs to be distinguished from other histiocytoses as the clinical manifestations and prognosis may differ significantly. In Langerhans cell histiocytosis, there are clusters or sheets of Langerhans cells with pale eosinophilic cytoplasm and reniform nuclei, often admixed with a large number of eosinophils. Both Langerhans cells and RD cells are positive for S100, whereas CD1a and langerin are expressed by Langerhans cells only. As mentioned above, foci of LCH may be present and do not exclude a diagnosis of C-RDD. Similarly, xanthogranuloma may enter the differential diagnosis when a conspicuous population of xanthomatous cells is present. Recognition of emperipolesis by RD cells, which may be aided by the use of S100 immunostain, should allow for the correct diagnosis of RDD. A comparison of RDD with other cutaneous histiocytoses is summarized in Table 13.3.

Histologic overlap between soft tissue RDD and inflammatory pseudotumor is known to be a diagnostic pitfall. Emperipolesis may be inconspicuous in the soft tissue as the RD cells tend to be more spindle and may be overshadowed by a dense inflammatory infiltrate, including numerous plasma cells which are also characteristic of inflammatory pseudotumor (Veinot et al. 1998; Kroumpouzos and Demierre 2002). Some authors have proposed a temporal sequence in which histiocyte-rich RDD may transform to fibroblast-rich inflammatory pseudotumor (Govender and Chetty 1997), a hypothesis that has not been proven. An S100 immunostain to highlight any RD cells is probably prudent before rendering a diagnosis of inflammatory pseudotumor in the soft tissue. Lastly, as with other plasma cell-rich conditions, illustration of polytypic light-chain expression by either immunohistochemistry or in situ hybridization would help to exclude a plasma cell or B-cell neoplasm.

Sarcoidosis

Introduction

Sarcoidosis is a multisystem granulomatous disorder. Its incidence is highest among African Americans and peaks in the third to fourth decades of life (Rybicki et al. 1997; Hosoda et al. 2002). The pathogenesis remains elusive, but current data point to immune dysregulation following exposure to certain antigens in genetically predisposed individuals. Due to the diverse clinical morphologies of cutaneous sarcoidosis, skin biopsy is important in excluding other dermatologic conditions. A confirmed diagnosis should prompt clinical evaluation for systemic involvement.

Clinical Features

Sarcoidosis mainly affects the lungs, lymph nodes, and skin, although virtually any organs may be affected. Cutaneous involvement is present in about 25 % of patients with sarcoidosis (Newman et al. 1997) and is the first presenting sign of systemic disease in a third of these patients (Costabel et al. 2007). Isolated cutaneous sarcoidosis without evidence of systemic involvement is less common. The skin lesions may present as maculopapules, infiltrated plaques, subcutaneous nodules, lupus pernio, or infiltrated scars (Mañá et al. 1997; Haimovic et al. 2012). Papular lesions typically occur on the face, while plaques are most commonly found on the buttocks, back, and other extensor surfaces (Elgart 1986). Lupus pernio refers to violaceous induration on the nose and cheeks which may result in significant disfiguration (James 1992). Verrucous sarcoidosis is an uncommon variant which may mimic squamous cell carcinoma clinically (Stockman et al. 2013). Another rare variant is syringotropic sarcoidosis, which presents as multiple erythematous patches or plaques on the lower extremities (Hayakawa et al. 2013). Interestingly, the sweating responses to thermal stress were reported to be markedly diminished in these cases. Other uncommon presentations include annular, photodistributed, ichthyosiform, atrophic, ulcerative, and hypopigmented forms (Haimovic et al. 2012).

Associations between sarcoidosis and various malignancies have been well documented. These include lymphoma, leukemia, cutaneous squamous cell carcinoma, lung cancer, and many others (Brincker and Wilbek 1974; Ji et al. 2009). Sarcoidosis precedes the diagnosis of malignancy by an average of 8 years (Alexandrescu et al. 2011). The risk is highest during the first year following hospitalization for sarcoidosis (Ji et al. 2009). The term "sarcoidosis-lymphoma syndrome" was used to describe the development of lymphoma within 2 years following the diagnosis of sarcoidosis (Brincker 1986). Other reported associations include primary biliary cirrhosis, interferon therapy, and hepatitis C (Kishor et al. 2008; Lee et al. 2011; North and Mully 2011).

Histopathology

Regardless of site, sarcoidosis is characterized by well-formed, non-necrotizing granulomas. The granulomas are usually numerous and extensively infiltrate the affected organ (Fig. 13.13). The discrete and rounded granulomas typically lack a significant lymphocytic infiltrate, hence the description of "naked granulomas" (Fig. 13.14). The granulomas are composed of predominantly epithelioid histiocytes admixed with scattered multinucleated foreign body-type giant cells (Fig. 13.15). The specificity of "asteroid body" in the giant cells is limited, as it may be encountered in sarcoidosis as well as other

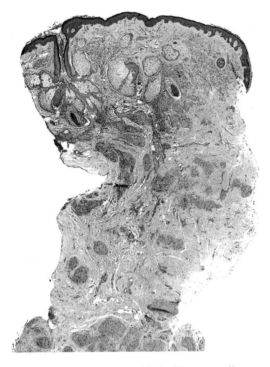

Fig. 13.13 Cutaneous sarcoidosis. Numerous discrete, rounded granulomas are present throughout the dermis

granulomatous conditions. The granulomas sometimes display a periadnexal and/or perivascular distribution (Mangas et al. 2006). Scar sarcoidosis refers to sarcoidosis involving a pre-existing scar, including post-herpes zoster scars (Selim et al. 2006). An interesting finding in the syringotropic variant was the profoundly decreased expression of dermcidin and aquaporin 5 in the affected sweat glands (Hayakawa et al. 2013). In verrucous sarcoidosis, there is verrucous pseudoepitheliomatous hyperplasia of the overlying epidermis (Stockman et al. 2013). A study has expanded the histologic spectrum of cutaneous sarcoidosis, including tuberculoid granulomas, interstitial granulomas, focal necrosis, and lichenoid inflammation (Ball et al. 2004). The exclusion of infection, however, is of paramount importance in light of these atypical presentations, despite an established diagnosis of systemic sarcoidosis in these patients.

Although once regarded as an excluding factor, polarizable foreign bodies are now recognized as a fairly common finding in sarcoidosis. Approximately 25 % of the cutaneous lesions of sarcoidosis may contain polarizable foreign bodies (Kim et al. 2000; Mangas et al. 2006). The foreign bodies are composed of calcium, phosphorus, silicon, and aluminum and are thought

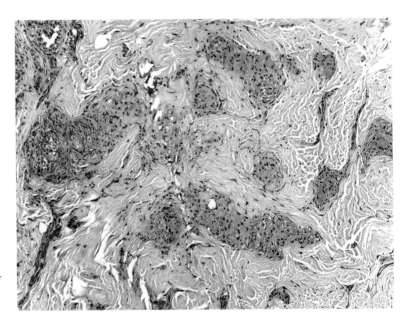

Fig. 13.14 Cutaneous sarcoidosis. The so-called naked granulomas are free of surrounding lymphocytic infiltrate

Fig. 13.15 Cutaneous sarcoidosis. Discrete sarcoidal granulomas are composed of epithelioid histiocytes and occasional foreign body-type giant cells

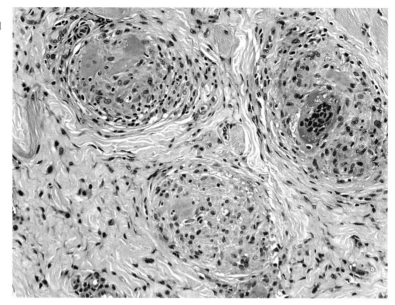

Fig. 13.16 Sarcoidal granulomatous reaction to tattoo pigment

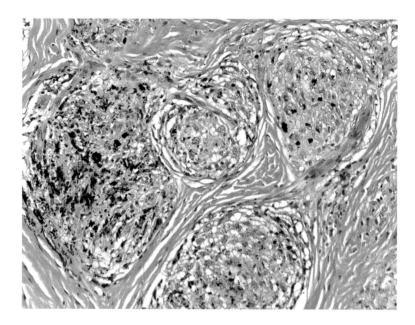

to serve as a nidus for granuloma formation secondary to an overactive cellular immune response in sarcoidosis patients (Walsh et al. 1993). Some cases of sarcoidal granulomatous response to tattoo granules (Fig. 13.16) or silicone implants may be followed by subsequent development of more widespread sarcoidosis, further supporting a systemic rather than localized disease in these patients (Hanada et al. 1985; Teuber et al. 1994).

Immunophenotype

The histiocytes in the sarcoidal granulomas are immunoreactive for CD68 and CD163. The lymphocytes present in sarcoidosis are predominantly CD3-positive and CD4-positive T-helper cells (de Jager et al. 2008). These findings are in keeping with the current understanding of the crucial role of T-cell activation in granuloma formation (Agostini et al. 2000; Chen and Moller 2008).

Genetics and Molecular Findings

The initial step in the formation of a sarcoidal granuloma involves recognition and phagocytosis of a putative antigen by the antigen-presenting cell (APC) (Co et al. 2004). The APC in turn presents any nondegradable particles to a T cell, a process that triggers a cellular immune response with the secretion of multiple cytokines including tumor necrosis factor (TNF-α), interleukins (IL-12, IL-15, and IL-18), and macrophage inflammatory protein (MIP-1), which drive the formation of granulomas (Agostini et al. 2000). The T cells in sarcoidosis are polyclonal (Pfaltz et al. 2011).

Familial clustering of sarcoidosis has been well documented (Iannuzzi 1998). Having a first-degree relative with sarcoidosis corresponds to a fivefold increase in one's risk of developing the disease (Rybicki et al. 2001). The most widely studied genes are those in the major histocompatibility complex on chromosome 6 which encode the human leukocyte antigens (HLAs). Various studies have correlated different HLA phenotypes with specific manifestations and severity of sarcoidosis. For example, HLA-B13 and HLA-B35 are associated with early disease onset, whereas HLA-A30, HLA-B8, HLA-DR3, and HLA-DR4 are associated with late disease onset (Smith et al. 2008). Studies on cytokine genes such as tumor necrosis factor (TNF) and interferon (IFN) and receptor genes such as Toll-like receptor (TRL4) and butyrophilin-like protein (BTNL2) also reveal possible links to sarcoidosis (Smith et al. 2008). The current data suggest a complex interplay between multiple genes and environmental factors in the pathogenesis of sarcoidosis, which makes genetic studies particularly challenging.

Prognosis or Course

While the majority of cases resolve spontaneously within 2–5 years, up to 10–30 % of cases may persist or progress (Hunninghake et al. 1999; Baughman et al. 2003). The maculopapular lesions have the best clinical outcome, whereas plaque-type lesions and lupus pernio usually run a chronic and progressive course (Veien et al. 1987;

James 1992; Samtsov 1992; Mañá et al. 1997). Fibrosis is an unfavorable and irreversible sequela of chronic sarcoidal granuloma.

Differential Diagnosis

Sarcoidosis remains a diagnosis of exclusion. The presence of sarcoidal granulomas in a biopsy should prompt a careful search for microorganisms, in particular fungi and mycobacteria, by Grocott's methenamine silver (GMS) and Ziehl-Neelsen or Fite stains. Although infectious granulomas are more likely to be necrotizing, suppurative, or "tuberculoid" (surrounded by lymphocytes), the absence of these features does not exclude an infectious etiology. Tissue culture is therefore advisable prior to the establishment of a diagnosis of sarcoidosis.

Foreign body granulomas may also mimic sarcoidosis. Examination of the tissue sections under polarized light is often helpful in identifying foreign materials. However, as discussed above, the presence of foreign bodies does not always exclude sarcoidosis. For cases in which the foreign body granulomas display a classic sarcoidal morphology, clinical work-up to rule out sarcoidosis should be considered.

Some cases of cutaneous T-cell lymphoma may consist of a prominent granulomatous component simulating sarcoidosis (Mainguene et al. 1993; Bessis et al. 1996; Telle et al. 1998). A high index of suspicion should be maintained when a lymphocytic infiltrate is present in addition to the epithelioid granulomas. Careful examination for epidermotropism and lymphocytic atypia, followed by immunophenotyping and/or molecular studies, will allow for correct diagnosis of granulomatous mycosis fungoides (Pfaltz et al. 2011). See Chaps. 4 and 6.

Granuloma Annulare

Introduction

Granuloma annulare is a relatively common and self-limited dermatologic condition characterized by palisaded granulomatous dermatitis and necrobiosis. Many possible pathogenic mechanisms have been proposed; however, none has been universally accepted (Dahl 1985). Cases may be subdivided into localized, generalized, subcutaneous, and perforating forms depending on their clinical and histopathologic presentations. Although most cases of granuloma annulare occur as an isolated phenomenon, its associations with a variety of medical and neoplastic conditions have also been described.

Clinical Features

Granuloma annulare has a predilection for females and young patients under 30 years of age (Dahl 1993; Zax and Callen 1990). In general, the hands and feet are most frequently affected, while the face is often spared; however, involvement of virtually any skin sites has been reported.

The *classic localized form* typically manifests as a limited number of asymptomatic, skin-colored, or pink papules or plaques with an annular or arcuate configuration in the absence of surface changes (Muhlbauer 1980). In the *generalized form*, there are over hundreds of small skin-colored papules widely distributed over the trunk and, to a lesser degree, the extremities (Dabski and Winkelmann 1989). The *subcutaneous form* typically occurs in children (Felner et al. 1997; Grogg and Nascimento 2001), although rarely it may also occur in adults (De Aloe et al. 2006; Salomon et al. 1986). It is characterized by larger and deeper nodules located on the extremities, the buttocks, and/or the scalp (Felner et al. 1997; Politz and Miller 1983). The rare *perforating form* accounts for approximately 5 % of cases and is more likely to affect older patients (Penas et al. 1997). The dorsal hands and other extensor surfaces of the extremities are the most common sites. These lesions often have a pustular or crusted surface owing to the perforating process.

The occurrence of granuloma annulare in patients with coexisting systemic diseases or malignancies has been well documented. Various studies have shown that approximately 10–20 % of patients with granuloma annulare also carry a diagnosis of diabetes (Dabski and Winkelmann 1989; Jelinek 1993; Studer et al. 1996). However, given the relatively high prevalence of diabetes in the general population, this may be a result of coincidence rather than true association (Smith et al. 1997). A different study failed to confirm any statistically significant association between granuloma annulare and type 2 diabetes (Nebesio et al. 2002). Another frequently reported association is human immunodeficiency virus infection (Cohen 1999; Ghadially et al. 1989; Jones and Harman 1989; O'Moore et al. 2000; Toro et al. 1999). Potential links to various neoplastic conditions have also been suggested. These include hematologic malignancies (both lymphomas and leukemias) and, less often, solid tumors (Barksdale et al. 1994; Cohen 2006). Although no definite association has been established, it is suggested that atypical presentation of granuloma annulare—such as those occurring on the face and in older patients—may warrant clinical work-up to exclude an underlying cancer (Li et al. 2003). Other less common associations include Sjögren's syndrome, autoimmune thyroiditis, uveitis, dyslipidemia, hypercalcemia, hepatitis C virus infection, BCG vaccination, and TNF-α treatment (Baker and Pehr 2006; Granel et al. 2000; Kakurai et al. 2001; Oz et al. 2003; Sumikawa et al. 2010; Vazquez-Lopez et al. 2003; Voulgari et al. 2008; Wu et al. 2012).

Histopathology

The histologic hallmark of granuloma annulare is palisading granuloma with central necrobiosis (Fig. 13.17). The histiocytes are typically spindle in appearance, although occasional multinucleated giant cells may also be seen (Fig. 13.18). The central necrobiotic zone is composed of degenerated collagen which tends to appear more eosinophilic, swollen, and/or fragmented compared to the normal dermal collagen (Figs. 13.18 and 13.19). A variable amount of mucin is usually present (Fig. 13.19). The histiocytes tend to infiltrate in between collagen bundles at the periphery of the granuloma giving rise to an interstitial pattern. "Interstitial granuloma annulare" is used to describe cases which demonstrate a prominent interstitial pattern in the absence of palisading or necrobiosis (Fig. 13.20). There is usually a mild perivascular lymphocytic infiltrate with or without a few admixed eosinophils.

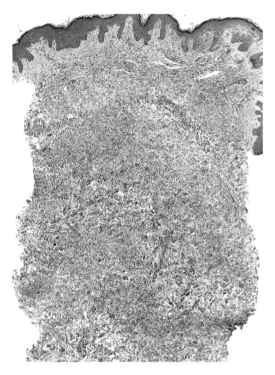

Fig. 13.17 Granuloma annulare. An annular infiltrate is present in the dermis

Sometimes a vaguely annular distribution of a mild perivascular lymphohistiocytic infiltrate may be the only clue to an early granuloma annulare. On rare occasions the lymphocytic infiltrate may be so brisk that it mimics a T-cell lymphoma (see section "Differential diagnosis" below) (Cota et al. 2012). Vascular changes including leukocytoclastic or granulomatous vasculitis and/or thrombogenic vasculopathy are found to be a marker for underlying systemic diseases (Magro et al. 1996). Cases associated with systemic diseases are also more likely to contain scattered extravascular neutrophils (Magro et al. 1996). Such cases are virtually indistinguishable from "interstitial granulomatous dermatitis" (Peroni et al. 2012) and "palisaded and neutrophilic granulomatous dermatitis" on histologic grounds (Chu et al. 1994).

In the perforating form, a well-developed palisading granuloma comes in direct contact with the overlying invaginated epidermis which has a disrupted basal layer. This forms a perforating channel permitting transepidermal elimination of the necrobiotic collagen (Fig. 13.21). Subcutaneous granuloma annulare is characterized by numerous palisading granulomas located primarily within the subcutaneous fat, with or without involvement of the overlying dermis (Fig. 13.22).

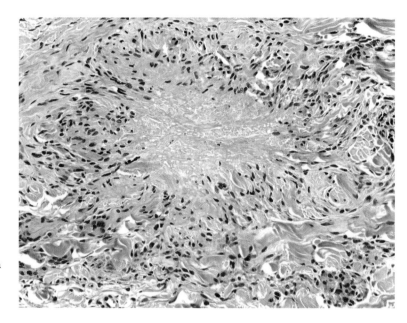

Fig. 13.18 Granuloma annulare. Spindle-shaped histiocytes palisade around a central zone of necrobiosis composed of swollen and degenerated collagen

Fig. 13.19 Granuloma annulare. The central necrobiotic zone consists of fragmented collagen and abundant mucin

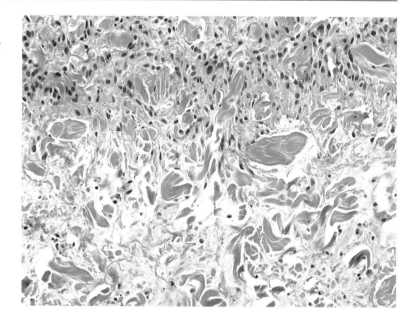

Fig. 13.20 Interstitial granuloma annulare. In this example the histiocytes percolate between collagen bundles without palisading around a central necrobiotic zone. A mild perivascular lymphocytic infiltrate is also present

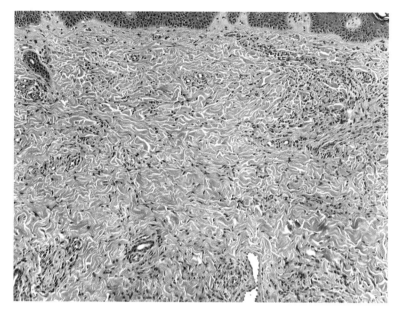

Immunophenotype

The histiocytes in granuloma annulare are immunoreactive for CD68 and CD163. Staining for lysozyme is variable (Stefanaki et al. 2007). The lymphocytic infiltrate is comprised of mostly T cells, with CD4 predominating over CD8 in most cases except in those associated with immunodeficiency (Morris et al. 2002; Stefanaki et al. 2007).

Genetics and Molecular Findings

A study has found clonal T cells in 2 of 15 cases (13 %) of granuloma annulare by T-cell receptor (TCR) gene rearrangement analysis (Pfaltz et al. 2011). Another study has detected T-cell clonality in 3 of 12 cases (25 %), but the clone was only demonstrable in one of the two biopsies obtained from the same patients (Dabiri et al. 2011).

Fig. 13.21 Perforating granuloma annulare. The palisading granuloma comes in direct contact with the invaginated epidermis, forming a perforating channel in the process of transepidermal elimination of the necrobiotic collagen

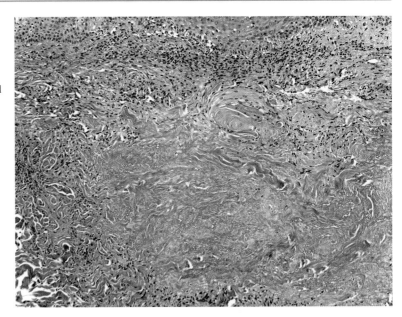

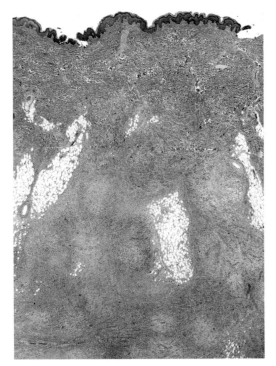

Fig. 13.22 Subcutaneous granuloma annulare. Numerous palisading granulomas are present exclusively in the subcutaneous tissue

This "dual TCR-PCR" approach supports a false-positive result in some cases of granuloma annulare and is helpful in distinguishing these cases from granulomatous T-cell lymphoma.

Prognosis and Course

More than half of the cases resolve spontaneously within 2 years of onset (Zax and Callen 1990; Dahl 1993). Recurrence at the same sites is not uncommon. The generalized form may result in anetoderma (Ozkan et al. 2000; Kiremitci et al. 2006). The possible role of biopsy in promoting resolution of granuloma annulare remains controversial (Levin et al. 2002; Wells and Smith 1963).

Differential Diagnosis

Necrobiosis lipoidica is another palisading granulomatous dermatitis which may be difficult to distinguish from granuloma annulare. Clinically, the classic presentation of an orange plaque on the shin favors necrobiosis lipoidica. The granulomas in necrobiosis lipoidica tend to be organized horizontally resulting in a "layered" appearance. There is usually more extensive and prominent eosinophilic necrobiosis than in granuloma annulare. Other findings in favor of necrobiosis lipoidica include a conspicuous plasma cell infiltrate, the lack of an interstitial pattern, and the paucity of mucin.

Cutaneous infections caused by certain organisms, such as *Mycobacterium marinum* and *Borrelia burgdorferi*, may elicit an interstitial granulomatous dermatitis simulating interstitial granuloma annulare (Barr et al. 2003; Moreno et al. 2003). Borrelial infection may demonstrate "histiocytic pseudorosettes." Work-up for an infectious cause should be considered in patients with atypical clinical presentations and/or under immunosuppression.

Mycosis fungoides (MF) may contain a reactive granulomatous component in addition to the neoplastic lymphocytic infiltrate (LeBoit et al. 1988). In particular, interstitial MF is a rare variant in which the prominent interstitial distribution of the infiltrate closely mimics that of interstitial granuloma annulare (Su et al. 2002). While some of these cases may be recognized histologically based on the findings of epidermotropism and lymphocytic atypia, others may require molecular analysis to confirm a neoplastic T-cell clone. A study suggested the presence of pseudovascular clefts with "free-floating" collagen fibers as a helpful clue in identifying interstitial MF (Ferrara et al. 2010). Of note, interstitial granuloma annulare may be seen in association with mycosis fungoides, which further adds to the diagnostic challenge (Koochek et al. 2012).

References

Agostini C, Adami F, Semenzato G. New pathogenetic insights into the sarcoid granuloma. Curr Opin Rheumatol. 2000;12(1):71–6.

Al-Daraji W, Anandan A, Klassen-Fischer M, Auerbach A, Marwaha JS, Fanburg-Smith JC. Soft tissue Rosai-Dorfman disease: 29 new lesions in 18 patients, with detection of polyomavirus antigen in 3 abdominal cases. Ann Diagn Pathol. 2010;14(5):309–16. doi:10.1016/j.anndiagpath.2010.05.006.

Alexandrescu DT, Kauffman CL, Ichim TE, Riordan NH, Kabigting F, Dasanu CA. Cutaneous sarcoidosis and malignancy: an association between sarcoidosis with skin manifestations and systemic neoplasia. Dermatol Online J. 2011;17(1):2.

Amir ARA, Amr SS, Sheikh SS. Kikuchi-Fujimoto's disease: report of familial occurrence in two human leucocyte antigen-identical non-twin sisters. J Intern Med. 2002;252(1):79–83.

Aqel N, Henry K, Woodrow D. Skin involvement in Kikuchi's disease: an immunocytochemical and immunofluorescence study. Virchows Arch. 1997;430(4):349–52.

Atwater AR, Longley BJ, Aughenbaugh WD. Kikuchi's disease: case report and a systemic review of cutaneous and histopathologic presentations. J Am Acad Dermatol. 2008;59(1):130–6. doi:10.1016/j.jaad.2008.03.012.

Baker K, Pehr K. Granuloma annulare associated with hypercalcemia secondary to hyperparathyroidism. Int J Dermatol. 2006;45(9):1118–20.

Ball NJ, Kho GT, Martinka M. The histologic spectrum of cutaneous sarcoidosis: a study of twenty-eight cases. J Cutan Pathol. 2004;31(2):160–8.

Barksdale SK, Perniciaro C, Halling KC, Strickler JG. Granuloma annulare in patients with malignant lymphoma: clinicopathologic study of thirteen new cases. J Am Acad Dermatol. 1994;31(1):42–8.

Barr KL, Lowe L, Su LD. Mycobacterium marinum infection simulating interstitial granuloma annulare: a report of two cases. Am J Dermatopathol. 2003;25(2):148–51.

Baughman RP, Lower EE, du Bois RM. Sarcoidosis. Lancet. 2003;361(9363):1111–8.

Bessis D, Sotto A, Farcet JP, Barneon G, Guilhou JJ. Granulomatous mycosis fungoides presenting as sarcoidosis. Dermatology. 1996;193(4):330–2.

Bonetti F, Chilosi M, Menestrina F, Scarpa A, Pelicci PG, Amorosi E, et al. Immunohistological analysis of Rosai-Dorfman histiocytosis. A disease of S-100+ CD1- histiocytes. Virchows Arch A Pathol Anat Histopathol. 1987;411(2):129–35.

Brenn T, Calonje E, Granter SR, Leonard N, Grayson W, Fletcher CD, et al. Cutaneous Rosai-Dorfman disease is a distinct clinical entity. Am J Dermatopathol. 2002;24(5):385–91.

Brincker H. The sarcoidosis-lymphoma syndrome. Br J Cancer. 1986;54(3):467–73.

Brincker H, Wilbek E. The incidence of malignant tumours in patients with respiratory sarcoidosis. Br J Cancer. 1974;29(3):247–51.

Cangelosi JJ, Prieto VG, Ivan D. Cutaneous Rosai-Dorfman disease with increased number of eosinophils: coincidence or histologic variant? Arch Pathol Lab Med. 2011;135(12):1597–600. doi:10.5858/arpa.2010-0554-CR.

Chappell JA, Burkemper NM, Frater JL, Hurley MY. Cutaneous Rosai-Dorfman disease and morphea: coincidence or association? Am J Dermatopathol. 2009;31(5):487–9. doi:10.1097/DAD.0b013e318196f883.

Chen ES, Moller DR. Etiology of sarcoidosis. Clin Chest Med. 2008;29(3):365–77. doi:10.1016/j.ccm.2008.03.011. vii.

Cheng CY, Sheng WH, Lo YC, Chung CS, Chen YC, Chang SC. Clinical presentations, laboratory results and outcomes of patients with Kikuchi's disease: emphasis on the association between recurrent Kikuchi's disease and autoimmune diseases. J Microbiol Immunol Infect. 2010;43(5):366–71. doi:10.1016/S1684-1182(10)60058-8.

Chu P, Connolly MK, LeBoit PE. The histopathologic spectrum of palisaded and neutrophilic granulomatous dermatitis in patients with collagen vascular disease. Arch Dermatol. 1994;130(10):1278–83.

Chu P, LeBoit PE. Histologic features of cutaneous sinus histiocytosis (Rosai-Dorfman disease): study of cases both with and without systemic involvement. J Cutan Pathol. 1992;19(2):201–6.

Co DO, Hogan LH, Il-Kim S, Sandor M. T cell contributions to the different phases of granuloma formation. Immunol Lett. 2004;92(1–2):135–42.

Cohen PR. Granuloma annulare: a mucocutaneous condition in human immunodeficiency virus-infected patients. Arch Dermatol. 1999;135(11):1404–7.

Cohen PR. Granuloma annulare, relapsing polychondritis, sarcoidosis, and systemic lupus erythematosus: conditions whose dermatologic manifestations may occur as hematologic malignancy-associated mucocutaneous paraneoplastic syndromes. Int J Dermatol. 2006;45(1):70–80.

Costabel U, Guzman J, Baughman RP. Systemic evaluation of a potential cutaneous sarcoidosis patient. Clin Dermatol. 2007;25(3):303–11.

Cota C, Ferrara G, Cerroni L. Granuloma annulare with prominent lymphoid infiltrates ("pseudolymphomatous" granuloma annulare). Am J Dermatopathol. 2012;34(3):259–62. doi:10.1097/DAD.0b013e31822a2aca.

Dabiri S, Morales A, Ma L, Sundram U, Kim YH, Arber DA, Kim J. The frequency of dual TCR-PCR clonality in granulomatous disorders. J Cutan Pathol. 2011;38(9):704–9. doi:10.1111/j.1600-0560.2011.01727.x.

Dabski K, Winkelmann RK. Generalized granuloma annulare: clinical and laboratory findings in 100 patients. J Am Acad Dermatol. 1989;20(1):39–47.

Dahl MV. Speculations on the pathogenesis of granuloma annulare. Australas J Dermatol. 1985;26(2):49–57.

Dahl MV. Granuloma annulare. In: Fitzpatrick TB, Eisen AZ, Wolff K, et al., editors. Dermatology in general medicine. New York: McGraw-Hill; 1993.

De Aloe G, Risulo M, Sbano P, De Nisi MC, Fimiani M. Subcutaneous granuloma annulare in an adult patient. J Eur Acad Dermatol Venereol. 2006;20(4):462–4.

de Jager M, Blokx W, Warris A, Bergers M, Link M, Weemaes C, et al. Immunohistochemical features of cutaneous granulomas in primary immunodeficiency disorders: a comparison with cutaneous sarcoidosis. J Cutan Pathol. 2008;35(5):467–72. doi:10.1111/j.1600-0560.2007.00854.x.

Elgart ML. Cutaneous sarcoidosis: definitions and types of lesions. Clin Dermatol. 1986;4(4):35–45.

Felner EI, Steinberg JB, Weinberg AG. Subcutaneous granuloma annulare: a review of 47 cases. Pediatrics. 1997;100(6):965–7.

Fernandez-Flores A, Bouso M, Alonso A, Manjon JA. The histiocytic component of cutaneous manifestations of Kikuchi disease expresses myeloperoxidase. Appl Immunohistochem Mol Morphol. 2008;16(2):202–3. doi:10.1097/PAI.0b013e318074c94c.

Ferrara G, Crisman G, Zalaudek I, Argenziano G, Stefanato CM. Free-floating collagen fibers in interstitial mycosis fungoides. Am J Dermatopathol. 2010;32(4):352–6. doi:10.1097/DAD.0b013e3181b876d7.

Foucar E, Rosai J, Dorfman RF, Eyman JM. Immunologic abnormalities and their significance in sinus histiocytosis with massive lymphadenopathy. Am J Clin Pathol. 1984;82(5):515–25.

Fujimoto Y, Kojima Y, Yamaguchi K. Cervical subacute lymphadenitis: a new clinicopathologic entity. Naika. 1972;20:920.

George TI, Jones CD, Zehnder JL, Warnke RA, Dorfman RF. Lack of human herpesvirus 8 and Epstein-Barr virus in Kikuchi's histiocytic necrotizing lymphadenitis. Hum Pathol. 2003;34(2):130–5.

Ghadially R, Sibbald RG, Walter JB, Haberman HF. Granuloma annulare in patients with human immunodeficiency virus infections. J Am Acad Dermatol. 1989;20(2 Pt 1):232–5.

Go EJ, Jung YJ, Han SB, Suh BK, Kang JH. A case of Kikuchi-Fujimoto disease with autoimmune thyroiditis. Korean J Paediatr. 2012;55(11):445–8. doi:10.3345/kjp.2012.55.11.445.

Govender D, Chetty R. Inflammatory pseudotumour and Rosai-Dorfman disease of soft tissue: a histological continuum? J Clin Pathol. 1997;50(1):79–81.

Granel B, Serratrice J, Rey J, Bouvier C, Weiller-Merli C, Disdier R, et al. Chronic hepatitis C virus infection associated with a generalized granuloma annulare. J Am Acad Dermatol. 2000;43(5 Pt 2):918–9.

Grogg KL, Nascimento AG. Subcutaneous granuloma annulare in childhood: clinicopathologic features in 34 cases. Pediatrics. 2001;107(3):E42.

Haimovic A, Sanchez M, Judson MA, Prystowski S. Sarcoidosis: a comprehensive review and update for the dermatologist: part I. Cutaneous disease. J Am Acad Dermatol. 2012;66(5):699.e1–18. doi:10.1016/j.jaad.2011.11.965.

Hanada K, Chiyoya S, Katabira Y. Systemic sarcoidal reaction in tattoo. Clin Exp Dermatol. 1985;10(5):479–84.

Hayakawa J, Mizukawa Y, Kurata M, Shiohara T. A syringotropic variant of cutaneous sarcoidosis: presentation of 3 cases exhibiting defective sweating responses. J Am Acad Dermatol. 2013;68(6):1016–21. doi:10.1016/j.jaad.2012.11.039.

Hollingsworth HC, Peiper SC, Weiss LM, Raffeld M, Jaffe ES. An investigation of the viral pathogenesis of Kikuchi-Fujimoto disease. Lack of evidence for Epstein-Barr virus or human herpesvirus type 6 as the causative agents. Arch Pathol Lab Med. 1994;118(2):134–40.

Hosoda Y, Sasagawa S, Yasuda N. Epidemiology of sarcoidosis: new frontiers to explore. Curr Opin Pulm Med. 2002;8(5):424–8.

Hunninghake GW, Costabel U, Ando M, Baughman R, Cordier JF, du Bois R, et al. ATS/ERS/WASOG statement on sarcoidosis. American Thoracic Society/European Respiratory Society/World Association of Sarcoidosis and other granulomatous disorders. Sarcoidosis Vasc Diffuse Lung Dis. 1999;16(2):149–73.

Iannuzzi MC. Genetics of sarcoidosis. Monaldi Arch Chest Dis. 1998;53(6):609–13.

Imanishi T, Akaza T, Kimura A, Tokunaga K, Gojobori T. Allele frequencies and haplotype frequencies for

HLA and complement loci in various ethnic groups. In: Tsuji K, Aizawa M, Sasazuki T, editors. HLA 1991, vol. 1. Oxford: Oxford University Press; 1992.

Jaffe R, DeVaughn D, Langhoff E. Fascin and the differential diagnosis of childhood histiocytic lesions. Pediatr Dev Pathol. 1998;1(3):216–21.

James DG. Lupus pernio. Lupus. 1992;1(3):129–31.

Jelinek JE. Dermatology. In: Levin ME, O'Neal LW, Bowker JH, editors. The diabetic foot. 5th ed. St. Louis: Mosby Year Book; 1993.

Ji J, Shu X, Li X, Sundquist K, Sundquist J, Hemminki K. Cancer risk in hospitalized sarcoidosis patients: a follow-up study in Sweden. Ann Oncol. 2009;20(6):1121–6. doi:10.1093/annonc/mdn767.

Jones SK, Harman RR. Atypical granuloma annulare in patients with the acquired immunodeficiency syndrome. J Am Acad Dermatol. 1989;20(2 Pt 1):299–300.

Kakurai M, Kiyosawa T, Ohtsuki M, Nakagawa H. Multiple lesions of granuloma annulare following BCG vaccination: case report and review of the literature. Int J Dermatol. 2001;40(9):579–81.

Kikuchi M. Lymphadenitis showing focal reticular cell hyperplasia with nuclear debris and phagocytosis. Acta Haematol Jpn. 1972;35:379–80.

Kim JH, Kim YB, In SI, Kim YC, Han JH. The cutaneous lesions of Kikuchi's disease: a comprehensive analysis of 16 cases based on the clinicopathologic, immunohistochemical, and immunofluorescence studies with an emphasis on the differential diagnosis. Hum Pathol. 2010;41(9):1245–54. doi:10.1016/j.humpath.2010.02.002.

Kim YC, Triffet MK, Gibson LE. Foreign bodies in sarcoidosis. Am J Dermatopathol. 2000;22(5):408–12.

Kiremitci U, Karagulle S, Topcu E, Gurel MS, Erdogan SS, Erdemir AT, et al. Generalized granuloma annulare resolving to anetoderma. Dermatol Online J. 2006;12(7):16.

Kishor S, Turner ML, Borg BB, Kleiner DE, Cowen EW. Cutaneous sarcoidosis and primary biliary cirrhosis: a chance association or related diseases? J Am Acad Dermatol. 2008;58(2):326–35. doi:10.1016/j.jaad.2007.07.031.

Kong YY, Kong JC, Shi DR, Lu HF, Zhu XZ, Wang J, et al. Cutaneous Rosai-Dorfman disease. A clinical and histopathologic study of 25 cases in China. Am J Surg Pathol. 2007;31(3):341–50.

Koochek A, Fink-Puches R, Cerroni L. Coexistence of patch stage mycosis fungoides and interstitial granuloma annulare in the same patient: a pitfall in the clinicopathologic diagnosis of mycosis fungoides. Am J Dermatopathol. 2012;34(2):198–202. doi:10.1097/DAD.0b013e318230ee1c.

Kroumpouzos G, Demierre MF. Cutaneous Rosai-Dorfman disease: histopathological presentation as inflammatory pseudotumor. A literature review. Acta Derm Venereol. 2002;82(4):292–6.

Kuo TT, Chen TC, Lee LY, Lu PH. IgG4-positive plasma cells in cutaneous Rosai-Dorfman disease: an additional immunohistochemical feature and possible relationship to IgG4-related sclerosing disease. J Cutan Pathol. 2009;36(10):1069–73. doi:10.1111/j.1600-0560.2008.01222.x.

LeBoit PE, Zackheim HS, White Jr CR. Granulomatous variants of cutaneous T-cell lymphoma. The histopathology of granulomatous mycosis fungoides and granulomatous slack skins. Am J Surg Pathol. 1988;12(2):83–95.

Lee YB, Lee JI, Park HJ, Cho BK, Oh ST. Interferon-alpha induced sarcoidosis with cutaneous involvement along the lines of venous drainage. Ann Dermatol. 2011;23(2):239–41. doi:10.5021/ad.2011.23.2.239.

Levin NA, Patterson JW, Yao LL, Wilson BB. Resolution of patch-type granuloma annulare lesions after biopsy. J Am Acad Dermatol. 2002;46(3):426–9.

Levine PH, Jahan N, Murari P, Manak M, Jaffe ES. Detection of human herpesvirus-6 in tissues involved by sinus histiocytosis with massive lymphadenopathy (Rosai-Dorfman disease). J Infect Dis. 1992;166(2):291–5.

Li A, Hogan DJ, Sanusi D, Smoller BR. Granuloma annulare and malignant neoplasms. Am J Dermatopathol. 2003;25(2):113–6.

Lin CW, Chang CL, Li CC, Chen YH, Lee WH, Hsu SM. Spontaneous regression of Kikuchi lymphadenopathy with oligoclonal T-cell populations favors a benign immune reaction over a T-cell lymphoma. Am J Clin Pathol. 2002;117(4):627–35.

Lu CI, Kuo TT, Wong WR, Hong HS. Clinical and histopathologic spectrum of cutaneous Rosai-Dorfman disease in Taiwan. J Am Acad Dermatol. 2004;51(6):931–9.

Luppi M, Barozzi P, Garber R, Maiorana A, Bonacorsi G, Artusi T, et al. Expression of human herpesvirus-6 antigens in benign and malignant lymphoproliferative diseases. Am J Pathol. 1998;153(3):815–23.

Magro CM, Crowson AN, Regauer S. Granuloma annulare and necrobiosis lipoidica tissue reactions as a manifestation of systemic disease. Hum Pathol. 1996;27(1):50–6.

Mainguene C, Picard O, Audouin J, Le Tourneau A, Jagueux M, Diebold J. An unusual case of mycosis fungoides presenting as sarcoidosis or granulomatous mycosis fungoides. Am J Clin Pathol. 1993;99(1):82–6.

Mangas C, Fernández-Figueras MT, Fité E, Fernández-Chico N, Sàbat M, Ferrándiz C. Clinical spectrum and histological analysis of 32 cases of specific cutaneous sarcoidosis. J Cutan Pathol. 2006;33(12):772–7.

Mañá J, Marcoval J, Graells J, Salazar A, Peyrí J, Pujol R. Cutaneous involvement in sarcoidosis. Relationship to systemic disease. Arch Dermatol. 1997;133(7):882–8.

Maric I, Pittaluga S, Dale JK, Niemela JE, Delsol G, Diment J, et al. Histologic features of sinus histiocytosis with massive lymphadenopathy in patients with autoimmune lymphoproliferative syndrome. Am J Surg Pathol. 2005;29(7):903–11.

Mehraein Y, Wagner M, Remberger K, Fuzesi L, Middel P, Kaptur S, et al. Parvovirus B19 detected in Rosai-

Dorfman disease in nodal and extranodal manifestations. J Clin Pathol. 2006;59(12):1320–6.

Moore JC, Zhao X, Nelson EL. Concomitant sinus histiocytosis with massive lymphadenopathy (Rosai-Dorfman Disease) and diffuse large B-cell lymphoma: a case report. J Med Case Rep. 2008;2:70. doi:10.1186/1752-1947-2-70.

Moreno C, Kutzner H, Palmedo G, Goerttler E, Carrasco L, Requena L. Interstitial granulomatous dermatitis with histiocytic pseudorosettes: a new histopathologic pattern in cutaneous borreliosis. Detection of Borrelia burgdorferi DNA sequences by a highly sensitive PCR-ELISA. J Am Acad Dermatol. 2003;48(3):376–84.

Morris SD, Cerio R, Paige DG. An unusual presentation of diffuse granuloma annulare in an HIV-positive patient – immunohistochemical evidence of predominant CD8 lymphocytes. Clin Exp Dermatol. 2002;27(3):205–8.

Motta L, McMenamin ME, Thomas MA, Calonje E. Crystal deposition in a case of cutaneous Rosai-Dorfman disease. Am J Dermatopathol. 2005;27(4):339–42.

Muhlbauer JE. Granuloma annulare. J Am Acad Dermatol. 1980;3(3):217–30.

Nebesio CL, Lewis C, Chuang TY. Lack of an association between granuloma annulare and type 2 diabetes mellitus. Br J Dermatol. 2002;146(1):122–4.

Newman LS, Rose CS, Maier LA. Sarcoidosis. N Engl J Med. 1997;336(17):1224–34.

North J, Mully T. Alpha-interferon induced sarcoidosis mimicking metastatic melanoma. J Cutan Pathol. 2011;38(7):585–9. doi:10.1111/j.1600-0560.2011.01702.x.

O'Malley DP, Duong A, Barry TS, Chen S, Hibbard MK, Ferry JA, et al. Co-occurrence of Langerhans cell histiocytosis and Rosai-Dorfman disease: possible relationship of two histiocytic disorders in rare cases. Mod Pathol. 2010;23(12):1616–23. doi:10.1038/modpathol.2010.157.

O'Moore EJ, Nandawni R, Uthayakumar S, Nayagam AT, Darley CR. HIV-associated granuloma annulare (HAGA): a report of six cases. Br J Dermatol. 2000;142(5):1054–6.

Ortonne N, Fillet AM, Kosuge H, Bagot M, Frances C, Wechsler J. Cutaneous Destombes-Rosai-Dorfman disease: absence of detection of HHV-6 and HHV-8 in skin. J Cutan Pathol. 2002;29(2):113–8.

Oz O, Tursen U, Yildirim O, Kaya TI, Ikizoglu G. Uveitis associated with granuloma annulare. Eur J Ophthalmol. 2003;13(1):93–5.

Ozkan S, Fetil E, Izler F, Pabucçuoğlu U, Yalçin N, Güneş AT. Anetoderma secondary to generalized granuloma annulare. J Am Acad Dermatol. 2000;42(2 Pt 2):335–8.

Papaioannou G, Speletas M, Kaloutsi V, Pavlitou-Tsiontsi A. Histiocytic necrotizing lymphadenitis (Kikuchi-Fujimoto disease) associated with antiphospholipid syndrome: case report and literature review. Ann Hematol. 2002;81(12):732–5.

Paradela S, Lorenzo J, Martínez-Gómez W, Yebra-Pimentel T, Valbuena L, Fonseca E. Interface dermatitis in skin lesions of Kikuchi-Fujimoto's disease: a histopathological marker of evolution into systemic lupus erythematosus? Lupus. 2008;17(12):1127–35. doi:10.1177/0961203308092161.

Paulli M, Bergamaschi G, Tonon L, Viglio A, Rosso R, Facchetti F, et al. Evidence for a polyclonal nature of the cell infiltrate in sinus histiocytosis with massive lymphadenopathy (Rosai-Dorfman disease). Br J Haematol. 1995;91(2):415–8.

Penas PF, Jones-Caballero M, Fraga J, Sánchez-Pérez J, García-Díez A. Perforating granuloma annulare. Int J Dermatol. 1997;36(5):340–8.

Peroni A, Colato C, Schena D, Gisondi P, Girolomoni G. Interstitial granulomatous dermatitis: a distinct entity with characteristic histological and clinical pattern. Br J Dermatol. 2012;166(4):775–83. doi:10.1111/j.1365-2133.2011.10727.x.

Perrin C, Michiels JF, Lacour JP, Chagnon A, Fuzibet JG. Sinus histiocytosis (Rosai-Dorfman disease) clinically limited to the skin. An immunohistochemical and ultrastructural study. J Cutan Pathol. 1993;20(4):368–74.

Pfaltz K, Kerl K, Palmedo G, Kutzner H, Kempf W. Clonality in sarcoidosis, granuloma annulare, and granulomatous mycosis fungoides. Am J Dermatopathol. 2011;33(7):659–62. doi:10.1097/DAD.0b013e318222f906.

Pileri SA, Facchetti F, Ascani S, Sabattini E, Poggi S, Piccioli M, et al. Myeloperoxidase expression by histiocytes in Kikuchi's and Kikuchi-like lymphadenopathy. Am J Pathol. 2001;159(3):915–24.

Pilichowska ME, Pinkus JL, Pinkus GS. Histiocytic necrotizing lymphadenitis (Kikuchi-Fujimoto disease): lesional cells exhibit an immature dendritic cell phenotype. Am J Clin Pathol. 2009;131(2):174–82. doi:10.1309/AJCP7V1QHJLOTKKJ.

Politz MJ, Miller ML. Subcutaneous granuloma annulare of the foot. An atypical case report. J Am Podiatry Assoc. 1983;73(3):146–52.

Quaglino P, Tomasini C, Novelli M, Colonna S, Bernengo MG. Immunohistologic findings and adhesion molecule pattern in primary pure cutaneous Rosai-Dorfman disease with xanthomatous features. Am J Dermatopathol. 1998;20(4):393–8.

Ratzinger G, Zelger BG, Zelger B. Is there a true association between Rosai-Dorfman disease and malignancy? Br J Dermatol. 2003;149(5):1085–6.

Rosai J, Dorfman RF. Sinus histiocytosis with massive lymphadenopathy: a newly recognized benign clinicopathologic entity. Arch Pathol. 1969;87(1):63–70.

Rosai J, Dorfman RF. Sinus histiocytosis with massive lymphadenopathy: a pseudolymphomatous benign disorder. Analysis of 34 cases. Cancer. 1972;30(5):1174–88.

Rybicki BA, Major M, Popovich Jr J, Maliarik MJ, Iannuzzi MC. Racial differences in sarcoidosis incidence: a 5-year study in a health maintenance organization. Am J Epidemiol. 1997;145(3):234–41.

Rybicki BA, Iannuzzi MC, Frederick MM, Thompson BW, Rossman MD, Bresnitz EA, et al. Familial aggregation of sarcoidosis: A Case Control Etiologic Study of Sarcoidosis (ACCESS). Am J Respir Crit Care Med. 2001;164(11):2085–91.

Salomon RJ, Gardepe SF, Woodley DR. Deep granuloma annulare in adults. Int J Dermatol. 1986;25(2):109–12.

Samtsov AV. Cutaneous sarcoidosis. Int J Dermatol. 1992;31(6):385–91.

Santana A, Lessa B, Galrão L, Lima I, Santiago M. Kikuchi-Fujimoto's disease associated with systemic lupus erythematosus: case report and review of the literature. Clin Rheumatol. 2005;24(1):60–3.

Selim A, Ehrsam E, Atassi MB, Khachemoune A. Scar sarcoidosis: a case report and brief review. Cutis. 2006;78(6):418–22.

Shusang V, Marelli L, Beynon H, Davies N, Patch D, Dhillon AP, et al. Autoimmune hepatitis associated with Kikuchi-Fujimoto's disease. Eur J Gastroenterol Hepatol. 2008;20(1):79–82.

Smith G, Brownell I, Sanchez M, Prystowsky S. Advances in the genetics of sarcoidosis. Clin Genet. 2008;73(5):401–12. doi:10.1111/j.1399-0004.2008.00970.x.

Smith MD, Downie JB, DiCostanzo D. Granuloma annulare. Int J Dermatol. 1997;36(5):326–33.

Song JY, Lee J, Park DW, Sohn JW, Suh SI, Kim IS, et al. Clinical outcome and predictive factors of recurrence among patients with Kikuchi's disease. Int J Infect Dis. 2009;13(3):322–6. doi:10.1016/j.ijid.2008.06.022.

Sopeña B, Rivera A, Vázquez-Triñanes C, Fluiters E, González-Carreró J, del Pozo M, et al. Semin Arthritis Rheum. 2012;41(6):900–6. doi: 10.1016/j.semarthrit.2011.11.001.

Spies J, Foucar K, Thompson CT, LeBoit PE. The histopathology of cutaneous lesions of Kikuchi's disease (necrotizing lymphadenitis): a report of five cases. Am J Surg Pathol. 1999;23(9):1040–7.

Stebbing C, van der Walt J, Ramadan G, Inusa B. Rosai-Dorfman disease: a previously unreported association with sickle cell disease. BMC Clin Pathol. 2007;7:3.

Stefanaki K, Tsivitanidou-Kakourou T, Stefanaki C, Valari M, Argyrakos T, Konstantinidou CV, et al. Histological and immunohistochemical study of granuloma annulare and subcutaneous granuloma annulare in children. J Cutan Pathol. 2007;34(5):392–6.

Stockman DL, Rosenberg J, Bengana C, Suster S, Plaza JA. Verrucous cutaneous sarcoidosis: case report and review of this unusual variant of cutaneous sarcoidosis. Am J Dermatopathol. 2013;35(2):273–6. doi:10.1097/DAD.0b013e318262ed4c.

Studer EM, Calza AM, Saurat JH. Precipitating factors and associated diseases in 84 patients with granuloma annulare: a retrospective study. Dermatology. 1996;193(4):364–8.

Su LD, Kim YH, LeBoit PE, Swetter SM, Kohler S. Interstitial mycosis fungoides: a variant of mycosis fungoides resembling granuloma annulare and inflammatory morphea. J Cutan Pathol. 2002;29(3):135–41.

Sumikawa Y, Ansai S, Kimura T, Nakamura J, Inui S, Katayama I. Interstitial type granuloma annulare associated with Sjogren's syndrome. J Dermatol. 2010;37(5):493–5. doi:10.1111/j.1346-8138.2010.00865.x.

Sumiyoshi Y, Kikuchi M, Oshima K, Yoneda S, Kobari S, Takeshita M, et al. Human herpesvirus-6 genomes in histiocytic necrotizing lymphadenitis (Kikuchi's disease) and other forms of lymphadenitis. Am J Clin Pathol. 1993;99(5):609–14.

Tanaka T, Ohmori M, Yasunaga S, Ohshima K, Kikuchi M, Sasazuki T. DNA typing of HLA class II genes (HLA-DR, -DQ, and –DP) in Japanese patients with histiocytic necrotizing lymphadenitis (Kikuchi's disease). Tissue Antigens. 1999;54(3):246–53.

Telle H, Koeppel MC, Jreissati M, Andrac L, Horschowski N, Sayag J. Granulomatous mycosis fungoides. Eur J Dermatol. 1998;8(7):506–10.

Teuber SS, Howell LP, Yoshida SH, Gershwin ME. Remission of sarcoidosis following removal of silicone gel breast implants. Int Arch Allergy Immunol. 1994;105(4):404–7.

Thawerani H, Sanchez RL, Rosai J, Dorfman RF. The cutaneous manifestations of sinus histiocytosis with massive lymphadenopathy. Arch Dermatol. 1978;114(2):191–7.

Toro JR, Chu P, Yen TS, LeBoit PE. Granuloma annulare and human immunodeficiency virus infection. Arch Dermatol. 1999;135(11):1341–6.

Vassilakopoulos TP, Pangalis GA, Siakantaris MP, Levidou G, Yiakoumis X, Floudas C, et al. Kikuchi's lymphadenopathy: a relative rare but important cause of lymphadenopathy in Greece, potentially associated with antiphospholipid syndrome. Rheumatol Int. 2010;30(7):925–32. doi:10.1007/s00296-009-1077-2.

Vazquez-Lopez F, Pereiro Jr M, Manjon Haces JA, Gonzalez Lopez MA, Soler Sanchez T, Fernandez Coto T, et al. Localized granuloma annulare and autoimmune thyroiditis in adult women: a case-control study. J Am Acad Dermatol. 2003;48(4):517–20.

Veien NK, Stahl D, Brodthagen H. Cutaneous sarcoidosis in Caucasians. J Am Acad Dermatol. 1987;16(3 pt 1):534–40.

Veinot JP, Eidus L, Jabi M. Soft tissue Rosai Dorfman disease mimicking inflammatory pseudotumor: a diagnostic pitfall. Pathology. 1998;30(1):14–6.

Voulgari PV, Markatseli TE, Exarchou SA, Zioga A, Drosos AA. Granuloma annulare induced by anti-tumour necrosis factor therapy. Ann Rheum Dis. 2008;67(4):567–70.

Walsh NM, Hanly JG, Tremaine R, Murray S. Cutaneous sarcoidosis and foreign bodies. Am J Dermatopathol. 1993;15(3):203–7.

Wang KH, Cheng CJ, Hu CH, Lee WR. Coexistence of localized Langerhans cell histiocytosis and cutaneous Rosai-Dorfman disease. Br J Dermatol. 2002;147(4):770–4.

Wang KH, Chen WY, Liu HN, Huang CC, Lee WR, Hu CH. Cutaneous Rosai-Dorfman disease: clinicopathological profiles, spectrum and evaluation of 21 lesions in six patients. Br J Dermatol. 2006;154(2):277–86.

Wells RS, Smith MA. The natural history of granuloma annulare. Br J Dermatol. 1963;75:199–205.

Wu W, Robinson-Bostom L, Kokkotou E, Jung HY, Kroumpouzos G. Dyslipidemia in granuloma annulare: a case-control study. Arch Dermatol. 2012;148(10):1131–6.

Yen A, Fearneyhough P, Raimer SS, Hudnall SD. EBV-associated Kikuchi's histiocytic necrotizing lymphadenitis with cutaneous manifestations. J Am Acad Dermatol. 1997;36(2 Pt 2):342–6.

Yu JB, Liu WP, Zuo Z, Tang Y, Liao DY, Ji H, et al. Rosai-Dorfman disease: clinicopathologic, immunohistochemical and etiologic study of 16 cases. Zhonghua Bing Li Xue Za Zhi. 2007;36(1):33–8.

Zax RH, Callen JP. Granulomatous reactions. In: Sams WM, Lynch PJ, editors. Principles and practice of dermatology. New York: Churchill Livingstone; 1990.

Zhang WP, Wang JH, Wang WQ, Chen XQ, Wang Z, Li YF, et al. An association between parvovirus B19 and Kikuchi-Fujimoto disease. Viral Immunol. 2007; 20(3):421–8.

Zhang X, Hyjek E, Vardiman J. A subset of Rosai-Dorfman disease exhibits features of IgG4-related disease. Am J Clin Pathol. 2013;139(5):622–32. doi:10.1309/AJCPARC3YQ0KLIOA.

Cutaneous Pathology of Emergent and Tropical Infections: Skin, Infectious Pathogens, and Emergent and Tropical Infections

Wun-Ju Shieh

Introduction to Cutaneous Infections

The skin is often a sentinel for many infectious diseases by being the primary site of involvement, by being the entry site of infectious pathogens, or by demonstrating lesions that result from toxin, inflammatory, or vascular-mediated changes associated with infection. Cutaneous lesions are one of the top medical concerns in travelers returning from tropical regions. According to previous studies (Caumes et al. 1995; Lederman et al. 2008), dermatological disorders were the third most common cause of health problems associated with returning travelers after systemic febrile illness and acute diarrhea. The majority of these lesions develop before the travelers return home and rarely require hospitalization; however, they often lead to medical evaluation.

Healthy and intact skin provides an effective barrier against invasion by microorganisms. Clinical infection usually results from breaks in the skin, loss of local immunity, and disturbances within the normal flora resident on skin surface. The cutaneous flora is relatively simple compared to the diverse variety of microorganisms that inhabits the oral cavity, digestive tract, and female genital tract. The skin flora is mainly composed of aerobic cocci, anaerobic coryneform bacteria, gram-negative bacteria, and yeasts. A major function of this flora is to prevent skin infections, both by providing ecological competition for pathogenic microorganisms and by hydrolyzing lipids of sebum to produce free fatty acids, which are toxic to many bacteria.

Although many pathogens can cause cutaneous infections, the skin has a limited number of responses to inflammatory or infectious processes. In approaching patients with possible infectious rashes or tropical exposures, there are three important steps to help triage the diagnostic possibilities. First, the patient's travel and exposure history needs to be fully obtained; the exposure history should include animal, vector, environment, social behavior, chemical substance, etc. Second, the rash should be accurately defined based on its gross morphology, location, distribution, and associated symptoms. Third, a complete medical history and physical examination needs to be integrated into other clinical information. The underlying immune status of the patient has important implications regarding the differential diagnosis. Immunosuppressed travelers may acquire emergent pathogens at a higher risk. Some infections acquired in the developing countries may have the potential for reactivation or dissemination years later, especially when the patient becomes immunocompromised. There are several factors commonly present among immunocompromised patients that enhance their risk to have cutaneous infections.

W.-J. Shieh, MD, MPH, PhD
Infectious Disease Pathology Branch, Centers for Disease Control and Prevention, 1600 Clifton Road, N.E., Mail Stop G-32, Atlanta, GA 30333, USA
e-mail: wshieh@cdc.gov; wbs9@cdc.gov

For example, medical interventions with needle punctures and catheters provide a ready route for microorganisms to go through the stratum corneum and enter the bloodstream. Chemotherapy and irradiation can cause hair loss, dryness, and loss of sweat production that disrupt the barrier of healthy skin with these radical changes. When the balance is lost between host defenses and commensal flora on the skin surface or around the hair follicle, the follicles can become inflamed and form a potential entry point of infection. Therefore, cutaneous infections, especially the emergent and tropical infections, pose a substantial threat to immunocompromised patients.

Bacterial Infections

A wide range of bacteria, including mycobacteria, rickettsiae, and spirochetes, can affect the skin and subcutaneous tissue. They represent the largest proportion of pathogens causing emergent and tropical cutaneous infections. A limited number of histopathologic patterns are seen with bacterial infections in the skin, and none of these reaction patterns are specific for any particular pathogens. Definitive diagnosis of most bacterial diseases depends on specific identification of the pathogenic organisms with appropriate cultures or molecular techniques. Cultures from actual biopsies have a higher yield than cultures from aspirates or superficial swabs. An ideal method to maximize the yield of etiologic diagnosis for deeper skin infections is to send half of the biopsy for culture and the other half for hematoxylin and eosin (H&E) and special stains (Maingi and Helm 1998). The location of the bacteria in the skin biopsy is important to note. Gram-positive cocci and coccobacilli, such as staphylococci and corynebacteria, are usually normal flora within the follicles or on the surface of crusted, eroded, or ulcerated conditions. On the contrary, gram-positive cocci in the dermis or subcutaneous tissue indicate a true significant infectious process such as cellulitis, panniculitis, or fasciitis. Special stains, including Gram stain, acid-fast bacillus (AFB) stain, and Warthin–Starry silver stain,

may help highlight certain bacteria, but none of them is specific. Immunohistochemical methods are available for the detection of some pathogens, while molecular technique offers a more sensitive and specific method for a definitive identification of etiologic agent. However, many of these applications are available only in research laboratories or in special facilities (Rapini 1991).

The following section describes some of the emerging or tropical pathogens that can cause significant skin infection.

Anthrax

Etiology and Epidemiology

Anthrax is an acute infection caused by *Bacillus anthracis*, a gram-positive rod that is enzootic in many countries, and human infections are usually associated with animal exposure (Godyn et al. 2004). It occurs occasionally among workers through handling infected hides, wool, or hair in wool-scouring mills and tanneries. However, the organism was used as a biological weapon in 2001 through mails intentionally contaminated with white powder containing spores of *Bacillus anthracis*. Before September 2001, cases of anthrax in the United States have been reported infrequently since the 1970s; the last reported case of inhalational anthrax occurred in 1976, while the last reported case of cutaneous anthrax occurred in the summer of 2001 (Tutrone et al. 2002). During the 2001 incidence, 11 confirmed inhalational anthrax with five deaths and 11 cutaneous anthrax with no fatality were identified from October to November (Jernigan et al. 2002; Shieh et al. 2003).

Clinical Features

The majority of natural human infections occur 1–7 days after primary inoculation of the skin with the bacteria from animals or animal products. Only a small proportion (~5 %) of human cases are inhalation anthrax or gastrointestinal disease from eating infected meat. The skin lesion usually starts as a red macule, sometimes pruritic, and evolves through papular and vesicular stages into hemorrhagic pustule. The pustule eventually ulcerates, and the lesion will be covered by a thick, black eschar (the name anthrax comes from the Greek word for "coal"). The eschar is usually surrounded by marked erythema and edema, which usually is more extensive on the head or neck than on the trunk or extremities. Characteristically, pain is mild or absent. Patients usually are afebrile, but tender regional lymphadenopathy, fatigue, fever, or chills may develop in some cases. The skin lesions usually heal spontaneously in 1–2 weeks, leaving very little scarring. Death from untreated cutaneous anthrax can be as high as 25 % but is near 0 % with appropriate early treatment. The bacteria grow readily in culture media, but the organisms may not be identified correctly if the laboratory is not alerted to the suspicion of anthrax. Confirmatory cultures, serologic assays, and polymerase chain reaction (PCR) testing are available through the public health network (Dauphin et al. 2012).

Histopathology

Histopathologic features can vary according to the stages of infection and sites of biopsy. Cultures and full-thickness punch biopsies should be taken from the edges of both vesicle and eschar, if present. At the site of the eschar, the epidermis is destroyed, and the ulcerated surface is covered with necrotic tissue. There is marked edema of the dermis with variable lymphocytes and neutrophils (Fig. 14.1). Vasculitis, vascular necrosis, and hemorrhage can be observed (Fig. 14.2).

In acute stage of untreated cases, bacilli with characteristic capsule are present in large numbers and can be recognized in sections stained with tissue Gram stain (Fig. 14.3). The organism is best demonstrated when the lesion is in the vesicular stage, so swab exudates for Gram stain and biopsy should be taken for suspect cases. The organisms are usually more abundant in upper dermis, especially in the necrotic tissue toward the ulcerated surface. However, typical bacilli are rarely seen in skin biopsies obtained from a later stage of cases with antibiotic treatment. In general, the longer the duration of illness and treatment course, the less chance of detecting *B. anthracis* organism by culture and special stains. Steiner's silver-impregnation stain appears to be more sensitive than Gram stain for demonstrating these bacilli in cutaneous lesion obtained at a later stage (Fig. 14.4) (Shieh et al. 2003).

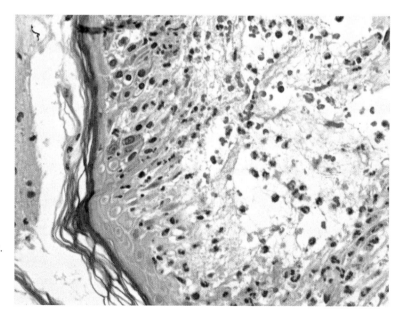

Fig. 14.1 Cutaneous anthrax. Marked edema of the dermis with neutrophils and lymphocytes (H&E, 200× original magnification)

Fig. 14.2 Cutaneous anthrax. Ulceration of epidermis and marked edema, necrosis, and hemorrhage in dermis (H&E, 50× original magnification)

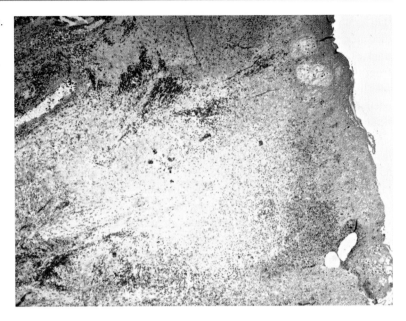

Fig. 14.3 Cutaneous anthrax. Bacilli with characteristic capsule, usually more abundant in upper dermis, especially in the necrotic tissue toward the ulcerated surface (Gram stain, 630× original magnification)

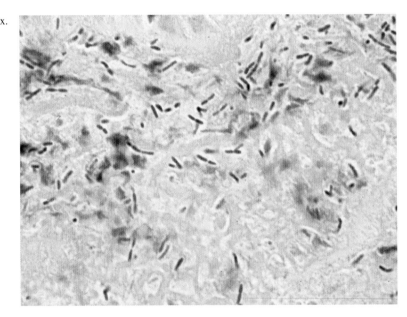

Immunohistochemical assay (IHC) provides a more sensitive and specific way to establish the diagnosis of cutaneous anthrax because of its capability to detect bacterial antigens in tissues regardless of the treatment (Fig. 14.5) (Shieh et al. 2003; Tatti et al. 2006).

Differential Diagnosis

Clinical lesions of anthrax may resemble impetigo, sporotrichosis, orf, arthropod bites, plague, rickettsialpox, scrub typhus, or tularemia. Painful pustules are more typical of impetigo caused by streptococcal or staphylococcal

Fig. 14.4 Cutaneous anthrax. Bacilli highlighted by Steiner silver stain (Steiner stain, 630× original magnification)

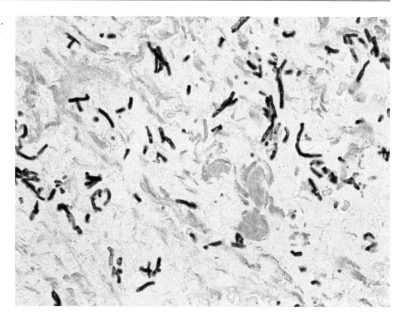

Fig. 14.5 Cutaneous anthrax. Immunostaining of *B. anthracis* antigens in dermis (IHC, 400× original magnification)

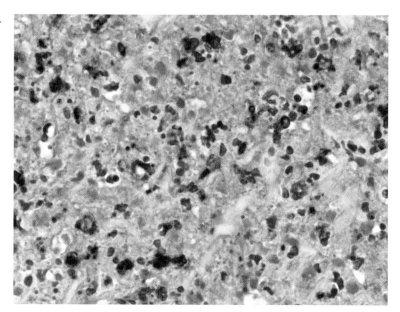

infections with prominent neutrophilic infiltrate in epidermis and dermis. Spider and other arthropod bites also are more likely to be painful with prominent eosinophilic infiltrate and vascular necrosis in dermis.

Plague

Etiology and Epidemiology

Plague is caused by *Yersinia pestis*, a small, gram-negative, non-sporing, and nonmotile bacillus. It is a zoonotic infection that affects a wide variety of rodents, particularly the urban and domestic rats, and the organisms are conveyed from infected rodents to humans by the bites of fleas. Human-to-human transmission rarely occurs in pneumonic plague through inhalation of infectious droplets or other contaminated material. Plague is still endemic in many regions of the world, including India and the Far East, and in Southern and Central Africa. Sporadic outbreaks occur in North Africa and the Middle East, and there are small endemic areas in the United States as well. Occasional cases have been reported elsewhere in travelers from the endemic areas. The potential use of plague as a biological weapon has been of recent interest (Inglesby et al. 2000).

Clinical Features

The incubation period is usually 3 or 4 days, but it may occasionally be longer than 7 days. Following inoculation of the organism by a flea bite, the regional lymph node becomes swollen (the classic presentation of bubonic plague), and systemic dissemination with a severe febrile illness can quickly develop, leading to death within days if untreated. Primary pulmonary infection (pneumonic plague) occurs in some cases, if *Y. pestis* is inhaled, which is almost always fatal within 3 or 4 days. In plague epidemics, mild bubonic infections with no systemic spread and subclinical infections both have been observed. Conversely, a patient may rapidly die of flea-transmitted plague without ever developing a bubo. Clinical cutaneous manifestations of plague are usually nonspecific. Although typically there is no distinct lesion at the site of the initial flea bite, an erythematous plaque may appear, which will become bullous and subsequently crusted like an eschar seen in cutaneous anthrax. Such primary cutaneous lesions may occur in 10 % of patients. The involved regional lymph nodes become painfully swollen several days later. During the bacteremic phase, a macular, erythematous, or petechial rash may develop and sometimes generalized purpuric rash may appear, thus the historic name of "black death."

Necrotic lesions that closely resemble ecthyma gangrenosum may develop. Aspiration of a bubo and direct examination of smears and culture confirm the diagnosis. The culture of blood and sputum should also be undertaken if septicemic or pneumonic plague is suspected. Serologic and PCR assays can also confirm the diagnosis.

Histopathology

The histopathologic features of the skin lesions are generally not diagnostic and vary according to the type of lesion associated with their clinical presentation. The purpuric and petechial lesions, especially in those associated with shock, may show vasculitis, vascular necrosis with microthrombi, hemorrhage, and other signs of disseminated intravascular coagulation (Fig. 14.6). The erythematous lesions appear to have a septal panniculitis. The morbilliform rash is associated with a perivascular lymphocytic infiltrate. Giemsa and Gram stain may highlight bacilli with characteristic bipolar staining. Bacilli are usually more abundant in vessels and perivascular areas in biopsy samples obtained at septicemic stage (Fig. 14.7). IHC with a specific anti-*Y. pestis* antibody provides a sensitive method for confirmatory diagnosis because of its capability to detect bacilliform and granular antigens in areas of inflammation and necrotic debris (Fig. 14.8) (Guarner et al. 2002, 2005).

Differential Diagnosis

Plague can mimic many other infectious diseases. Since clinical and histopathologic features of skin lesions are both nonspecific, only definitive serology or cultures allow a confirmed diagnosis of *Y. pestis* infection.

Tularemia

Etiology and Epidemiology

Tularemia is caused by *Francisella tularensis*, a small, gram-negative, pleomorphic coccobacillus. Human infection is usually acquired through direct contact with animal reservoirs harboring the bacteria. The disease can also be transmitted

Fig. 14.6 Cutaneous plague. Vasculitis and vascular necrosis with mixed inflammatory infiltrate (H&E, 100× original magnification)

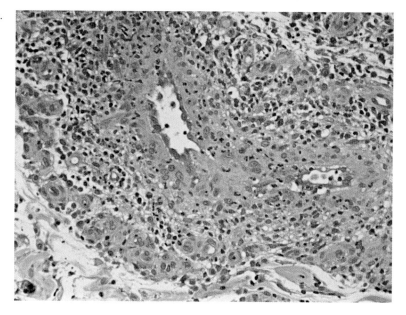

Fig. 14.7 Septicemic plague. Abundant gram-negative bacilli in a dermal vessel (Gram stain, 400× original magnification)

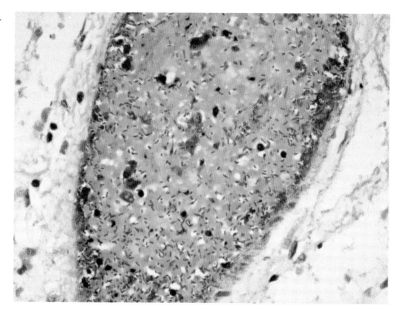

by insects, such as mosquitoes, ticks, deer flies, etc. The disease is endemic in North America and parts of Europe and Asia. The bacterium has several subspecies with varying degrees of virulence. The most important one is *F. tularensis tularensis* (type A), which is found in lagomorphs, such as rabbits and other similar animals in North America, and it is highly pathogenic in humans

Fig. 14.8 Septicemic plague.
Immunostaining of *Y. pestis*
antigens in a large vascular
thrombus (IHC, 400× original
magnification)

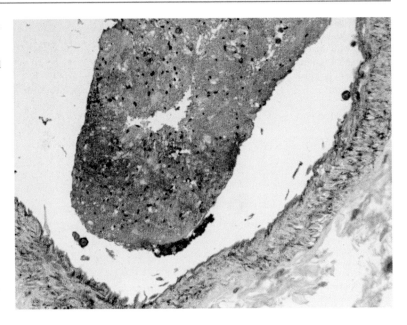

and domestic rabbits. *F. tularensis palaearctica* (type B) occurs mainly in aquatic rodents, such as beavers and muskrats in North America, and in hares and small rodents in northern Eurasia. It is less virulent for humans and rabbits (Eliasson et al. 2006).

Clinical Features

The disease can occur as sporadic cases or small epidemics. The usual incubation period is 3–5 days. The characteristic clinical presentation of this disease is the so-called ulceroglandular tularemia, which represents about 80 % of cases (Syrjala et al. 1984). Usually, the finger or hand is the primary site of the inoculation, where a rapidly growing papulonodular lesion develops followed by painful ulceration and necrosis. Tender subcutaneous nodes may form along the lymph vessels that drain the primary lesion. There is considerable swelling of the regional lymph nodes with marked constitutional symptoms. A black eschar appears within 3–5 days after contact. Complete healing of the lesion may take place in 2–5 weeks. Other important forms of tularemia include oculoglandular, oropharyngeal, gastrointestinal, pulmonary, and typhoidal. Mortality of pneumonic tularemia ranges from 30 % to 60 % if untreated. Culture of the organism can confirm the diagnosis but laboratory biosafety is a concern, while serologic diagnosis is safer and more effective. PCR testing also provides a sensitive and rapid method for confirmatory diagnosis (Splettstoesser et al. 2005).

Histopathology

Skin biopsies typically show ulceration, extravasated erythrocytes, and necrosis surrounded by palisading neutrophils. Suppurative granuloma formation eventually develops with central necrosis and nuclear debris (Fig. 14.9). Some of them may appear with caseous necrosis similar to mycobacterial infections. In some cases, only a moderate number of epithelioid cells and a few giant cells are observed. The tender nodes that may be found along lymph vessels show multiple necrotizing granulomas deep in the dermis and extending into the subcutaneous tissue (Fig. 14.10). Organisms are rarely demonstrated with the Gram stain. Steiner or Warthin–Starry silver-impregnation stain may be more sensitive in demonstrating the organisms. IHC with a specific anti-*F. tularensis* antibody provides a sensitive method for confirmatory diagnosis because of its capability to detect bacterial antigens in skin and lymph node biopsies (Fig. 14.11) (Lamps et al. 2004; Asano et al. 2012).

Fig. 14.9 Ulceroglandular tularemia. Suppurative granulomatous inflammation with necrosis and nuclear debris (H&E, 100× original magnification)

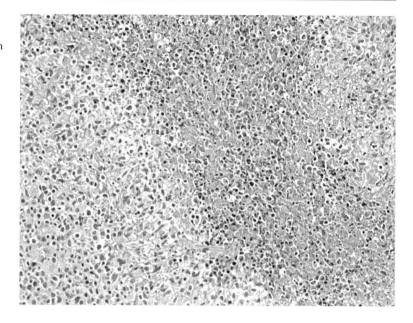

Fig. 14.10 Subcutaneous lymphadenitis of tularemia. Necrotizing granuloma in dermis extending into the subcutaneous tissue (H&E, 50× original magnification)

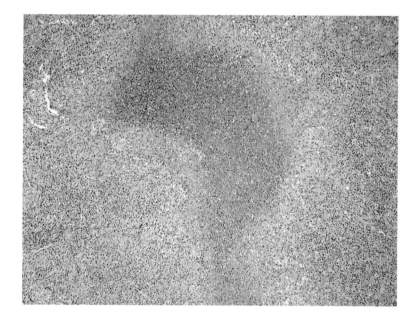

Differential Diagnosis

A good clinical history and physical findings usually can point toward the diagnosis. Clinical lesions of cutaneous tularemia, especially with eschar formation, may resemble impetigo, anthrax, sporotrichosis, orf, arthropod bites, plague, rickettsialpox, and scrub typhus. Histologically, mycobacterial infections, cat-scratch disease, leishmaniasis, sporotrichosis, and other fungal infections should be considered when prominent granulomatous inflammation is observed.

Fig. 14.11 Ulceroglandular tularemia. Immunostaining of *F. tularensis* antigens in areas of necrosis (IHC, 400× original magnification)

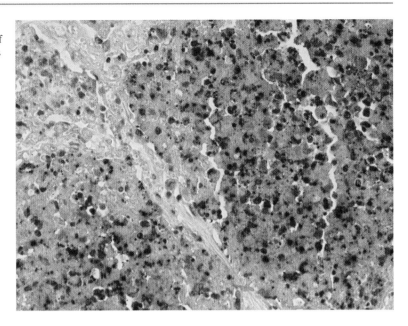

Cat-Scratch Disease

Etiology and Epidemiology

Cat-scratch disease is caused by *Bartonella henselae*, a gram-negative bacillus similar to that of bacillary angiomatosis. It is closely related to *Bartonella quintana*, the etiologic agent of louse-borne trench fever. The cat was recognized as the natural reservoir of the disease in 1950. The causative organism was first thought to be *Afipia felis*, but this was disproved by immunological studies demonstrating that cat-scratch fever patients developed antibodies to other organisms, especially *B. henselae* (Bergmans et al. 1995). Kittens are more likely to carry the bacteria in their blood and may therefore be more likely to transmit the disease than adult cats. From many studies, it is believed that a likely pathway of transmission of *B. henselae* from cats to humans may be inoculation with flea feces containing bacteria through a contaminated cat-scratch wound or across a mucosal surface (Murakawa 1997).

Clinical Features

The organism is carried in the blood and oral cavities of cats. The skin lesion develops 2–4 days after a scratch or bite from a cat; it may resemble an insect bite but does not itch. The lesion may appear as macular, papular, or nodular lesions, usually on the forearm or hand. A single or a group of large, tender swelling lymph nodes develops in the drainage area of the scratch 2–3 weeks later. The scratch skin lesion heals in a normal fashion, but the affected lymph nodes may become fluctuant as a result of suppuration (Chian et al. 2002; Pierard-Franchimont et al. 2010). Most cases are mild and resolve spontaneously, but lymphadenopathy may persist for several months after other symptoms disappear. The average duration of lymphadenopathy is 2 months. About one-third of patients develop fever or constitutional symptoms. In immunocompromised patients more severe complications sometimes occur. Other clinical forms of *B. henselae* infections include bacillary angiomatosis, bacillary peliosis, optic neuritis, and acute encephalopathy. Bacillary angiomatosis is primarily a vascular skin lesion more commonly associated with HIV or severe immunocompromised patients. The infection may extend to bone or other areas of the body. The diagnosis may be established by the cat-scratch skin test (Hanger-Rose test).

Fig. 14.12 Cat-scratch disease. Variable shapes of necrosis in the dermis (H&E, 100× original magnification)

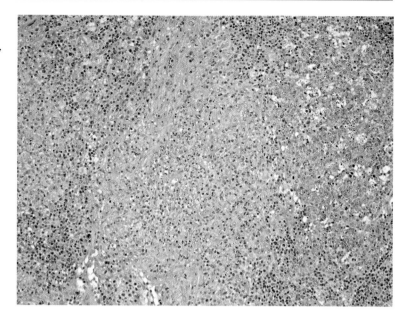

Fig. 14.13 Cat-scratch disease. Lymphohistiocytic and epithelioid cells surrounding the dermal necrosis with palisading arrangement (H&E, 400× original magnification)

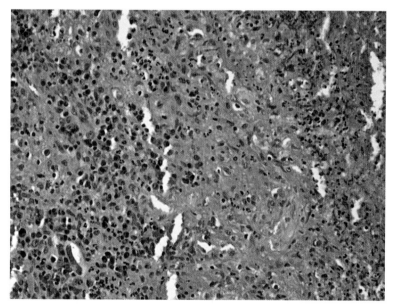

The skin test is reliable when performed 1 week after infection; however, it is not readily available and is not standardized. The organism is extremely difficult to culture. Serologic and PCR assays have been used to confirm the diagnosis (Maass et al. 1992; Hansmann et al. 2005).

Histopathology

Biopsies of the primary papular lesion at the site of the scratch show palisading granulomas around necrobiotic foci. Basically, one or several areas of necrosis in the dermis with variable shapes, including round, triangular, or stellate are seen (Fig. 14.12). There are usually several layers of lymphohistiocytic and epithelioid cells surrounding the necrosis, with the innermost layer exhibiting a palisading arrangement (Fig. 14.13). The periphery of the epithelioid cell reaction is surrounded by a zone of lymphocytes, plasma cells, and eosinophils. Scattered multinucleated

Fig. 14.14 Cat-scratch disease. Lichenoid lympho-plasmacytic infiltrate in dermis (H&E, 50× original magnification)

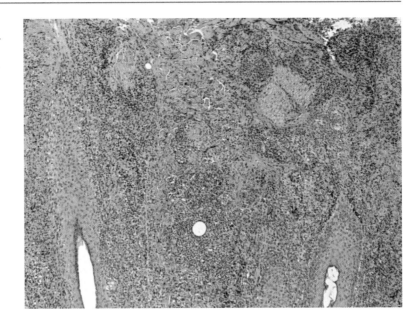

Fig. 14.15 Cat-scratch disease. Small, pleomorphic coccobacilli highlighted by Warthin–Starry silver stain at the periphery of necrosis (Warthin–Starry stain, 400× original magnification)

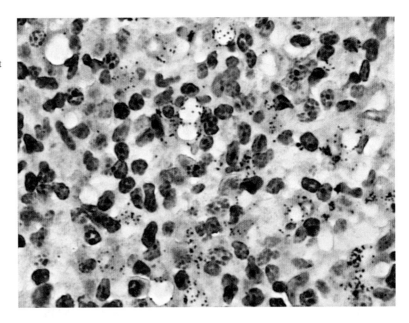

giant cells may be present. Other microscopic features, such as perivascular or lichenoid lymphoplasmacytic or neutrophilic infiltrates, can also present (Fig. 14.14) (Czarnetzki et al. 1975).

The reaction in the lymph nodes is similar to that observed in the skin, except microabscess formation in the central necrotic areas of the epithelioid granulomas is more commonly present due to the accumulation of numerous neutrophils. As the abscesses enlarge, they become confluent. Warthin–Starry silver-impregnation stain may occasionally demonstrate the small, pleomorphic, gram-negative bacilli at the periphery of central necrosis in involved skin and lymph nodes (Fig. 14.15). IHC is an excellent method to demonstrate the coccobacilli and bacterial antigens in

Fig. 14.16 Cat-scratch disease. Immunostaining of *B. henselae* antigens in areas of inflammation and necrosis (IHC, 400× original magnification)

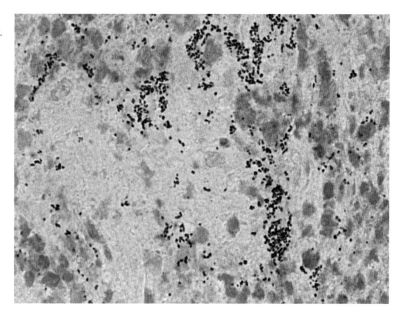

tissues (Fig. 14.16). PCR can be performed on paraffin-embedded skin biopsies to confirm the diagnosis (Maass et al. 1992; Scott et al. 1996).

Differential Diagnosis

The palisading granulomas in the skin lesions of patients with cat-scratch disease need to be differentiated with granulomatous inflammation caused by other infectious agents, such as mycobacteria, fungi, *Leishmania* spp., *F. tularensis*, etc. However, a careful history and the clinical presentations usually allow distinction of cat-scratch disease from other infectious diseases.

Rickettsial and Rickettsia-Like Infections

Rickettsiae are obligate intracellular parasites that are transmitted to humans from infected arthropods. *Rickettsia* species infect and damage endothelial cells, leading to cutaneous and systemic lymphohistiocytic vasculitis, the hallmark and major pathogenetic lesion of vasculotropic rickettsioses. New species and new strains of existing species are being characterized, and there is also reemergence of older organisms. The *Rickettsia*

organisms are divided into the spotted fever group and the typhus group. Other rickettsia-like organisms include *Orientia tsutsugamushi* (scrub typhus), *Coxiella burnetii* (Q fever), *Ehrlichia chaffeensis* (ehrlichiosis), and *Anaplasma phagocytophilum* (human granulocytic anaplasmosis). Skin lesions are more commonly seen in infections associated with spotted fever group rickettsiae and *Orientia tsutsugamushi*.

Spotted Fever Group Rickettsioses
Etiology and Epidemiology

There are many diseases caused by spotted fever group rickettsiae depending on the vectors and geographic areas. The more common ones include the following: (1) Rocky Mountain spotted fever (RMSF) caused by *Rickettsia rickettsii*, (2) Mediterranean spotted fever or boutonneuse fever caused by *R. conorii*, (3) African tick-bite fever caused by *R. africae*, (4) maculatum disease caused by *R. parkeri*, and (5) rickettsialpox caused by *R. akari*. The rickettsial disease of greatest importance in the United States is RMSF (Walker 1995; Chapman et al. 2006b), which is acquired after the bite of infected Dermacentor subspecies ticks. The disease is encountered most commonly in the southeast of the United States

Fig. 14.17 Spotted fever group rickettsioses. Mild to moderate lymphohistiocytic perivascular infiltrate in dermis; acantholysis and focal necrosis in epidermis (H&E, 50× original magnification)

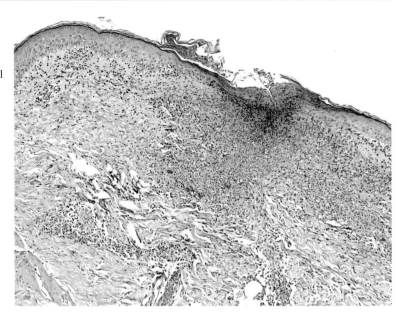

and has been reported even within New York City. Mediterranean spotted fever is widespread in Mediterranean basin, Africa, and Asia (Cascio and Iaria 2006). African tick-bite fever occurs mainly in sub-Saharan Africa and the Caribbean (Althaus et al. 2010). Maculatum disease occurs in North and South America (Paddock et al. 2008). Rickettsialpox is unique because the bacteria is transmitted to humans from a bite by infected mite, not tick. It has been reported from the United States, Ukraine, Croatia, Turkey, and Mexico (Koss et al. 2003).

Clinical Features

The vasculotropic rickettsioses share many similar clinical features. In RMSF, after an incubation period of 1–2 weeks after the tick bite, a short period of malaise and headache is followed by high fever and chills (Walker 1995; Sexton and Kaye 2002). After 3 or 4 days, a maculopapular eruption appears on the wrists and ankles and soon spreads centrally to limbs, trunk, and face. The palms and soles are usually involved. The lesions at first are macular to papular but become purpuric within 2–3 days. The degree of cutaneous involvement is highly variable and sometimes transient; approximately 10–15 % of infected patients do not develop a prominent rash

(Sexton and Corey 1992). There may be only petechiae, but in fatal cases widespread ecchymoses are common. Acral gangrene may result from small vessel occlusion. Because the diagnosis may not be made in the beginning and the course may be rapid, mortality exceeds 10 %, despite the effectiveness of antibiotics. Whenever a diagnosis of RMSF is suspected, a search should be made for an eschar indicating the site of a tick bite. Eschar is usually more prominent in Mediterranean spotted fever, African tick-bite fever, and rickettsialpox. Although serologic assay has been used for clinical diagnosis, the titer may not rise in the acute phase up to 10 days. PCR testing is a more sensitive and rapid method to confirm the diagnosis (Dumler and Walker 1994; Chapman et al. 2006a).

Histopathology

The histopathologic features are similar among the vasculotropic rickettsioses. Significant findings are confined mostly within the dermis. The early changes include a mild to moderate mixed lymphohistiocytic infiltrate that surrounds and penetrates into the walls of the dermal vessels (Fig. 14.17). Erythrocyte extravasation (Fig. 14.18) endothelial swelling (Fig. 14.19), and edema are commonly seen. Later (usually after 1 week),

Fig. 14.18 Spotted fever group rickettsioses. Erythrocyte extravasation, edema, and vasculitis in dermis (H&E, 100× original magnification)

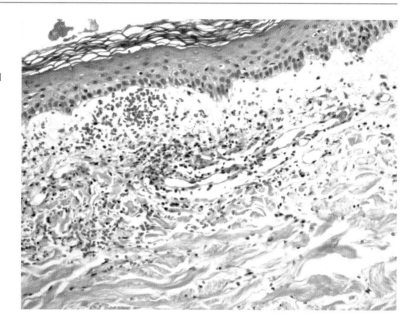

Fig. 14.19 Spotted fever group rickettsioses. Endothelial swelling and lymphohistiocytic perivascular infiltrate in dermis (H&E, 400× original magnification)

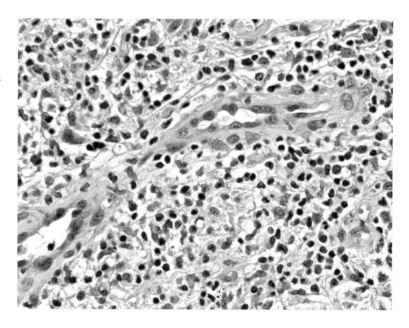

vascular damage with leukocytoclastic vasculitis frequently occurs; the infiltrate is predominantly lymphohistiocytic with occasional neutrophilic infiltrate and karyorrhectic nuclear debris. These later lesions are often associated clinically with nonblanching petechiae or hemorrhagic, purpuric rashes. Some of these lesions contain micro-thrombi and vessel wall necrosis (Fig. 14.20). In the advanced stage there is dermal and epidermal necrosis (Fig. 14.21) (Walker et al. 1987; Kao et al. 1997). The causative organism, which usually measures 0.3 by 1 μm, is too small to be visible by light microscopy using regular stains. IHC can readily demonstrate rickettsial antigen in

Fig. 14.20 Spotted fever
group rickettsioses.
Microthrombi and vessel wall
necrosis (H&E, 400× original
magnification)

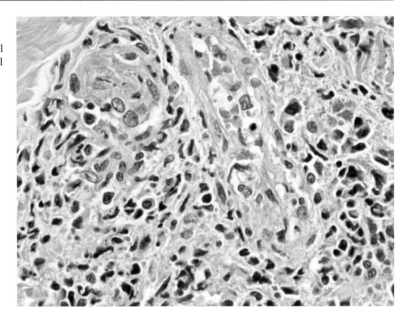

Fig. 14.21 Spotted fever
group rickettsioses. Eschar
formation with extensive
epidermal and dermal
necrosis (H&E, 50× original
magnification)

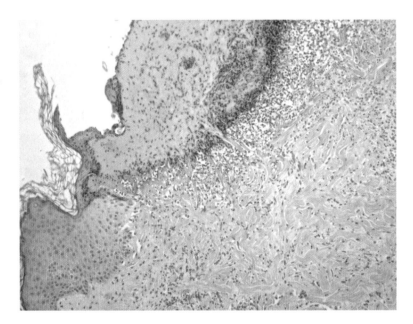

endothelial cells in association with perivascular lymphocytic infiltration (Fig. 14.22) (Dumler et al. 1990; Paddock et al. 1999).

Differential Diagnosis

The histologic differential diagnosis includes diseases associated with vascular or capillary inflammation, such as insect bite reaction, drug reaction, septic vasculitis secondary to disseminated intravascular coagulation (DIC), collagen vascular diseases, and many other autoimmune disorders with vasculitis. Many of the lesions can be differentiated by other laboratory or histologic methods, including culture or special stains for specific infectious agents.

Fig. 14.22 Spotted fever group rickettsioses. Immunostaining of rickettsial antigens in endothelial cells of dermal vessels (IHC, 400× original magnification)

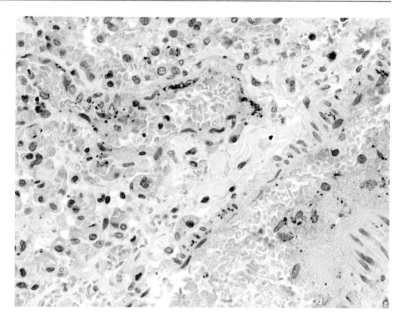

Scrub Typhus

Etiology and Epidemiology

Scrub typhus is caused by *Orientia (formerly Rickettsia) tsutsugamushi* and transmitted from its natural rodent reservoir by the bites of the mites, *Trombicula akamushi* and *T. deliensis*. It is a common disease in endemic areas of Southeast Asia and western Pacific islands. During the Vietnam War, it was the second or third most common cause of fever in American soldiers (Seong et al. 2001).

Clinical Features

Scrub typhus usually presents as an acute febrile illness after an incubation period of about 10 days (6–21 days). Fever, headache, and conjunctivitis accompany the development of the primary skin lesion. The primary eschar lesion is a firm papule surmounted by a vesicle, which dries to form a black crust. The regional lymph nodes are enlarged and tender. A generalized macular or maculopapular eruption develops after about a week and may fade rapidly or persist for 7–10 days. More severe clinical manifestations, such as pneumonitis and myocarditis, can occur and the mortality in cases without treatment can reach 60 % (Lee et al. 2013). In mild or treated cases, the fever subsides and recovery occurs during the second or third week. Serologic and PCR assays have been used for confirmatory diagnosis.

Histopathology

Eschar lesion exhibits ulceration with prominent coagulative necrosis of the epidermis and underlying dermis (Fig. 14.23). A lymphocytic vasculitis of small vessels with microthrombi and vascular necrosis is typically present in the dermis (Fig. 14.24). Various degrees of perivascular infiltrate with lymphocytes and occasional neutrophils are seen. IHC assay can demonstrate the organisms in endothelial cells and macrophages (Allen and Spitz 1945; Park and Hart 1946).

If immunohistochemistry for lymphoma is performed, CD30 positive immunoblasts may be seen raising concern for a CD30 + skin lymphomas (Lee et al. 2009).

Differential Diagnosis

Eschar lesions of scrub typhus may resemble impetigo, anthrax, sporotrichosis, orf, arthropod bites, plague, rickettsialpox, or tularemia. Travel history to endemic areas should raise the index of suspicion.

Fig. 14.23 Scrub typhus. Eschar lesion with ulceration and prominent coagulative necrosis in epidermis and underlying dermis (H&E, 50× original magnification)

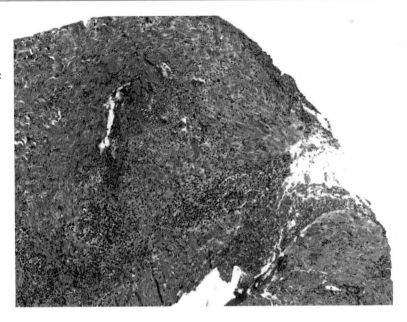

Fig. 14.24 Scrub typhus. Vasculitis of small vessels with microthrombi and vascular necrosis in dermis (H&E, 400× original magnification)

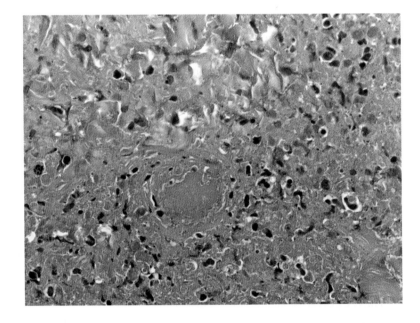

Mycobacterial Infections

The mycobacteria can be divided into two major groups based on their culture growth and biochemical characteristics. The slow growers include *Mycobacterium tuberculosis*, *M. avium* complex, *M. kansasii*, *M. marinum*, and *M. ulcerans*. The rapid growers include *M. fortuitum* and *M. chelonei*. *M. leprae is* not included in this classification because it cannot be grown in culture. *M. tuberculosis* and *M. leprae* are intracellular parasites usually confined to the tissues of humans and animals; therefore they are mainly transmitted by exposure to infected hosts. Other mycobacteria are present in soil and water, and the exposure of persons to these bacteria is widespread but usually is not associated with significant clinical disease. Because of the large number of mycobacterial species and wide spectrum of associated illness, only the following are described in this chapter: (1) cutaneous tuberculosis caused by *M. tuberculosis complex*, including BCG; (2) atypical mycobacteria, such as *M. avium complex*, *M. kansasii complex*, *M. Marinum*, *M. ulcerans*, and *M. haemophilum*; and (3) leprosy caused by *M. leprae*.

Cutaneous Tuberculosis
Etiology and Epidemiology
Mycobacterium tuberculosis primarily affects the lungs, but skin and many other organs may also be involved. The incidence of tuberculosis (TB) was decreasing in North America and Europe until the advent of AIDS. It has been estimated that almost 50 % of the earth's population is infected with *M. tuberculosis*, and the infection is responsible for 6 % of all deaths worldwide. The strains with antibiotics resistance have been a growing concern. Majority of individuals who are infected recover completely from their primary TB in the lung, with no further evidence of active disease. However, immunosuppression or any deterioration in health status may allow the bacteria proliferate from their quiescent status within macrophages to cause clinical disease.

In some parts of the world, immunity results from vaccination with bacille Calmette-Guérin (BCG). Skin testing with tuberculin purified-protein derivative is commonly used in patients who have not been vaccinated with BCG as a reliable means of confirming previous mycobacterial infection. Cultures and acid-fast stains of biopsies, sputum, or other fluids are required to make a diagnosis of active disease. When these results are negative, PCR testing may be helpful (Penneys et al. 1993; Degitz 1996).

Clinical Features
Cutaneous TB almost always means long-standing active disease elsewhere, with the rare exception of primary inoculation TB. There are many different types of cutaneous tuberculosis; their clinical features are summarized in Table 14.1 (Beyt et al. 1981; Kakakhel and Fritsch 1989; Sehgal et al. 1989; Inwald et al. 1994; Chong and Lo 1995; Farina et al. 1995; Kothavade et al. 2013).

Histopathology
TB typically causes caseating granulomas, but granulomas do not caseate in some forms, and suppuration or purulence may be more prominent, depending on the stage of lesion and patient's immune status. There are common histopathologic features as well as different patterns among various clinical forms; the features are summarized in Table 14.1 (Figs. 14.25, 14.26, 14.27, 14.28, 14.29, and 14.30) (Kakakhel and Fritsch 1989; Inwald et al. 1994; Jordaan et al. 1994; Farina et al. 1995; Mahaisavariya et al. 2004; Min et al. 2012).

Differential Diagnosis
The differential diagnosis includes other granulomatous conditions, such as atypical mycobacteriosis, leprosy, deep fungal infections, Treponema infections, cat-scratch disease, granuloma inguinale, lymphogranuloma venereum, tularemia, brucellosis, leishmaniasis, and other noninfectious granulomas.

Atypical Mycobacteriosis
Etiology and Epidemiology
There are many different Mycobacterium species that may infect humans besides *M. tuberculosis* and *M. leprae*. Common organisms include *M. marinum* ("swimming pool granuloma") (Bonamonte et al. 2013), *M. ulcerans* (Buruli ulcer in Central Africa), *M. avium-intracellulare* (MAI, especially with AIDS) (Cole and Gebhard 1979), and *M. fortuitum* and *M. chelonei* (rapid growers) (Kothavade et al. 2013). Unlike *M. tuberculosis*, which is transmitted from person to person, nontuberculosis mycobacteria are abundant in nature, in soil and water, and contact is frequent in most zones of the world. These skin infections may be acquired by direct inoculation into the skin or by hematogenous spread from

Table 14.1 Clinical and histopathologic features of various cutaneous tuberculosis

Disease	Clinical features	Histopathologic features
Primary inoculation	Rare crusted ulcer with regional adenopathy following infection of the skin by laboratory accidents, trauma, performance of autopsies, or tattooing	Variable epidermal ulceration. Diffuse mixed infiltrate with many neutrophils in early phase. Variable granulomatous components with epithelioid cells and multinucleated giant cells. Caseation more prominent in later stage. Acid-fast bacilli often present, particularly in areas of necrosis
Miliary	Rare papulopustular eruption as a result of widespread hematogenous dissemination owing to poor immunity or steroid treatment	Similar as the above. In severe form, microabscess at center of the papule with abundant neutrophils, cellular debris, and numerous acid-fast bacilli. In mild form, acid-fast bacilli less appreciable
TB cutis orificialis	Mucosal ulcers in patients with poor immunity	Similar as primary inoculation
Scrofuloderma	Nodular swelling or ulceration resulting from direct extension of underlying bone or lymph node TB	Similar as primary inoculation. Central abscess formation or ulceration more prominent
TB verrucosa cutis	Solitary purulent verrucous plaque seen in patients with high immunity	Hyperkeratosis, papillomatosis, acanthosis. Sometimes neutrophilic microabscesses in the epidermis. Diffuse mixed infiltrate in the dermis with prominent neutrophils. Tuberculoid granulomas, sometimes with caseation. Acid-fast bacilli may or may not present
Lupus vulgaris	Reddish brown apple jelly patches or plaques, usually on the head or neck, resulting from reactivation in a patient with good immunity	Secondary changes in the epidermis common, such as epidermal atrophy, hyperplasia, or ulceration. Tuberculoid granulomas in the superficial dermis with minimal or no caseation. Abundant Langhans-type giant cells. Acid-fast bacilli usually absent
Tuberculids (hypersensitivity reactions to active TB elsewhere)	Papulonecrotic tuberculid: multiple erythematous or crusted papules, usually on the limbs in a symmetrical distribution	Papulonecrotic tuberculid: lymphocytic or neutrophilic vasculitis. Fibrinoid necrosis of vessels with microthrombi frequently observed. Wedge of dermal necrosis. Acid-fast bacilli negative
	Lichen scrofulosorum: lichenoid papules, sometimes follicular or annular, mostly on the trunk	Lichen scrofulosorum: superficial dermal granulomas with or without caseation. Often around follicles or sweat ducts. Acid-fast bacilli negative

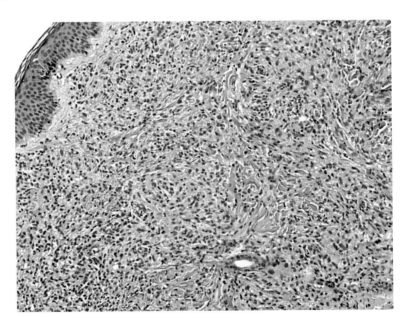

Fig. 14.25 Cutaneous tuberculosis. Diffuse mixed inflammatory infiltrate in dermis with variable epithelioid cells and multinucleated giant cells (H&E, 200× original magnification)

Fig. 14.26 Cutaneous
tuberculosis. Noncaseating
granuloma with epithelioid
cells and lymphohistiocytic
infiltrate (H&E, 400× original
magnification)

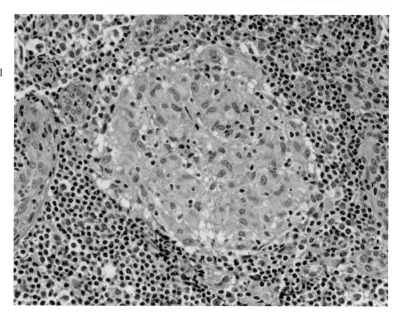

Fig. 14.27 Scrofuloderma.
Prominent epidermal
ulceration, abscess formation,
and caseating necrosis in
dermis (H&E, 50× original
magnification)

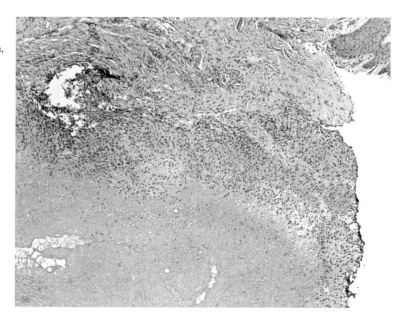

other visceral foci (Dodiuk-Gad et al. 2007).
Increased use of immunosuppression in medicine
such as those for organ transplant and cancer chemotherapy and the pandemic of HIV/AIDS have
resulted in many more mycobacterial skin infections (Mahaisavariya et al. 2003; Lee et al. 2010).

Clinical Features

Clinical lesions are variable, including solitary
or multiple erythematous nodules, abscesses,
ulcers, verrucous plaques, cysts, or sinus tracts.
Sometimes lesions spread in a sporotrichoid
pattern. In most cases, an infection is clinically

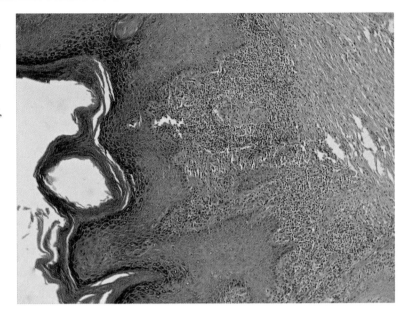

Fig. 14.28 Tuberculosis verrucosa cutis. Hyperkeratosis, papillomatosis, acanthosis, and neutrophilic microabscesses in epidermis. Diffuse mixed infiltrate in dermis with prominent neutrophils (H&E, 50× original magnification)

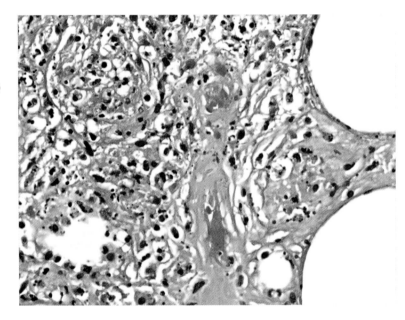

Fig. 14.29 Papulonecrotic tuberculid. Lymphocytic or neutrophilic vasculitis, fibrinoid necrosis of vessels with microthrombi (H&E, 400× original magnification)

appreciable, but some cases of prurigo nodularis and other chronic skin disorders have been found to be related to mycobacterial infection only when the skin lesions are tested by culture, biopsy, or molecular techniques. Their clinical features are summarized in Table 14.2 (Eckman 1981; Dodiuk-Gad et al. 2007; Elston 2009).

Multiple PCR assays have been established for the detection of a variety of mycobacterial organisms (Cook et al. 1994).

Histopathologic Features
The histopathologic picture in atypical mycobacterioses is just as variable as the clinical picture

Fig. 14.30 Cutaneous tuberculosis. Acid-fast bacilli in areas of lymphohistiocytic inflammation and necrosis (Ziehl–Neelsen acid-fast stain, 630× original magnification)

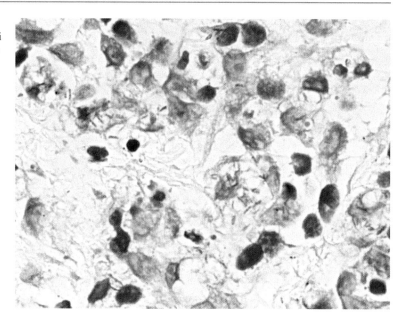

Table 14.2 Clinical and histopathologic features of various atypical mycobacteriosis

Disease	Clinical features	Histopathologic features
M. avium-intracellulare infection	Hematogenously borne lesions in skin and subcutis in patients with HIV/AIDS or other immunosuppressing diseases	Granulomatous or mixed acute and chronically inflammatory, as with tuberculosis. Sometimes may resemble lepromatous leprosy. Abundant acid-fast bacilli in areas without necrosis
M. marinum infection	Infections contracted through minor abrasions incurred while bathing in contaminated swimming pools or in ocean or lake water. Solitary indolent, dusky red, hyperkeratotic, papillomatous papules, nodules, or plaques. Fingers, knees, elbows, and feet most commonly affected	Early lesions: a nonspecific inflammatory infiltrate composed of neutrophils, monocytes, and macrophages. Acid-fast bacilli usually present Older lesions: a few multinucleated giant cells and small epithelioid cell granulomas with occasional necrosis. Marked hyperkeratosis with an acute inflammatory infiltrate and ulceration in epidermis. Acid-fast bacilli usually not appreciable
Buruli ulcer (*M. ulcerans* infection)	Endemic in West and Central Africa, Central America, China, and South Australia. Organism identified in nature, near inland water and rivers. Infections directly implanted or via an aquatic insect bite. Palpable cutaneous nodule usually on the extremities, buttocks, trunk, or face; progresses to painless ulceration with extensive undermining of the epidermis and extension of the necrosis down to fascia and even bone	Begins as a subcutaneous nodule exhibiting dermal collagen and fat necrosis with deposition of fibrin and extracellular clumps of acid-fast bacilli. Extensive ulceration with a variable degree of neutrophil infiltration and thrombosis of vessels. Variable nonspecific granulation tissue or a granulomatous reaction throughout the lesion
Other atypical Mycobacterioses: *M. chelonei, M. fortuitum, M. abscessus, M. haemophilum*	Commonly iatrogenic, associated with medical injections through unsterile contaminated needles and cannulae	Usually a mixed acute (neutrophilic) and chronic (granulomatous) inflammatory response, with various numbers of acid-fast bacilli

Fig. 14.31 *Mycobacterium marinum* infection. Mixed inflammatory infiltrate composed of neutrophils, monocytes, and macrophages in early lesion (H&E, 400× original magnification)

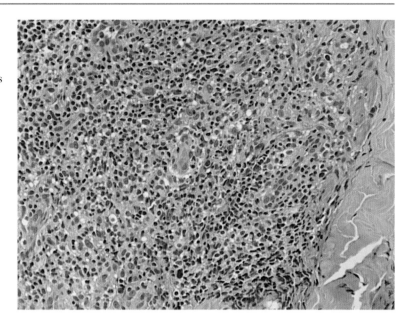

Fig. 14.32 *Mycobacterium marinum* infection. Epidermal ulceration, dense mixed inflammatory infiltrate, and scattered small epithelioid cell granulomas with multinucleated giant cells and occasional necrosis in later lesion (H&E, 100× original magnification)

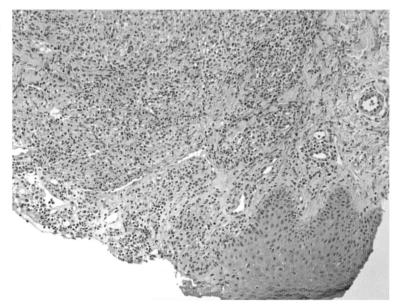

and may present nonspecific acute and chronic inflammation, suppuration, and abscess formation or tuberculoid granulomas with or without caseation. Coagulative necrosis is more prominent in the case of *M. ulcerans*. The epidermis may be hyperplastic or ulcerated. Fibrosis and granulation tissue may be prominent. The presence or absence of acid-fast bacilli depends on the tissue reaction. In suppurative lesions, numerous acid-fast bacilli often can be found. Various modifications of the Ziehl–Neelsen acid-fast stain or Fite stain may reveal the AFB. The AFB are most frequently found in microabscesses or within vacuoles in the sections rather than within multinucleated giant cells. The features are summarized in Table 14.2 (Hayman and McQueen 1985; Travis et al. 1985; Hanke et al. 1987; Hayman 1993; Mahaisavariya et al. 2004; Song et al. 2009; Min et al. 2012) (Figs. 14.31, 14.32, 14.33, 14.34, and 14.35).

Fig. 14.33 *Mycobacterium marinum* infection. Abundant immunostaining of mycobacteria in areas of lymphohistiocytic inflammation and necrosis (IHC, 630× original magnification)

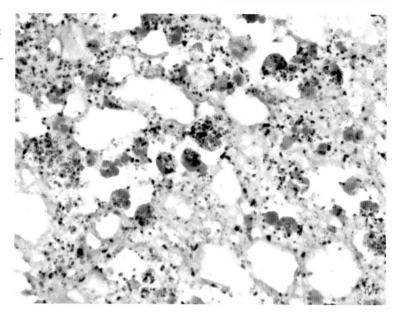

Fig. 14.34 *Mycobacterium haemophilum* infection. Lymphohistiocytic inflammation and necrosis in dermis (H&E, 400× original magnification)

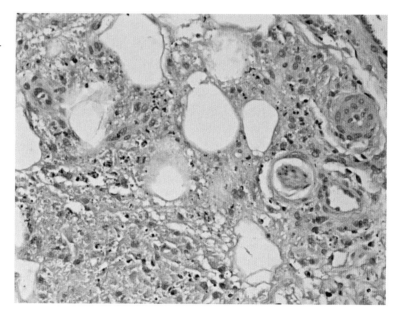

Differential Diagnosis

Other diseases associated with granulomas as described with cutaneous tuberculosis.

Leprosy (Hansen Disease)
Etiology and Epidemiology

Hansen disease, caused by *M. leprae*, affects millions of people worldwide. The disease is endemic in many tropical and subtropical countries but is declining in prevalence as a result of multidrug therapy (Noordeen 1995; Declercq 2001; Britton and Lockwood 2004). The Indian subcontinent, Southeast Asia, sub-Saharan countries in Africa, and Brazil comprise the areas most affected at present. In the United States, it occurs mainly in immigrants from endemic areas,

Fig. 14.35 *Mycobacterium ulcerans* infection. Prominent coagulative necrosis in dermis (H&E, 100× original magnification)

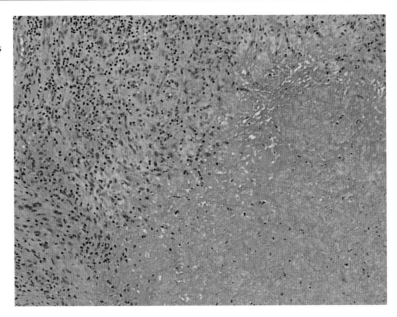

but some cases have been reported in Texas and Louisiana, perhaps from armadillo exposure. Leprosy affects multiple organs of the body, but clinical disease is most apparent in the skin, eyes, and peripheral nerves. Neuropathies may result in deformities of the distal extremities. The mode of transmission of leprosy is largely unknown; however, the bacilli may be inhaled from the nasal excretion of a multibacillary patient or possibly implanted from organisms in the soil. Direct person-to-person infection through skin contact occurs rarely. After inhalation, it is likely that bacilli pass through the blood to peripheral and cutaneous nerves, where infection and host reaction occurs.

Clinical Features

Leprosy is divided into several types in the Ridley–Jopling classification system based on the immune status of the patient (Ridley and Jopling 1966; Skinsnes 1973). Patients with lepromatous leprosy are anergic, and they tend to develop widespread cutaneous lesions. Lepromatous leprosy initially has cutaneous and mucosal lesions, with neural changes occurring later. The lesions usually are numerous and are symmetrically arranged. Although they are less

likely to have hypoesthesia in the lesions, the peripheral nerves may still be enlarged with consequent neuropathies. Lepromatous lesions include hypopigmented or erythematous macules, infiltrated erythematous nodules or plaques, leonine (lionlike) facies with a loss of eyebrows and eyelashes, and diffuse macular involvement of the skin resulting in a smooth surface. A distinctive variant of lepromatous leprosy, the histoid type, is characterized by the occurrence of well-demarcated cutaneous and subcutaneous nodules resembling dermatofibromas. It frequently follows incomplete chemotherapy or acquired drug resistance, leading to bacterial relapse.

The skin lesions of tuberculoid leprosy are scanty, dry, erythematous, hypopigmented papules, or plaques with sharply defined edges. The tuberculoid form occurs in those with intact immunity, and patients tend to develop one or a few lesions with prominent hypoesthesia and palpable thickened peripheral nerves. In borderline leprosy, combined features of tuberculoid and lepromatous disease are seen. The lesions are less numerous and less symmetrical than lepromatous leprosy lesions and often display some central dimples. Indeterminate leprosy represents early disease in patients living in populations where leprosy is prevalent; it is difficult to establish a definite diagnosis in some of these patients. The earliest detectable skin lesion may present as one or a few hypopigmented macules with variable loss of sensation. Any part of the body may be affected and the disease may heal spontaneously or may evolve into one of the other forms.

There are three types of reactional leprosy, and they usually occur as a result of a change in the patient's immune status, with or without treatment (Skinsnes 1973; Rea and Modlin 1991; Ottenhoff 1994; Pardillo et al. 2007). The type I reaction (lepra reaction) is called a reversal reaction when the patient is under treatment and has shifted toward the tuberculoid spectrum with greater immunity. On the contrary, it is considered as a downgrading reaction when untreated patients shift toward the lepromatous spectrum. Type I reactions involve swelling of previously existing cutaneous and neural lesions with associated constitutional symptoms. Type II reactions (erythema nodosum leprosum) occur most commonly in lepromatous leprosy and less frequently in borderline lepromatous leprosy. Clinically, the reaction has a greater resemblance to erythema multiforme than to erythema nodosum. Tender new red plaques and nodules develop on normal skin. The eruption is widespread and is accompanied by fever, malaise, arthralgia, and leukocytosis. This type of reaction involves immune complexes. Type III reactions (Lucio phenomenon) occur only in patients with the diffuse form of lepromatous leprosy. Hemorrhagic plaques occur on the legs, arms, or buttocks. These may ulcerate eventually. There are usually no constitutional symptoms.

Histopathology

The histopathologic findings vary in different forms and are summarized in Table 14.3 (Figs. 14.36, 14.37, 14.38, 14.39, 14.40, 14.41, and 14.42) (Ridley 1974; Modlin and Rea 1988; Fine et al. 1993). The Fite stain is recommended because the conventional AFB stain methods,

Table 14.3 Clinical and histopathologic features of various types of leprosy

Type	Clinical features	Histopathologic features
Lepromatous	Cutaneous and mucosal lesions with multiple erythematous or hypopigmented smooth patches, plaques, or nodules, sometimes leonine facies with a loss of eyebrows and eyelashes	Diffuse dermal infiltrate of foamy macrophages with grenz zone separating the macrophages from the epidermis; numerous acid-fast bacilli, often in clumps or in endothelial cells
Tuberculoid	Hypopigmented scaly or annular patches or plaques, smaller in number than lepromatous, more hypoesthesia in the lesions	Tuberculoid (epithelioid) granulomas without grenz zone; granulomas often linear, following nerves; Langhans giant cells typically absent; acid-fast bacilli rare or absent
Borderline	Features intermediate between lepromatous and tuberculoid	Histology in between lepromatous and tuberculoid
Indeterminate	Early hypopigmented or erythematous macules	Perivascular and perineural lymphohistiocytic inflammation. Few or no acid-fast bacilli
Lepra reaction (type I reaction)	Acute redness or pain in previously existing lesions with associated constitutional symptoms	Histology as in borderline leprosy
Erythema nodosum leprosum (type II reaction)	Acute onset of erythematous nodules in new sites not previously involved with associated constitutional symptoms	Lepromatous leprosy plus leukocytoclastic vasculitis
Lucio phenomenon (type III reaction)	Occurs exclusively in diffuse lepromatous leprosy with acute onset of hemorrhagic plaques or ulcers and no associated constitutional symptoms	Similar to type II, with greater tendency of endothelial proliferation leading to vascular obliteration, thrombosis, necrosis, and ulceration; dense aggregates of acid-fast bacilli in vascular walls and the endothelium

Fig. 14.36 Lepromatous leprosy. Diffuse dermal infiltrate of lymphocytes and macrophages with grenz zone separating the infiltrate from the epidermis (H&E, 50× original magnification)

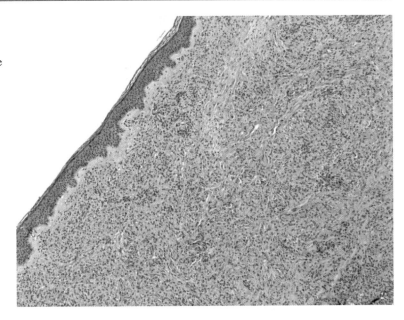

Fig. 14.37 Lepromatous leprosy. Dermal infiltrate with abundant foamy macrophages underneath the narrow grenz zone (H&E, 400× original magnification)

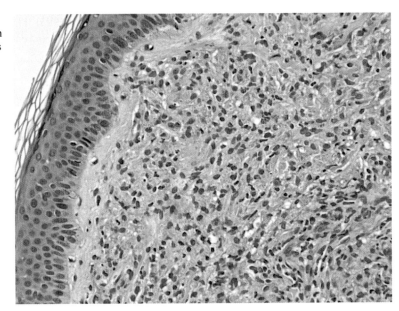

such as Ziehl–Neelsen stain, do not work as well (Fig. 14.39). Immunostaining for AFBs can enhance the ability to diagnose lesions containing few bacilli (Fig. 14.40). In situ hybridization and PCR analysis of specimens are more sensitive and are available at a few specialized laboratories (Fleury and Bacchi 1987; de Wit et al. 1991; Nishimura et al. 1994).

Differential Diagnosis

These include other granulomatous conditions, such as cutaneous tuberculosis, atypical mycobacteriosis, deep fungal infections, Treponema infections, cat-scratch disease, granuloma inguinale, lymphogranuloma venereum, tularemia, brucellosis, leishmaniasis, and other noninfectious granulomas.

Fig. 14.38 Lepromatous leprosy. Diffuse infiltrate of lymphocytes and macrophages in deep dermis and subcutaneous tissue with scattered multinucleated cells (H&E, 50× original magnification)

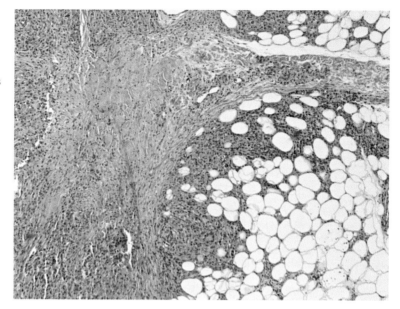

Fig. 14.39 Lepromatous leprosy. Abundant acid-fast bacilli highlighted by Fite acid-fast stain in dermis (Fite stain, 630× original magnification)

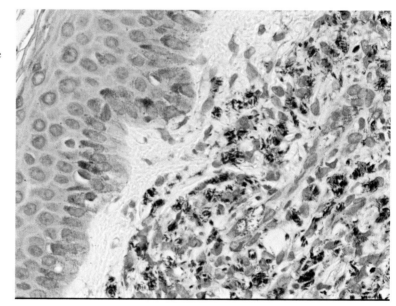

Treponemal Diseases

The venereal and nonvenereal treponemal diseases are caused by motile bacteria of the family Spirochaetaceae. Accurate recognition of spirochetal infection requires correlation of the patient's travel and medical history to a detailed knowledge of the clinical and histologic expression of each

pathogen. The pathogenic treponemes measure 6–20 by 0.10–0.18 μm, are coiled with regular periodicity, have a high degree of DNA sequence homology, and react with silver stains in darkfield and biopsy material (Hook and Marra 1992). The nonvenereal treponematoses include endemic syphilis, yaws, and pinta (Antal et al. 2002). The use of polymerase chain reaction (PCR)

Fig. 14.40 Lepromatous leprosy. Abundant immunostaining of *M. leprae* in foamy macrophages (IHC, 400× original magnification)

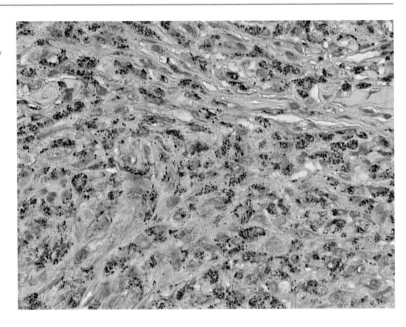

Fig. 14.41 Tuberculoid leprosy. Linear epithelioid granulomas following distribution of nerves (H&E, 50× original magnification)

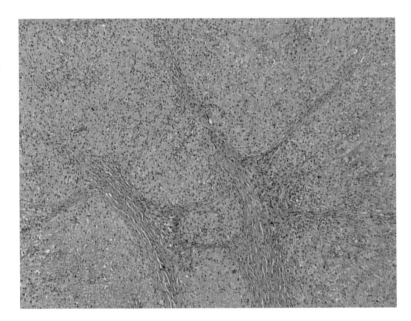

methodologies and restriction polymorphism analysis has allowed the identification of at least 27 distinct strains of pathogenic treponemal species (Centurion-Lara et al. 2006). Many studies suggest that these organisms have evolved from a common ancestor to cause different diseases in the modern era.

Venereal Syphilis
Etiology and Epidemiology

Venereal syphilis, caused by Treponema pallidum, has afflicted humanity since at least the fifteenth century. It was a significant cause of morbidity and mortality in the early twentieth century, although its incidence in the developed

Fig. 14.42 Tuberculoid leprosy. Epithelioid granulomas with no conspicuous Langhans giant cells (H&E, 200× original magnification)

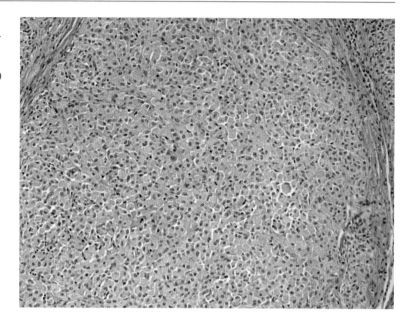

world has diminished due to public health programs and the advent of antibiotics (Goh 2005). Recently, the incidence of venereal syphilis has been steadily increasing, in part reflecting the epidemic of human immunodeficiency virus infection, with which venereal syphilis is linked epidemiologically. In 1990, the incidence was 20 per 100,000 in the United States and 360 per 100,000 in parts of Africa. New diagnoses of syphilis increased eightfold in the United Kingdom between 1997 and 2002. By 2003, more than 60 % of all reported cases of syphilis were believed to occur in men who have had sex with men (Heffelfinger et al. 2007).

Clinical Features

Spread of *T. pallidum* usually occurs by contact between an infectious lesion and disrupted epithelium, either at sites of trauma occurred during sexual intercourse or at sites of concurrent chancroid and other genital sores. Primary syphilis is defined by a skin lesion, or chancre, in which organisms are identified. It typically arises three weeks after exposure at the inoculation site and is classically a painless, brown-red, indurated, round papule, nodule, or plaque 1–2 cm in diameter. Lesions may be multiple or ulcerative, and

the regional lymph nodes may be enlarged (Goh 2005; Lautenschlager 2006; Bjekić et al. 2012).

Secondary syphilis occurs after hematogenous dissemination of organisms, resulting in widespread disease with constitutional symptoms. Fever, malaise, and generalized lymphadenopathy can occur; a disseminated eruption of red-brown macules, papules, papulosquamous lesions, and pustules may appear (Noppakun et al. 1987; Lawrence and Saxe 1992). Lesions may be follicular-based, annular, or serpiginous, particularly in recurrent attacks of secondary syphilis. Other cutaneous manifestations include alopecia and condylomata lata, the latter comprising confluent gray papules in anogenital areas and pitted hyperkeratotic palmoplantar papules, or in severe cases, ulcerative lesions of lues maligna may develop. Shallow, painless ulcers sometimes are seen in mucosal surfaces (Lautenschlager 2006; Arias-Santiago et al. 2009; Pföhler et al. 2011; Sezer et al. 2011; Villaseñor-Park et al. 2011).

Primary- and secondary-stage lesions may resolve without therapy or go unnoticed by the patient, who then develops into a latent phase, consisting of an early and late stage. The Centers for Disease Control and Prevention bases its

Fig. 14.43 Cutaneous syphilis. Typical feature with perivascular infiltrate composed of lymphoid cells, especially prominent plasma cells (H&E, 400× original magnification)

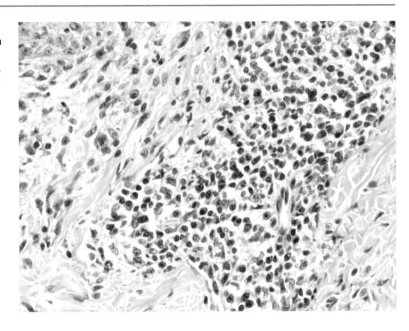

distinction on whether the duration of the infection is less or more than 1 year: the early (infectious) latent stage if less than a year and the late (noninfectious) latent stage if more than year.

After a variable period of latency, the patient enters the tertiary stage. Tertiary syphilis can present as gummatous skin and mucosal lesions, as well as involves cardiovascular and neurologic systems (Schoutens et al. 1996; Chudomirova et al. 2009). Skin lesions are solitary or multiple and consist of superficial nodular and deep gummatous subtypes. Superficial nodular type has smooth, atrophic centers with raised, serpiginous borders; deep gummatous type appears as ulcerative subcutaneous swellings. Congenital syphilis arises through transplacental infection and affects more than 50 % of infants born to mothers with primary or secondary syphilis, roughly 40 % of those born to mothers in the early latent stage, and only 10 % of those born to mothers with late latent infections (Sanchez 1992). Most HIV-infected patients exhibit a normal serologic response to *T. pallidum* infection; however, in some HIV-positive patients, both treponemal (FTA-ABS, MHA-TP, HATTS) and nontreponemal (VDRL, RPR) test results for syphilis have been reported as negative (Terry et al. 1988). The diagnosis of syphilis

in seronegative HIV-infected patients depends on dark-field microscopy, fluorescent antibody, and histopathology with conventional silver-impregnation stains or IHC (Guarner et al. 1999).

Histopathology

Cutaneous syphilis presents as a perivascular infiltrate composed of lymphoid cells, especially prominent plasma cells (Fig. 14.43). The late secondary and tertiary stages also show infiltrates of epithelioid histiocytes and occasional giant cells. In all stages, endothelial swelling and proliferation are apparent.

Primary Syphilis

The primary syphilitic chancre presents a variety of histopathology, depending on the location of lesion that is biopsied. The epidermis at the periphery of the syphilitic chancre reveals changes comparable to those observed in lesions of secondary syphilis, mainly acanthosis, spongiosis, and exocytosis of lymphocytes and neutrophils (Fig. 14.44). Toward the center, the epidermis becomes thinned, edematous, and permeated by inflammatory cells (Fig. 14.45). In the center, the epidermis may be absent. The papillary dermis is edematous, and a dense dermal perivascular and interstitial lymphohistiocytic and plasmacellular

Fig. 14.44 Primary syphilis. Acanthosis, spongiosis, dermal edema, and exocytosis of lymphocytes and neutrophils at the periphery of the chancre (H&E, 50× original magnification)

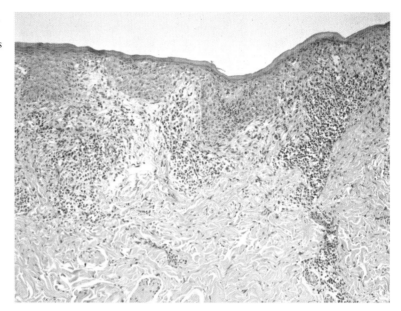

Fig. 14.45 Primary syphilis. Thinned and ulcerated epidermis with inflammatory infiltrate toward the center of chancre (H&E, 50× original magnification)

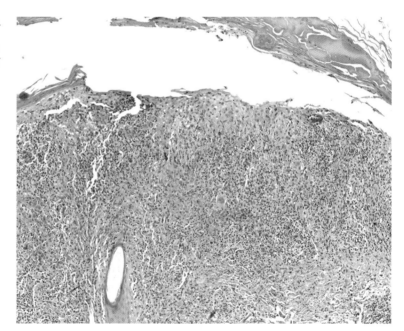

infiltrate is present (Fig. 14.43). Neutrophils are often admixed. Endarteritis obliterans characterized by endothelial swelling and mural edema may be observed (Engelkens et al. 1991b). With silver-impregnation stains or IHC techniques, spirochetes are usually seen within and around blood vessels and along the dermal–epidermal junction (Figs. 14.46 and 14.47). Warthin–Starry silver stain and Steiner silver stain must be interpreted with caution in evaluating biopsy specimens because other cellular structures and artifacts may resemble *T. pallidum*.

Fig. 14.46 Primary syphilis. Abundant spirochetes highlighted by Warthin–Starry silver stain along the dermal–epidermal junction (Warthin–Starry stain, 630× original magnification)

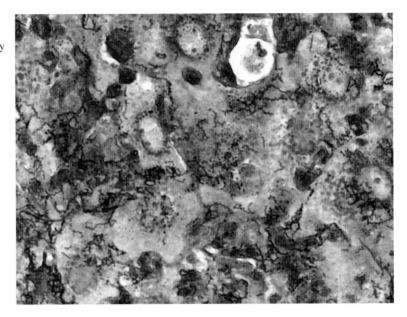

Fig. 14.47 Primary syphilis. Abundant immunostaining of *T. pallidum* in epidermis and dermal–epidermal junction (IHC, 400× original magnification)

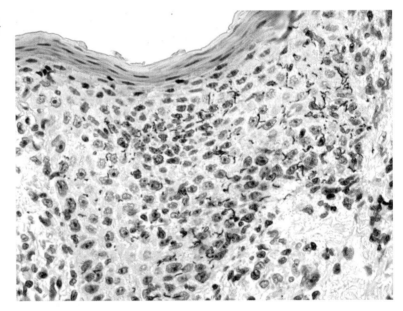

Secondary Syphilis

In secondary syphilis, skin biopsies generally reveal variable epithelial changes in the macular, papular, and papulosquamous eruptions (Jeerapaet and Ackerman 1973; Abell et al. 1975; Cochran et al. 1976; Engelkens et al. 1991b). There is considerable histologic overlap among the various clinical forms of secondary syphilis; however, epidermal changes are least pronounced in the macular type and most pronounced in papulosquamous lesions. Biopsies generally reveal psoriasiform hyperplasia, often with spongiosis and basilar vacuolar alteration and often with edema of the papillary dermis (Fig. 14.48).

Fig. 14.48 Secondary syphilis. Psoriasiform hyperplasia, spongiosis, edema of the papillary dermis, and dense dermal inflammatory infiltrate (H&E, 50× original magnification)

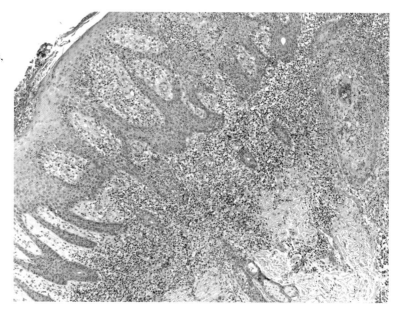

Exocytosis of lymphocytes, spongiform pustulation, and parakeratosis also may be observed. Patchy or confluent parakeratosis may be present, sometimes accompanied by intracorneal neutrophilic abscesses. Ulceration is not a feature, except in patients with lues maligna. The dermal changes include marked papillary dermal edema and a perivascular and/or periadnexal infiltrate that may be lymphocyte predominant, lymphohistiocytic, histiocytic predominant, or frankly granulomatous and that is of greatest intensity in the papillary (Sezer et al. 2011). Atypical lymphoid forms, representing a type of lymphomatoid hypersensitivity, may suggest the possibility of mycosis fungoides or non-Hodgkin lymphoma. Plasma cells are inconspicuous or absent in 25 % of patients. Eosinophils are usually absent. Endothelial cell swelling and mural edema are seen in only 50 % of patients, and mural necrosis is rare. Silver stains show spirochetes in only one-third of patients and are best visualized within the epidermis and around the superficial blood vessels (Poulsen et al. 1986).

Tertiary Syphilis

Tertiary syphilis includes a wide spectrum of clinical manifestations, including nodular tertiary syphilis confined to the skin; benign gummatous syphilis principally affecting skin, bone, and liver; cardiovascular syphilis; neurosyphilis; and syphilitic hepatic cirrhosis. In nodular tertiary syphilis, granulomas are small and limited to the dermis, in which scattered, nested epithelioid cells are admixed with a few multinucleated giant cells and lymphoplasmacytic cells (Fig. 14.49). Granulomas may be absent and necrosis is usually inconspicuous. The vessels may show endothelial swelling. Benign gummatous syphilis shows granulomatous inflammation with central zones of acellular necrosis in involved organs. In cutaneous lesions, blood vessels throughout the dermis and subcutaneous fat exhibit endarteritis obliterans, with variable angiocentric plasma cell infiltrates (Schoutens et al. 1996; Wu et al. 2000; Rocha et al. 2004; Chudomirova et al. 2009).

Differential Diagnosis

Lesions of chancroid caused by *Haemophilus ducreyi* are the most difficult to differentiate clinically from a syphilitic chancre. The characteristic histopathology of chancroid is one of dense lymphohistiocytic infiltrates with a paucity of plasma cells and a granulomatous vasculitis. An epidermal reaction pattern similar to the syphilitic chancre is observed, namely, psoriasiform epidermal hyperplasia and spongiform

Fig. 14.49 Tertiary syphilis. Small granulomas limited to the dermis with scattered, nested epithelioid cells admixed with lymphoplasma-cytic cells and occasional multinucleated cells (H&E, 400× original magnification)

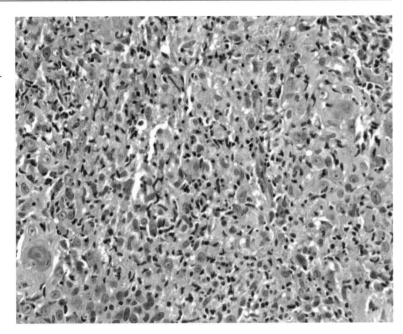

pustulation. A Giemsa, Alcian blue, or periodic acid–Schiff stain reveals coccobacillary forms between keratinocytes and along the dermal–epidermal junction. Spirochetes may coinfect chancroid lesions.

The differential diagnosis of lesions of secondary syphilis includes other causes of lichenoid dermatitis including lichen planus, a lichenoid hypersensitivity reaction, pityriasis lichenoides and connective tissue disease, sarcoidosis, psoriasis, and psoriasiform drug eruptions.

The differential diagnosis of lesions of tertiary syphilis depends on the involved organ system. The cutaneous lesions need to be differentiated with other granulomatous diseases.

Nonvenereal Treponematoses
Yaws
Etiology and Epidemiology
Yaws is caused by *T. pallidum pertenue*, which is indistinguishable microscopically from *T. pallidum subspecies pallidum* but has been shown to be genetically distinctive by molecular methods (Noordhoek et al. 1989; Wicher et al. 2000). Yaws is spread by casual contact between primary or secondary lesions and abraded skin.

The infection classically affects the buttocks, legs, and feet of children and is most prevalent in warm, moist tropical climates (Engelkens et al. 1991a). Despite only minor sequence variation between the organisms, there are distinct differences between disease expressions and host immunologic responses of yaws and syphilis (Noordhoek et al. 1990). Infants born to mothers with yaws do not produce IgM antibodies, and no spirochete is found in their organs. These findings strongly support the dermotropic nature of *T. pallidum pertenue*, as opposed to organotropic property of *T. pallidum subspecies pallidum*.

Clinical Features
Primary yaws usually starts as an erythematous papule, or mother yaws, roughly 21 days after inoculation. The lesion enlarges peripherally to form a 1–5-cm nodule, with an amber crust and adjacent satellite pustules. Lesions heal as pitted, hypopigmented scars. Fever, arthralgia, or lymphadenopathy may develop during the course.

Secondary yaws is characterized by involvement of skin, bones, joints, and cerebrospinal fluid. Skin lesions, or daughter yaws, resemble the mother yaw but are smaller and more numerous.

Fig. 14.50 Primary yaws. Epidermal acanthosis, papillomatosis, spongiosis, and neutrophilic exocytosis with microabscesses (H&E, 200× original magnification)

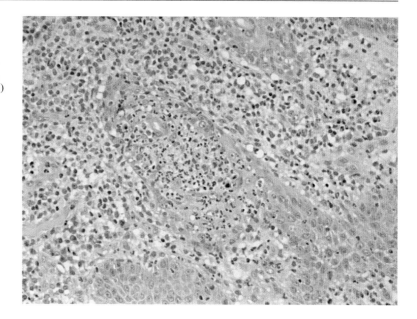

Although periorificial lesions may resemble venereal syphilis, a circinate appearance may mimic fungal infection. A morbilliform eruption or condylomatous vegetations involving the axillae and groin may occur. Macular, hyperkeratotic, and papillomatous lesions may be seen on palmoplantar surfaces and may cause the patient to walk with a painful, crablike gait (crab yaws). Papillomatous nail fold lesions may give rise to pianic onychia. Bone lesions consist of painful, sometimes palpable periosteal thickening of arms and legs (Engelkens et al. 1991a; Antal et al. 2002).

Skin manifestations in tertiary yaws include subcutaneous abscesses, coalescing serpiginous ulcers, keratoderma, keloids, and palmoplantar hyperkeratosis. The bone and joint involvements include osteomyelitis, hypertrophic or gummatous periostitis, and chronic tibial osteitis. Obstructive hypertrophy of the nasal maxillary processes produces the rare but characteristic goundou. Another otorhinolaryngologic complication, termed gangosa, consists of nasal septal or palatal perforation.

Histopathology

Primary lesions show epidermal acanthosis, papillomatosis, spongiosis, and neutrophilic exocytosis with microabscesses (Fig. 14.50).

A diffuse dermal infiltrate of plasma cells, lymphocytes, histiocytes, and granulocytes is seen. Prominent eosinophils can also be present in some cases (Fig. 14.51). Unlike syphilis, little or no endothelial proliferation is present. Secondary lesions may resemble condylomata lata in their epidermal changes but differ with a diffuse dermal infiltrate. The ulcerative lesions of tertiary yaws histologically resemble those of late syphilis. Spirochetes are demonstrated in primary and secondary lesions by dark-field examination and silver stains. Unlike *T. pallidum*, which can also been found in the dermis, *T. pertenue* is almost entirely seen in epidermis (Hasselmann 1957).

Differential Diagnosis

The distinction of yaws from syphilis is based on clinical features, although localization of the organism in a skin biopsy may be helpful.

Other Nonvenereal Treponematoses

These diseases are rare and confined to small endemic areas (Antal et al. 2002). Pinta is caused by *T. carateum*, and the involvement is usually confined to the skin with hypopigmentation being the only significant sequela. Pinta is endemic to Central America and is not observed outside the Western Hemisphere. It affects all age groups with a mild

Fig. 14.51 Primary yaws. Diffuse dermal infiltrate of plasma cells, lymphocytes, histiocytes, and granulocytes with prominent eosinophils in some cases (H&E, 400× original magnification)

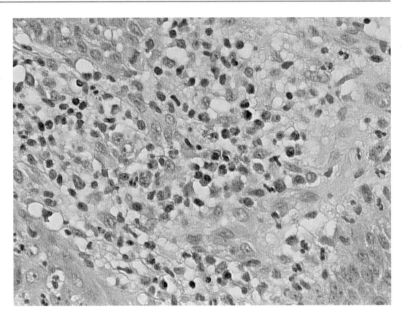

clinical course and is declining in incidence. Transmission appears to be from lesion to skin, usually between family members. Endemic syphilis, or bejel, is thought to affect about 2.5 million people. It is caused by *T. pallidum endemicum*, and the disease is largely confined to the arid Arabian peninsula and the southern border of the Sahara Desert. Children are the principal reservoir for a disease spread by skin-to-skin contact or via fomites such as communal pipes or drinking vessels. The rare primary-stage skin lesions usually go unnoticed, or appear as stomatitis at the angles of the lips. These painless lesions may resolve spontaneously but are usually followed by papulosquamous and erosive papular lesions of the trunk and extremities that are similar to yaws (Engelkens et al.1991c).

Viral Infections

Many viral infections have prominent skin manifestations. Certain characteristic skin lesions suggest a specific viral illness and the diagnosis can be confirmed by appropriate laboratory testing, such as cell culture, serology, electron microscopy, and PCR-based molecular assays. Viruses are obligatory intracellular organisms that need to use the metabolic machinery of the host cells for replica-tion. Viral infection of the host cells induces alterations of cellular functions, inflammatory responses, and apoptosis that lead to the manifestations of viral illness. Viruses attach themselves to specific receptors on the surface before entering a host cell; therefore, virus infection is a receptor-mediated, species-type-specific, and cell-type-specific process. Viral infections of the skin are of increased significance and frequency in immunocompromised patients. Some of the common skin diseases, such as those caused by herpes simplex virus, herpes zoster virus, or enteroviruses will not be discussed in this chapter.

Acquired Immunodeficiency Syndrome

Etiology and Epidemiology

Acquired immune deficiency syndrome (AIDS) is an infectious disease caused by the human immunodeficiency virus (HIV). AIDS was first recognized in the United States in 1981 and is the advanced form of infection with the HIV virus. Early HIV infection may not cause recognizable disease for a long period after the initial exposure. AIDS is considered one of the most devastating public health problems in recent history. AIDS can be transmitted in several ways, and the risk factors for HIV include sexual contact, vertical transmission in pregnancy, exposure to contaminated blood or blood products, and needle sticks among healthcare professionals or drug abusers.

Clinical Features

HIV infects predominantly CD4+ cells, mainly T-helper cells, and leads to a profound alteration of immune system function that predisposes patients to numerous opportunistic infections, malignancies, and neurologic diseases. HIV itself produces cutaneous lesions shortly after exposure. More than 50 % of patients report cutaneous symptoms of acute HIV infection, approximately 2–6 weeks following HIV exposure. These usually present as a macular or morbilliform rash involving the trunk. Pruritic papular eruption is the most common cutaneous manifestation in HIV-infected patients (Kaplan et al. 1987; Hevia et al. 1991; Zalla et al. 1992; Ray and Gately 1994).

Several skin diseases occur almost exclusively in HIV-infected individuals, such as oral hairy leukoplakia, bacillary angiomatosis, and Kaposi's sarcoma. Approximately 25 % of HIV-infected individuals may be affected with oral hairy leukoplakia. These are white, verrucous, confluent plaques most commonly located on the lateral aspects of the tongue, which do not scrape off with a tongue depressor. EBV infection plays an important role in production of this lesion, although HPV and Candida are also frequently present (Ficarra et al. 1988; Scully et al. 1998; Patton 2013). Bacillary angiomatosis is a systemic infections caused by *Bartonella henselae* or *B. quintana*. Patients may have palpable painful subcutaneous nodules, which may resemble Kaposi's sarcoma or hemangioma but resolve with appropriate antibiotic therapy (Plettenberg et al. 2000; Grilo et al. 2009). Kaposi's sarcoma is the most common AIDS-associated cancer in the United States. Over 95 % of all Kaposi's sarcoma lesions have been associated with HHV-8 infections (Kemény et al. 1996). Skin lesions of Kaposi's sarcoma typically present with asymptomatic reddish-purple patches that may progress to raised plaques or nodules. One-third of patients also experience oral cavity lesions characterized by red-to-purple plaques or nodules (Ball 2003; Grayson and Pantanowitz 2008; O'Donnell et al. 2010).

Gradual deterioration of the immune system makes HIV-infected patients susceptible to many cutaneous viral diseases, such as those caused by herpesviruses (HSV, VZV, EBV, CMV) and human papillomavirus. Patients with HIV are also subject to fungal, protozoa, and arthropod infections that produce mucocutaneous lesions.

Histopathology

The histopathologic finding of the acute exanthema of HIV infection is nonspecific and mainly shows a dense perivascular infiltrate of lymphocytes in the dermis. Epidermal changes are usually mild, but may include spongiosis, vacuolar change, and keratinocyte apoptosis. The papular eruption of AIDS may show nonspecific perivascular eosinophils with mild folliculitis, although occasional epithelioid cell granulomas have also been reported (Smith et al. 1993a, b).

The lesions of oral hairy leukoplakia show irregular keratin projections, parakeratosis, and acanthosis (Fig. 14.52). Vacuolar change of superficial keratinocytes is a characteristic finding within the epithelium (Ficarra et al. 1988).

Skin biopsies of bacillary angiomatosis show single or multinodular proliferations of capillaries in the dermis accompanied by an inflammatory infiltrate that includes variable numbers of neutrophils, eosinophils, and mononuclear cells (Fig. 14.53). Leukocytoclasia and edema are frequently observed. Characteristic extracellular deposits of palely hematoxyphilic granular material containing dense masses of short bacilli can be observed and further highlighted with Warthin–Starry silver staining. These bacilli may also be delineated as gram-negative bacilli by modified Gram stains such as the Brown–Hopps stain (LeBoit et al. 1989; Cockerell 1990; Cockerell et al. 1991).

Differential Diagnosis

The acute exanthema of HIV infection can mimic many other skin lesions. Since there is no specific histopathologic finding to suggest the etiologic diagnosis, other confirmatory laboratory tests must be performed when there is a high index of suspicion.

Fig. 14.52 Oral hairy leukoplakia. Irregular keratin projections, parakeratosis, acanthosis, and mild to moderate inflammatory infiltrate in dermis (H&E, 100× original magnification)

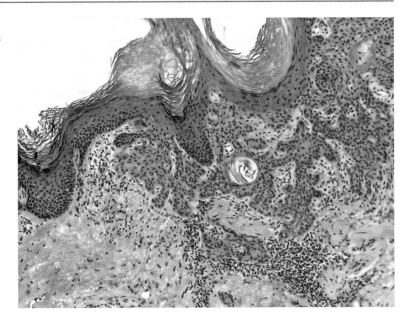

Fig. 14.53 Bacillary angiomatosis. Proliferations of capillaries in dermis accompanied by an inflammatory infiltrate, including variable numbers of neutrophils, eosinophils, and mononuclear cells (H&E, 200× original magnification)

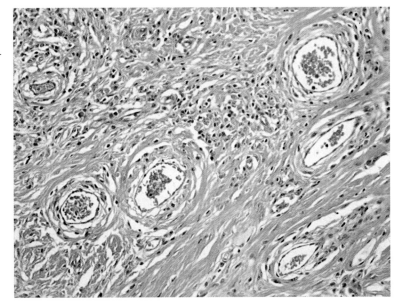

Poxvirus Infections

The Poxviridae are double-stranded DNA viruses with two subfamilies that can infect both vertebrate and invertebrate animals. Four genera of poxviruses may infect humans: (1) orthopoxviruses such as variola (smallpox), monkeypox, and vaccinia, which are ovoid and 300 by 250 nm in diameter; (2) parapoxviruses such as those cause orf (ecthyma contagiosum) and milker's nodule, which are cylindrical and 260 by 160 nm in diameter; (3) Molluscipoxvirus, mainly molluscum contagiosum virus, which has an oval bullet shape and is 275 by 200 nm in diameter; and (4) Yatapoxviruses, such as tanapox, which is somewhat similar to the parapoxviruses.

These are complex DNA viruses that replicate in the cytoplasm and are adapted to proliferation in keratinocytes. Spread is primarily by direct contact with infectious material from an infected individual or animal or via fomites, although variola is spread via aerosolized droplets.

After the eradication of smallpox (Bhattacharya 2008), the most common poxvirus infections in humans are vaccinia (in Indian subcontinent), orf, and molluscum contagiosum; however, monkeypox (in West and Central African rain forest countries) and some unusual parapoxvirus infections have become emerging diseases with public health concern.

Monkeypox

Etiology and Epidemiology

Monkeypox virus belongs to the genus *Orthopoxvirus*. It is a zoonotic pathogen that causes a febrile rash disease in humans (Di Giulio and Eckburg 2004). It was first identified as a pathogen of laboratory macaque monkeys in 1958, but the first human cases were not reported until 1970, in Democratic Republic of the Congo. More than 400 cases in humans were reported between 1970 and 1995, and sporadic cases continue to be reported in several health districts within Democratic Republic of the Congo (Levine et al. 2007). Several studies showed that a variety of African mammals had serological evidence of previous infections with an Orthopoxvirus, and some of these species could serve as a natural reservoir for monkeypox virus in its endemic range. Humans and monkeys were possibly infected incidentally and did not readily transmit infection to others (Fleischauer et al. 2005). The first reported outbreak in the United States occurred in 2003 in several midwestern states (Centers for Disease Control and Prevention CDC 2003; Reed et al. 2004). Most of the patients became sick after having contact with pet prairie dogs infected with monkeypox virus, through contact with imported rodents from Ghana.

Clinical Features

Monkeypox has a mean incubation period of approximately 12 days, with a range of 7–17 days. The signs and symptoms of monkeypox in humans are similar to those of smallpox, but usually milder. Clinical manifestations often start with several days of high fever, general malaise, muscle aches, and headache followed by the development of a maculopapular rash. Similar to smallpox, the rash appears first on the mucosa of oropharynx, the face, and the forearms and spreads to the trunk and legs. The lesions usually develop through several stages before crusting and detaching. Within 1–2 days of appearance, the rash becomes vesicular and then pustular. The illness typically lasts for 2–4 weeks. The main distinguishing characteristic between monkeypox and smallpox is the prominent involvement of lymph nodes in monkeypox. Generalized or regional lymphadenopathy can appear and usually develops concurrently with or shortly after the onset of the prodromal fever. The involved lymph nodes are 1–2 cm in diameter and are firm with tenderness. Most of the monkeypox cases resolve spontaneously within 2–4 weeks. However, a small number of patients, especially in pediatric population, may present with a more severe course with respiratory distress or neurologic deterioration. Complications reported from African outbreaks include deforming scars, bronchopneumonia, secondary bacterial infection with septicemia, respiratory failure, ulcerative keratitis, blindness, and encephalitis (McCollum and Damon 2013). PCR assays have been developed to provide a rapid confirmatory diagnosis as well as speciation (Putkuri et al. 2009).

Histopathology

The skin lesion shows a spectrum of changes corresponding to the progression of disease (Stagles et al. 1985). At early stage, a mildly acantholytic epidermis with spongiosis and ballooning degeneration of basal keratinocytes is seen (Fig. 14.54). The changes progress to marked acantholysis and full-thickness necrosis of epidermis later (Fig. 14.55). A mixed inflammatory cell infiltrate is usually present around the vascular areas, eccrine glands, and follicles in the epidermis and dermis. Viral cytopathic effect is present with multinucleated syncytial keratinocytes with eosinophilic intracytoplasmic inclusions (Fig. 14.56). IHC demonstrates viral

Fig. 14.54 Monkeypox. Epidermis with mild acantholysis, spongiosis, and ballooning degeneration of basal keratinocytes at early stage of infection (H&E, 100× original magnification)

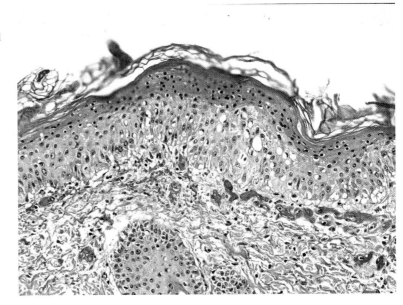

Fig. 14.55 Monkeypox. Marked acantholysis and full-thickness necrosis of epidermis at later stage of infection (H&E, 50× original magnification)

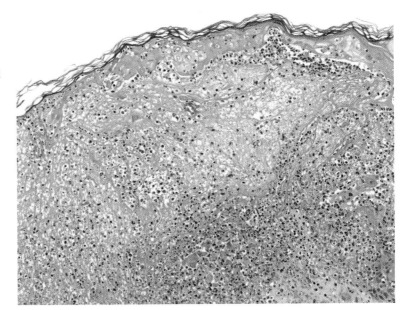

antigens within the infected keratinocytes and dermal adnexa (Fig. 14.57) (Guarner et al. 2004).

Differential Diagnosis

Skin lesions of monkeypox have to be differentiated from other vesicular pustular rash illnesses, such as varicella, impetigo, erythema multiforme, enteroviral infections, disseminated herpes simplex, and molluscum contagiosum.

Parapoxvirus Infections
Etiology and Epidemiology

Parapoxviruses infect many vertebrates, such as cows, sheep, goats, and red squirrels worldwide

Fig. 14.56 Monkeypox. Viral cytopathic effect in keratinocytes with eosinophilic intracytoplasmic inclusions (H&E, 630× original magnification)

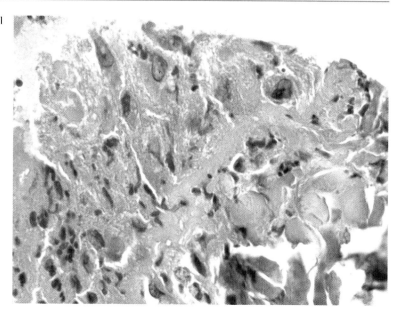

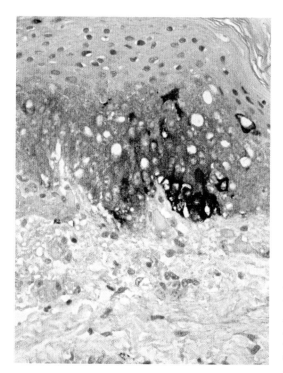

Fig. 14.57 Monkeypox. Immunostaining of *orthopoxvirus* antigens in the infected keratinocytes (IHC, 400× original magnification)

(Hessami et al. 1979). They cause skin lesions with a wide spectrum of clinical presentations that vary in size and location. Orf and Milker's nodule

are the two most common human infections caused by parapoxvirus. There are many emerging parapoxviruses identified in the past decade because of increasing awareness and availability of molecular assays (Tondury et al. 2010).

Clinical Features

Orf virus is widespread in sheep and goats. Human lesions are caused by direct inoculation of infected material and are more common among shepherds, veterinary surgeons, and other individuals with exposure to animals. Butchers, meat porters, and cooks are sometimes infected from infected carcasses. There is an incubation period of 5–6 days, after which a small, firm, red, or reddish-blue papule enlarges to form an umbilicated hemorrhagic pustule or bulla. In the fully developed lesion, which is usually 2 or 3 cm in diameter but may be as large as 5 cm, the central crust is surrounded by a grayish to violaceous ring further encircled by a zone of erythema. The lesions are usually solitary or few in number and are located most commonly on the fingers, hands, or forearms. There may be tenderness and associated lymphangitis and regional lymphadenitis with mild fever. Spontaneous recovery usually occurs within 3–6 weeks (Leavell et al. 1968; Johannessen et al. 1975).

Fig. 14.58 Orf. Prominent parakeratosis, marked inter- and intracellular edema, vacuolization, ballooning degeneration, epidermolysis, and focal necrosis in epidermis (H&E, 50× original magnification)

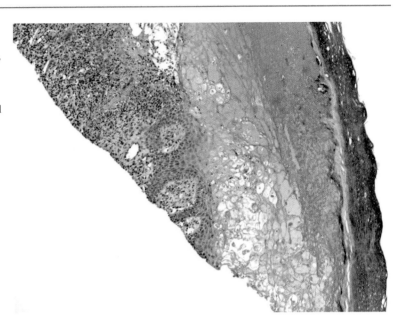

Milker's nodule is caused by a parapoxvirus that most commonly leads to infection of the teats and mouths of cattle. Milkers, farmers, and veterinarians with a direct exposure to these lesions are accidental hosts. After an incubation period of about 5 days to 2 weeks, flat, red papules are formed. Within a week they appear as reddish-blue, firm, slightly tender nodules. The epidermis becomes opaque and grayish, and soon after, a crust develops centrally. As with orf, central umbilication is usually present. Many cases develop lymphangitis, but there are rarely any constitutional symptoms. Lesions resolve over 4–6 weeks without scarring. In contrast to orf, lesions are usually multiple. The most common sites of involvement are the hands and fingers. Rarely, a more widespread papulovesicular eruption of the hands, arms, legs, and neck may develop (Kuokkanen et al. 1976; Groves et al. 1991).

Histopathology

Parapoxvirus infections share some common histopathologic features. The epidermis usually shows prominent parakeratosis, marked inter- and intracellular edema, vacuolization, ballooning degeneration, epidermolysis, and focal necrosis (Fig. 14.58). Keratinocytes with eosinophilic cytoplasmic and intranuclear inclusions can be observed (Fig. 14.59). A dense infiltrate is present in the dermis that consists mainly of histiocytes at the center with lymphocytes and plasma cells at the periphery. There are usually very few neutrophils. The dermis may contain many newly formed, dilated capillaries with perivascular mononuclear infiltrate (Leavell et al. 1968; Evins et al. 1971; Groves et al. 1991). IHC is a useful ancillary assay that can highlight the parapoxviruses in skin biopsies to establish the diagnosis (Fig. 14.60) (Sanchez et al. 1985).

Differential Diagnosis

Each of the parapoxvirus infections must be distinguished from the others by clinical history and number of lesions. Other acute inflammatory infections that may resemble parapoxvirus infections include primary tuberculosis, sporotrichosis, pyogenic granulomas, anthrax, impetigo, arthropod bites, plague, rickettsialpox, scrub typhus, and tularemia. These lesions can usually be differentiated by histopathologic examination. Arthropod bites reaction, if persistent, raise a differential of T cell lymphoma and T cell pseudolymphoma. If immunohistochemistry for lymphoma is performed, CD30 positive immunoblasts may be seen raising concern for a CD30 + skin lymphomas (Rose et al. 1999).

Fig. 14.59 Orf.
Keratinocytes with vacuolization, ballooning degeneration,
and eosinophilic cytoplasmic
and intranuclear inclusions
(H&E, 630× original
magnification)

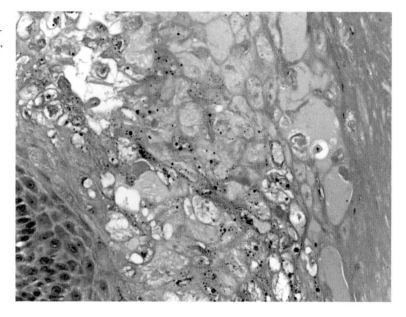

Fig. 14.60 Orf.
Immunostaining of *parapox-*
virus antigens in the infected
keratinocytes (IHC, 200×
original magnification)

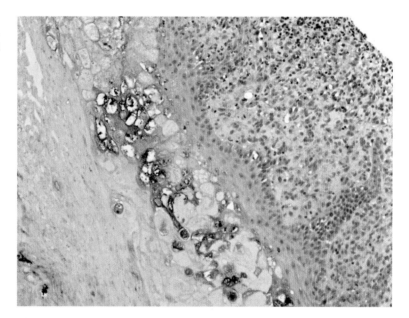

Viral Hemorrhagic Fevers

Etiology and Epidemiology

Although viral hemorrhagic fevers (VHF) are
generally regarded as emerging diseases, they
have existed for many years in different parts of
the world. This designation does not mean to
imply that they are newly recognized, but rather
that the human exposure to the causative viruses
has been increasing to an alarming level. These
viruses are maintained in different species of
reservoir in nature, such as insect, arthropod, or
animal populations. They are transmitted from
these reservoir populations to humans by direct

Fig. 14.61 Ebola hemorrhagic fever. Immunostaining
of *Ebola* virus antigens in
dermis, usually with no
prominent inflammation
(IHC, 400× original
magnification)

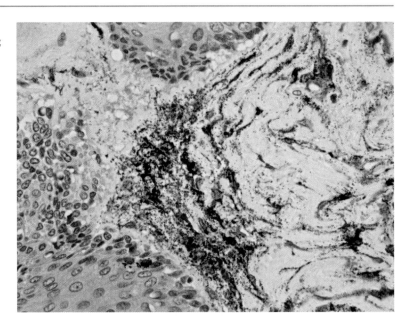

or indirect exposure. Hemorrhagic fevers are usually endemic or linked to specific locations. The
incidence and prevalence varies widely due to
many factors, such as the reservoir and human
population density, mode of transmission, environmental changes, geoclimateric alterations,
and virulence of viruses (Guerrant et al. 2011;
Singh and Ruzek 2013).

The viruses that cause hemorrhagic fevers are
found most commonly in tropical locations; however, some of them can exist in cooler climates.
Typical disease vectors include rodents, ticks, or
mosquitoes, but person-to-person transmission in
health-care settings or through sexual contact can
also occur. The major viruses causing hemorrhagic fever belong to the following four families:
(1) Filoviridae, such as Ebola virus and Marburg
virus; (2) Arenaviridae, such as Lassa virus (Lassa
HF), Junin virus (Argentinian HF), Machupo
virus (Bolivian HF), and Guanarito virus
(Venezuelan HF); (3) Flaviviridae, such as yellow
fever virus and dengue virus; and (4) Bunyaviridae,
such as Rift Valley fever virus (RVF), Crimean–
Congo hemorrhagic fever virus (CCHF), and
hantavirus (HF with renal syndrome and hantavirus pulmonary syndrome).

Since dengue virus infection has a much
higher incidence with a more profound public

health impact than other hemorrhagic fever
viruses, it will be discussed in more detail later.

Clinical Features

The incubation period of these VHFs varies from
3 days to 3 weeks. The clinical symptoms and
signs are nonspecific and usually start as flulike
illness with fever, headache, backache, and generalized muscle and joint pain. These symptoms
may be accompanied by nausea, vomiting, diarrhea, and abdominal pain. Hemorrhagic manifestations can appear early as petechiae, purpura,
subconjunctival hemorrhage, or mucosal bleeding
in oral cavity and gastrointestinal tract. Case fatality varies widely according to the different family
of viruses, ranging from 15 to >90 %.

Histopathology

There is no specific histopathologic finding in
skin biopsies of VHFs. Occasionally, mild perivascular lymphocytic infiltrate and subtle endothelial hyperplasia may be seen, but they do not
provide any diagnostic value. IHC assay is a sensitive method for diagnosis of Ebola virus infection in skin biopsies; (Fig. 14.61) (Zaki et al.
1999) however, the sensitivity for other VHFs
using skin biopsy as test sample is generally
very low.

Differential Diagnosis

The petechial or purpural lesions should be differentiated with meningococcemia, bacterial sepsis, RMSF, and other forms of vasculitis and within the category of VHF itself.

Dengue Fever

Etiology and Epidemiology

Dengue fever (DF) and dengue hemorrhagic fever (DHF) are caused by arthropod-borne viruses in the Flaviviridae family. They are single-stranded RNA viruses with four antigenically distinct members in the subgroup. Dengue viruses are transmitted by mosquitoes of the genus *Aedes* (e.g., *A. aegypti* and *A. albopictus*). The principal vector, *A. aegypti*, is found worldwide in the tropics and subtropics. Dengue virus infection has been reported in over 100 countries and has become one of the world's major emerging infectious diseases. About 100 million cases of DF, 250,000 cases of DHF, and 25,000 fatal cases are estimated to occur annually. DF is diagnosed in an increasing proportion of febrile travelers returning from the tropics, ranging from 2 % in the early 1990s to 16 % more recently. In some case series, DF now presents as the second most frequent cause of hospitalization (after malaria) in travelers returning from the tropics. There are now small endemic areas of disease in the United States as well. The majority of DHF cases are reported from Asian countries, where it is a leading cause of hospitalization and death among children. In the American tropics, DHF was once a rare disease but has been reported with a significantly increasing incidence since the 1980s, especially in the Caribbean, Central America, and South America (McBride and Bielefeldt-Ohmann 2000; Halstead 2008; Whitehorn and Farrar 2010).

Clinical Features

The incubation period is 2–8 days after a mosquito bite. The onset of the infection usually starts with abrupt fever, chills, headache, conjunctival injection, severe bone pain ("break bone fever"), generalized myalgias, arthralgias, and cutaneous exanthem. The exanthem is morbilliform and central in distribution. Petechiae and thrombocytopenia may be seen with initial infections, although hemorrhagic manifestations are seen more commonly in DHF. Hemorrhagic manifestations include petechiae, purpura, and bleeding of the gums, nose, and GI tract. Uncomplicated DF resolves within 5–7 days, whereas DHF carries mortality rate as high as 20 %. According to WHO criteria, the diagnosis of DHF is made based on the combination of hemorrhagic manifestations, with platelet count <100,000/mm^3, and objective evidence of plasma leakage, shown by either increased packed cell volume >20 % during the course of illness or hematocrit >45 % and clinical signs of plasma leakage, such as pleural effusion, ascites, or hypoproteinemia.

Histopathology

The morbilliform eruption appears similar to other viral exanthems with mild to moderate perivascular infiltrate of lymphocytes and slight spongiosis. Skin biopsies of hemorrhagic dengue show abundant extravasated erythrocytes. Occasionally, endothelial hyperplasia and thrombosis may be seen in vessels. None of the histopathologic changes are specific and there was no apparent correlation between histopathologic features and prognosis (Thomas et al. 2007; Saadiah et al. 2008; Saleem and Shaikh 2008). Although IHC with specific anti-dengue virus antibody can demonstrate viral antigens in endothelial cells or circulating monocytes (Fig. 14.62), the sensitivity is too low in skin biopsies to be a useful diagnostic method (Boonpucknavig et al. 1979; de Andino et al. 1985; Saadiah et al. 2008).

Differential Diagnosis

The differential diagnosis varies depending on which type of skin eruption is present. For the morbilliform eruption, scarlet fever, measles, rubella, toxoplasmosis, syphilis, drug eruption, and the acute HIV seroconversion reaction must be distinguished. For petechiae or purpura, meningococcemia, bacterial sepsis, RMSF, other hemorrhagic fever viruses, and other forms of vasculitis have to be considered.

Fig. 14.62 Dengue hemorrhagic fever. Immunostaining of *dengue* virus antigens in endothelial cells (IHC, 400× original magnification)

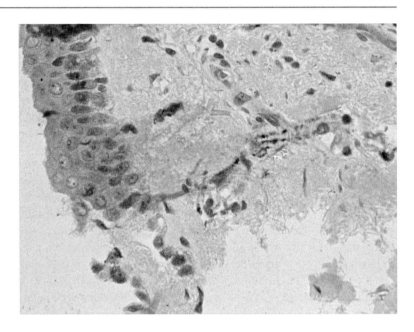

Parasitic Infections

Protozoal Diseases

Protozoa may cause cutaneous lesions as a primary, secondary, or incidental infection. Leishmaniasis is the most common form of protozoal dermatitis and affects millions of people in the tropical and subtropical belts of the world. Free-living ameba such as *Acanthamoeba* species and *Balamuthia mandrillaris* have become emerging organisms associated with both immunocompromised and immunocompetent patients. Many protozoal infections can cause cutaneous immune reactions without the presence of organisms in the skin.

Leishmaniasis
Etiology and Epidemiology
Leishmaniasis is caused by the protozoon *Leishmania* with a wide spectrum of clinical illness, including cutaneous, mucosal, or visceral diseases. Leishmaniasis is one of the most common infectious diseases globally with a prevalence of 12 million cases and annual incidence of more than two million cases worldwide. The disease is more prevalent in countries with warmer climate, such as those around the Mediterranean

coast, North Africa, South America, Central America, and Central Asia. There are many species of *Leishmania*, but most cases seen in travelers returning from tropical areas are due to *L. tropica*, *L. major*, and *L. aethiopica* (Grevelink and Lerner 1996; Choi and Lerner 2001; Weina et al. 2004; Rastogi and Nirwan 2007; Pavli and Maltezou 2010).

Leishmania spp. have both flagellar (promastigote) and aflagellar (amastigote) stages during their life cycle. The organisms are present at the elongated motile promastigote stage with an anterior flagellum in sandfly or in artificial culture media. Human infection is transmitted by the bite of the sandfly, usually at night and outdoors. After the promastigotes have entered the skin of the human host via the bite of infected sandflies, they transform into amastigotes, which primarily affect cells of mononuclear phagocytic system in its vertebrate host. If the host response to *Leishmania* spp. is confined to the skin, cutaneous lesions develop; however, if dissemination of the protozoa occurs, internal organs will become involved. The amastigote is round or oval, 2–3 μm in diameter, with no protruding flagellum. The nucleus and kinetoplast stain deeply with the Romanovsky stains, giving the organism its characteristic appearance. The infection is commonly zoonotic; one species of *Leishmania* may be associated with

Table 14.4 Etiologic organisms and histopathologic features of various types of cutaneous leishmaniasis

Type	New World parasites	Old World parasites	Histopathologic features
Localized acute cutaneous leishmaniasis	*L. b. braziliensis* *L. b. guyanensis* *L. b. panamensis* *L. m. mexicana* *L. m. amazonensis* *L. donovani chagasi*	*L. major* *L. tropica* *L. aethiopica* *L. infantum*	A dense and diffuse lymphohistiocytic infiltrate throughout the dermis with varying numbers of organisms. Amastigotes (Leishman–Donovan bodies) with dull blue-gray, round to oval bodies measuring 2–4 μm in diameter are seen in the cytoplasm of the histiocytes. Typical organisms also show a round basophilic nucleus and a rod-shaped paranuclear kinetoplast. These intracellular bodies stain red or dark blue with Giemsa stain but not with PAS or GMS stains. A granulomatous reaction containing epithelioid cells and multinucleated giant cells develops at later stages
Diffuse acute cutaneous leishmaniasis	*L. m. amazonensis* *L. mexicana* *L. m. pifanoi*	*L. aethiopica*	Similar as those seen in localized acute cutaneous leishmaniasis except for more abundant Leishman–Donovan bodies and a relative lack of accompanying lymphocytes. Eosinophils are prominent in the rare ulcerated lesions
Chronic cutaneous leishmaniasis (Leishmaniasis recidivans)	*L. braziliensis*	*L. tropica*	The histopathologic hallmark is a dense, diffuse, or nodular infiltrate composed of epithelioid cell granulomas within the superficial and deep dermis. The granulomas made up of epithelioid histiocytes and Langerhans giant cells surrounded by lymphocytes and plasma cells
Mucocutaneous leishmaniasis	*L. b. braziliensis*		In the early edematous phase, parasites are scant, a lymphohistiocytic infiltrate with admixed plasma cells in the superficial and deep dermis is present. At proliferative phase, parasites become obvious and granulomas can be seen. In necrotizing phase, areas of necrosis with numerous neutrophils and abundant Leishman–Donovan bodies are present
Post-kala-azar dermal leishmaniasis	*L. donovani chagasi*	*L. donovani* *L. tropica* *L. infantum*	The amount of epidermal melanin is decreased. Dermis shows superficial perivascular lymphocytic infiltrate with admixed plasma cells without evidence of granuloma formation
Visceral leishmaniasis	*L. donovani chagasi*	*L. donovani* *L. infantum* *L. tropica*	The cutaneous lesions, if present, are nonspecific and consist of a perivascular lymphohistiocytic infiltrate within the superficial dermis

one or many natural vertebrate hosts, which provide the reservoir of infection. Humans are usually accidental hosts (Ryan et al. 2012).

Clinical Features

Leishmaniasis used to be classified into a cutaneous, mucocutaneous, and visceral form; however, this simplistic classification has been abandoned in favor of a classification that recognizes the overlap in the clinical spectrum of various types of leishmaniasis (Sangueza et al. 1993; Pearson and Sousa 1996; Samady et al. 1996). Each form of leishmaniasis is associated with a different type of *Leishmania* spp. and has a specific predilection for a geographic location. These different forms include (1) localized acute cutaneous leishmaniasis; (2) diffuse acute cutaneous leishmaniasis; (3) chronic cutaneous leishmaniasis, including leishmaniasis recidivans (lupoid leishmaniasis); (4) mucocutaneous leishmaniasis; (5) post-kala-azar dermal leishmaniasis; and (6) visceral leishmaniasis. Because of the wide spectrum of clinical manifestations and complexity of host–vector–parasite relationship associated with these different forms, a detailed description of each form is beyond the scope of this chapter. The causative organisms and main histopathologic features are summarized in Table 14.4. The following description will only focus on the most common form of skin involvement, i.e., localized acute cutaneous leishmaniasis. This form usually affects the exposed parts of the body, such as face, scalp, and arms. It appears initially as a painless, erythematous papule which enlarges over a period of 4–12 weeks to a nodule or a plaque measuring up to 2 cm in diameter. Ulceration is common. After several months the lesion spontaneously regresses, starting from the center and progressing outward. The end stage is represented by a scar accompanied by hypo- or hyperpigmentation. New World leishmaniasis commonly presents with a single lesion, while Old World leishmaniasis with multiple lesions (Goihman-Yahr 1994; Samady et al. 1996; Salman et al. 1999; Scarisbrick et al. 2006). The diagnosis of leishmaniasis depends on isolation or identification of the organism from tissue (Sharquie et al. 2002; Gazozai et al. 2010). Species-specific PCR assays have been developed to provide a rapid confirmatory diagnosis, especially in lesions that organisms cannot be identified in histologic sections (Safaei et al. 2002).

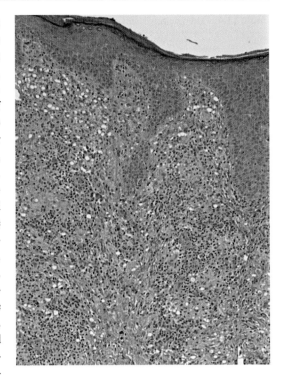

Fig. 14.63 Leishmaniasis. Dense and diffuse lymphohistiocytic infiltrate throughout the dermis (H&E, 100× original magnification)

Histopathology

The characteristic histopathologic change is a dense and diffuse lymphohistiocytic infiltrate throughout the dermis with varying numbers of organisms (Fig. 14.63). Eosinophils and neutrophils are rare and more commonly seen in ulcerated lesion. In routine H&E sections, amastigotes (Leishman–Donovan bodies) with dull blue-gray, round to oval bodies measuring 2–4 μm in diameter are seen in the cytoplasm of the histiocytes (Fig. 14.64). Typical organisms also show a round basophilic nucleus and a rod-shaped paranuclear kinetoplast, a specialized mitochondrial structure containing extracellular DNA (Fig. 14.65). These intracellular bodies stain red or dark blue with Giemsa stain but not with PAS or GMS stains. Organisms vary in number depending on the stage of the lesion and the immunologic status of the host. They are more abundant in early lesions and in immunocompromised hosts. Extracellular distribution can be observed when there are numerous organisms. As the lesions progress, the number of both organisms and histiocytes tend to

gradually reduce. A granulomatous reaction containing epithelioid cells and multinucleated giant cells develops (Fig. 14.66); caseous necrosis is notably absent. The epidermal changes are nonspecific and consist of hyperkeratosis, parakeratosis, and epidermal atrophy or hyperplasia. Ulceration can be seen in some cases (Kurban et al. 1966; Gutierrez et al. 1991; Peltier et al. 1996; Botelho et al. 1998; Mehregan et al. 1999).

IHC with specific anti-*Leishmania* antibodies is a useful assay that can highlight *Leishmania* in skin biopsy samples to establish the diagnosis (Fig. 14.67) (Kenner et al. 1999). It is also a valuable tool for identifying organisms in unusual histopathological manifestations of leishmaniasis. Extracellular parasites can be noted in the connective tissue or in capillary lumens. Furthermore, immunolocalization of the antigens provides insightful information to understand the pathogenesis of leishmaniasis.

Fig. 14.64 Leishmaniasis. Amastigotes (Leishman–Donovan bodies) with dull blue-gray, round to oval bodies in the cytoplasm of the histiocytes (H&E, 400× original magnification)

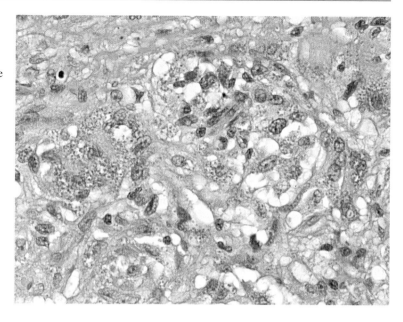

Fig. 14.65 Leishmaniasis. Amastigotes with a round basophilic nucleus and a rod-shaped paranuclear kinetoplast (H&E, 630× original magnification)

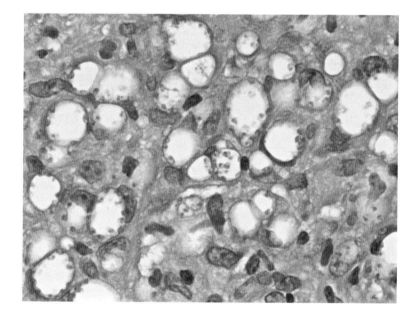

Differential Diagnosis

The morphology of intracytoplasmic amastigotes can appear similar to organisms of histoplasmosis, toxoplasmosis, and Chagas disease. *Histoplasma capsulatum* does not exhibit a kinetoplast and does stain with PAS and GMS. *Toxoplasma gondii* and *Trypanosoma cruzi* rarely cause skin lesions.

Fig. 14.66 Leishmaniasis. A granulomatous reaction containing epithelioid cells and multinucleated giant cells at later stage of infection (H&E, 100× original magnification)

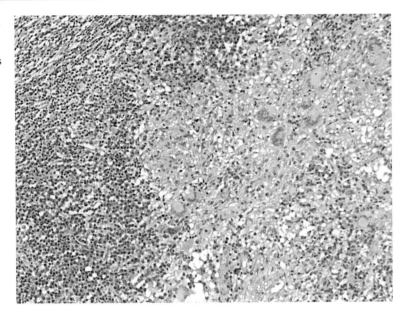

Fig. 14.67 Leishmaniasis. Immunostaining of leishmanial antigens in histiocytes (IHC, 630× original magnification)

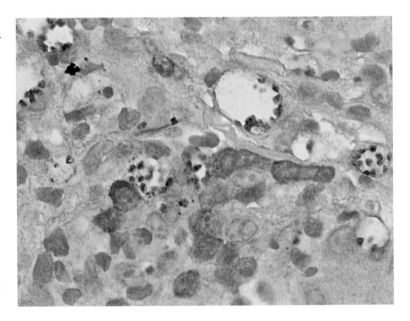

Free-Living Amebic Infections

Free-living amebae are important causes of disease in humans and animals. These organisms are commonly found in soil and water throughout the world. Species that are able to tolerate temperatures above 37 °C are most likely to cause human disease.

Cutaneous Acanthamebiasis

Etiology and Epidemiology

Among the free-living amebic organisms capable of producing cutaneous lesions, acanthamebiasis recently surfaced as the most common one, especially among HIV, organ transplant, and other immunocompromised patients (Helton et al.

Fig. 14.68 Acanthamebiasis. Diffuse perivascular inflammatory infiltrate composed mainly of neutrophils and histiocytes admixed with extensive tissue necrosis, sometimes evolving into abscess formation (H&E, 50× original magnification)

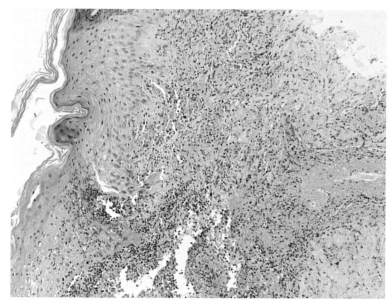

1993; Tan et al. 1993; Deluol et al. 1996). *Acanthamoeba* spp. can be isolated from soil, dust, air, natural and treated water, etc. These organisms can also be found in nasal and pharyngeal mucosa of healthy individuals. They have a worldwide distribution with many species that can cause skin infections. Most infections are caused by three or four genotypes; T4 is the most common genotype in the environment and causes most cases of corneal and cutaneous infections. Multiplication occurs in the trophozoite stage by binary fission. *Acanthamoeba* spp. exists in two forms. The amebic cysts, measuring 12–20 μm in diameter, are resistant to desiccation and transform to trophozoites only in a favorable environment. Trophozoites, measuring between 15 and 45 μm in size, represent the infectious and invasive form of the organism. Both cyst and trophozoite stages exist in nature and can be identified in tissue sections. Transmission occurs via the respiratory mucosa or contamination of skin lesions. The organisms can infect other organs through hematogenous spread.

Clinical Features

The cutaneous lesions in acanthamebiasis are nonspecific and may present as macules, papules, nodules, or chronic nonhealing ulcers. The ulcers are poorly demarcated with elevated borders that may form eschar and eventually heal. The lesions are usually multiple as well as multifocal and may appear in crops involving the trunk, face, and extremities. Disseminated form has been reported in transplant patients. The skin may serve either as the initial port of entry or may become secondarily involved via hematogenous spread (Gullett et al. 1979; Wortman 1996; Galarza et al. 2009).

Other clinical diseases caused by acanthamebic infection include granulomatous amebic encephalitis, pneumonitis, keratitis, and osteomyelitis. Clinical laboratory diagnosis can be made by culture, DFA, or PCR assays.

Histopathology

The skin biopsies usually demonstrate multifocal or diffuse perivascular inflammatory infiltrate composed mostly of neutrophils and histiocytes admixed with extensive tissue necrosis, sometimes evolving into abscess formation (Fig. 14.68). A predominant neutrophilic infiltrate may be present in the pustules, acute ulcers, or abscesses. Leukocytoclastic vasculitis with fibrin deposits within the vessel wall and vascular necrosis can also be observed. Lobular panniculitis with necrotizing vasculitis has been reported

Fig. 14.69 Acanthamebiasis. Variable numbers of amebic organisms throughout the skin lesion, often more abundant in perivascular areas (H&E, 200× original magnification)

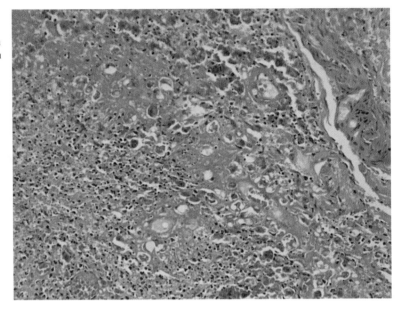

Fig. 14.70 Acanthamebiasis. Round trophozoites with projecting acanthopodia, vacuolated cytoplasm, and a centrally placed large nucleus with a single prominent nucleolus (karyosome) mixed within the inflammatory infiltrate (H&E, 630× original magnification)

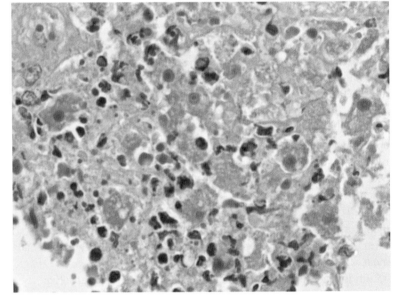

in cases with deep dermal and subcutaneous lesions. Skin lesions in severely immunocompromised hosts show an altered tissue response with lack of giant cells and only poorly formed granulomas (Helton et al. 1993; Rosenberg and Morgan 2001; Galarza et al. 2009).

Variable numbers of amebic organisms are seen throughout the skin lesion and often more abundant in perivascular areas (Fig. 14.69). The round trophozoites usually present with projecting acanthopodia, vacuolated cytoplasm, and a centrally placed large nucleus with a single prominent nucleolus (karyosome) mixed within the inflammatory infiltrate (Fig. 14.70). Despite often being numerous, the trophozoite forms are relatively inconspicuous and can be missed easily, because their morphology closely resembles macrophages. The cyst forms display a double

Fig. 14.71 Acanthamebiasis. Immunostaining of antigens in amebic cysts with outer wavy and wrinkled wall (IHC, 630× original magnification)

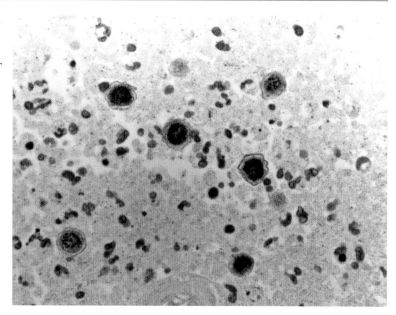

wall, with the outer wall wavy and wrinkled in appearance and the inner wall shallow and scalloped surrounding the cytoplasm (Fig. 14.71). The cyst walls can be highlighted with PAS and GMS. The genus and species cannot be determined by morphologic features. IHC is a useful ancillary assay to help highlight the amebic organisms in tissue samples, especially amid abundant macrophages with similar morphology (Fig. 14.71) (Guarner et al. 2007).

Differential Diagnosis

In immunocompromised hosts, *Acanthamoeba* infection must be differentiated from other skin lesions caused by many parasitic, fungal, bacterial, and viral infections. Most of these can be ruled out by clinical history, biopsy, direct examination, culture, or molecular testing of material from the lesion. *Entamoeba histolytica* produces painful ulcers that are seen most often in the perineal or perianal areas rather than on the face or extremities. The trophozoites of *E. histolytica* have similar size range with *Acanthamoeba* species, but they have a smaller nucleus with a vaguely perceptible karyosome. No cyst form of *E. histolytica* is present in tissue. *Acanthamoeba* cysts may be confused with *Blastomyces dermatitidis*; the yeast is

slightly smaller with no prominent karyosome and has characteristically thick cell walls with broad-based budding.

Cutaneous *Balamuthia mandrillaris* Infection

Etiology and Epidemiology

B. mandrillaris, formerly referred to as leptomyxid ameba, is the only known species of this genus and was originally isolated from the brain of a mandrill baboon (Visvesvara et al. 1993). *B. mandrillaris* is found in the environment and can infect human beings through skin wounds or by inhaling the dust containing the organisms. Though *B. mandrillaris* infects animals and humans worldwide, it has only rarely been isolated from the soil and water, presumptively because it does not grow on conventional culture media. The life cycle consists of the trophozoite and cyst stages, both of which are infectious. *B. mandrillaris* trophozoites have a mean diameter of 30 μm (range 12–60 μm) and are uninucleate. Cysts have a mean diameter of 15 μm (range 12–30 μm) with a wavy and irregular outer wall that is composed of three layers. On H&E-stained slides, the organism cannot be reliably differentiated from *Acanthamoeba* (Lobo et al. 2013).

Fig. 14.72 *Balamuthia mandrillaris* infection. Diffuse inflammatory infiltrate in dermis and subcutaneous tissue with a mixture of neutrophils, lymphocytes, histiocytes, and scattered multinucleated giant cells (H&E, 50× original magnification)

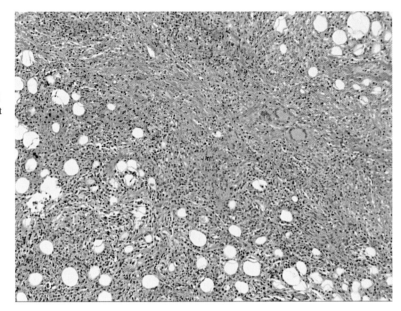

Fig. 14.73 *Balamuthia mandrillaris* infection. Perivascular inflammatory infiltrate, vasculitis, and vascular necrosis in dermis (H&E, 400× original magnification)

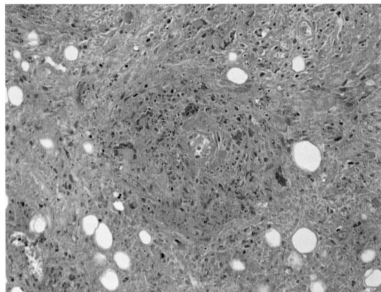

Clinical Features

Balamuthia can cause disease in both immunocompetent and immunocompromised hosts. Subacute or chronic granulomatous meningoencephalitis is the most common clinical presentation with a high mortality rate (Bravo et al. 2011). Balamuthiasis also sometimes manifests with skin lesions, particularly common in Peruvian patients (Martinez et al. 2010). These skin lesions are usually solitary and nodular and often appear on the central face, although other locations such as the lower face, abdomen, and extremities have been reported. Balamuthia skin lesions frequently precede CNS involvement. Clinical laboratory diagnosis can be made by DFA or PCR assays (Qvarnstrom et al. 2006).

Histopathology

The skin lesions caused by *B. mandrillaris* are similar to those caused by *Acanthamoeba* species with a broader spectrum. The inflammatory responses can range from an acute or neutrophilic infiltrate to a lymphocytic or granulomatous response (Fig. 14.72). Perivascular inflammatory infiltrate, vasculitis, and vascular necrosis are observed (Fig. 14.73). Unlike CNS infection, cysts and trophozoites of *B. mandrillaris* are not readily appreciable (Pritzker et al. 2004; Guarner et al. 2007). IHC is a useful ancillary assay to help highlight the antigens of *B. Mandrillaris* in skin biopsy samples for etiologic diagnosis.

Differential Diagnosis

Similar to cutaneous Acanthamebiasis, the skin infection caused by *B. mandrillaris* must be differentiated from other infectious skin lesions. Most of these can be ruled out by clinical history, biopsy, direct examination, culture, or molecular testing of material from the lesion.

Helminthic Diseases

Skin lesions caused by endemic helminth infections are still prevalent in many tropical rural regions. These lesions can occasionally be seen in the United States and Europe as imported cases. Skin biopsies taken from such lesions are usually sent to a parasitologist for consultation; however, because such specimens usually demonstrate a limited spectrum of specific morphologic criteria, any pathologist should be able to arrive at a precise etiologic diagnosis with information on patient's travel or exposure history. The life cycles of these helminth worms may be complex, but humans can only be infected in three manners: (1) ingestion of eggs or larvae, (2) skin penetration of larvae, or (3) a bite or sting of an insect vector.

When a suspected helminth structure is seen microscopically, the first differential diagnosis should be the possibility of plant material, insect, or other foreign bodies. Plant cells can usually be recognized by their rigid and refringent cell walls with prominent glycogen granules. Intact insect cuticles are thick, chitinous, and pigmented with elaborate appendages. Nevertheless, a partially destroyed worm or helminth egg can be confused with plant material or insect, and the distinction between these materials can be very difficult. Once the helminth structures are determined, a taxonomic differentiation should be made to further categorize the organisms in the order of roundworms (nematodes), tapeworms (cestodes), or flukes (trematodes). The main morphologic features of differentiation are summarized in Table 14.5 (Chiodini et al. 2001; Satoskar et al. 2009).

Onchocerciasis
Etiology and Epidemiology

Onchocerciasis is caused by the filarial nematode *Onchocerca volvulus*. The cutaneous lesion is a chronic dermatitis accompanied by progressive keratitis, uveitis, and loss of vision (river blindness). It is transmitted by black flies of the genus *Simulium*, which breed in fast-flowing rivers. Onchocerciasis is endemic in the savannahs and rain forests of subequatorial Africa and in Yemen, Central America, and the Amazon basin of South America (Gibson et al. 1989).

Clinical Features

The adult worms live in the deep dermis and subcutis and become clinically apparent as asymptomatic subcutaneous nodules. These nodules are discrete, movable, ranging in size from 0.5 to 2.0 cm, and often located close to the bony prominences. The adult worms do not cause any detrimental host response; on the contrary, their progeny, consisting of numerous microfilariae, can provoke intense inflammatory changes in the dermis and the aqueous humor of the eyes. Endemic onchocercal dermatitis is predominantly papular and lichenoid and intensely itchy. The appearance of skin lesions varies according to their duration; they can be spotty and depigmented ("leopard skin"), scaly and atrophic ("lizard skin"), or thickened and hyperkeratotic ("elephant skin"). Inguinal lymphadenopathy and lymphedema of the groin ("hanging groin") may occur in advanced disease (Edungbola et al. 1987; Gibson et al. 1989; Murdoch et al. 1993; Somo et al. 1993; Abanobi et al. 1994). Onchocerciasis acquired by travelers to endemic regions can be seen up to 2 years later as an itchy rash with marked peripheral eosinophilia. In the eyes, keratitis, iridocyclitis, chorioretinitis, and optic atrophy can occur, leading to eventual blindness.

Histopathology

The cutaneous nodules show a chronic inflammatory infiltrate and fibrosis at their peripheries.

Table 14.5 Main morphologic features for differentiation of helminths

Helminth	Nematode		Trematode		Cestode
Stage in cutaneous lesion	Adult	Larva	Adult or larva	Ova	Larva
Common species	*Dracunculus, Onchocerca, Wuchereria, Brugia, Mansonella, Loa Loa, Dirofilaria*	*Ankylostoma, Onchocerca, Mansonella, Gnathostoma*	*Schistosoma, Fasciola*	*Schistosoma, Paragonimus, Fasciola*	*Cysticercus, Sparganum*
Size and shape	2 mm to 35 cm, round and slender	500 μm in length; no more than 10–30 μm in cross section	Variable size; leaf shaped	Variable sizes up to 140 μm in greatest diameter, round or elliptical shells	1–10 cm, rounded cysts
Detailed structures	Nonsegmented body with a true collagenous epicuticle surrounding a coelomic cavity that contains their sexually differentiated reproductive organs, as well as a digestive tract with a distinct proximal esophageal segment and with both buccal and anal openings	No sexual differentiation; tiny, basophilic, dot-like nuclei.	Nonsegmented body with a syncytial, noncollagenous tegument with spines or tubercles; ventral sucker plates; a primitive gut ending in two blind bifurcations (ceca); hermaphroditic or sexually dimorphic reproductive organs with prominently granulated vitellaria Larvae: smaller with no true cuticle; syncytial, noncollagenous tegument; larger and more distinct nuclei than roundworm larvae		Hyaline wall containing an inwardly protruding embryo lined by a noncollagenous syncytial tegument with a brush border; scolex or scolices possess arrays of sucker plates and shark tooth-shaped hooklets

Their centers consist of dense fibrous tissue containing long, tangled, and coiled worms of both sexes (Fig. 14.74). The transverse and diagonal sections of adult worms measure from 125 to 450 μm in transverse diameter and up to 500 mm in length in females and 42 mm in males. Adult worms are embedded in dense granulation tissue and in mixed inflammatory cells, including macrophages and multinuclear giant cells of the foreign body type (Fig. 14.75). Microfilariae are occasionally observed within lymphatic vessels of the cutaneous lesions. Their size ranges from 5 to 9 μm in diameter and from 220 to 360 μm in length. In early, untreated onchocercal dermatitis, many undulating microfilariae are present within the upper dermis with minimal inflammatory response around intact microfilariae. Their number decreases greatly with time and may be

Fig. 14.74 Onchocerciasis. Chronic inflammatory infiltrate, fibrosis, and dense fibrous tissue containing long, tangled, and coiled worms of both sexes (H&E, 50× original magnification)

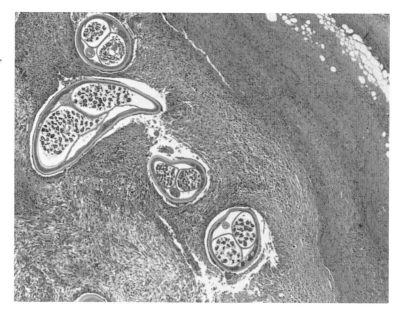

Fig. 14.75 Onchocerciasis. Adult worms embedded in dense granulation tissue and mixed inflammatory cells, including macrophages and multinuclear giant cells (H&E, 200× original magnification)

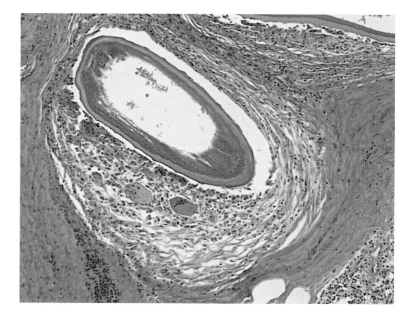

difficult to find in old lesions. In early infections, reactive changes in the dermis are minimal, but, in the course of years, mixed inflammatory cells including eosinophils accumulate around the vessels, and, ultimately, fibrosis of the dermis results, especially in the perivascular areas (Fig. 14.76). Hyperorthokeratosis, parakeratosis, epidermal hyperplasia (in the late-stage flattening

Fig. 14.76 Onchocerciasis. Mixed inflammatory cells including eosinophils around the vessels and diffuse fibrosis of dermis, especially in the perivascular areas (H&E, 50× original magnification)

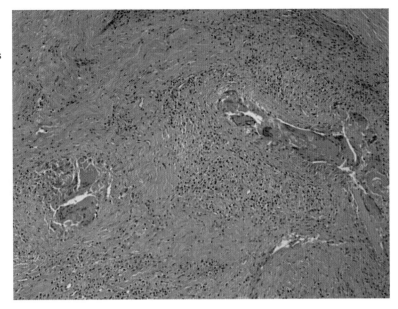

of the epidermis), tortuosity of dermal vessels, and pigment incontinence are other features of long-standing onchocercal dermatitis (Benitez Soto 1947; Bonucci et al. 1979; Langham and Richardson 1981; Taylor et al. 1987).

Schistosomiasis
Etiology and Epidemiology
Schistosomiasis is a widespread chronic endemic infection by sexually dimorphic trematodes of the genus *Schistosoma*. The disease affects 180–200 million people in more than 80 countries, thereby making it the most important trematode pathogenic to humans worldwide. Human skin lesions can be caused by animal schistosomes or one of the schistosome species, most commonly *Schistosoma mansoni*, *S. haematobium*, or *S. japonicum*. *S. mansoni* is common in the Caribbean islands and in northeastern South America; *S. japonicum* is found in Eastern Asia; and *S. haematobium* is common in the Middle East and in Africa. The infection is usually acquired through exposure to skin-penetrating cercariae, a stage in the life cycle of the parasite. The cercariae emerge from a freshwater snail which functions as an obligate intermediate host to the fluke. The cercariae burrow through the

skin and migrate to venous plexuses in various organs, where they mature into adult worms. *S. mansoni* and *S. japonicum* can cause portal hypertension and esophageal varices through lesions in the liver, and *S. haematobium* may lead to hematuria and hydronephrosis with involvement in the bladder. In Africa, mixed infections with both *S. mansoni* and *S. haematobium* are not uncommon (Secor and 2006; Meltzer and Schwartz 2013).

Clinical Features
The cutaneous manifestations of schistosomiasis can be divided into three types depending on the life cycle of the trematode. A pruritic, maculopapular erythematous skin rash called swimmers' itch (*dermatitis schistosomica*) occurs after penetration of the human skin by human or nonhuman cercarial larvae. This rash is self-healing within hours or days. Cercariae of nonhuman *Schistosoma* species exposed to human tissue always die at an early developmental stage (El-Mofty and Cahill 1964; El-Mofty and Nada 1975). More rarely, a similar rash occurs soon after exposure to cercariae of any of the major human-adapted schistosomes. This rash is usually mild and is seen more frequently in adult

Fig. 14.77 Schistosomiasis. Necrotizing granulomatous inflammation in dermis with complete or degenerated schistosomal ova located in the center of necrosis (H&E, 630× original magnification)

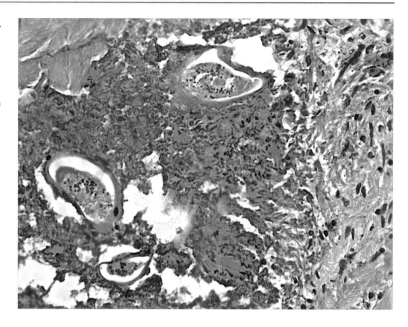

travelers to the tropics than in residents of the endemic zone. The initial skin penetration of cercariae is followed by full-scale systemic reactions including fever, urticaria, and sometimes purpura known as Katayama syndrome in Japan and Yangtze fever in China (Marotto et al. 1995; Rocha et al. 1995; Doherty et al. 1996). This usually occurs within a few weeks due to release of numerous eggs into the blood stream by adult female worms. Another rare type of skin lesions is due to ectopic deposition of eggs within the dermis (known as *bilharziasis cutanea tarda*) by established schistosome worms during the chronic phase of infection (MacDonald and Morrison 1976; Wood et al. 1976). These lesions are most commonly seen in *S. haematobium* infection and presents as papular, verrucous, ulcerative, or granulomatous lesions in the genital or perianal skin.

Histopathology

The skin lesion of swimmers' itch is rarely biopsied. The chronic lesion of Bilharziasis cutanea tarda represents the main persistent cutaneous pathology of schistosomiasis. The histopathologic features comprise a palisading, necrotizing granulomatous inflammation within the dermis with complete or degenerated schistosomal ova located in the center of necrosis (Fig. 14.77). These ova are usually surrounded by histiocytes, lymphocytes, plasma cells, and occasional multinucleated giant cells. Prominent eosinophils can be observed in some lesions as part of the inflammation. Calcification of the eggs surrounded by fibrosis is a common finding in older lesions. The overlying epidermis often reveals pseudopapillomatous hyperplasia (Uthman et al. 1990; Kick et al. 2000).

The ova measure up to 120 μm in greatest dimension and possess a chitinous outer shell that stains positively with PAS. The presence and position of a spine on the shell of the ova allow their classification within the tissue. The spine of *S. mansoni* ova is on the lateral aspect, whereas *S. haematobium* ova have a spine in the apical position, and *S. japonicum* ova have no prominent spine. However, the morphology of these ova is often too distorted to discern the characteristic spines in paraffin-embedded sections. *S. mansoni* and *S. japonicum* eggs are acid fast by the Ziehl–Neelsen method, while *S. haematobium* eggs are negative.

Differential Diagnosis

Acute cercarial dermatitis should be differentiated from other allergic and pruritic skin lesions based on clinical evaluation and serologic testing. Patients with chronic skin lesions due to deposition of schistosome eggs usually also excrete eggs in the feces or urine or present with clinical evidence of urinary or hepatointestinal schistosome pathology.

Fungal Infections

The primary cutaneous fungal pathogens can be divided into two groups according to their nature and locations of the lesions they produced: those tend to cause superficial infections and those mainly cause deep infections. Another group of cutaneous fungal pathogens are more commonly seen in immunocompromised patients. These infections only involve the skin secondarily as part of systemic disease. The basic histopathologic pattern of cutaneous fungal infection is relatively uniform within each of these three groups because of similar host responses.

The degree of inflammatory response varies according to the host immune status. For example, infections with organisms causing superficial dermatomycoses, such as the dermatophytes, *Candida* species, or *Malassezia furfur*, are generally characterized by hyphae or pseudohyphae and sometimes yeast cells in the keratin layer of the epidermis and in follicles. The intensity of the tissue reaction in the epidermis and follicular epithelium ranges from no response to a mild or moderate lymphocytic infiltrate with chronic spongiotic-psoriasiform pattern. These organisms are usually not found in the dermis except in the case of follicular rupture.

Deep cutaneous fungal infections are clinically more significant because of their detrimental local or systemic consequence. These infections typically demonstrate a mixed dermal inflammatory infiltrate associated with pseudo-epitheliomatous hyperplasia and occasionally with dermal fibrosis. Deep cutaneous fungal infections have also been associated with traumatic wound or iatrogenic injection. These rare instances are caused by environmental fungi that penetrate into host tissue due to breakdown of cutaneous barrier.

The laboratory diagnosis of fungal infections relies on culture, histopathologic evaluation, and other ancillary tests, such as special stains, IHC, ISH, and PCR assays.

Multiple special stains have been used to highlight certain fungal elements. These techniques can be helpful especially when the overall histologic pattern is suspicious for a fungal infection, but fungi are not conspicuous on routine H&E-stained sections. These special stains include periodic acid–Schiff (PAS), Grocott's methenamine silver impregnation (GMS), Gram, Fontana–Masson, mucicarmine, Alcian blue, India ink, and acid-fast stains. Immunohistochemical assays with relevant antibodies, in situ hybridization with pertinent probes, and PCR assays with specific primers have been developed to provide more sensitive and specific diagnosis for fungal infections in tissue samples.

It is beyond the scope of this chapter to describe these fungal infections individually in detail; the epidemiologic, clinical, morphologic, and histopathologic features of primary deep fungal infections and secondary cutaneous infections are summarized in Table 14.6 (Figs. 14.78, 14.79, 14.80, 14.81, 14.82, 14.83, 14.84, 14.85, 14.86, 14.87, 14.88, 14.89, 14.90, 14.91, 14.92, 14.93, 14.94, 14.95, 14.96, 14.97, 14.98, 14.99, and 14.100) (Chapman and Daniel 1994; Symposium 2002; Dismukes et al. 2003; Kauffman et al. 2011).

Table 14.6 Clinical, epidemiological, and histopathologic features of deep and secondary dermatomycoses

Disease	Etiology and epidemiology	Clinical features	Fungal size and morphology	Histopathologic features
Alternariosis (Figs. 14.78 and 14.79)	*Alternaria* species; ubiquitous saprophytic fungi in natural soil and plants	Exogenous form: ulcers and warty and granulomatous plaques. Endogenous form: deep dermis and subcutis involvement by hematogenous spread in immunocompromised patients	5–7 μm septate hyphae with variable branching and brown pigmentation; 3–10 μm round to oval spores, often with double contours	Suppurative and granulomatous dermatitis or panniculitis
Aspergillosis (Fig. 14.80)	*Aspergillus* species; *A. fumigatus* is the most common human pathogen of the genus; ubiquitous saprophytes found in soil, air, and decaying organic matter	Leading cause of opportunistic infection among immunocompromised patients, especially those with leukemia and solid organ or bone marrow transplant recipients	2–4 μm septate hyphae with dichotomous branching at 45° angle	Primary infection: granulomatous infiltrate. Secondary infection: angioinvasion, ischemic necrosis, and hemorrhage
Blastomycosis, North American (Figs. 14.81 and 14.82)	*Blastomyces dermatitidis*; in acidic soil of wooded areas near Mississippi and Ohio River valleys, South America, Europe, and Africa	Cutaneous infection occurs from hematogenous spread in 70 % of patients with disseminated blastomycosis; primary cutaneous infection is rare with ulcerated verrucous plaque at the inoculation site followed by lymphangitis and nodules spreading in a sporotrichoid distribution	5–15 μm thick-walled spores with single broad-based buds	Pseudoepitheliomatous hyperplasia with intraepidermal microabscesses. Suppurative granulomatous dermal infiltrate with giant cells
Candidiasis (Figs. 14.83 and 14.84)	Mainly *C. albicans, C. glabrata, C. parapsilosis, C. tropicalis,* and *C. krusei; C. albicans* is part of the normal flora of the GI tract, oral cavity, and vagina	Clinical forms: acute mucocutaneous, chronic mucocutaneous, and disseminated	3–7 μm yeast cells; hyphae 3–5 μm wide; pseudohyphae with chains of cells formed by repeated budding of blastoconidia	Subcorneal pustules, pustules in dermis, variable acute and chronic dermal infiltrate with occasional granulomas
Chromoblastomycosis	*Fonsecaea pedrosoi* (most common), *Phialophora verrucosa, Cladophialophora carrionii, Fonsecaea compacta, Rhinocladiella aquaspersa,* endemic in decaying wood or soil in tropical and subtropical regions	Erythematous papule that subsequently develops into one or multiple coalescing warty papules or plaques, typically occur on an extremity.	6–12 μm thick-walled, dark brown spores, often in clusters; some cells possess central septation and cross walls (*Medlar bodies, sclerotic bodies*)	Hyperkeratosis and epidermal hyperplasia, often with a pseudoepitheliomatous pattern, overlying a suppurative and granulomatous dermatitis

(continued)

Table 14.6 (continued)

Disease	Etiology and epidemiology	Clinical features	Fungal size and morphology	Histopathologic features
Coccidioidomycosis (Fig. 14.85)	*Coccidioides immitis* and *C. posadasii*; endemic in the arid and semiarid regions of the southwestern United States and northern Mexico, also occurs in parts of Central and South America	Clinical forms: pulmonary, cutaneous inoculation, and systemic; primary cutaneous infection shows verrucous plaques often associated with lymphangitis and lymphadenitis	20–80 μm thick-walled sporangia spores with granular cytoplasm; 1–4 um endospores in spherules	Primary inoculation: mixed dermal infiltrate with granulocytes, lymphocytes, and occasional histiocytic giant cells Systemic: acanthosis and formation of intraepidermal microabscesses with granulomas
Cryptococcosis (Figs. 14.86 and 14.87)	*Cryptococcus neoformans and C. gattii*; in soil contaminated with bird and bat excreta	Skin involvement variable with papules, pustules, nodules, plaques, and cellulitis; most common systemic fungal infection in AIDS patients	5–15 μm spore with wide capsule in gelatinous reaction. 2–4 μm spore in granulomatous reaction	Gelatinous reaction with many spores Granulomatous reaction with fewer spores
Eumycetoma (Figs. 14.88 and 14.89)	*Madurella mycetomatis*: the most prevalent dematiaceous fungal agent. Many other etiologic fungi. Endemic in equatorial Africa, the Middle East, India, and Mexico; etiologic agents usually associated with woody plants and soil	Inoculation into skin after trauma; localized infection of skin, subcutis, fascia, and bone; tumefactive nodules, ulceration, and draining sinuses with extrusion of sclerotia (grains, granules) in exudates; bone involvement often extensive	0.5–2.0 mm sulfur granules composed of 4–5 μm thick septate hyphae	Aggregate of microorganisms (grain) in a microabscess surrounded by granulation tissue and fibrosis; numerous neutrophils with granulomatous inflammation
Histoplasmosis, African	*H. capsulatum var. duboisii*; endemic in Central and West Africa and on the island of Madagascar	Localized form: chronic illness involving the skin, bone, and lymph nodes Disseminated form: involves the liver, spleen, and other organs in addition to the features of the localized form and often fatal	8–15 μm ovoid spores in macrophages and free in tissue	Granulomatous dermal infiltrate with focal suppuration
Histoplasmosis, classic (Figs. 14.90 and 14.91)	*H. capsulatum var. capsulatum*, worldwide in soil containing bird excreta, common in Southeastern and Midwestern United States, Central America, parts of Southeast Asia, and the Mediterranean basin	Clinical forms: pulmonary, cutaneous inoculation, and systemic. Primary cutaneous infection presents as a chancriform ulcer with associated regional lymphadenopathy	2–4 μm round, narrow-necked budding spores with clear halo in the cytoplasm of large histiocytes	Suppurative granulomatous infiltrate in ulcerative skin lesions, neutrophils and eosinophils in oral lesions; histiocytes contain variable numbers of organisms
Hyalohyphomycosis (Figs. 14.92 and 14.93)	*Fusarium, Acremonium, Paecilomyces, Scedosporium, and Trichoderma* species; ubiquitous saprophytic organisms found in soil	Cutaneous infection may develop as a complication of ulcers, surgical trauma, and burns; disseminated infection may arise after pulmonary inhalation or as a result of spread of cutaneous disease	Septate, 2–4 μm-diameter hyalinized hyphae with branching at an acute angle	Cutaneous plaques, ulceration, and subcutaneous abscesses

Disease	Etiology and epidemiology	Clinical features	Fungal size and morphology	Histopathologic features
Lobomycosis (keloidal blastomycosis)	*Lacazia loboi*; endemic in South America near Amazon and Orinoco Rivers	Slowly growing cutaneous and subcutaneous keloidal nodules and plaques that occur on the cooler regions of the body, such as the ears, face, arms, and legs	6–12 μm thick double wall spherical spores with single or multiple budding, often in chains or beaded appearance	Atrophic epidermis with dermal macrophage and giant cells; nodules with numerous intracellular organisms and fibroblastic proliferation
Paracoccidioidomycosis (South American blastomycosis)	*Paracoccidioides brasiliensis*; endemic in the humid mountain forests of South and Central America	Cutaneous infection typically developed by dissemination from primary pulmonary infection; acneiform papules or nodules slowly develop into crusted plaques with well-defined, raised borders	6–20 μm thick-walled, refractile yeasts with narrow-necked, single or multiple buds	Similar to North American blastomycosis
Penicilliosis (Fig. 14.94)	*Penicillium marneffei*; endemic in Southeast Asia; the third most common opportunistic infection after tuberculosis and cryptococcosis in AIDS patients in northern Thailand	Significant cause of disseminated infection in HIV-infected patients residing or traveling to endemic area. Papular skin eruptions progress to necrotic cutaneous ulcers and abscesses, generalized lymphadenopathy, and hepatosplenomegaly, which can be fatal	Resembles *H. capsulatum*, except yeast cells multiply by binary fission rather than by budding	Granulomatous inflammation with foci of suppuration or necrosis
Phaeohyphomycosis (Figs. 14.95 and 14.96)	The most common fungi in this group are *Exophiala jeanselmei* and *Wangiella dermatitidis*; others include *Cladophialophora bantiana*, *Bipolaris spicifera*, *Exophiala* species, *Wangiella dermatitidis*, *Ramichloridium obovoideum*, and *Chaetomium atrobrunneum*	Subcutaneous pseudocysts, ulcerated and verrucous lesions	Loosely arranged, septate, occasionally branching pigmented hyphae varying from 2 to 25 μm diameter, budding spores often producing chains	Deep, coalescing, suppurative granulomas with multinucleated giant cells, fibrous encapsulation of cystlike lesions, pseudoepitheliomatous hyperplasia and intradermal neutrophilic microabscesses at the surface of nodules or verrucous plaques
Rhinosporidiosis (Fig. 14.97)	*Rhinosporidium seeberi*; highest prevalence in India and Sri Lanka, also reported in Americas, Africa, and Europe	Large polypoid growths usually involve the nasal (70 %), ocular, nasopharyngeal mucosa or skin	Sporangia up to 300 μm; 7–12 μm endospores within sporangia	Hyperplastic epithelium with papillomatosis, deep invagination with pseudocysts, submucosal infiltrate of neutrophils, lymphocytes, histiocytes, plasma cells, and multinucleated giant cells

(continued)

Table 14.6 (continued)

Disease	Etiology and epidemiology	Clinical features	Fungal size and morphology	Histopathologic features
Sporotrichosis (Figs. 14.98 and 14.99)	*Sporothrix schenckii*, saprophytic mold in soil, wood, and decaying vegetative matter; widely distributed in the United States, Central and South America, Australia, Asia, and South Africa	Clinical forms: lymphocutaneous, fixed cutaneous, and disseminated. Inoculation into skin with trauma, cutaneous and subcutaneous nodules with frequent involvement of lymphatics	4–6 μm round to oval spores, cigar-shaped forms; single or uncommon multiple buds, rare branching, nonseptate hyphae	Cutaneous lesions: epidermal hyperplasia with intraepidermal abscesses, suppurative granulomatous dermal infiltrate, occasional asteroid bodies Subcutaneous nodules: central zone of neutrophils surrounded by zones of epithelioid macrophages and round cells
Zygomycosis (mucormycosis) (Fig. 14.100)	Order Mucorales: *Rhizopus, Mucor, Absidia, Rhizomucor, Apophysomyces,* and *Cunninghamella bertholletiae* Order Entomophthorales: *Conidiobolus* and *Basidiobolus*; ubiquitous saprophytic organisms found in soil and on decomposing organic material	Clinical forms: rhinocerebral, pulmonary, GI, cutaneous, and disseminated	8–30 μm hyphae with pauciseptation and branching at haphazardly arranged angles. Variably thin, often collapsed or twisted walls	Angioinvasion with thrombosis, infarction, necrosis, and variable, mild, neutrophilic infiltrate

Fig. 14.78 Alternariosis. Suppurative and granulomatous inflammation in dermis, sometimes extending into subcutaneous tissue (H&E, 50× original magnification)

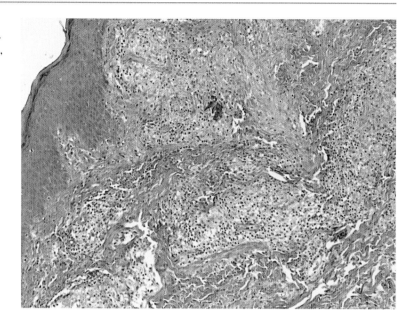

Fig. 14.79 Alternariosis. Septate hyphae with variable branching and brown pigmentation and round to oval spores, often with double contours (Grocott's methenamine silver stain, 1,000× original magnification)

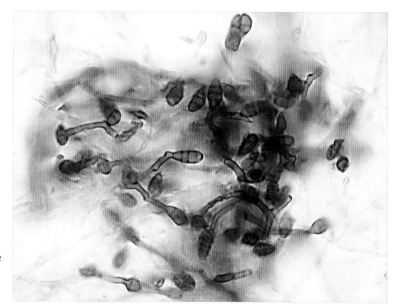

Fig. 14.80 Aspergillosis. Septate hyphae with dichotomous branching at 45° angle in areas of granulomatous infiltrate or in areas with angioinvasion and ischemic necrosis (H&E, 630× original magnification)

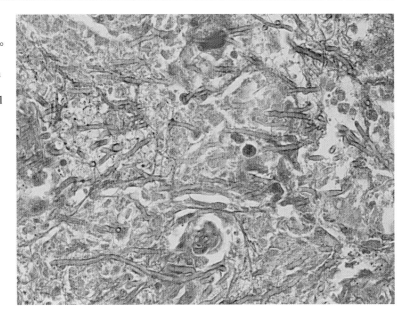

Fig. 14.81 Blastomycosis. Pseudoepitheliomatous hyperplasia with intraepidermal microabscesses and granulomatous dermal infiltrate (H&E, 50× original magnification)

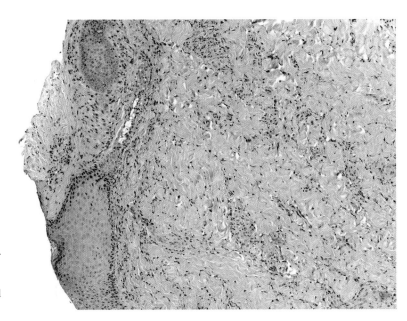

Fig. 14.82 Blastomycosis. Thick-walled spores with single broad-based buds in areas of inflammation (Grocott's methenamine silver stain, 1,000× original magnification)

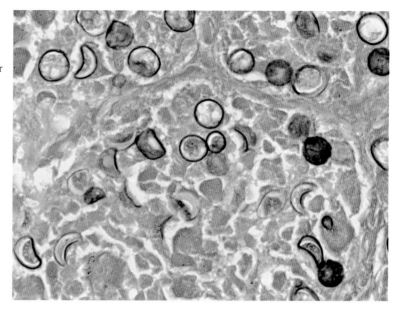

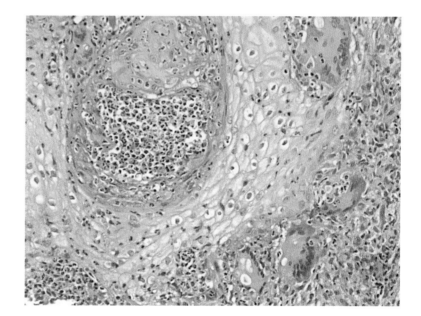

Fig. 14.83 Candidiasis. Pustules beneath stratum corneum and in dermis, variable acute and chronic dermal infiltrate with granulomas (H&E, 400× original magnification)

Fig. 14.84 Candidiasis. Yeast cells with budding of blastoconidia (Grocott's methenamine silver stain, 630× original magnification)

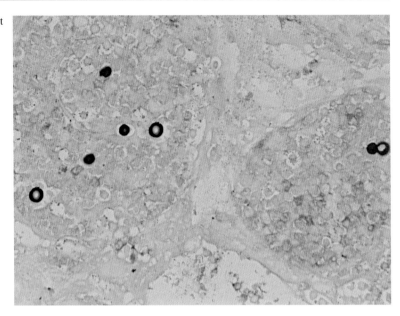

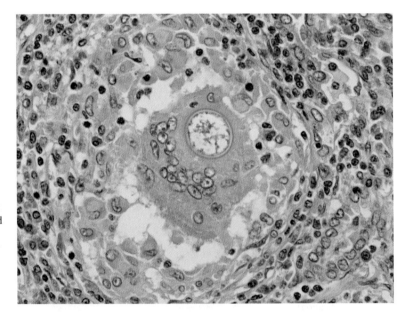

Fig. 14.85 Coccidioido-mycosis. Spherule with thick wall, granular cytoplasm, and endospores in a multinucle-ated giant cell surrounded by mixed infiltrate of granulo-cytes, lymphocytes, and plasma cells (H&E, 630× original magnification)

Fig. 14.86 Cryptococcosis. Gelatinous reaction in dermis with mixed inflammatory infiltrate and many yeasts (H&E, 200× original magnification)

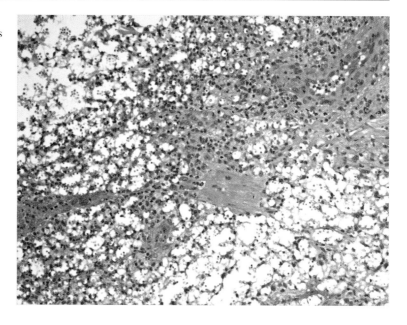

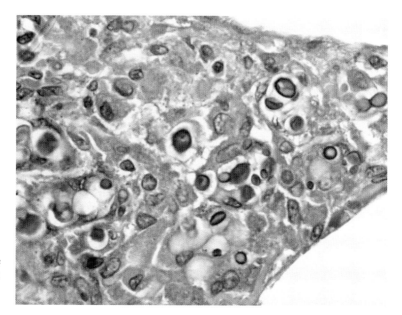

Fig. 14.87 Cryptococcosis. Yeast cells with wide capsule in dermal gelatinous reaction (Mucicarmine stain, 1,000× original magnification)

Fig. 14.88 Eumycetoma.
Aggregate of microorganisms
in a microabscess surrounded
by granulation tissue, fibrosis,
numerous neutrophils, and
granulomatous inflammation
(H&E, 50× original
magnification)

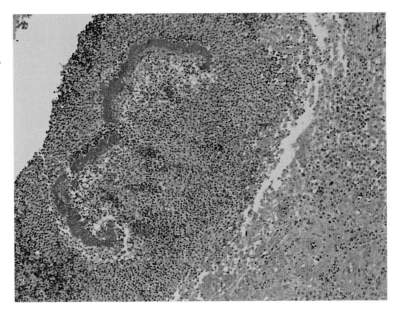

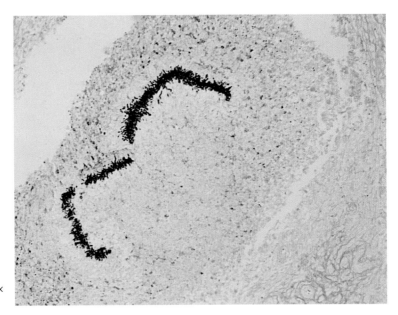

Fig. 14.89 Eumycetoma.
Numerous septate hyphae in
microabscess (Grocott's
methenamine silver stain, 50×
original magnification)

Fig. 14.90 Classic histoplasmosis. Suppurative granulomatous inflammation with abundant yeasts in large histiocytes (H&E, 630× original magnification)

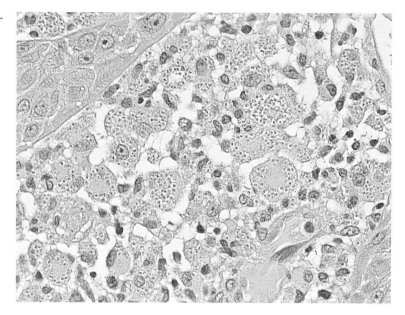

Fig. 14.91 Classic histoplasmosis. Small round, narrow-necked budding yeasts with clear halo in the cytoplasm of histiocytes (Grocott's methenamine silver stain, 630× original magnification)

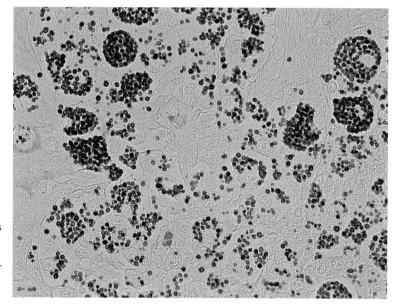

Fig. 14.92 Hyalohypho-
mycosis. Ulceration, dermal
hemorrhage, mixed inflammatory infiltrate, and subcutaneous abscesses (H&E, 50×
original magnification)

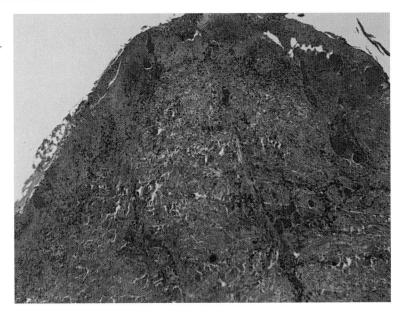

Fig. 14.93 Hyalohypho-
mycosis. Septate, hyalinized
hyphae with branching at an
acute angle and many
intercalated spores (H&E,
200× original magnification)

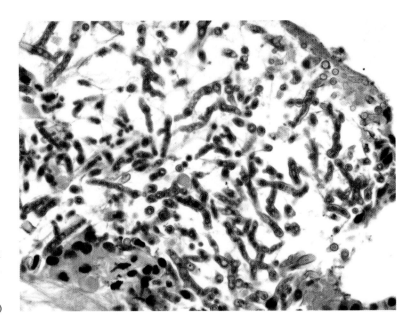

Fig. 14.94 Penicilliosis. Granulomatous inflammation and small round yeasts with clear halo in the cytoplasm of large histiocytes (H&E, 630× original magnification)

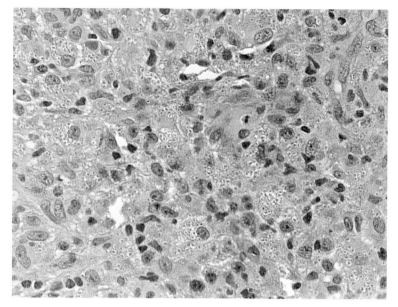

Fig. 14.95 Phaeohypho-mycosis. Coalescing, suppurative granulomas with multinucleated giant cells in dermis (H&E, 400× original magnification)

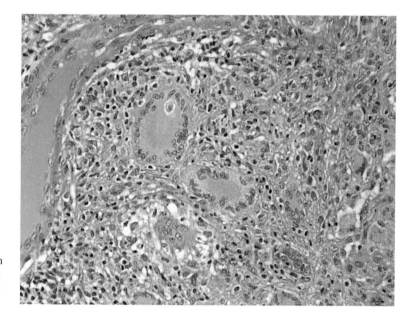

Fig. 14.96 Phaeohypho-
mycosis. Loosely arranged,
septate, occasionally
branching pigmented hyphae
with budding spores in chains
(Grocott's methenamine silver
stain, 630× original
magnification)

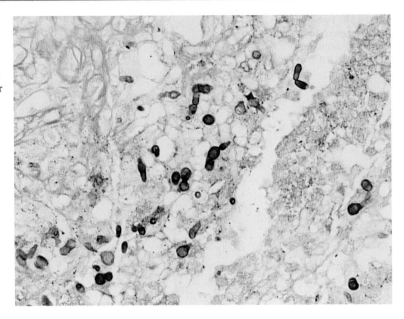

Fig. 14.97 Rhinosporidiosis.
Hyperplastic epithelium and
mixed inflammatory infiltrate
in dermis with multiple
various-sized sporangia
containing endospores (H&E,
400× original magnification)

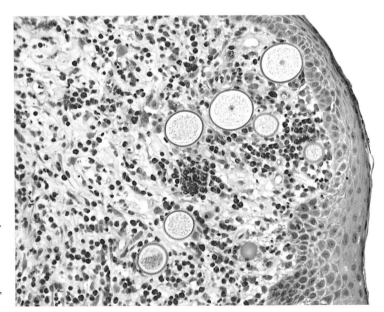

Fig. 14.98 Sporotrichosis. Intraepidermal abscesses and suppurative granulomatous inflammation in dermis (H&E, 50× original magnification)

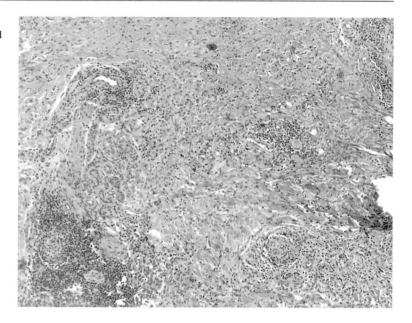

Fig. 14.99 Sporotrichosis. Suppurative granulomatous inflammation in dermis with occasional asteroid bodies (H&E, 400× original magnification)

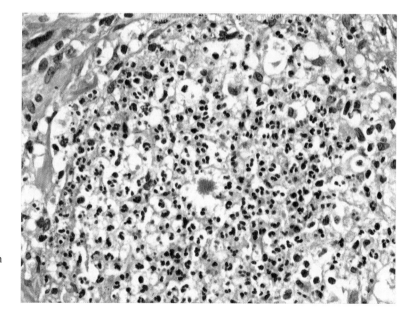

Fig. 14.100 Zygomycosis (mucormycosis). Thrombosis, infarction, and necrosis caused by angioinvasion of hyphae with pauciseptation and branching at haphazardly arranged angles (H&E, 630× original magnification)

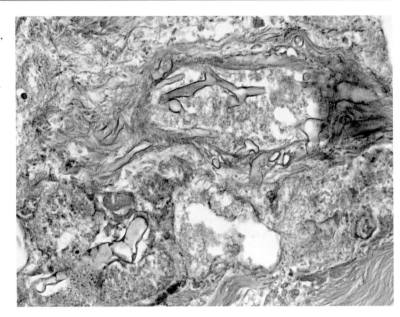

References

Abanobi OC, Edungbola LD, Nwoke BE, Mencias BS, Nkwogu FU, Njoku AJ. Validity of leopard skin manifestation in community diagnosis of human onchocerciasis infection. Appl Parasitol. 1994;35(1):8–11. 1994 ed.

Abell E, Marks R, Jones EW. Secondary syphilis: a clinico-pathological review. Br J Dermatol. 1975;93(1):53–61. 1975 ed.

Allen AC, Spitz S. A comparative study of the pathology of scrub typhus (Tsutsugamushi disease) and other rickettsial diseases. Am J Pathol. 1945;21(4):603–81. 1945 ed.

Althaus F, Greub G, Raoult D, Genton B. African tick-bite fever: a new entity in the differential diagnosis of multiple eschars in travelers. Description of five cases imported from South Africa to Switzerland. Int J Infect Dis. 2010;14 Suppl 3:e274–6. 2010 ed.

Antal GM, Lukehart SA, Meheus AZ. The endemic treponematoses. Microbes Infect. 2002;4(1):83–94. 2002nd ed.

Arias-Santiago S, Arrabal-Polo MA, Hernández-Quero J, Naranjo-Sintes R. Multiple cutaneous ulcerations: secondary syphilis in an HIV-positive patient. Int J Infect Dis. 2009;13(5):e337.

Asano S, Mori K, Yamazaki K, Sata T, Kanno T, Sato Y, et al. Temporal differences of onset between primary skin lesions and regional lymph node lesions for tularemia in Japan: a clinicopathologic and immunohistochemical study of 19 skin cases and 54 lymph node cases. Virchows Arch. 2012;460(6):651–8. 2012 ed.

Ball SC. Kaposi sarcoma and its changing course in HIV infection. AIDS Read. 2003;13(10):470–5, 4766–9.

Benitez Soto L. Histological studies in biopsy skin specimens taken from patients with onchocerciasis and in onchocercomas. Lab Dig. 1947;11(4):1–5. 1947 ed.

Bergmans AM, Groothedde JW, Schellekens JF, van Embden JD, Ossewaarde JM, Schouls LM. Etiology of cat scratch disease: comparison of polymerase chain reaction detection of Bartonella (formerly Rochalimaea) and Afipia felis DNA with serology and skin tests. J Infect Dis. 1995;171(4):916–23. 1995 ed.

Beyt BEJ, Ortbals DW, Santa Cruz DJ, Kobayashi GS, Eisen AZ, Medoff G. Cutaneous mycobacteriosis: analysis of 34 cases with a new classification of the disease. Medicine (Baltimore). 1981;60(2):95–109. 1981st ed.

Bhattacharya S. The World Health Organization and global smallpox eradication. J Epidemiol Community Health. 2008;62(10):909–12. 2008 ed.

Bjekić M, Marković M, Sipetić S. Clinical manifestations of primary syphilis in homosexual men. Braz J Infect Dis. 2012;16(4):387–9.

Bonamonte D, De Vito D, Vestita M, Delvecchio S, Ranieri LD, Santantonio M, et al. Aquarium-borne Mycobacterium marinum skin infection. Report of 15 cases and review of the literature. Eur J Dermatol. 2013;23(4):510–6. 2013 ed.

Bonucci E, Brinkmann UK, Onori E. A histological investigation of skin lesions in onchocerciasis patients from Southern Togo. Tropenmed Parasitol. 1979;30(4):489–98. 1979 ed.

Boonpucknavig S, Boonpucknavig V, Bhamarapravati N, Nimmannitya S. Immunofluorescence study of skin rash in patients with dengue hemorrhagic fever. Arch Pathol Lab Med. 1979;103(9):463–6. 1979 ed.

Botelho AC, Tafuri WL, Genaro O, Mayrink W. Histopathology of human American cutaneous leishmaniasis before and after treatment. Rev Soc Bras Med Trop. 1998;31(1):11–8. 1998 ed.

Bravo FG, Alvarez PJ, Gotuzzo E. Balamuthia mandrillaris infection of the skin and central nervous system: an emerging disease of concern to many specialties in medicine. Curr Opin Infect Dis. 2011;24(2):112–7. 2010 ed.

Britton WJ, Lockwood DN. Leprosy. Lancet. 2004;363(9416):1209–19. 2004 ed.

Cascio A, Iaria C. Epidemiology and clinical features of Mediterranean spotted fever in Italy. Parassitologia. 2006;48(1–2):131–3. 2006 ed.

Caumes E, Carrière J, Guermonprez G, Bricaire F, Danis M, Gentilini M. Dermatoses associated with travel to tropical countries: a prospective study of the diagnosis and management of 269 patients presenting to a tropical disease unit. Clin Infect Dis. 1995;20(3):542–8.

Centers for Disease Control and Prevention CDC. Multistate outbreak of monkeypox – Illinois, Indiana, and Wisconsin, 2003. MMWR Morb Mortal Wkly Rep. 2003;52(23):537–40.

Centurion-Lara A, Molini BJ, Godornes C, Sun E, Hevner K, Van Voorhis WC, et al. Molecular differentiation of Treponema pallidum subspecies. J Clin Microbiol. 2006;44(9):3377–80. 2006 ed.

Chapman AS, Bakken JS, Folk SM, Paddock CD, Bloch KC, Krusell A, et al. Diagnosis and management of tickborne rickettsial diseases: Rocky Mountain spotted fever, ehrlichioses, and anaplasmosis – United States: a practical guide for physicians and other health-care and public health professionals. MMWR Recomm Rep. 2006a;55(RR-4):1–27. 2006 ed.

Chapman AS, Murphy SM, Demma LJ, Holman RC, Curns AT, McQuiston JH, et al. Rocky Mountain spotted fever in the United States, 1997–2002. Vector Borne Zoonotic Dis. 2006b;6(2):170–8. 2006 ed.

Chapman SW, Daniel 3rd CR. Cutaneous manifestations of fungal infection. Infect Dis Clin N Am. 1994;8(4):879–910. 1994 ed.

Chian CA, Arrese JE, Pierard GE. Skin manifestations of Bartonella infections. Int J Dermatol. 2002;41(8): 461–6. 2002nd ed.

Chiodini PL, Moody AH, Manser DW. Atlas of medical helminthology and protozoology. 4th ed. Edinburg: Churchill Livingstone; 2001.

Choi CM, Lerner EA. Leishmaniasis as an emerging infection. J Investig Dermatol Symp Proc. 2001;6(3):175–82. 2002nd ed.

Chong LY, Lo KK. Cutaneous tuberculosis in Hong Kong: a 10-year retrospective study. Int J Dermatol. 1995;34(1):26–9. 1995 ed.

Chudomirova K, Chapkanov A, Abadjieva T, Popov S. Gummatous cutaneous syphilis. Sex Transm Dis. 2009;36(4):239–40.

Cochran RE, Thomson J, Fleming KA, Strong AM. Histology simulating reticulosis in secondary syphilis. Br J Dermatol. 1976;95(3):251–4. 1976 ed.

Cockerell CJ. The clinicopathologic spectrum of bacillary (epithelioid) angiomatosis. Prog AIDS Pathol. 1990; 2:111–26.

Cockerell CJ, Tierno PM, Friedman-Kien AE, Kim KS. Clinical, histologic, microbiologic, and biochemical characterization of the causative agent of bacillary (epithelioid) angiomatosis: a rickettsial illness with features of bartonellosis. J Invest Dermatol. 1991;97(5):812–7.

Cole GW, Gebhard J. Mycobacterium avium infection of the skin resembling lepromatous leprosy. Br J Dermatol. 1979;101(1):71–4. 1979 ed.

Cook SM, Bartos RE, Pierson CL, Frank TS. Detection and characterization of atypical mycobacteria by the polymerase chain reaction. Diagn Mol Pathol. 1994;3(1):53–8. 1994 ed.

Czarnetzki BM, Pomeranz JR, Khandekar PK, Wolinsky E, Belcher RW. Cat-scratch disease skin test. Studies of specificity and histopathologic features. Arch Dermatol. 1975;111(6):736–9.

Dauphin LA, Marston CK, Bhullar V, Baker D, Rahman M, Hossain MJ, et al. Swab protocol for rapid laboratory diagnosis of cutaneous anthrax. J Clin Microbiol. 2012;50(12):3960–7.

de Andino RM, Botet MV, Gubler DJ, Garcia C, Laboy E, Espada F, et al. The absence of dengue virus in the skin lesions of dengue fever. Int J Dermatol. 1985;24(1):48–51. 1985 ed.

de Wit MY, Faber WR, Krieg SR, Douglas JT, Lucas SB, Montreewasuwat N, et al. Application of a polymerase chain reaction for the detection of Mycobacterium leprae in skin tissues. J Clin Microbiol. 1991;29(5):906–10. 1991st ed.

Declercq E. Guide to eliminating leprosy as a public health problem. Lepr Rev. 2001;72(1):106–7. 2001st ed.

Degitz K. Detection of mycobacterial DNA in the skin. Etiologic insights and diagnostic perspectives. Arch Dermatol. 1996;132(1):71–5. 1996 ed.

Deluol AM, Teilhac MF, Poirot JL, Maslo C, Luboinski J, Rozenbaum W, et al. Cutaneous lesions due to Acanthamoeba sp in a patient with AIDS. J Eukaryot Microbiol. 1996;43(5):130S–1. 1996 ed.

Di Giulio DB, Eckburg PB. Human monkeypox: an emerging zoonosis. Lancet Infect Dis. 2004;4(1): 15–25. 2004 ed.

Dismukes WE, Pappas PG, Sobel JD. Clinical mycology. New York: Oxford University Press; 2003.

Dodiuk-Gad R, Dyachenko P, Ziv M, Shani-Adir A, Oren Y, Mendelovici S, et al. Nontuberculous mycobacterial infections of the skin: a retrospective study of 25 cases. J Am Acad Dermatol. 2007;57(3):413–20. 2007 ed.

Doherty JF, Moody AH, Wright SG. Katayama fever: an acute manifestation of schistosomiasis. BMJ. 1996;313(7064):1071–2.

Dumler JS, Gage WR, Pettis GL, Azad AF, Kuhadja FP. Rapid immunoperoxidase demonstration of Rickettsia rickettsii in fixed cutaneous specimens from patients with Rocky Mountain spotted fever. Am J Clin Pathol. 1990;93(3):410–4. 1990 ed.

Dumler JS, Walker DH. Diagnostic tests for Rocky Mountain spotted fever and other rickettsial diseases. Dermatol Clin. 1994;12(1):25–36. 1994 ed.

Eckman MR. Nontuberculous mycobacterial skin infections. Ann Intern Med. 1981;94(3):414–5. 1981st ed.

Edungbola LD, Alabi TO, Oni GA, Asaolu SO, Ogunbanjo BO, Parakoyi BD. "Leopard skin" as a rapid diagnostic index for estimating the endemicity of African onchocerciasis. Int J Epidemiol. 1987;16(4):590–4. 1987 ed.

Eliasson H, Broman T, Forsman M, Bäck E. Tularemia: current epidemiology and disease management. Infect Dis Clin N Am. 2006;20(2):311, ix.

El-Mofty AM, Cahill KM. Cutaneous manifestations of schistosomiasis. Dermatol Trop Ecol Geogr. 1964;30:157–61. 1964 ed.

El-Mofty AM, Nada M. Cutaneous schistosomiasis. Egypt J Bilharz. 1975;2(1):23–30. 1975 ed.

Elston D. Nontuberculous mycobacterial skin infections: recognition and management. Am J Clin Dermatol. 2009;10(5):281–5. 2009 ed.

Engelkens HJ, Judanarso J, Oranje AP, Vuzevski VD, Niemel PL, van der Sluis JJ, et al. Endemic treponematoses. Part I. Yaws. Int J Dermatol. 1991a;30(2):77–83. 1991st ed.

Engelkens HJ, ten Kate FJ, Vuzevski VD, van der Sluis JJ, Stolz E. Primary and secondary syphilis: a histopathological study. Int J STD AIDS. 1991b;2(4):280–4.

Engelkens HJ, Niemel PL, van der Sluis JJ, Meheus A, Stolz E. Endemic treponematoses. Part II. Pinta and endemic syphilis. Int J Dermatol. 1991c;30(4):231–8. 1991st ed.

Evins S, Leavell UWJ, Phillips IA. Intranuclear inclusions in milker's nodules. Arch Dermatol. 1971;103(1):91–3. 1971st ed.

Farina MC, Gegundez MI, Pique E, Esteban J, Martin L, Requena L, et al. Cutaneous tuberculosis: a clinical, histopathologic, and bacteriologic study. J Am Acad Dermatol. 1995;33(3):433–40. 1995 ed.

Ficarra G, Barone R, Gaglioti D, Milo D, Riccardi R, Romagnoli P, et al. Oral hairy leukoplakia among HIV-positive intravenous drug abusers: a clinicopathologic and ultrastructural study. Oral Surg Oral Med Oral Pathol. 1988;65(4):421–6.

Fine PE, Job CK, Lucas SB, Meyers WM, Ponnighaus JM, Sterne JA. Extent, origin, and implications of observer variation in the histopathological diagnosis of suspected leprosy. Int J Lepr Other Mycobact Dis. 1993;61(2):270–82. 1993rd ed.

Fleischauer AT, Kile JC, Davidson M, Fischer M, Karem KL, Teclaw R, et al. Evaluation of human-to-human transmission of monkeypox from infected patients to health care workers. Clin Infect Dis. 2005;40(5):689–94. 2005 ed.

Fleury RN, Bacchi CE. S-100 protein and immunoperoxidase technique as an aid in the histopathologic diagnosis of leprosy. Int J Lepr Other Mycobact Dis. 1987;55(2):338–44. 1987 ed.

Galarza C, Ramos W, Gutierrez EL, Ronceros G, Teran M, Uribe M, et al. Cutaneous acanthamebiasis infection in immunocompetent and immunocompromised patients. Int J Dermatol. 2009;48(12):1324–9.

Gazozai S, Iqbal J, Bukhari I, Bashir S. Comparison of diagnostic methods in cutaneous leishmaniasis (histopathology compared to skin smears). Pak J Pharm Sci. 2010;23(4):363–6. 2010 ed.

Gibson DW, Duke BO, Connor DH. Onchocerciasis: a review of clinical, pathologic and chemotherapeutic aspects, and vector control program. Prog Clin Parasitol. 1989;1:57–103.

Godyn JJ, Siderits R, Dzaman J. Cutaneous anthrax. Arch Pathol Lab Med. 2004;128(6):709–10. 2004 ed.

Goh BT. Syphilis in adults. Sex Transm Infect. 2005;81(6):448–52. 2005 ed.

Goihman-Yahr M. American mucocutaneous leishmaniasis. Dermatol Clin. 1994;12(4):703–12. 1994 ed.

Grayson W, Pantanowitz L. Histological variants of cutaneous Kaposi sarcoma. Diagn Pathol. 2008;3:31.

Grevelink SA, Lerner EA. Leishmaniasis. J Am Acad Dermatol. 1996;34(2 Pt 1):257–72. 1996 ed.

Grilo N, Modi D, Barrow P. Cutaneous bacillary angiomatosis: a marker of systemic disease in HIV. S Afr Med J. 2009;99(4):220–1.

Groves RW, Wilson-Jones E, MacDonald DM. Human orf and milkers' nodule: a clinicopathologic study. J Am Acad Dermatol. 1991;25(4):706–11. 1991st ed.

Guarner J, Bartlett J, Shieh W-J, Paddock CD, Visvesvara GS, Zaki SR. Histopathologic spectrum and immunohistochemical diagnosis of amebic meningoencephalitis. Mod Pathol. 2007;20(12):1230–7.

Guarner J, Greer PW, Bartlett J, Ferebee T, Fears M, Pope V, et al. Congenital syphilis in a newborn: an immunopathologic study. Mod Pathol. 1999;12(1):82–7. 1999 ed.

Guarner J, Johnson BJ, Paddock CD, Shieh W-J, Goldsmith CS, Reynolds MG, et al. Monkeypox transmission and pathogenesis in prairie dogs. Emerg Infect Dis. 2004;10(3):426–31.

Guarner J, Shieh W-J, Chu M, Perlman DC, Kool J, Gage KL, et al. Persistent Yersinia pestis antigens in ischemic tissues of a patient with septicemic plague. Hum Pathol. 2005;36(7):850–3.

Guarner J, Shieh W-J, Greer PW, Gabastou J-M, Chu M, Hayes E, et al. Immunohistochemical detection of Yersinia pestis in formalin-fixed, paraffin-embedded tissue. Am J Clin Pathol. 2002;117(2):205–9.

Guerrant RL, Walker DH, Weller PF. Tropical infectious diseases: principles, pathogens and practice. Edinburgh: Saunders/Elsevier; 2011.

Gullett J, Mills J, Hadley K, Podemski B, Pitts L, Gelber R. Disseminated granulomatous acanthamoeba infection presenting as an unusual skin lesion. Am J Med. 1979;67(5):891–6. 1979 ed.

Gutierrez Y, Salinas GH, Palma G, Valderrama LB, Santrich CV, Saravia NG. Correlation between histopathology, immune response, clinical presentation, and evolution in Leishmania braziliensis infection. Am J Trop Med Hyg. 1991;45(3):281–9. 1991st ed.

Halstead SB. Dengue. Imperial College Pr; 2008.

Hanke CW, Temofeew RK, Slama SL. Mycobacterium kansasii infection with multiple cutaneous lesions. J Am Acad Dermatol. 1987;16(5 Pt 2):1122–8. 1987 ed.

Hansmann Y, DeMartino S, Piemont Y, Meyer N, Mariet P, Heller R, et al. Diagnosis of cat scratch disease with detection of *Bartonella henselae* by PCR: a study of patients with lymph node enlargement. J Clin Microbiol. 2005;43(8):3800–6. 2005 ed.

Hasselmann CM. Comparative studies on the histopathology of syphilis, yaws, and pinta. Br J Vener Dis. 1957;33(1):5–12. 1957 ed.

Hayman J. Out of Africa: observations on the histopathology of Mycobacterium ulcerans infection. J Clin Pathol. 1993;46(1):5–9. 1993rd ed.

Hayman J, McQueen A. The pathology of Mycobacterium ulcerans infection. Pathology. 1985;17(4):594–600. 1985 ed.

Heffelfinger JD, Swint EB, Berman SM, Weinstock HS. Trends in primary and secondary syphilis among men who have sex with men in the United States. Am J Public Health. 2007;97(6):1076–83. 2007 ed.

Helton J, Loveless M, White CRJ. Cutaneous acanthamoeba infection associated with leukocytoclastic vasculitis in an AIDS patient. Am J Dermatopathol. 1993;15(2):146–9. 1993rd ed.

Hessami M, Keney DA, Pearson LD, Storz J. Isolation of parapox viruses from man and animals: cultivation and cellular changes in bovine fetal spleen cells. Comp Immunol Microbiol Infect Dis. 1979;2(1):1–7.

Hevia O, Jimenez-Acosta F, Ceballos PI, Gould EW, Penneys NS. Pruritic papular eruption of the acquired immunodeficiency syndrome: a clinicopathologic study. J Am Acad Dermatol. 1991;24(2 Pt 1):231–5.

Hook 3rd EW, Marra CM. Acquired syphilis in adults. N Engl J Med. 1992;326(16):1060–9. 1992nd ed.

Inglesby TV, Dennis DT, Henderson DA, Bartlett JG, Ascher MS, Eitzen E, et al. Plague as a biological weapon: medical and public health management. Working Group on civilian biodefense. JAMA. 2000;283:2281–90.

Inwald D, Nelson M, Cramp M, Francis N, Gazzard B. Cutaneous manifestations of mycobacterial infection in patients with AIDS. Br J Dermatol. 1994;130(1):111–4. 1994 ed.

Jeerapaet P, Ackerman AB. Histologic patterns of secondary syphilis. Arch Dermatol. 1973;107(3):373–7. 1973rd ed.

Jernigan DB, Raghunathan PL, Bell BP, Brechner R, Bresnitz EA, Butler JC, et al. Investigation of bioterrorism-related anthrax, United States, 2001: epidemiologic findings. Emerg Infect Dis. 2002;8(10):1019–28.

Johannessen JV, Krogh HK, Solberg I, Dalen A, van Wijngaarden H, Johansen B. Human orf. J Cutan Pathol. 1975;2(6):265–83. 1975 ed.

Jordaan HF, Van Niekerk DJ, Louw M. Papulonecrotic tuberculid. A clinical, histopathological, and immunohistochemical study of 15 patients. Am J Dermatopathol. 1994;16(5):474–85. 1994 ed.

Kakakhel KU, Fritsch P. Cutaneous tuberculosis. Int J Dermatol. 1989;28(6):355–62. 1989 ed.

Kao GF, Evancho CD, Ioffe O, Lowitt MH, Dumler JS. Cutaneous histopathology of Rocky Mountain spotted fever. J Cutan Pathol. 1997;24(10):604–10. 1998 ed.

Kaplan MH, Sadick N, McNutt NS, Meltzer M, Sarngadharan MG, Pahwa S. Dermatologic findings and manifestations of acquired immunodeficiency syndrome (AIDS). J Am Acad Dermatol. 1987;16(3 Pt 1):485–506.

Kauffman CA, Pappas PG, Sobel JD. Essentials of clinical mycology. New York: Springer; 2011.

Kemény L, Kiss M, Gyulai R, Kenderessy AS, Adám E, Nagy F, et al. Human herpesvirus 8 in classic Kaposi sarcoma. Acta Microbiol Immunol Hung. 1996;43(4):391–5.

Kenner JR, Aronson NE, Bratthauer GL, Turnicky RP, Jackson JE, Tang DB, et al. Immunohistochemistry to identify Leishmania parasites in fixed tissues. J Cutan Pathol. 1999;26(3):130–6. 1999 ed.

Kick G, Schaller M, Korting HC. Late cutaneous schistosomiasis representing an isolated skin manifestation of schistosoma mansoni infection. Dermatology. 2000;200(2):144–6. 2000 ed.

Koss T, Carter EL, Grossman ME, Silvers DN, Rabinowitz AD, Singleton JJ, et al. Increased detection of rickettsialpox in a New York City hospital following the anthrax outbreak of 2001: use of immunohistochemistry for the rapid confirmation of cases in an era of bioterrorism. Arch Dermatol. 2003;139(12):1545–52. 2003rd ed.

Kothavade RJ, Dhurat RS, Mishra SN, Kothavade UR. Clinical and laboratory aspects of the diagnosis and management of cutaneous and subcutaneous infections caused by rapidly growing mycobacteria. Eur J Clin Microbiol Infect Dis. 2013;32(2):161–88. 2012 ed.

Kuokkanen K, Launis J, Mörttinen A. Erythema nodosum and erythema multiforme associated with milker's nodules. Acta Derm Venereol. 1976;56(1):69–72.

Kurban AK, Malak JA, Farah FS, Chaglassian HT. Histopathology of cutaneous leishmaniasis. Arch Dermatol. 1966;93(4):396–401. 1965 ed.

Lamps LW, Havens JM, Sjostedt A, Page DL, Scott MA. Histologic and molecular diagnosis of tularemia: a potential bioterrorism agent endemic to North America. Mod Pathol. 2004;17(5):489–95.

Langham ME, Richardson R. Onchocerciasis diagnosis and the probability of visual loss in patients with skin snips negative for Onchocerca volvulus microfilariae. Tropenmed Parasitol. 1981;32(3):171–80. 1981st ed.

Lautenschlager S. Cutaneous manifestations of syphilis: recognition and management. Am J Clin Dermatol. 2006;7(5):291–304.

Lawrence P, Saxe N. Bullous secondary syphilis. Clin Exp Dermatol. 1992;17(1):44–6. 1992nd ed.

Leavell UWJ, McNamara MJ, Muelling R, Talbert WM, Rucker RC, Dalton AJ. Orf. Report of 19 human cases with clinical and pathological observations. JAMA. 1968;204(8):657–64. 1968 ed.

LeBoit PE, Berger TG, Egbert BM, Beckstead JH, Yen TS, Stoler MH. Bacillary angiomatosis. The histopathology and differential diagnosis of a pseudoneoplastic infection in patients with human immunodeficiency virus disease. Am J Surg Pathol. 1989;13(11):909–20.

Lederman ER, Weld LH, Elyazar IRF, von Sonnenburg F, Loutan L, Schwartz E, et al. Dermatologic conditions of the ill returned traveler: an analysis from the

GeoSentinel Surveillance Network. Int J Infect Dis. 2008;12(6):593–602.

Lee J-H, Lee J-H, Chung KM, Kim ES, Kwak YG, Moon C, et al. Dynamics of clinical symptoms in patients with scrub typhus. Jpn J Infect Dis. 2013;66(2):155–7.

Lee JS, Park MY, Kim YJ, Kil HI, Choi YH, Kim YC. Histopathological features in both the eschar and erythematous lesions of Tsutsugamushi disease: identification of CD30+ cell infiltration in Tsutsugamushi disease. Am J Dermatopathol. 2009;31(6):551–6.

Lee WJ, Kang SM, Sung H, Won CH, Chang SE, Lee MW, et al. Non-tuberculous mycobacterial infections of the skin: a retrospective study of 29 cases. J Dermatol. 2010;37(11):965–72. 2010 ed.

Levine RS, Peterson AT, Yorita KL, Carroll D, Damon IK, Reynolds MG. Ecological niche and geographic distribution of human monkeypox in Africa. PLoS ONE. 2007;2(1):e176. 2007 ed.

Lobo SA, Patil K, Jain S, Marks S, Visvesvara GS, Tenner M, et al. Diagnostic challenges in Balamuthia mandrillaris infections. Parasitol Res. 2013;112(12):4015–9.

Maass M, Schreiber M, Knobloch J. Detection of Bartonella bacilliformis in cultures, blood, and formalin preserved skin biopsies by use of the polymerase chain reaction. Trop Med Parasitol. 1992;43(3):191–4. 1992nd ed.

MacDonald DM, Morrison JG. Cutaneous ectopic schistosomiasis. Br Med J. 1976;2(6036):619–20. 1976 ed.

Mahaisavariya P, Chaiprasert A, Khemngern S, Manonukul J, Gengviniij N, Ubol PN, et al. Nontuberculous mycobacterial skin infections: clinical and bacteriological studies. J Med Assoc Thai. 2003;86(1):52–60. 2003rd ed.

Mahaisavariya P, Manonukul J, Khemngern S, Chaiprasert A. Mycobacterial skin infections: comparison between histopathologic features and detection of acid fast bacilli in pathologic section. J Med Assoc Thai. 2004;87(6):709–12.

Maingi CP, Helm KF. Utility of deeper sections and special stains for dermatopathology specimens. J Cutan Pathol. 1998;25(3):171–5.

Marotto PC, Michalany NS, Vilela MP, Mendes NF, Mendes E. Cutaneous immediate and late phase reactions to schistosomin in schistosomiasis patients. J Investig Allergol Clin Immunol. 1995;5(5):269–71. 1995 ed.

Martinez DY, Seas C, Bravo F, Legua P, Ramos C, Cabello AM, et al. Successful treatment of Balamuthia mandrillaris amoebic infection with extensive neurological and cutaneous involvement. Clin Infect Dis. 2010;51(2):e7–11. 2010 ed.

McBride WJ, Bielefeldt-Ohmann H. Dengue viral infections; pathogenesis and epidemiology. Microbes Infect. 2000;2(9):1041–50.

McCollum AM, Damon IK. Human monkeypox. Clin Infect Dis. 2014;58(2):260–7.

Mehregan DR, Mehregan AH, Mehregan DA. Histologic diagnosis of cutaneous leishmaniasis. Clin Dermatol. 1999;17(3):297–304. 1999 ed.

Meltzer E, Schwartz E. Schistosomiasis: current epidemiology and management in travelers. Curr Infect Dis Rep. 2013;15(3):211–5.

Min K-W, Ko JY, Park CK. Histopathological spectrum of cutaneous tuberculosis and non-tuberculous mycobacterial infections. J Cutan Pathol. 2012;39(6):582–95.

Modlin RL, Rea TH. Immunopathology of leprosy granulomas. Springer Semin Immunopathol. 1988;10(4):359–74. 1988 ed.

Murakawa GJ. American Academy of Dermatology 1997 awards for young investigators in dermatology. Pathogenesis of Bartonella henselae in cutaneous and systemic disease. J Am Acad Dermatol. 1997;37(5 Pt 1):775–6. 1997 ed.

Murdoch ME, Hay RJ, Mackenzie CD, Williams JF, Ghalib HW, Cousens S, et al. A clinical classification and grading system of the cutaneous changes in onchocerciasis. Br J Dermatol. 1993;129(3):260–9. 1993rd ed.

Nishimura M, Kwon KS, Shibuta K, Yoshikawa Y, Oh CK, Suzuki T, et al. Methods in pathology. An improved method for DNA diagnosis of leprosy using formaldehyde-fixed, paraffin-embedded skin biopsies. Mod Pathol. 1994;7(2):253–6. 1994 ed.

Noordeen SK. Eliminating leprosy as a public health problem; why the optimism is justified. Int J Lepr Other Mycobact Dis. 1995;63(4):559–66. 1995 ed.

Noordhoek GT, Cockayne A, Schouls LM, Meloen RH, Stolz E, van Embden JD. A new attempt to distinguish serologically the subspecies of Treponema pallidum causing syphilis and yaws. J Clin Microbiol. 1990;28(7):1600–7. 1990 ed.

Noordhoek GT, Hermans PW, Paul AN, Schouls LM, van der Sluis JJ, van Embden JD. Treponema pallidum subspecies pallidum (Nichols) and Treponema pallidum subspecies pertenue (CDC 2575) differ in at least one nucleotide: comparison of two homologous antigens. Microb Pathog. 1989;6(1):29–42. 1989 ed.

Noppakun N, Dinehart SM, Solomon AR. Pustular secondary syphilis. Int J Dermatol. 1987;26(2):112–4. 1987 ed.

O'Donnell PJ, Pantanowitz L, Grayson W. Unique histologic variants of cutaneous Kaposi sarcoma. Am J Dermatopathol. 2010;32(3):244–50.

Ottenhoff TH. Immunology of leprosy: lessons from and for leprosy. Int J Lepr Other Mycobact Dis. 1994;62(1):108–21. 1994 ed.

Paddock CD, Finley RW, Wright CS, Robinson HN, Schrodt BJ, Lane CC, et al. Rickettsia parkeri rickettsiosis and its clinical distinction from Rocky Mountain spotted fever. Clin Infect Dis. 2008;47(9):1188–96. 2008 ed.

Paddock CD, Greer PW, Ferebee TL, Singleton J, McKechnie DB, Treadwell TA, et al. Hidden mortality attributable to Rocky Mountain spotted fever: immunohistochemical detection of fatal, serologically unconfirmed disease. J Infect Dis. 1999;179(6):1469–76.

Pardillo FE, Fajardo TT, Abalos RM, Scollard D, Gelber RH. Methods for the classification of leprosy for treatment purposes. Clin Infect Dis. 2007;44(8):1096–9. 2007 ed.

Park JH, Hart MS. The pathology of scrub typhus. Am J Clin Pathol. 1946;16:139–49. 1946 ed.

Patton LL. Oral lesions associated with human immunodeficiency virus disease. Dent Clin N Am. 2013;57(4):673–98.

Pavli A, Maltezou HC. Leishmaniasis, an emerging infection in travelers. Int J Infect Dis. 2010;14(12):e1032–9. 2010 ed.

Pearson RD, Sousa AQ. Clinical spectrum of leishmaniasis. Clin Infect Dis. 1996;22(1):1–13. 1996 ed.

Peltier E, Wolkenstein P, Deniau M, Zafrani ES, Wechsler J. Caseous necrosis in cutaneous leishmaniasis. J Clin Pathol. 1996;49(6):517–9. 1996 ed.

Penneys NS, Leonardi CL, Cook S, Blauvelt A, Rosenberg S, Eells LD, et al. Identification of Mycobacterium tuberculosis DNA in five different types of cutaneous lesions by the polymerase chain reaction. Arch Dermatol. 1993;129(12):1594–8. 1993rd ed.

Pföhler C, Koerner R, Müller von L, Vogt T, Müller CSL. Lues maligna in a patient with unknown HIV infection. BMJ Case Rep. 2011;27:1–4.

Pierard-Franchimont C, Quatresooz P, Pierard GE. Skin diseases associated with Bartonella infection: facts and controversies. Clin Dermatol. 2010;28(5):483–8. 2010 ed.

Plettenberg A, Lorenzen T, Burtsche BT, Rasokat H, Kaliebe T, Albrecht H, et al. Bacillary angiomatosis in HIV-infected patients – an epidemiological and clinical study. Dermatology. 2000;201(4):326–31.

Poulsen A, Kobayasi T, Secher L, Weismann K. Treponema pallidum in macular and papular secondary syphilitic skin eruptions. Acta Derm Venereol. 1986;66(3):251–8.

Pritzker AS, Kim BK, Agrawal D, Southern PMJ, Pandya AG. Fatal granulomatous amebic encephalitis caused by Balamuthia mandrillaris presenting as a skin lesion. J Am Acad Dermatol. 2004;50(2 Suppl):S38–41. 2004 ed.

Putkuri N, Piiparinen H, Vaheri A, Vapalahti O. Detection of human orthopoxvirus infections and differentiation of smallpox virus with real-time PCR. J Med Virol. 2009;81(1):146–52. 2008 ed.

Qvarnstrom Y, Visvesvara GS, Sriram R, da Silva AJ. Multiplex real-time PCR assay for simultaneous detection of Acanthamoeba spp., Balamuthia mandrillaris, and Naegleria fowleri. J Clin Microbiol. 2006;44(10):3589–95.

Rapini RP. Overview of new dermatopathology techniques. Clin Dermatol. 1991;9(2):115–7.

Rastogi V, Nirwan PS. Cutaneous leishmaniasis: an emerging infection in a non-endemic area and a brief update. Indian J Med Microbiol. 2007;25(3):272–5. 2007 ed.

Ray MC, Gately LE. Dermatologic manifestations of HIV infection and AIDS. Infect Dis Clin N Am. 1994;8(3):583–605.

Rea TH, Modlin RL. Immunopathology of leprosy skin lesions. Semin Dermatol. 1991;10(3):188–93. 1991st ed.

Reed KD, Melski JW, Graham MB, Regnery RL, Sotir MJ, Wegner MV, et al. The detection of monkeypox in humans in the western hemisphere. N Engl J Med. 2004;350(4):342–50. 2004 ed.

Ridley DS. Histological classification and the immunological spectrum of leprosy. Bull World Health Organ. 1974;51(5):451–65. 1974 ed.

Ridley DS, Jopling WH. Classification of leprosy according to immunity. A five-group system. Int J Lepr Other Mycobact Dis. 1966;34(3):255–73. 1966 ed.

Rocha MO, Greco DB, Pedroso ER, Lambertucci JR, Rocha RL, Rezende DF, et al. Secondary cutaneous manifestations of acute schistosomiasis mansoni. Ann Trop Med Parasitol. 1995;89(4):425–30. 1995 ed.

Rocha N, Horta M, Sanches M, Lima O, Massa A. Syphilitic gumma – cutaneous tertiary syphilis. J Eur Acad Dermatol Venereol. 2004;18(4):517–8.

Rose C, Starostik P, Bröcker EB. Infection with parapoxvirus induces CD30-positive cutaneous infiltrates in humans. J Cutan Pathol. 1999;26(10):520–2.

Rosenberg AS, Morgan MB. Disseminated acanthamoebiasis presenting as lobular panniculitis with necrotizing vasculitis in a patient with AIDS. J Cutan Pathol. 2001;28(6):307–13. 2001st ed.

Ryan ET, Maguire JH, Strickland GT, Solomon T, Hill DR. Hunter's tropical medicine and emerging infectious disease. London: Saunders/Elsevier; 2012.

Saadiah S, Sharifah BI, Robson A, Greaves MW. Skin histopathology and immunopathology are not of prognostic value in dengue haemorrhagic fever. Br J Dermatol. 2008;158(4):836–7.

Safaei A, Motazedian MH, Vasei M. Polymerase chain reaction for diagnosis of cutaneous leishmaniasis in histologically positive, suspicious and negative skin biopsies. Dermatology. 2002;205(1):18–24. 2002nd ed.

Saleem K, Shaikh I. Skin lesions in hospitalized cases of dengue fever. J Coll Physicians Surg Pak. 2008;18(10):608–11. 2008 ed.

Salman SM, Rubeiz NG, Kibbi AG. Cutaneous leishmaniasis: clinical features and diagnosis. Clin Dermatol. 1999;17(3):291–6. 1999 ed.

Samady JA, Janniger CK, Schwartz RA. Cutaneous and mucocutaneous leishmaniasis. Cutis. 1996;57(1):13–20. 1996 ed.

Sanchez PJ. Congenital syphilis. Adv Pediatr Infect Dis. 1992;7:161–80. 1992nd ed.

Sanchez RL, Hebert A, Lucia H, Swedo J. Orf. A case report with histologic, electron microscopic, and immunoperoxidase studies. Arch Pathol Lab Med. 1985;109(2):166–70. 1985 ed.

Sangueza OP, Sangueza JM, Stiller MJ, Sangueza P. Mucocutaneous leishmaniasis: a clinicopathologic classification. J Am Acad Dermatol. 1993;28(6):927–32. 1993rd ed.

Satoskar AR, Simon G, Hotez PJ, Tsuji M. Medical parasitology. Landes Bioscience. Austin, Texas, USA; 2009.

Scarisbrick JJ, Chiodini PL, Watson J, Moody A, Armstrong M, Lockwood D, et al. Clinical features and diagnosis of 42 travellers with cutaneous leishmaniasis. Travel Med Infect Dis. 2006;4(1):14–21. 2006 ed.

Schoutens C, Boute V, Govaerts D, De Dobbeleer G. Late cutaneous syphilis and neurosyphilis. Dermatology. 1996;192(4):403–5.

Scott MA, McCurley TL, Vnencak-Jones CL, Hager C, McCoy JA, Anderson B, et al. Cat scratch disease: detection of Bartonella henselae DNA in archival biopsies from patients with clinically, serologically, and histologically defined disease. Am J Pathol. 1996;149(6):2161–7. 1996 ed.

Scully C, Porter SR, Di Alberti L, Jalal M, Maitland N. Detection of Epstein-Barr virus in oral scrapes in HIV infection, in hairy leukoplakia, and in healthy non-HIV-infected people. J Oral Pathol Med. 1998; 27(10):480–2.

Secor WE, Colley DG. Schistosomiasis. Boston: Springer; 2006.

Sehgal VN, Jain MK, Srivastava G. Changing pattern of cutaneous tuberculosis. A prospective study. Int J Dermatol. 1989;28(4):231–6. 1989 ed.

Seong SY, Choi MS, Kim IS. Orientia tsutsugamushi infection: overview and immune responses. Microbes Infect. 2001;3(1):11–21.

Sexton DJ, Corey GR. Rocky Mountain "spotless" and "almost spotless" fever: a wolf in sheep's clothing. Clin Infect Dis. 1992;15(3):439–48.

Sexton DJ, Kaye KS. Rocky Mountain spotted fever. Med Clin N Am. 2002;86(2):351–60, vii–viii. 2002nd ed.

Sezer E, Luzar B, Calonje E. Secondary syphilis with an interstitial granuloma annulare-like histopathologic pattern. J Cutan Pathol. 2011;38(5):439–42.

Sharquie KE, Hassen AS, Hassan SA, Al-Hamami IA. Evaluation of diagnosis of cutaneous leishmaniasis by direct smear, culture and histopathology. Saudi Med J. 2002;23(8):925–8. 2002nd ed.

Shieh W-J, Guarner J, Paddock C, Greer P, Tatti K, Fischer M, et al. The critical role of pathology in the investigation of bioterrorism-related cutaneous anthrax. Am J Pathol. 2003;163(5):1901–10.

Singh SK, Ruzek D. Viral hemorrhagic fevers. Boca Raton, Florida: CRC Press; 2013.

Skinsnes OK. Immuno-pathology of leprosy: the century in review. Pathology, pathogenesis, and the development of classification. Int J Lepr Other Mycobact Dis. 1973;41(3):329–60. 1973rd ed.

Smith KJ, Skelton HG, Yeager J, Angritt P, Frisman D, Wagner KF, et al. Histopathologic and immunohistochemical findings associated with inflammatory dermatoses in human immunodeficiency virus type 1 disease and their correlation with Walter Reed stage. Military Medical Consortium for applied retroviral research. J Am Acad Dermatol. 1993a;28(2 Pt 1): 174–84.

Smith KJ, Skelton HG, Yeager J, Angritt P, Wagner KF. Histologic features of foreign body reactions in patients infected with human immunodeficiency virus type 1. The Military Medical Consortium for applied retroviral research. J Am Acad Dermatol. 1993b; 28(3):470–6.

Somo RM, Enyong PA, Fobi G, Dinga JS, Lafleur C, Agnamey P, et al. A study of onchocerciasis with severe skin and eye lesions in a hyperendemic zone in the forest of Southwestern Cameroon: clinical, parasi-tologic, and entomologic findings. Am J Trop Med Hyg. 1993;48(1):14–9. 1993rd ed.

Song H, Lee H, Choi G, Shin J. Cutaneous nontuberculous mycobacterial infection: a clinicopathological study of 7 cases. Am J Dermatopathol. 2009;31(3):227–31.

Splettstoesser WD, Tomaso H, Dahouk Al S, Neubauer H, Schuff-Werner P. Diagnostic procedures in tularaemia with special focus on molecular and immunological techniques. J Vet Med B Infect Dis Vet Public Health. 2005;52(6):249–61.

Stagles MJ, Watson AA, Boyd JF, More IA, McSeveney D. The histopathology and electron microscopy of a human monkeypox lesion. Trans R Soc Trop Med Hyg. 1985;79(2):192–202. 1985 ed.

Symposium BMS. Tropical mycology. CABI; 2002.

Syrjala H, Karvonen J, Salminen A. Skin manifestations of tularemia: a study of 88 cases in northern Finland during 16 years (1967–1983). Acta Derm Venereol. 1984;64(6):513–6. 1984 ed.

Tan B, Weldon-Linne CM, Rhone DP, Penning CL, Visvesvara GS. Acanthamoeba infection presenting as skin lesions in patients with the acquired immunodeficiency syndrome. Arch Pathol Lab Med. 1993;117(10):1043–6. 1993rd ed.

Tatti KM, Greer P, White E, Shieh W-J, Guarner J, Ferebee-Harris T, et al. Morphologic, immunologic, and molecular methods to detect bacillus anthracis in formalin-fixed tissues. Appl Immunohistochem Mol Morphol. 2006;14(2):234–43.

Taylor HR, Keyvan-Larijani E, Newland HS, White AT, Greene BM. Sensitivity of skin snips in the diagnosis of onchocerciasis. Trop Med Parasitol. 1987; 38(2):145–7. 1987 ed.

Terry PM, Page ML, Goldmeier D. Are serological tests of value in diagnosing and monitoring response to treatment of syphilis in patients infected with human immunodeficiency virus? Genitourin Med. 1988;64(4):219–22.

Thomas EA, John M, Bhatia A. Cutaneous manifestations of dengue viral infection in Punjab (North India). Int J Dermatol. 2007;46(7):715–9. 2007 ed.

Tondury B, Kuhne A, Kutzner H, Palmedo G, Lautenschlager S, Borelli S. Molecular diagnostics of parapox virus infections. J Dtsch Dermatol Ges. 2010;8(9):681–4. 2010 ed.

Travis WD, Travis LB, Roberts GD, Su DW, Weiland LW. The histopathologic spectrum in mycobacterium marinum infection. Arch Pathol Lab Med. 1985;109(12):1109–13. 1985 ed.

Tutrone WD, Scheinfeld NS, Weinberg JM. Cutaneous anthrax: a concise review. Cutis. 2002;69(1):27–33. 2002nd ed.

Uthman MA, Mostafa WZ, Satti MB. Cutaneous schistosomal granuloma. Int J Dermatol. 1990;29(9):659–60.

Villaseñor-Park J, Clark E, Ho J, English JC. Folliculotropic non-alopecic secondary syphilis. J Am Acad Dermatol. 2011;65(3):686–7.

Visvesvara GS, Schuster FL, Martinez AJ. Balamuthia mandrillaris, N. G., N. Sp., agent of amebic meningoencephalitis in humans and other animals. J Eukaryot Microbiol. 1993;40(4):504–14.

Walker DH. Rocky Mountain spotted fever: a seasonal alert. Clin Infect Dis. 1995;20(5):1111–7. 1995 ed.

Walker DH, Herrero-Herrero JI, Ruiz-Beltran R, Bullon-Sopelana A, Ramos-Hidalgo A. The pathology of fatal Mediterranean spotted fever. Am J Clin Pathol. 1987;87(5):669–72. 1987 ed.

Weina PJ, Neafie RC, Wortmann G, Polhemus M, Aronson NE. Old world leishmaniasis: an emerging infection among deployed US military and civilian workers. Clin Infect Dis. 2004;39(11):1674–80. 2004 ed.

Whitehorn J, Farrar J. Dengue. Br Med Bull. 2010;95:161–73.

Wicher K, Wicher V, Abbruscato F, Baughn RE. Treponema pallidum subsp. pertenue displays pathogenic properties different from those of T. pallidum subsp. pallidum. Infect Immun. 2000;68(6):3219–25. 2000 ed.

Wood MG, Srolovitz H, Schetman D. Schistosomiasis. Paraplegia and ectopic skin lesions as admission symptoms. Arch Dermatol. 1976;112(5):690–5. 1976 ed.

Wortman PD. Acanthamoeba infection. Int J Dermatol. 1996;35(1):48–51. 1996 ed.

Wu SJ, Nguyen EQ, Nielsen TA, Pellegrini AE. Nodular tertiary syphilis mimicking granuloma annulare. J Am Acad Dermatol. 2000;42(2 Pt 2):378–80.

Zaki SR, Shieh WJ, Greer PW, Goldsmith CS, Ferebee T, Katshitshi J, et al. A novel immunohistochemical assay for the detection of Ebola virus in skin: implications for diagnosis, spread, and surveillance of Ebola hemorrhagic fever. Commission de Lutte contre les Epidémies à Kikwit. J Infect Dis. 1999;179 Suppl 1: S36–47.

Zalla MJ, Su WP, Fransway AF. Dermatologic manifestations of human immunodeficiency virus infection. Mayo Clin Proc. 1992;67(11):1089–108.

Cutaneous Lymphoid Infiltrates in Patients Receiving Biologic Modifiers

15

Jonathan J. Lee and Mai P. Hoang

Introduction

Over the past few decades, the introduction of new biologic agents, such as tumor necrosis factor-alpha inhibitors, has resulted in potent disease-modifying effects in a variety of immune-mediated diseases. There have also been major advancements in cancer chemotherapy with the recent addition of granulocyte colony-stimulating factor, interferon, kinase inhibitors, and CD20 and CD52 inhibitors for the treatment of hematologic malignancies as well as solid tumors. However, a variety of toxicities, including adverse cutaneous reactions, are seen in association with these agents. Awareness of these cutaneous toxicities and recognition of corresponding histologic features is of diagnostic and therapeutic importance.

TNF-α Inhibitors

Tumor necrosis factor-α (TNF-α) is a powerful proinflammatory cytokine that is a central player to the activation of inflammation (Parameswaran and Patial 2010). Lymphocytes, macrophages,

endothelial cells, Langerhans cells, as well as keratinocytes, melanocytes, and many others are capable of producing TNF-α (Deng et al. 2006). It is rapidly released in response to trauma, infection, or exposure to toxins wherein it functions as the "master regulator" of proinflammatory cytokine production (Parameswaran and Patial 2010). Despite its role in the normal host defense response, TNF-α is also central to the pathogenesis of several chronic inflammatory conditions and autoimmune disorders, including rheumatoid arthritis, psoriasis, inflammatory bowel disease, and ankylosing spondylitis (Kollias et al. 1999; Moustou et al. 2009).

Biologic antibody inhibitors of TNF-α, including infliximab (Remicade, Centocor, USA), etanercept (Enbrel, Immunex, USA), adalimumab (Humira), and certolizumab pegol (Cimzia), have been used with success in the treatment of these disorders. Nevertheless, their use has been associated with class-wide adverse reactions events, including opportunistic infections (Kim and Solomon 2010), reactivation of latent tuberculosis (Keane et al. 2001), lupus-like syndrome (Williams and Cohen 2011), demyelinating disease (Omair et al. 2012), exacerbation of heart failure (Colombel et al. 2004), and lymphoma (Adams et al. 2004). Cutaneous adverse events of antitumor necrosis factor therapy include infusion and injection site reactions, psoriasiform eruptions, granulomatous dermatitis, lupus-like disorders, vasculitis, cutaneous infections, and cutaneous neoplasms (Moustou et al. 2009; Bovenschen et al. 2006; Esser et al. 2004; Deng et al. 2006) (Table 15.1).

J.J. Lee, BA
Department of Pathology, Harvard Medical School, Boston, MA, USA

M.P. Hoang, MD (✉)
Department of Pathology, Harvard Medical School, Massachusetts General Hospital,
55 Fruit Street, Warren 820, Boston, MA 02114, USA
e-mail: mhoang@mgh.harvard.edu

H.D. Cualing et al. (eds.), *Cutaneous Hematopathology*,
DOI 10.1007/978-1-4939-0950-6_15, © Springer Science+Business Media New York 2014

Table 15.1 Cutaneous reactions associated with TNF-α (Moustou et al. 2009; Deng et al. 2006; Voulgari et al. 2008; Bovenschen et al. 2006; Esser et al. 2004)

Infusion and injection site reactions
Psoriasis and psoriasiform dermatitis
Eczematous dermatitis
Lupus erythematosus-like eruption
Leukocytoclastic vasculitis
Lichenoid dermatitis
Granuloma annulare/interstitial granulomatous dermatitis
Cutaneous infections
Cutaneous lymphomas
Multiple lentigines or eruptive melanocytic nevi
Multiple keratoacanthomas

Granuloma Annulare/Interstitial Granulomatous Dermatitis

TNF-α inhibitor-associated granulomatous reactions, including interstitial granulomatous dermatitis and granuloma annulare (GA), are rare cutaneous lymphoid reactions that have only recently been reported in the literature (Deng et al. 2006; Voulgari et al. 2008).

Clinical Presentation

Granulomatous adverse cutaneous reactions may occur anywhere from 1 month to over 1 year after initiating anti-TNF-α therapy and may occur after treatment with any of the aforementioned agents (Deng et al. 2006; Voulgari et al. 2008). Cases of interstitial granulomatous dermatitis presented with rapid-onset, asymptomatic to mildly pruritic, 1–4 cm macules or indurated papules or plaques, many of which are annular in morphology, that occur on the trunk, shoulders, and upper extremities (Deng et al. 2006). In the first reported series, this reaction led to the discontinuation of treatment in four of five patients (Deng et al. 2006). Of these four patients, the eruption cleared or improved within 2 months of discontinuation (Deng et al. 2006). One patient had to be maintained on therapy due to the severity of underlying rheumatoid arthritis, and the lesions persisted at 3-month follow-up (Deng et al. 2006).

TNF-α inhibitor-induced GA presented with erythematous skin eruptions covering the fingers, hands, and forearms (Voulgari et al. 2008). In the largest report in the literature, nine such cases were reported among 197 patients (incidence, 4.5 %) undergoing anti-TNF therapy for the treatment of rheumatoid arthritis (Voulgari et al. 2008). Biologic therapy was maintained on seven of nine of these cases (Voulgari et al. 2008). Lesions were treated with topical corticosteroids with resolution of eruption after 3–4 weeks (Voulgari et al. 2008).

Histology Features

Histopathologic examination of TNF-α inhibitor-associated GA is characterized by palisading granulomas surrounding an area of necrobiosis and mucin deposition (Voulgari et al. 2008; Stewart et al. 2011) (Fig. 15.1). The histology of interstitial granulomatous dermatitis is characterized by a diffuse interstitial infiltrate of histiocytes and lymphocytes that palisade around partially degenerated or "piecemeal"-fragmented collagen, resulting in granulomatous foci in the mid and deep dermis (Deng et al. 2006). Eosinophils, neutrophils, and multinucleated giant cells may be present in scant numbers (Deng et al. 2006).

Pathogenesis

The precise pathomechanism underlying TNF-α inhibitor-induced GA is not known, but evidence suggests that anti-TNF therapy may induce autoreactive T cells (Sfikakis and Kollias 2003). Paradoxically, infliximab has been reported to have led to the rapid improvement of disseminated GA (Hertl et al. 2005). Chu et al. (1994) postulated that the granulomatous infiltrate in interstitial granulomatous dermatitis is a secondary reaction to dermal collagen damage induced initially by the deposition of immune complexes in dermal vessels and subsequent ischemia, followed by complement and neutrophil activation. It is known that interstitial granulomatous dermatitis can present in association with rheumatoid arthritis, lupus erythematosus, and other systemic disorders (Long et al. 1996) and may also be induced by other medications, including calcium channel blockers, lipid-lowering agents, and others (Magro et al. 1998).

Fig. 15.1 A 50-year-old female on Humira for Crohn's disease presented with a pruritic and indurated plaques and papules on her left leg. A skin biopsy shows an interstitial and perivascular infiltrate of histiocytes and lymphocytes consistent with an interstitial granulomatous dermatitis

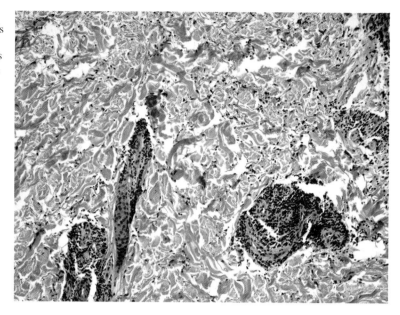

Enbrel (Etanercept): Urticaria and Cellulitis

Urticaria and cellulitis are the most commonly reported cutaneous toxicity associated with Enbrel/etanercept, although it is not frequently biopsied.

Clinical Presentation

Etanercept-induced urticaria or urticaria-like reactions typically present 3–4 months after receiving twice-weekly subcutaneous etanercept injections (Skytta et al. 2000; Borrás-Blasco et al. 2009). After the inciting injection, an erythematous, macular, papular, or plaque-like urticarial lesion with or without central clearing develops initially on the extensor surfaces of the elbows and, subsequently, on the extensor surfaces of the knees (Borrás-Blasco et al. 2009). Lesions may also appear elsewhere on the body, such as the buttocks, trunk, proximal limbs, or ears (Skytta et al. 2000; Borrás-Blasco et al. 2009). Laboratory abnormalities, including eosinophilia, are typically absent (Skytta et al. 2000). These lesions have been reported to resolve after cessation of etanercept treatment (Skytta et al. 2000) or a course of steroid (Borrás-Blasco et al. 2009).

Reactions at the injection site can be urticarial reactions (Batycka-Baran et al. 2012) or eosinophilic cellulitis-like reaction (Winfield et al. 2006). Typically within 24 h of receiving the first dose, the patient developed evanescent, pruritic, slightly indurated, and erythematous plaques surrounding the injection site. These lesions resolved upon treatment with antihistamines and prednisone (Winfield et al. 2006) or topical steroids (Batycka-Baran et al. 2012).

Histologic Features

Histopathologic examination of the etanercept injection site urticarial lesions reveals a perivascular inflammatory infiltrate composed predominantly of neutrophils without eosinophils (Batycka-Baran et al. 2012). Immunophenotypic study may reveal either CD8+ (Zeltser et al. 2001) or CD4+ (González-López et al. 2007) predominance of T lymphocytes within the dermal infiltrate. Histology of the eosinophilic cellulitis-like injection site reaction to etanercept demonstrates an unremarkable epidermis and underling perivascular and interstitial lymphocytic infiltrates with numerous eosinophils with associated edema in the dermis (Winfield et al. 2006) (Fig. 15.2). Other notable features are multiple foci of hypereosinophilic collagen surrounded by eosinophils in the dermis as well as flame figures (Winfield et al. 2006).

Fig. 15.2 A 47-year-old male with a history of psoriasis and on Enbrel treatment developed a lesion at the injection site on his right upper arm. A skin biopsy revealed an interstitial and perivascular infiltrate (**a**) of lymphocytes, histiocytes, and many eosinophils (**b**) in the dermis consistent with a hypersensitivity reaction

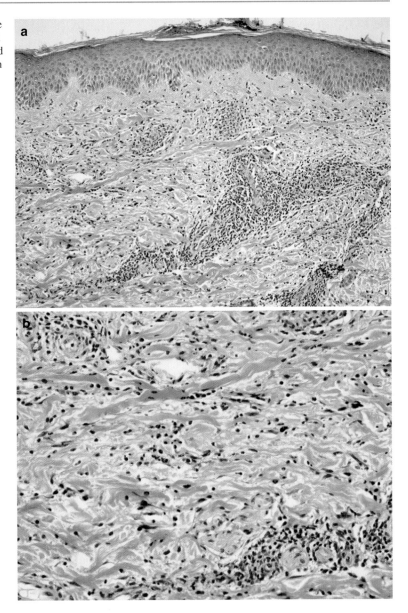

Pathogenesis

Batycka-Baran et al. (2012) proposed that the kinetics of the reaction, as revealed by the time course between the injection and onset of cutaneous eruption, may provide insight into the mechanism. It is thought that injection site reactions occurring rapidly after the first injection are due to an irritative mechanism and may not require discontinuation of treatment (Batycka-Baran et al. 2012). Urticarial lesions that occur within hours of the second or later injection with etanercept may reflect an immediate type I, IgE-mediated hypersensitivity reaction that would require stopping the medication and close monitoring for possible anaphylaxis (Batycka-Baran et al. 2012). Finally, reactions that occur hours after the injection and persist for several days may reflect an Arthus-like type III hypersensitivity reaction, mediated in part by the recruitment of neutrophilic granulocytes (Batycka-Baran et al. 2012).

G-CSF: Neutrophilic Dermatoses

Granulocyte colony-stimulating factor (G-CSF) is a neutrophil-specific growth factor that promotes the survival, proliferation, and maturation of neutrophil progenitors (Kaushansky 2006). This cytokine also enhances their phagocytic capacity, superoxide anion production, and bacterial killing mechanisms (Spiekermann et al. 1997). In contrast, granulocyte-macrophage colony-stimulating factor (GM-CSF) stimulates the production and activation of eosinophils, basophils, monocytes, and dendritic cells in addition to neutrophils.

G-CSF is used clinically to treat neutropenia associated with chemotherapy, myelodysplasia, or aplastic anemia as well as to reduce infections in patients with congenital, idiopathic, or cyclic neutropenia (Prendiville et al. 2001). Mild adverse effects include transient bone pain, edema, arthralgias, and myalgias as well as elevations in serum lactate dehydrogenase (LDH), alanine aminotransferase (ALT), aspartate aminotransferase (AST), and alkaline phosphatase (AP) levels (Paydas et al. 1993). It has also been found to increase the risk of treatment-related acute myelogenous leukemia, particularly in those with congenital neutropenia, wherein approximately 10 % will develop a malignant myeloid disorder (Kaushansky 2006; Dong et al. 1995).

Adverse cutaneous effects of G-CSF (Table 15.2) include diffuse eruption or reaction at injection site (Alvarez-Ruiz et al. 2004; Valks et al. 1998). Skin biopsies show an increase in the number of dermal macrophages, often enlarged

Table 15.2 Cutaneous reactions associated with G-CSF (Alvarez-Ruiz et al. 2004; Valks et al. 1998; Prendiville et al. 2001; Johnson and Grimwood 1994; Ross et al. 1991; Paydas et al. 1993; Fukutoku et al. 1994; Jain 1994; Ostlere et al. 1992)

Generalized or diffuse eruption
Local cutaneous reaction
Neutrophilic dermatoses
Sweet syndrome
Pyoderma gangrenosum
Vasculitis
Folliculitis

in size (Alvarez-Ruiz et al. 2004; Valks et al. 1998). Neutrophilic dermatoses (Prendiville et al. 2001; Johnson and Grimwood 1994), including pyoderma gangrenosum (Ross et al. 1991) and Sweet syndrome (Paydas et al. 1993; Fukutoku et al. 1994), rare cases of vasculitis (Jain 1994; Couderc et al. 1995), and folliculitis (Ostlere et al. 1992) have been reported in association with G-CSF.

Sweet Syndrome Associated with G-CSF

Sweet syndrome, first documented by RD Sweet in (1964), is characterized by a pentad of findings, including fever, neutrophilia, multiple erythematous and painful cutaneous papules or nodules, dense dermal infiltrate of neutrophils, and rapid response to steroid therapy (Paydas et al. 1993). Cases of Sweet syndrome are categorized based on etiology into classical/idiopathic, malignancy-associated, and drug-induced (Cohen 2007). Classical Sweet syndrome is associated with upper respiratory tract and gastrointestinal infections, inflammatory bowel disease, and pregnancy (Cohen 2007). Malignancy-associated Sweet syndrome is most commonly caused by hematologic malignancies (especially acute myelogenous leukemia), but solid tumors of the genitourinary and gastrointestinal tracts and breast have also been associated. A wide variety of medications have been associated with drug-induced Sweet syndrome, including antibiotics such as trimethoprim-sulfamethoxazole, all-trans retinoic acid, and antineoplastic agents such as Imatinib (Cohen 2007). However, G-CSF is the most frequently and widely implicated medications in causing Sweet syndrome (White et al. 2006).

Walker and Cohen (1996) put forth the following diagnostic criteria for drug-induced Sweet syndrome: (1) abrupt onset of painful erythematous plaques or nodules, (2) histopathologic evidence of a dense neutrophilic infiltrate without evidence of leukocytoclastic vasculitis, (3) fever >38 °C, (4) temporal relationship between drug ingestion and clinical presentation or temporally related recurrence after reintroduction of drug, and (5) temporally related resolution of lesions after drug withdrawal or treatment with systemic corticosteroids. Drug-induced Sweet syndrome typically affects patients between 29 and 68 years of age (mean, 45 years) and presents anywhere from days to weeks (mean, 7.5 days) after initiation of drug therapy. It is characterized by the development of fever, arthralgias, and diffuse, erythematous, painful papules, plaques, or nodules found most commonly in the upper extremities (71 %) but may also affect the chest (50 %), head and neck (43 %), lower extremities (36 %), or oral mucous membranes (7 %) (Walker and Cohen 1996). Lesions on the face may follow a periorbital or periauricular distribution (Bidyasar et al. 2008). Cutaneous lesions in a photodistributed pattern (Walker and Cohen 1996) as well as lesions that develop clinical features of necrosis (Fukutoku et al. 1994) have also been described. Ocular manifestations, characterized by "bilateral conjunctivitis" or "conjunctival lesions," have also been documented in case reports (Bidyasar et al. 2008; Paydas et al. 1993).

Histopathologic examination of these cutaneous lesions reveals superficial edema and an underlying dense infiltrate of neutrophils in the dermis (Walker and Cohen 1996) (Fig. 15.3).

Nuclear features of apoptosis such as karyorrhexis and an absence of vasculitis and pathogenic microbes are typical features (Bidyasar et al. 2008; Walker and Cohen 1996). The histologic differential diagnosis for drug-induced Sweet syndrome includes Sweet syndrome proper, abscess/cellulitis, granuloma faciale, leukemia cutis, lobular neutrophilic panniculitis, rheumatoid neutrophilic dermatitis, and pyoderma gangrenosum (Cohen et al. 2007).

Laboratory abnormalities include neutrophilia, although this is much less common with drug-induced Sweet syndrome, especially that associated with G-CSF, than it is with Sweet syndrome proper (Walker and Cohen 1996). The cutaneous lesions in G-CSF associated Sweet syndrome may appear with the rise or normalization of neutrophil counts (Walker and Cohen 1996) and may disappear when they fall (van Kamp et al. 1994). Elevations in the erythrocyte sedimentation rate, anemia, and thrombocytosis have also been documented (Walker and Cohen 1996).

The mainstay of treatment for all forms of drug-induced Sweet syndrome is removal of the offending agent, after which the lesions typically resolve within 1–2 weeks (Walker and Cohen 1996). Clinical improvements in both cutaneous

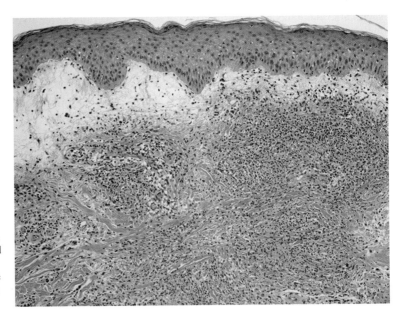

Fig. 15.3 A 51-year-old female on granulocyte colony-stimulating factor presented with erythematous plaques on her left upper arm. A skin biopsy showed marked papillary dermal edema and underlying band-like infiltrate of neutrophils consistent with Sweet syndrome

lesions and the overall condition have been achieved with low-dose systemic steroids alone (Bidyasar et al. 2008) as well as in combination with colchicine (van Kamp et al. 1994). Remission of the myeloid disorder, such as acute myeloid leukemia or myelodysplastic syndrome, also results in resolution of Sweet syndrome.

The precise etiology and pathogenic mechanism underlying all forms of Sweet syndrome is currently unknown. Elevated levels of G-CSF and interleukin-6 have been documented in a G-CSF-naïve patient with myelodysplastic syndrome-associated Sweet syndrome (Reuss-Borst et al. 1993). G-CSF, a cytokine, likely plays a direct pathogenic role, given that serum levels appear to directly correlate with dermatosis activity (Kawakami et al. 2004).

Pyoderma Gangrenosum Associated with G-CSF

The first case of biopsy-proven neutrophilic dermatosis without vasculitis was reported by Ross et al. (1991) in a 50-year-old woman who underwent G-CSF therapy for neutropenia related to chemotherapy for metastatic small cell lung cancer. Since this initial report, few additional cases of pyoderma gangrenosum associated with G-CSF and pegylated G-CSF therapy have been reported in the literature (Lewerin et al. 1997; Miall et al. 2006). G-CSF-associated pyoderma gangrenosum typically presents days to weeks after starting G-CSF therapy (Lewerin et al. 1997). It is characterized by the simultaneous onset of fever and erythematous plaques that can appear anywhere on the body, such as the face, trunk, upper, and lower extremities (Miall et al. 2006). The lesions rapidly progresses in size, swiftly develop blue or black edematous central regions of necrosis, and may appear clinically as a hemorrhagic blister, earning the name "bullous pyoderma gangrenosum" (Lewerin et al. 1997). There does not appear to be a correlation between the dosage or duration of therapy and the severity of this adverse cutaneous reaction (Ross et al. 1991).

Histopathologic examination reveals typical features of pyoderma gangrenosum characterized by a dense neutrophilic dermal infiltrate (Lewerin et al. 1997). Features of vasculitis are typically absent but have been described in association with this lesion (Miall et al. 2005; Lewerin et al. 1997). Studies for acid-fast bacilli, bacteria, and fungi are typically negative (Ross et al. 1991).

It appears that this adverse cutaneous reaction may not resolve with simple withdrawal of G-CSF (Lewerin et al. 1997). Treatment success has been reported with cyclosporin A (Lewerin et al. 1997). Others have had success with high-dose steroids in combination with dapsone (an anti-neutrophil agent) and topical tacrolimus (Miall et al. 2005). Interestingly, there was also a recent report of a case of Crohn's-associated pyoderma gangrenosum that was successfully treated with perilesional granulocyte-macrophage colony-stimulating factor (GM-CSF) (Shpiro et al. 1998).

Classic pyoderma gangrenosum is most commonly associated with inflammatory bowel disease, rheumatologic disorders, or malignancy. The pathogenesis of this condition is poorly understood but thought to be related to loss of altered neutrophil trafficking and chemotaxis, genetic variations, and dysregulation of the innate immune system (Ahronowitz et al. 2012).

Interferon: Lymphocutaneous Injection Site Reactions

Interferon is a complex family of host-derived glycoproteins produced and secreted by eukaryotic cells in response to viruses, antigens, and mitogens (Baron et al. 1991). During their study of cellular viral infections, Isaacs and Lindemann (1957) identified a protein produced by cells infected by the virus that interfered with the virus' ability to infect other cells. It is now known that interferons, of which there are three main groups (IFN-α, IFN-β, IFN-γ), have intrinsic antiviral, antimicrobial, immunomodulatory, and antiproliferative properties (Baron et al. 1991). Thus, today they are used to treat a variety of malignancies, viral infections, and inflammatory conditions, including hairy cell leukemia (IFN-α2b), chronic hepatitis C infection (IFN-α2b),

Table 15.3 Cutaneous reactions associated with interferon

Injection site reaction
Local necrotizing
Granulomatous and suppurative
Lupus erythematosus-like
Embolia cutis medicamentosa
Local alopecia
Eczematous drug eruption
Sarcoidosis
Leukocytoclastic vasculitis
Alopecia
Vitiligo
Fixed drug eruption
Lupus erythematosus

multiple sclerosis (IFN-β1a), and chronic granulomatous disease (IFN-γ1b).

Despite their therapeutic yield, the doses required are frequently associated with significant side effects, including flu-like symptoms, weight loss, depression, as well as neurologic toxicity (Krainick et al. 1998). Moreover, interferon is believed to precipitate autoimmune disorders such as type I diabetes, thyroid disease, and systemic lupus erythematosus and may also worsen certain granulomatous diseases (Selmi et al. 2006).

Psoriasis was one of the early cutaneous reactions (Table 15.3) developed in association with interferon treatment (Quesada and Gutterman 1986), and there have been multiple subsequent reports in the literature (Ketikoglou et al. 2005). Eczematous drug eruptions associated with interferon, which often present as ill-defined clusters of coalescing, erythematous, blanchable, pruritic papules often on the extremities and trunk, have also been described (Dereure et al. 2002; Moore et al. 2004). Sarcoidosis has been described in patients receiving interferon treatment for hepatitis C as well as in a patient receiving adjuvant interferon-alpha immunotherapy for melanoma (Fantini et al. 2009; Alonso-Perez et al. 2006).

Alopecia has been reported in up to 19 % of patients treated with combination interferon and ribavirin, including alopecia areata (Agesta et al. 2002) and alopecia universalis (Demirturk et al. 2006). Vitiligo has been reported in a number of patients who were treated for hepatitis C with interferon (Tomasiewicz et al. 2006). Cases of cutaneous necrosis (Dalmau et al. 2005), fixed drug eruption (Tai and Tam 2005), lichenoid eruption (Pinto et al. 2003), lupus erythematosus (Fukuyama et al. 2000), indurated erythema (Detmar et al. 1989), leukocytoclastic vasculitis (Christian et al. 1997), as well as pyoderma gangrenosum (Montoto et al. 1998) have been reported in association with interferon.

Delivered through the intramuscular or subcutaneous route, interferon has also been associated with local injection site reactions in just under 5 % of patients, including local necrotizing (Krainick et al. 1998), granulomatous and suppurative (Sanders et al. 2002), lupus erythematosus-like (Arrue et al. 2007), embolia cutis medicamentosa (Koontz and Alshekhlee 2007), and local alopecia (Lang et al. 1999) lesions. The pathogenesis of these reactions remains uncertain. Multiple mechanisms have been proposed, and these, in addition to the basic clinical presentation and histopathology, are summarized by each pattern of reaction below. Whether there is a common underlying mode of pathogenesis underlying these reactions is yet to be determined, but interferon's role in modulating multiple inflammatory pathways is likely central to the explanation.

Local Cutaneous Necrotizing Lesions

Krainick et al. (1998) described seven cases of local, painful cutaneous necrotizing lesions that arose in patients undergoing intramuscular or subcutaneous interferon therapy for Philadelphia chromosome-positive chronic myelogenous leukemia (CML). They occurred without correlation to specific stage of disease, course of illness, or interferon type. The lesions arose anywhere from 3 to 108 months after initiating interferon therapy. The lesions were described as necrotizing ulcers or abscess with surrounding erythematous, painful induration. Low-grade fever was commonly present. Microbiologic culture of the lesion was most commonly sterile and ultrasound findings were consistent with cellulitis.

Histopathologic examination revealed ulceration with underlying inflamed granulation tissue with scattered eosinophils in the dermis. One case was managed with reconstructive surgery, another with local surgical debridement and topical antibiotics, while the others generally resolved with more conservative measures even while maintained on therapy. The pathogenesis of these ulcers remains uncertain, but it is believed that local interferon-mediated keratinocyte toxicity, immune complex formation, and/or ischemia through multiple mechanisms, including interferon-mediated inhibition of angiogenesis, endothelial cell disruption, vasospasm, and intravascular thrombosis are involved (Sanders et al. 2002).

Granulomatous and Suppurative Dermatitis

Sanders et al. (2002) describe two cases wherein dusky, violaceous, multilobulated papules or indurated plaques and nodules with central ulceration developed at interferon injection sites in one patient undergoing treatment for non-remitting metastatic renal cell carcinoma (RCC) and another for metastatic melanoma. Histopathologic examination revealed suppurative and granulomatous dermatitis involving the superficial and deep dermis. The inflammatory cells were composed of neutrophils and histiocytes. Noninflammatory intravascular thrombosis was noted in the second case. Special stains for acid-fast bacilli, fungi, and bacteria were negative. Culture of lesions in one case was sterile and cultures from the second case contained surface colonization of bacteria that were not known to cause granulomas. Both patients' injection site reactions resolved with conservative management, and one was maintained on therapy.

The authors proposed that a pathogenic mechanism involving tissue ischemia and intravascular thrombi may play a role in interferon-induced granulomatous and suppurative dermatitis, citing morphologic and biochemical similarities with pyoderma gangrenosum and cutaneous Crohn's disease (Sanders et al. 2002).

Lupus Erythematosus-Like Reaction at Injection Site

Arrue et al. (2007) described five cases of cutaneous lesions at the interferon inoculation site with a lupus erythematosus-like histopathologic pattern. Three patients underwent treatment for metastatic melanoma and two patients for multiple sclerosis. The lesions generally occurred anywhere from days to years after inoculation with interferon and were described as painful erythematous nodules or exudative, infiltrated plaques that resolved spontaneously or with minimal treatment within 2–3 weeks. These patients had no history of prior lupus erythematosus, and serum studies conducted after the development of the lesions generally revealed negative antinuclear and deoxyribonucleic acid (DNA) antibodies and normal complement levels.

Histopathologic examination of biopsy specimens revealed prominent dermal mucin deposition highlighted by colloidal iron stain, perivascular and periadnexal infiltrate, and interface changes at the dermal follicular epithelium junction, while the epidermis exhibited only mild acanthosis and parakeratosis. In three of the cases, there was complete destruction of the folliculosebaceous unit, which was replaced by an inflammatory reaction or mucin pools.

While the pathogenesis of this adverse cutaneous reaction is uncertain, the authors of the case report postulate that abnormalities in platelet activation as well as the ability of interferon to transform fibroblast growth factor-β1, a cytokine that stimulates fibroblasts and, thus, increases the dermal mucin production, may play a role (Arrue et al. 2007).

Embolia Cutis Medicamentosa

Koontz and Alshekhlee (2007) reported a case of a 55-year-old man undergoing treatment with subcutaneous IFN-β1a who subsequently developed multiple painful necrotic skin lesions at the injection sites in various stages of healing. The diagnosis of embolia cutis medicamentosa was made based on the histologic findings of a thrombotic vasculopathy characterized by thrombotic occlusion of numerous capillaries. The authors hypothesized that patient self-administration of the medication resulted in inadvertent, deeper administration of the medication, leading to accidental arterial or periarterial injection of the agent. Their hypothesis is supported by the observation that after the patient was switched to an auto-injector, which controlled needle depth, no new lesions developed (Koontz and Alsshekhlee 2007).

Embolia cutis medicamentosa (Nicolau syndrome) was first described by Nicolau and Freudenthal in 1924 when they observed this phenomenon after an injection of bismuth salts in patients being treated for syphilis (Koontz and Alsshekhlee 2007). This adverse cutaneous effect is thought to be due to ischemic necrosis secondary to occlusion of the microvasculature (Luton et al. 2006). Proposed pathogenic mechanisms include intra-arterial, periarterial, or perivenous phenomenon wherein embolic or crystal occlusion by the injected agent, pain and sympathetically mediated vasospasm, or vascular trauma-induced thrombosis disrupts the microcirculation (Luton et al. 2006).

Alopecia

Lang et al. (1999) described three cases of transient, localized hair loss at IFN-α2b injection sites in patients undergoing treatment for chronic hepatitis C infection. The lesions were described as patches of non-scarring alopecia with or without perifollicular erythema or papules. Histopathologic examination revealed a non-scarring alopecia with perifollicular and perivascular lymphohistiocytic infiltrate at the infundibulum and isthmus. It is believed that multiple mechanisms may be at play in this reaction, including the formation of autoantibodies directed against follicular epithelium through interferon-mediated induction of previously masked surface antigens, and direct replicative inhibition of germinative hair cells (Lang et al. 1999).

Kinase Inhibitor (Sorafenib, Sunitinib): Hand-Foot Skin Reaction

Sorafenib and sunitinib are two novel, rationally designed, orally available, multikinase inhibitors (MKIs) used in the treatment of various malignancies for their anti-angiogenic and antiproliferative properties. Initially identified as a Raf-kinase inhibitor, sorafenib has also been shown to inhibit vascular endothelial growth factor receptor (VEGFR) 2–3, platelet-derived growth factor receptor (PDGFR)-β, Fms-like tyrosine kinase 3 (Flt-3), RET, c-KIT, p38α (member of the MAP-kinase family), and B-Raf (Wilhelm and Chien 2002). Sunitinib targets VEGFR 1–3, PDGFR-α, c-Kit, Flt-3, colony-stimulating factor receptor-1, and the glial cell line-derived neurotrophic factor receptor (Chow and Eckhardt 2007). Sorafenib is currently approved for the treatment of metastatic renal cell carcinoma (RCC) (Singer et al. 2012) but has also been shown to be effective in treating hepatocellular carcinoma (HCC) (Kokudo et al. 2012). Sunitinib has been approved for the treatment of gastrointestinal stromal tumor (GIST) as well as advanced RCC but has also been shown to be affective against neuroendocrine, colon, and breast cancers in phase II studies (Chow and Eckhardt 2007).

Significant cutaneous adverse events are present in up to 80 % of patients undergoing treatment with kinase inhibitors, of which the hand-foot skin reaction (HFSR) may be the most significant cutaneous toxicity. In a retrospective review of 109 patients on sorafenib for RCC or HCC and 119 patients receiving sunitinib for RCC or GIST, Lee et al. (2009) identified that HFSR was the most commonly observed cutaneous toxicity, seen in 48 % of patients on sorafenib and 36 % of patients on sunitinib. Moreover, HFSR is regarded as the most clinically significant dermatologic toxicity of sorafenib and sunitinib therapy, given the severity of symptoms and the potential for consequent chemotherapeutic dose modification (Chu et al. 2008; Lacouture et al. 2008).

Besides HFSR, a variety of other cutaneous reactions and neoplasms has been reported in

Table 15.4 Cutaneous reactions associated with multikinase inhibitors (sorafenib, sunitinib) (Robert et al. 2005, 2011; Smith et al. 2009; Raymond et al. 2010; Bovenschen et al. 2006; Kong et al. 2008; Rosenbaum et al. 2008; Chu et al. 2008; Lacouture et al. 2008)

Hand-foot skin reaction (47–83 %)
Nonspecific rash (19–40 %)
Hair and nail changes (27 %)
Mucositis (20 %)
Xerosis (16 %)
Xerostomia (11 %)
Multiple keratoacanthoma-type squamous cell carcinoma
Eruptive melanocytic nevi

association with sorafenib and sunitinib (Table 15.4) (Robert et al. 2005, 2011; Smith et al. 2009; Raymond et al. 2010; Bovenschen et al. 2006; Kong et al. 2008; Rosenbaum et al. 2008; Chu et al. 2008; Lacouture et al. 2008). Smith et al. (2009) reported 15 patients who developed keratoacanthoma-type squamous cell carcinomas associated with sorafenib treatment. Regional squamous cell carcinoma has also been recently reported to develop following limb infusion of sorafenib (Raymond et al. 2010). Rapid development of pigmented lesions has been reported in association with blistering disorders, immunodeficiency, and chemotherapeutic agents (Bovenschen et al. 2006). Kong et al. (2008) reported eruptive melanocytic nevi in two patients receiving sorafenib for treatment of metastatic RCC. Other skin changes associated with kinase inhibitors include nonspecific rash, skin discoloration, xerosis, hair color changes, alopecia, and nail changes (Rosenbaum et al. 2008).

Clinical Presentation

The hand-foot skin reaction (HFSR) is a distinct set of palmoplantar lesions in areas of frequent trauma or friction. They can develop anytime from 3 to 56 days (median, 18.4 days) after or within 4 weeks (83 %) of initiating therapy with sorafenib or sunitinib (Lee et al. 2009). These lesions are characterized by multiple, scaly, keratotic plaques on the knuckles of the dorsal hand, hyperkeratotic callus-like lesions on pressure areas of the sole, and/or yellow-colored blisters surrounded by an erythematous halo on fingers and palm (Lee et al. 2009). They are commonly associated with significant tenderness and paresthesias and result in significant alterations in quality of life (Lacouture et al. 2008).

Histologic Features

Skin biopsies from seven patients with HFSR associated with sorafenib or sunitinib showed band-like foci of necrotic keratinocytes in all seven, with two resulting in blister formation (Lacouture et al. 2008). All specimens showed superficial telangiectasia, sparse perivascular lymphocytic infiltrates, and subtle dilatation and cystic degeneration of eccrine glands (Lacouture et al. 2008). Dermal eosinophils are not prominent. The extent of this epidermal change appears to correlate with the duration of therapy with the multikinase inhibitor; less than 30 days of exposure was associated with only intraepidermal changes, while longer exposure times led to changes in the outermost stratum corneum, evident as hyperkeratosis and parakeratosis (Lacouture et al. 2008). In a case series by Lee et al. (2009), similar changes were noted in the skin biopsies from six patients. The general histopathologic pattern is an interface dermatitis with some degree of epidermal necrosis or vesiculation, as noted in some cases (Fig. 15.4) (Lacouture et al. 2008; Lee et al. 2009).

Differential Diagnosis/Pathogenesis

The differential diagnosis for hand-foot skin reaction (HFSR) includes hand-foot syndrome (HFS), palmoplantar keratoderma, radiation recall dermatitis, localized epidermal necrolysis, generalized epidermal necrolysis, and acute graft-versus-host disease (Lacouture et al. 2008; Nagore et al. 2000).

Fig. 15.4 A 51-year-old woman with hepatitis C and hepatocellular carcinoma on sorafenib treatment presented with bilateral vesicles and bullae on her feet. These blisters resolved after cessation of sorafenib treatment. A skin biopsy from her left dorsal foot showed focal epidermal necrosis and necrotic keratinocyte within the epidermis. There is papillary dermal edema and a perivascular lymphocytic infiltrate in the dermis

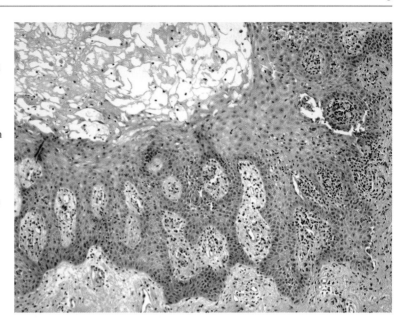

The pathogenesis of this adverse cutaneous reaction is uncertain. The most widely accepted theory is direct toxicity of chemotherapeutic agents against acral epithelium, which may occur through inhibition of the keratinocyte c-Kit receptor (Chu et al. 2008). Other direct cytotoxic agents have been hypothesized to inflict direct keratinocyte toxicity through eccrine sweat gland excretion (Jacobi et al. 2005). Chu et al. (2008) has suggested that direct effect of sorafenib on eccrine gland receptors may also play a pathogenic role. The histologic findings of apoptotic keratinocytes with satellitosis of lymphocytes led Beard et al. (1993) to propose the host-versus-altered-host response. Despite these suggestions, sorafenib and sunitinib's inhibitory effect on vascular endothelial growth factor (VEGF) and platelet-derived growth factor at the capillary and vascular endothelial level is likely central to the explanation, given that this reaction occurs in areas exposed to repeated trauma such as the palms and soles (Lacouture et al. 2008). Alas, direct VEGF inhibitor (bevacizumab) use does appear to associate with more severe sorafenib-associated HFSR (Azad et al. 2009). However, given that HFSR incidence is rare with isolated bevacizumab use (Chu et al. 2008), sorafenib and sunitinib's inhibitory effect on multiple kinase pathways suggests that there are multiple conspiring mechanisms underlying this reaction.

Treatment

There have been no randomized trials comparing the efficacy of various agents in the treatment of hand-foot skin reaction (HFSR) to multikinase inhibitors. The literature to date supports the use of supportive podiatric measures, including a variety of moisturizers, cotton socks, shock absorbers, and soft shoes that minimize pressure points (Chu et al. 2008). Lacouture et al. (2008) obtained significant clinical improvement in treating sorafenib- and sunitinib-induced HFSR with topical urea (keratolytic that supports skin integrity) alongside tazarotene (reduces epidermal proliferation and dermal inflammation) and/or topical fluorouracil.

CD20 Inhibitors: Urticaria and Infusion Reactions

In 1997, rituximab (Rituxan, IDEC-C2B8) became the first monoclonal antibody product approved in the United States for the treatment of a malignancy (Dillman 1999). Rituximab is a chimeric monoclonal antibody composed of human immunoglobulin G1 heavy-chain sequences and murine immunoglobulin variable regions that targets the human CD20 antigen (Maloney 2012). CD20 is a multimeric, cell-surface complex antigen that is specific to B cells (Maloney 2012). Physiologically, CD20 regulates transcellular calcium transport and is involved in the regulation of B-cell activation and proliferation (Maloney 2012). Anti-CD20 antibodies such as rituximab are thought to contribute to B-cell-specific destruction through a combination of synergistic mechanisms including complement-dependent cytotoxicity, antibody-dependent cell-mediated cytotoxicity, direct antiproliferative effect, and the induction of apoptosis (Maloney 2012).

Originally approved by the Food and Drug Administration for the treatment of follicular B-cell lymphoma, rituximab is one of the most widely used anticancer drugs in the United States. It is currently used to treat an array of malignancies and several inflammatory conditions, including chronic lymphocytic leukemia (Bauer et al. 2012), B-cell lymphomas (Maloney 2012), as well as rheumatoid arthritis (Moots and Naisbett-Groet 2012), systemic lupus erythematosus (Coca and Sanz 2012), and refractory nephrotic syndrome (van Husen and Kemper 2011). Additional anti-CD20 antibodies, including ofatumumab (human antibody), tositumomab (murine antibody), and obinutuzumab (human antibody), have been developed, but their use has been less well documented (Maloney 2012).

Rituximab is typically administered by intravenous infusion (Maloney 2012). Infusion-related reactions occur at an incidence rate of up to 14 %, as documented in clinical trials (Maloney 2012). To date, there have been three case reports of rituximab infusion-related urticarial reactions in patients undergoing treatment for follicular B-cell lymphoma, despite premedication with diphenhydramine, acetaminophen, and steroids (Heinzerling et al. 2000; Errante et al. 2006; Rey et al. 2009). This cutaneous reaction typically occurs 1 h after the first infusion and is characterized by a pruritic, erythematous to violaceous, well-demarcated, irregularly shaped plaques that develop at the site of existing or previously excised tumors (Errante et al. 2006). The lesions spontaneously regress one to two hours after stopping the infusion (Rey et al. 2009; Errante et al. 2006). Formal histopathologic descriptions of these lesions have yet to be described in the

literature, as biopsies of this rapidly resolving reaction may not be readily taken.

Infusion-related localized urticaria is thought to be an epiphenomenon of malignant B-cell destruction as opposed to a true hypersensitivity reaction (Errante et al. 2006). Because it occurs within an hour after the very first infusion further supports this hypothesis (Rey et al. 2009). Van der Kolk et al. (2001) have previously demonstrated that complement activation and subsequent release of tumor necrosis factor-α, interleukin (IL)-6, and IL-8 correlate with the severity of rituximab-related side effects. As such, cytokine release may be involved in the pathomechanism of infusion-related urticaria (Errante et al. 2006). Interestingly, all three reported cases of rituximab infusion-induced urticaria have been in patients undergoing treatment for follicular B-cell lymphoma, which is known to be sensitive to rituximab (Rey et al. 2009).

Other infusion-related adverse effects include fever, chills, nausea, and headache (Maloney 2012; Errante et al. 2006). More serious adverse reactions, including cytokine-release syndrome associated with lymphopenia, thrombocytopenia, and hepatotoxicity (Winkler et al. 1999), potentially life-threatening noninfectious pulmonary toxicity (Hadjinicolaou et al. 2012), and cardiac arrhythmias and acute coronary syndromes (Lee and Kukreti 2012), have been described in the literature. A single case report of Stevens-Johnson syndrome associated with rituximab therapy has been described (Lowndes et al. 2002). Otherwise, cutaneous adverse reactions are characterized predominantly by lesion-localized urticaria.

Alemtuzumab (Campath-1H): Richter's Syndrome

Alemtuzumab (Campath-1H) is a humanized, monoclonal antibody that targets CD52, a cell-surface peptide antigen expressed on normal and malignant B and T lymphocytes (Hale et al. 1985). Approved as salvage therapy for patients with chronic lymphocytic leukemia (CLL) and cutaneous T-cell lymphoma who have failed purine analogue treatment, alemtuzumab induces more prolonged depletion of CD4 and CD8 T-cell subpopulations (Keating et al. 2002). Adverse events associated with alemtuzumab include infusion-related rigors, fever, nausea, vomiting, and rash (Keating et al. 2002). Opportunistic infections, cardiac toxicity, and neutropenia may also occur (Keating et al. 2002; Lenihan et al. 2004).

Richter's syndrome (RS) refers to the development of a second, more aggressive lymphoma in a patient with CLL (Richter 1928). The secondary lymphoma is usually a diffuse large B-cell lymphoma (DLBCL), but the development of Hodgkin's lymphoma (Jamroziak et al. 2012) and T-cell lymphoma (Lee et al. 1995) after CLL has also been described. Studies to date have estimated that Richter's syndrome occurs in anywhere from 1 to 10 % of patients with CLL (Robertson et al. 1993). Clinically, RS is characterized by sudden clinical deterioration with rapid increase in lymphadenopathy or extranodal involvement and less commonly the presence of a monoclonal gammopathy, lytic bone lesions, and multiple cytogenetic changes (Robertson et al. 1993). Molecular analyses of immunoglobulin heavy- and light-chain rearrangements suggest that the secondary lymphoma generally arises from a transformation of the underlying CLL cell (Robertson et al. 1993). However, biclonal origin in RS has been described in the literature (Tohda et al. 1990).

To date, there have been two reported cases in the literature that describe Richter's or Richter's-like transformation associated primarily with alemtuzumab therapy (Janssens et al. 2006; Faguer et al. 2007). A long-term follow-up, retrospective study of 38 patients with CLL who underwent alemtuzumab therapy found that there was an increased but statistically insignificant risk of developing Richter's syndrome in patients on alemtuzumab therapy (16 %, 6/38) compared with consecutive historical controls who underwent alternative salvage therapy (12 %, 9/75) (Karlsson et al. 2006). In their report on 39 patients who developed Richter's syndrome, Robertson et al. (1993) noted that most of those that had developed the transformation had active and more advanced disease. Thus,

whether alemtuzumab therapy poses a true risk for the development of Richter's syndrome is still to be determined. Nonetheless, a summary of the reported clinical and pathologic features and a discussion of proposed pathogenic mechanisms of alemtuzumab-induced Richter's syndrome are noted below.

Clinical Presentation/Histologic Features

Janssens et al. (2006) report the case of a patient with B-CLL who after failing treatment with chlorambucil was started on alemtuzumab. Three months after initiating alemtuzumab therapy, the patient developed a fever and rapidly increasing lactate dehydrogenase (LDH), with recurrent thrombocytopenia and autoimmune hemolytic anemia, which had previously precluded her from fludarabine. Bone marrow biopsy led to a diagnosis of large B-cell lymphoma, revealing the Richter's transformation. Molecular microbiologic studies documented a negative Epstein-Barr virus (EBV) status. Molecular analysis of the immunoglobulin heavy chain confirmed that the CLL and the RS were of different clonal origin, and further analyses revealed that, in fact, the RS cells had evolved from a clone that was present 2 years before the clinical appearance of RS.

Faguer et al. (2007) report the case of a patient with cutaneous T-cell lymphoma (CTCL) who, 2 months after initiating alemtuzumab therapy, developed high fever, night sweats, and dramatic diffuse enlargement of lymph nodes and left temporal cutaneous tumor. A month prior to this presentation, the patient had developed febrile CMV viremia, which after treatment with ganciclovir and prophylaxis with valganciclovir, became and remained negative. Biopsy disclosed a transformed CTCL with CD30+ T cells, revealing a Richter's syndrome-like phenomenon. Rising titers of EBV virus were documented at this time, but in situ hybridization with EBV-specific EBER probes on the biopsy specimen were negative. The patient was treated with a separate course of chemotherapy with no obvious clinical response.

Pathogenesis

It is known that in typical RS, acquisition of TP53 mutations and/or 17p deletions are frequent molecular events (Rossi and Gaidano 2009). However, whether these mutations are sufficient to lead to the disease remains to be determined. The authors of both case reports above are in agreement that alemtuzumab may have promoted the uncontrolled growth of a novel, Richter's clone by eradicating the initial B-CLL or CTCL efficiently and by inducing T-cell depletion with consequent impairment of immunosurveillance (Janssens et al. 2006; Faguer et al. 2007). However, the relationship between chemotherapy-induced immunosuppression and the development of RS remains a controversial issue (Cohen et al. 2002).

Previous studies have emphasized the role of circulating natural killer lymphocytes in the cytotoxic response against Sézary cells (Bouaziz et al. 2005). The transformation of CLL into diffuse large B-cell lymphoma has also been reported after rituximab (Cohen et al. 2002). A very recent case was also reported by Salihoglu et al. (2013 in press) of a CLL patient who developed diffuse large B-cell lymphoma after treatment with rituximab, alemtuzumab, and reduced-intensity conditioning allogenic stem cell transplantation. However, considering the advanced stage of disease, it is still possible that this transformation reflects the natural history of the disease process itself as opposed to being a direct result of chemotherapeutics (Cohen et al. 2002). Further study and experience with alemtuzumab may reveal further insight.

Chronic Hydroxyurea: Pseudodermatomyositis

Hydroxyurea is a cytostatic, antineoplastic agent that interrupts the formation of deoxyribonucleotides from ribonucleotides by inhibiting the enzyme ribonucleotide diphosphate reductase. It is used to treat myeloproliferative disorders such as chronic myelogenous leukemia (CML),

Table 15.5 Mucocutaneous complications of hydroxyurea (Rocamora et al. 2000; Saraceno et al. 2008; Papi et al. 1993; Stasi et al. 1992; Hagen et al. 2012; Richard et al. 1989; Senet et al. 1995; Sigal et al. 1984)

Pseudodermatomyositis
Skin hyperpigmentation
Nail pigmentation
Traumatic or spontaneous ulceration
Alopecia
Stomatitis with ulceration
Plantar keratoderma
Non-melanoma skin cancer
Multiple actinic keratoses

essential thrombocythemia, polycythemia vera, as well as sickle cell anemia and severe, refractory psoriasis (Richard et al. 1989; Halverstam et al. 2008).

Major adverse reactions include bone marrow suppression (Oskay et al. 2002) and life-threatening alveolitis (Dacey and Callen 2003; Senet et al. 1995) as well as an elevated risk of multiple actinic keratoses and non-melanoma skin cancers, which is thought to be related to the inhibition of DNA damage repair mechanisms (Rocamora et al. 2000; Saraceno et al. 2008; Papi et al. 1993; Stasi et al. 1992). Documented adverse cutaneous effects associated with long-term hydroxyurea therapy include xerosis, hyperpigmentation, atrophy, lower extremity ulcerations, partial alopecia, and chromonychia (Hagen et al. 2012; Richard et al. 1989) (Table 15.5), but these effects are also common with use of other chemotherapeutic agents such as cytarabine, doxorubicin, busulfan, and bleomycin (Senet et al. 1995).

Pseudodermatomyositis is a cutaneous reaction unique to long-term hydroxyurea therapy that was first described in 1975 by Kennedy et al. who documented three patients undergoing said treatment for chronic myelogenous leukemia that developed erythematous lesions, violaceous papules, and atrophy involving the dorsa of the metacarpophalangeal and interphalangeal joints. Sigal et al. (1984) later described the eruption as dermatomyositis-like but ultimately eliminated the diagnosis because of the absence of muscular abnormalities. Interestingly, this rare but characteristic cutaneous side effect has not been documented in psoriatic patients treated with hydroxyurea, but this may be related to the shorter duration of therapy (Senet et al. 1995).

Clinical Presentation

Pseudodermatomyositis typically presents after years (2–10) of hydroxyurea therapy with scaly, linear, and erythematous plaques on the dorsa of the hands (Kennedy et al. 1975) that may or may not be tender (Suehiro et al. 1998). These lesions may strongly resemble the Gottron's sign of dermatomyositis proper (Rocamora et al. 2000). Associated findings include localized atrophy, nails telangiectatic changes, scaly poikilodermatous plaques, or violaceous papules on the feet, elbows, palms, or face (Hagen et al. 2012). The violaceous and erythematous lesions, which can appear around the eyelids and elsewhere on the face, resemble the heliotrope rash of dermatomyositis (Oskay et al. 2002). However, there are typically no signs of proximal muscle weakness or muscle enzymes and electromyography abnormalities (Senet et al. 1995). Furthermore, laboratory evaluation typically reveals negative antinuclear antibody as well as normal aldolase creatine kinase levels (Dacey and Callen 2003). Unlike in dermatomyositis proper, there is little data to suggest that pseudodermatomyositis is associated with any underlying malignancy (Robinson and Reed 2011).

Histologic Features

Histopathologic examination of skin biopsies shows hyperkeratosis, epidermal atrophy, vacuolar changes in the basal layer, and perivascular lymphohistiocytic infiltrate in the superficial dermis (Bahadoran et al. 1996; Senet et al. 1995). Variations on this common theme include focal lichenoid reactions, dyskeratotic cells, dermal mucin deposition, and dermal telangiectasia (Dacey and Callen 2003). Direct immunofluorescence studies have been reportedly negative (Senet et al. 1995).

Differential Diagnosis/Pathogenesis

The histologic differential diagnosis includes dermatomyositis, poikiloderma, lichenoid dermatitis, and graft-versus-host disease (Hagen et al. 2012). The mechanism underlying this reaction is not known at this time. Chronic, cumulative cytologic and selective DNA damage to the basal layer and epidermis is likely involved and may be related to the accumulation of the drug or one of its metabolites (Richard et al. 1989; Senet et al. 1995; Dacey and Callen 2003). Given that leg ulceration is another common adverse event associated with long-term hydroxyurea use, Suehiro et al. (1998) have postulated that chronic cumulative toxicity of the drug on the dividing cells of the basal epidermal layer may play a pathogenic role.

Treatment

Pseudodermatomyositis is a mild eruption that resolves without treatment between 10 days and 18 months after discontinuation of hydroxyurea but runs a benign course even if the medication is continued (Senet et al. 1995).

References

Adams AE, Zwicker J, Curiel C, Kadin ME, Falchuk KR, Drews R, Kupper TS. Aggressive cutaneous T-cell lymphomas after TNF-alpha blockade. J Am Acad Dermatol. 2004;51(4):660–2.

Agesta N, Zabala R, Diaz-Perez JL. Alopecia areata during interferon alpha-2b/ribavirin therapy. Dermatology. 2002;205(3):300–1.

Ahronowitz I, Harp J, Shinkai K. Etiology and management of pyoderma gangrenosum: a comprehensive review. Am J Clin Dermatol. 2012;13(3):191–211. doi:10.2165/11595240-000000000-00000.

Alonso-Perez A, Ballestero-Diez M, Fraga J, Garcia-Diez A, Fernandez-Herrera J. Cutaneous sarcoidosis by interferon therapy in a patient with melanoma. J Eur Acad Dermatol Venereol. 2006;20(10):1328–9.

Alvarez-Ruiz S, Penas PF, Fernandez-Herrera J, Sanchez-Perez J, Fraga J, Garcia-Diez A. Maculopapular eruption with enlarged macrophages in eight patients receiving G-CSF or GM-CSF. J Eur Acad Dermatol Venereol. 2004;18(3):310–3.

Arrue I, Saiz A, Ortiz-Romero PL, Rodriguez-Peralto JL. Lupus-like reaction to interferon at the injection site:

report of five cases. J Cutan Pathol. 2007;34 Suppl 1:18–21.

Azad NS, Aragon-Ching JB, Dahut WL, Gutierrez M, Figg WD, Jain L, et al. Hand-foot skin reaction increases with cumulative sorafenib dose and with combination anti-vascular endothelial growth factor therapy. Clin Cancer Res. 2009;15(4):1411–6. doi:10.1158/1078-0432.CCR-08-1141.

Bahadoran P, Castanet J, Lacour JP, Perrin C, Del Giudice P, Mannocci N, et al. Pseudo-dermatomyositis induced by long-term hydroxyurea therapy: report of two cases. Br J Dermatol. 1996;134(6):1161–3.

Baron S, Tyring SK, Fleischmann Jr WR, Coppenhaver DH, Niesel DW, Klimpel GR, et al. The interferons. Mechanisms of action and clinical applications. JAMA. 1991;266(10):1375–83.

Batycka-Baran A, Flaig M, Molin S, Ruzicka T, Prinz JC. Etanercept-induced injection site reactions: potential pathomechanisms and clinical assessment. Expert Opin Drug Saf. 2012;11(6):911–21. doi:10.1517/1474 0338.2012.727796.

Bauer K, Rancea M, Roloff V, Elter T, Hallek M, Engert A, Skoetz N. Rituximab, ofatumumab and other monoclonal anti-CD20 antibodies for chronic lymphocytic leukaemia. Cochrane Database Syst Rev. 2012;11:CD008079. doi:10.1002/14651858. CD008079.pub2.

Beard JS, Smith KJ, Skelton HG. Combination chemotherapy with 5-fluorouracil, folinic acid, and alpha-interferon producing histologic feature of graft-versus-host disease. J Am Acad Dermatol. 1993;29(2 Pt 2):325–30.

Bidyasar S, Montoya M, Suleman K, Markowitz AB. Sweet syndrome associated with granulocyte colony-stimulating factor. J Clin Oncol. 2008;26(26):4355–6. doi:10.1200/JCO.2008.16.2933.

Borrás-Blasco J, Gracia-Perez A, Rosique-Robles JD, Nuñez-Cornejo C, Casterá MD, Abad FJ. Urticaria due to etanercept in a patient with psoriatic arthritis. South Med J. 2009;102(3):304–5. doi:10.1097/ SMJ.0b013e31819450e7.

Bouaziz JD, Ortonne N, Giustiniani J, Schiavon V, Huet D, Bagot M, Bensussan A. Circulating natural killer lymphocytes are potential cytotoxic effectors against autologous malignant cells in sezary syndrome patients. J Invest Dermatol. 2005;125(6):1273–8.

Bovenschen HJ, Tjioe M, Vermaat H, de Hoop D, Witteman BM, Janssens RW, et al. Induction of eruptive benign melanocytic naevi by immune suppressive agents, including biologicals. Br J Dermatol. 2006;154:880–4.

Chow LQ, Eckhardt SG. Sunitinib: from rational design to clinical efficacy. J Clin Oncol. 2007;25(7):884–96.

Christian MM, Diven DG, Sanchez RL, Soloway RD. Injection site vasculitis in a patient receiving interferon alfa for chronic hepatitis C. J Am Acad Dermatol. 1997;37(1):118–20.

Chu D, Lacouture ME, Fillos T, Wu S. Risk of hand-foot skin reaction with sorafenib: a systematic review and meta-analysis. Acta Oncol. 2008;47(2):176–86. doi:10.1080/02841860701765675.

Chu P, Connolly MK, LeBoit PE. The histopathologic spectrum of palisaded neutrophilic and granulomatous dermatitis in patients with collagen vascular disease. Arch Dermatol. 1994;130(10):1278–83.

Coca A, Sanz I. Updates on B-cell immunotherapies for systemic lupus erythematosus and Sjogren's syndrome. Curr Opin Rheumatol. 2012;24(5):451–6. doi:10.1097/BOR.0b013e32835707e4.

Cohen PR. Sweet's syndrome – a comprehensive review of an acute febrile neutrophilic dermatosis. Orphanet J Rare Dis. 2007;2:34.

Cohen Y, Da'as N, Libster D, Amir G, Berrebi A, Polliack A. Large – cell transformation of chronic lymphocytic leukemia and follicular lymphoma during or soon after treatment with fludarabine-rituximab-containing regimens: natural history- or therapy-related complication? Eur J Haematol. 2002;68(2):80–3.

Colombel JF, Loftus Jr EV, Tremaine WJ, Egan LJ, Harmsen WS, Schleck CD, et al. The safety profile of infliximab in patients with Crohn's disease: the Mayo clinic experience in 500 patients. Gastroenterology. 2004;126(1):19–31.

Couderc LJ, Philippe B, Franck N, Balloul-Delclaux E, Lessana-Leibowitch M. Necrotizing vasculitis and exacerbation of psoriasis after granulocyte colony-stimulating factor for small cell lung carcinoma. Respir Med. 1995;89(3):237–8.

Dacey MJ, Callen JP. Hydroxyurea-induced dermatomyositis-like eruption. J Am Acad Dermatol. 2003;48(3):439–41.

Dalmau J, Pimentel CL, Puig L, Peramiquel L, Roe E, Alomar A. Cutaneous necrosis after injection of polyethylene glycol-modified interferon alfa. J Am Acad Dermatol. 2005;53(1):62–6.

Demirturk N, Aykin N, Demirdal T, Cevik F. Alopecia universalis: a rare side effect seen on chronic hepatitis C treatment with peg-INF and ribavirin. Eur J Dermatol. 2006;16(5):579–80.

Deng A, Harvey V, Sina B, Strobel D, Badros A, Junkins-Hopkins JM, et al. Interstitial granulomatous dermatitis associated with the use of tumor necrosis factor alpha inhibitors. Arch Dermatol. 2006;142(2):198–202.

Dereure O, Rason-Peyron N, Larrey D, Blanc F, Guilhou JJ. Diffuse inflammatory lesions in patients treated with interferon alpha and ribavirin for hepatitis C: a series of 20 patients. Br J Dermatol. 2002;147(6):1142–6.

Detmar U, Agathos M, Nerl C. Allergy of delayed type to recombinant interferon alpha 2c. Contact Dermatitis. 1989;20(2):149–50.

Dillman RO. Infusion reactions associated with the therapeutic use of monoclonal antibodies in the treatment of malignancy. Cancer Metastasis Rev. 1999;18(4):465–71.

Dong F, Brynes RK, Tidow N, Welte K, Löwenberg B, Touw IP. Mutations in the gene for the granulocyte colony-stimulating-factor receptor in patients with acute myeloid leukemia preceded by severe congenital neutropenia. N Engl J Med. 1995;333(8):487–93.

Errante D, Bernardi D, Bianco A, De Nardi S, Salvagno L. Rituximab-related urticarial reaction in a patient treated for primary cutaneous B-cell lymphoma. Ann Oncol. 2006;17(11):1720–1.

Esser AC, Abril A, Fayne S, Doyle JA. Acute development of multiple keratoacanthomas and squamous cell carcinomas after treatment with infliximab. J Am Acad Dermatol. 2004;50(5 Suppl):S75–7.

Faguer S, Launay F, Ysebaert L, Mailhol C, Estines-Chartier O, Lamant L, Paul C. Acute cutaneous T-cell lymphoma transformation during treatment with alemtuzumab. Br J Dermatol. 2007;157(4):841–2.

Fantini F, Padalino C, Gualdi G, Monari P, Giannetti A. Cutaneous lesions as initial signs of interferon alpha-induced sarcoidosis: report of three new cases and review of the literature. Dermatol Ther. 2009;22 Suppl 1:S1–7. doi:10.1111/j.1529-8019.2009.01263.x.

Fukutoku M, Shimizu S, Ogawa Y, Takeshita S, Masaki Y, Arai T, et al. Sweet's syndrome during therapy with granulocyte colony-stimulating factor in a patient with aplastic anaemia. Br J Haematol. 1994;86(3): 645–8.

Fukuyama S, Kajiwara E, Suzuki N, Miyazaki N, Sadoshima S, Onoyama K. Systemic lupus erythematosus after alpha-interferon therapy for chronic hepatitis C: a case report and review of the literature. Am J Gastroenterol. 2000;95(1):310–2.

González-López MA, Martínez-Taboada VM, González-Vela MC, Blanco R, Fernández-Llaca H, Rodríguez-Valverde V, Val-Bernal JF. Recall injection-site reactions associated with etanercept therapy: report of two new cases with immunohistochemical analysis. Clin Exp Dermatol. 2007;32(6):672–4.

Hadjinicolaou AV, Nisar MK, Parfrey H, Chilvers ER, Ostör AJ. Non-infectious pulmonary toxicity of rituximab: a systematic review. Rheumatology (Oxford). 2012;51(4):653–62. doi:10.1093/rheumatology/ker290.

Hagen JW, Magro CM, Crowson AN. Emerging adverse cutaneous drug reactions. Dermatol Clin. 2012;30(4):695–730. doi:10.1016/j.det.2012.06.016.

Hale G, Swirsky D, Waldmann H, Chan LC. Reactivity of rat monoclonal antibody CAMPATH-1 with human leukaemia cells and its possible application for autologous bone marrow transplantation. Br J Haematol. 1985;60(1):41–8.

Halverstam CP, Lebwohl M. Nonstandard and off-label therapies for psoriasis. Clin Dermatol. 2008;26(5):546–53. doi:10.1016/j.clindermatol.2007.10.023.

Heinzerling LM, Urbanek M, Funk JO, Peker S, Bleck O, Neuber K, et al. Reduction of tumor burden and stabilization of disease by systemic therapy with anti-CD20 antibody (rituximab) in patients with primary cutaneous B-cell lymphoma. Cancer. 2000;89(8):1835–44.

Hertl MS, Haendle I, Schuler G, Hertl M. Rapid improvement of recalcitrant disseminated granuloma annulare upon treatment with the tumour necrosis factor-alpha inhibitor, infliximab. Br J Dermatol. 2005;152(3):552–5.

Isaacs A, Lindemann J. Virus interference. I. The interferon. Proc R Soc Lond B Biol Sci. 1957;147(927): 258–67.

Jacobi U, Waibler E, Schulze P, Sehouli J, Oskay-Ozcelik G, Schmook T, et al. Release of doxorubicin in sweat:

first step to induce the palmar-plantar erythrodysesthesia syndrome? Ann Oncol. 2005;16(7):1210–1.

Jain KK. Cutaneous vasculitis associated with granulocyte colony-stimulating factor. J Am Acad Dermatol. 1994;31(2 Pt 1):213–5.

Jamroziak K, Grzybowska-Izydorczyk O, Jesionek-Kupnicka D, Gora-Tybor J, Robak T. Poor prognosis of Hodgkin variant of Richter transformation in chronic lymphocytic leukemia treated with cladribine. Br J Haematol. 2012;158(2):286–8; author reply 289. doi:10.1111/j.1365-2141.2012.09127.x.

Janssens A, Berth M, De Paepe P, Verhasselt B, Van Roy N, Noens L, et al. EBV negative Richter's syndrome from a coexistent clone after savage treatment with alemtuzumab in a CLL patient. Am J Hematol. 2006;81(9):706–12.

Johnson ML, Grimwood RE. Leukocyte colony-stimulating factors. A review of associated neutrophilic dermatoses and vasculitides. Arch Dermatol. 1994;130(1):77–81.

Karlsson C, Norin S, Kimby E, Sander B, Porwit Macdonald A, et al. Alemtuzumab as first-line therapy for B-cell chronic lymphocytic leukemia: long-term follow-up of clinical effects, infectious complications and risk of Richter transformation. Leukemia. 2006;20(12):2204–7.

Kaushansky K. Lineage-specific hematopoietic growth factors. N Engl J Med. 2006;354(19):2034–45.

Kawakami T, Ohashi S, Kawa Y, Takahama H, Ito M, Soma Y, Mizoguchi M. Elevated serum granulocyte colony-stimulating factor levels in patients with active phase of sweet syndrome and patients with active behcet disease: implication in neutrophil apoptosis dysfunction. Arch Dermatol. 2004;140(5):570–4.

Keane J, Gershon S, Wise RP, Mirabile-Levens E, Kasznica J, Schwieterman WD, et al. Tuberculosis associated with infliximab, a tumor necrosis factor alpha-neutralizing agent. N Engl J Med. 2001;345(15):1098–104.

Keating MJ, Flinn I, Jain V, Binet JL, Hillmen P, Byrd J, et al. Therapeutic role of alemtuzumab (Campath-1H) in patients who have failed fludarabine: results of a large international study. Blood. 2002;99(10):3554–61.

Kennedy BJ, Smith LR, Goltz RW. Skin changes secondary to hydroxyurea therapy. Arch Dermatol. 1975;111(2):183–7.

Ketikoglou I, Karatapanis S, Elefsiniotis I, Kafiri G, Moulakakis A. Extensive psoriasis induced by pegylated interferon alpha-2b treatment for Hepatitis B. Eur J Dermatol. 2005;15(2):107–9.

Kim SY, Solomon DH. Tumor necrosis factor blockade and the risk of viral infection. Nat Rev Rheumatol. 2010;6(3):165–74. doi:10.1038/nrrheum.2009.279.

Kokudo N, Nakajima J, Hatano E, Numata K. Current status of hepatocellular carcinoma treatment in Japan: practical use of sorafenib (Nexavar®). Clin Drug Investig. 2012;32 Suppl 2:25–35. doi:10.2165/1163023-S0-000000000-00000.

Kollias G, Douni E, Kassiotis G, Kontoyiannis D. The function of tumour necrosis factor and receptors in models of multi-organ inflammation, rheumatoid arthritis, multiple sclerosis and inflammatory bowel disease. Ann Rheum Dis. 1999;58 Suppl 1:I32–9.

Kong HH, Sibaud V, Chanco Turner ML, Fojo T, Hornyak TJ, Chevreau C. Sorafenib-induced eruptive melanocytic lesions. Arch Dermatol. 2008;144(6):820–2. doi:10.1001/archderm.144.6.820.

Koontz D, Alshekhlee A. Embolia cutis medicamentosa following interferon beta injection. Mult Scler. 2007;13(9):1203–4.

Krainick U, Kantarjian H, Broussard S, Talpaz M. Local cutaneous necrotizing lesions associated with interferon injections. J Interferon Cytokine Res. 1998;18(10):823–7.

Lacouture ME, Reilly LM, Gerami P, Guitart J. Hand foot skin reaction in cancer patients treated with the multikinase inhibitors sorafenib and sunitinib. Ann Oncol. 2008;19(11):1955–61. doi:10.1093/annonc/mdn389.

Lang AM, Norland AM, Schuneman RL, Tope WD. Localized interferon alfa-2b-induced alopecia. Arch Dermatol. 1999;135(9):1126–8.

Lee L, Kukreti V. Rituximab-induced coronary vasospasm. Case Rep Hematol. 2012;2012:984986. doi:10.1155/2012/984986.

Lee A, Skelly ME, Kingma DW, Medeiros LJ. B-cell chronic lymphocytic leukemia followed by high grade T-cell lymphoma. An unusual variant of Richter's syndrome. Am J Clin Pathol. 1995;103(3):348–52.

Lee WJ, Lee JL, Chang SE, Lee MW, Kang YK, Choi JH, et al. Cutaneous adverse effects in patients treated with the multitargeted kinase inhibitors sorafenib and sunitinib. Br J Dermatol. 2009;161(5):1045–51. doi:10.1111/j.1365-2133.2009.09290.x.

Lenihan DJ, Alencar AJ, Yang D, Kurzrock R, Keating MJ, Duvic M. Cardiac toxicity of alemtuzumab in patients with mycosis fungoides/Sézary syndrome. Blood. 2004;104(3):655–8.

Lewerin C, Mobacken H, Nilsson-Ehle H, Swolin B. Bullous pyoderma gangrenosum in a patient with myelodysplastic syndrome during granulocyte colony-stimulating factor therapy. Leuk Lymphoma. 1997;26(5–6):629–32.

Long D, Thiboutot DM, Majeski JT, Vasily DB, Helm KF. Interstitial granulomatous dermatitis with arthritis. J Am Acad Dermatol. 1996;34(6):957–61.

Lowndes S, Darby A, Mead G, Lister A. Stevens-Johnson syndrome after treatment with rituximab. Ann Oncol. 2002;13(12):1948–50.

Luton K, Garcia C, Poletti E, Koester G. Nicolau syndrome: three cases and review. Int J Dermatol. 2006;45(11):1326–8.

Magro CM, Crowson AN, Schapiro BL. The interstitial granulomatous drug reaction: a distinctive clinical and pathological entity. J Cutan Pathol. 1998;25(2):72–8.

Maloney DG. Anti-CD20 antibody therapy for B-cell lymphomas. N Engl J Med. 2012;366(21):2008–16. doi:10.1056/NEJMct1114348.

Miall FM, Harman K, Kennedy B, Dyer MJ. Pyoderma gangrenosum complicating pegylated granulocyte colony-stimulating factor in Hodgkin lymphoma. Br J Haematol. 2006;132(1):115–6.

Montoto S, Bosch F, Estrach T, Blade J, Nomdedeu B, Nontserrat E. Pyoderma gangrenosum triggered by alpha2b-interferron in a patient with chronic granulocytic leukemia. Leuk Lymphoma. 1998;30(1–2):199–202.

Moore MM, Elpern DJ, Carter DJ. Severe, generalized nummular eczema secondary to interferon alfa-2b plus ribavirin combination therapy in a patient with chronic hepatitis C virus infection. Arch Dermatol. 2004;140(2):215–7.

Moots RJ, Naisbett-Groet B. The efficacy of biologic agents in patients with rheumatoid arthritis and an inadequate response to tumour necrosis factor inhibitors: a systematic review. Rheumatology (Oxford). 2012;51(12):2252–61. doi:10.1093/rheumatology/kes217.

Moustou AE, Matelovits A, Dessinioti C, Antoniou C, Sfikakis PP, Stratigos AJ. Cutaneous side effects of anti-tumor necrosis factor biologic therapy: a clinical review. J Am Acad Dermatol. 2009;61(3):486–504. doi:10.1016/j.jaad.2008.10.060.

Nagore E, Insa A, Sanmartin O. Antineoplastic therapy-induced palmar plantar erythrodysesthesia ('hand-foot') syndrome. Incidence, recognition and management. Am J Clin Dermatol. 2000;1(4):225–34.

Omair MA, Alnaqbi KA, Lee P. Rituximab in a patient with ankylosing spondylitis with demyelinating disease: a case report and review of the literature. Clin Rheumatol. 2012;31(8):1259–61. doi:10.1007/s10067-012-2002-8.

Oskay T, Kutluay L, Ozyilkan O. Dermatomyositis-like eruption after long-term hydroxyurea therapy for polycythemia vera. Eur J Dermatol. 2002;12(6):586–8.

Ostlere LS, Harris D, Prentice HG, Rustin MHA. Widespread folliculitis induced by human granulocyte-colony stimulating factor therapy [Letter]. Br J Dermatol. 1992;127:193.

Papi M, Didona B, DePita O, Abruzzese E, Stasi R, Papa G, Cavalieri R. Multiple skin tumors on light-exposed areas during long-term treatment with hydroxyurea. J Am Acad Dermatol. 1993;28(3):485–6.

Parameswaran N, Patial S. Tumor necrosis factor-α signaling in macrophages. Crit Rev Eukaryot Gene Expr. 2010;20(2):87–103.

Paydas S, Sahin B, Seyrek E, Soylu M, Gonlusen G, Acar A, Tuncer I. Sweet syndrome associated with G-CSF. Br J Dermatol. 1993;85(1):191–2.

Pinto JM, Marques MS, Correia TE. Lichen planus and leukocytoclastic vasculitis induced by interferon alpha-2b in a subject with HCV-related chronic active hepatitis. J Eur Acad Dermatol. 2003;17(2):193–5.

Prendiville J, Thiessen P, Mallory SB. Neutrophilic dermatoses in two children with idiopathic neutropenia: association with granulocyte colony-stimulating factor (G-CSF) therapy. Pediatr Dermatol. 2001;18(5):417–21.

Quesada JR, Gutterman JU. Psoriasis and alpha-interferon. Lancet. 1986;1(8496):1466–8.

Raymond AK, Puri PK, Selim MA, Tyler DS, Nelson KC. Regional squamous cell carcinomas following sorafenib therapy and isolated limb infusion for regionally advanced metastatic melanoma of the limb. Arch Dermatol. 2010;146(12):1438–9. doi:10.1001/archdermatol.2010.367.

Reuss-Borst MA, Pawelec G, Saal JG, Horny HP, Müller CA, Waller HD. Sweet's syndrome associated with myelodysplasia: possible role of cytokines in the pathogenesis of the disease. Br J Haematol. 1993;84(2):356–8.

Rey J, Wickenhauser S, Ivanov V, Coso D, Gastaut JA, Bouabdallah R. A case of rituximab-related urticarial reaction in cutaneous B-cell lymphoma. J Eur Acad Dermatol Venereol. 2009;23(2):210. doi:10.1111/j.1468-3083.2008.02792.x.

Richard M, Truchetet F, Friedel J, Leclech C, Heid E. Skin lesions simulating chronic dermatomyositis during long-term hydroxyurea therapy. J Am Acad Dermatol. 1989;21(4 Pt 1):797–9.

Richter MN. Generalized reticular cell sarcoma of lymph nodes associated with lymphatic leukemia. Am J Pathol. 1928;4(4):285–92.7.

Robert C, Soria JC, Spatz A, Le Cesne A, Malka D, Pautier P, et al. Cutaneous side-effects of kinase inhibitors and blocking antibodies. Lancet Oncol. 2005;6(7):491–500.

Robert C, Arnault JP, Mateus C. RAF inhibition and induction of cutaneous squamous cell carcinoma. Curr Opin Oncol. 2011;23(2):177–82. doi:10.1097/CCO.0b013e3283436e8c.

Robertson LE, Pugh W, O'Brien S, Kantarjian H, Hirsch-Ginsberg C, Cork A, et al. Richter's syndrome: a report on 39 patients. J Clin Oncol. 1993;11(10):1985–9.

Robinson AB, Reed AM. Clinical features, pathogenesis and treatment of juvenile and adult dermatomyositis. Nat Rev Rheumatol. 2011;7(11):664–75. doi:10.1038/nrrheum.2011.139.

Rocamora V, Puig L, Alomar A. Dermatomyositis-like eruption following hydroxyurea therapy. J Eur Acad Dermatol Venereol. 2000;14(3):227–8.

Rosenbaum SE, Wu S, Newman MA, West DP, Kuzel T, Lacouture ME. Dermatological reactions to the multi-targeted tyrosine kinase inhibitor sunitinib. Support Care Cancer. 2008;16(6):557–66. doi:10.1007/s00520-008-0409-1.

Ross HJ, Moy LA, Kaplan R, Figlin RA. Bullous pyoderma gangrenosum after granulocyte colony-stimulating factor treatment. Cancer. 1991;68(2):441–3.

Rossi D, Gaidano G. Richter syndrome: molecular insights and clinical perspectives. Hematol Oncol. 2009;27(1):1–10. doi:10.1002/hon.880.

Salihoglu A, Ozbalak M, Keskin D, Tecimer T, Soysal T, Ferhanoglu B. An unusual presentation of a chronic lymphocytic leukemia patient with 17p deletion after reduced-intensity transplantation: Richter syndrome and concomitant graft-versus-host disease-case report. Transplant Proc. 2013;S0041-1345(12):1304–8. doi:10.1016/j.transproceed.2012.12.001.

Sanders S, Busam K, Tahan SR, Johnson RA, Sachs D. Granulomatous and suppurative dermatitis at inter-

feron alfa injection sites: report of 2 cases. J Am Acad Dermatol. 2002;46(4):611–6.

Saraceno R, Teoli M, Chimenti S. Hydroxyurea associated with concomitant occurrence of diffuse longitudinal melanonychia and multiple squamous cell carcinomas in an elderly subject. Clin Ther. 2008;30(7):1324–9.

Selmi C, Lleo A, Zuin M, Podda M, Rossaro L, Gershwin ME. Interferon alpha and its contribution to autoimmunity. Curr Opin Investig Drugs. 2006;7(5):451–6.

Senet P, Aractingi S, Porneuf M, Perrin P, Duterque M. Hydroxyurea-induced dermatomyositis-like eruption. Br J Dermatol. 1995;133(3):455–9.

Sfikakis PP, Kollias G. Tumor necrosis factor biology in experimental and clinical arthritis. Curr Opin Rheumatol. 2003;15(4):380–6.

Shpiro D, Gilat D, Fisher-Feld L, Shemer A, Gold I, Trau H. Pyoderma gangrenosum successfully treated with perilesional granulocyte-macrophage colony stimulating factor. Br J Dermatol. 1998;138(2):368–9.

Sigal M, Crickx B, Blanchet P, Perron J, Simony J, Belaïch S. Cutaneous lesions induced by long-term use of hydroxyurea. Ann Dermatol Venereol. 1984;111(10):895–900 [Article in French].

Singer EA, Gupta GN, Srinivasan R. Targeted therapeutic strategies for the management of renal cell carcinoma. Curr Opin Oncol. 2012;24(3):284–90. doi:10.1097/CCO.0b013e328351c646.

Skytta E, Phjankoski H, Savolainen A. Etanercept and urticaria in patients with juvenile idiopathic arthritis. Clin Exp Rheumatol. 2000;18:533–4.

Smith KJ, Haley H, Hamza S, Skelton HG. Eruptive keratoacanthoma-type squamous cell carcinomas in patients taking sorafenib for the treatment of solid tumors. Dermatol Surg. 2009;35(11):1766–70. doi:10.1111/j.1524-4725.2009.01289.x.

Spiekermann K, Roesler J, Emmendoerffer A, Elsner J, Welte K. Functional features of neutrophils induced by G-CSF and GM-CSF treatment: differential effects and clinical implications. Leukemia. 1997;11(4):466–78.

Stasi R, Cantonetti M, Abruzzesse E, Papi M, Didona B, Cavalieri R, Papa G. Multiple skin tumors in long-term treatment with hydroxyurea. Eur J Dermatol. 1992;48(2):121–2.

Stewart LR, George S, Hamacher KL, Hsu S. Granuloma annulare of the palms. Dermatol Online J. 2011;17(5):7.

Suehiro M, Kishimoto S, Wakabayashi T, Ikeuchi A, Miyake H, Takenaka H, et al. Hydroxyurea dermopathy with a dermatomyositis-like eruption and a large leg ulcer. Br J Dermatol. 1998;139(4):748–9.

Sweet RD. An acute febrile neutrophilic dermatosis. Br J Dermatol. 1964;76:349–56.

Tai YJ, Tam M. Fixed drug eruption with interferon-beta-1b. Australas J Dermatol. 2005;46(3):154–7.

Tohda S, Morio T, Suzuki T, Nagata K, Kamiyama T, Imai Y, et al. Richter syndrome with two B cell clones possessing different surface immunoglobulins and immunoglobulin gene rearrangements. Am J Hematol. 1990;35(1):32–6.

Tomasiewicz K, Modzewska R, Semczuk G. Vitiligo associated with pegylated interferon and ribavirin treatment of patients with chronic hepatitis C: a case report. Adv Ther. 2006;23(1):139–42.

Valks R, Vargas E, Munoz E, Fernandez-Herrera J, Garcia-Diez A, Fraga J. Dermal infiltrate of enlarged macrophages in patients receiving chemotherapy. J Cutan Pathol. 1998;25(5):259–64.

Van der Kolk LE, Grillo-Lopez AJ, Baars JW, Hack CE, van Oers MH. Complement activation plays a key role in the side-effects of rituximab treatment. Br J Haematol. 2001;115(4):807–11.

van Husen M, Kemper MJ. New therapies in steroid-sensitive and steroid-resistant idiopathic nephrotic syndrome. Pediatr Nephrol. 2011;26(6):881–92. doi:10.1007/s00467-010-1717-5. Epub 2011 Jan 13.

van Kamp H, van den Berg E, Timens W, Kraaijenbrink RA, Halie MR, Daenen SM. Sweet's syndrome in myeloid malignancy: a report of two cases. Br J Haematol. 1994;86(2):415–7.

Voulgari PV, Markatseli TE, Exarchou SA, Zioga A, Drosos AA. Granuloma annulare induced by anti-tumour necrosis factor therapy. Ann Rheum Dis. 2008;67(4):567–70.

Walker DC, Cohen PR. Trimethoprim-sulfamethoxazole-associated acute febrile neutrophilic dermatosis: case report and review of drug-induced Sweet's syndrome. J Am Acad Dermatol. 1996;34(5 Pt 2):918–23.

White JM, Mufti GJ, Salisbury JR, du Vivier AW. Cutaneous manifestations of granulocyte colony-stimulating factor. Clin Exp Dermatol. 2006;31(2):206–7.

Wilhelm S, Chien DS. Bay 43-9006: preclinical data. Curr Pharm Des. 2002;8(25):2255–7.

Williams VL, Cohen PR. TNF alpha antagonist-induced lupus-like syndrome: report and review of the literature with implications for treatment with alternative TNF alpha antagonists. Int J Dermatol. 2011;50(5):619–25. doi:10.1111/j.1365-4632.2011.04871.x.

Winfield H, Lain E, Horn T, Hoskyn J. Eosinophilic cellulitis-like reaction to subcutaneous etanercept injection. Arch Dermatol. 2006;142:218–20.

Winkler U, Jensen M, Manzke O, Schulz H, Diehl V, Engert A. Cytokine-release syndrome in patients with B-cell chronic lymphocytic leukemia and high lymphocyte counts after treatment with an anti-CD20 monoclonal antibody (rituximab, IDEC-C2B8). Blood. 1999;94(7):2217–24.

Zeltser R, Valle L, Tanck C, Holyst M, Ritchlin C, Gaspari AA. Clinical, histological, and immunophenotypic characteristics of injection site reactions associated with etanercept: a recombinant tumor necrosis factor alpha receptor: Fc fusion protein. Arch Dermatol. 2001;137(7):893–9.

Cutaneous Myelomonocytic Infiltrates

Samir Dalia, Lubomir Sokol, and Hernani D. Cualing

Introduction

Although extremely rare, myelomonocytic infiltrates can be found on the skin. Distinguishing different types is important since these infiltrates vary from benign to malignant in nature. Myelomonocytic skin lesions may be the first signs of a systemic disease amenable to systemic therapy or may be localized lesions that can be controlled with skin-directed therapy (Haniffa et al. 2006). Clinical features, cytomorphology, and immunophenotype are all important facets helpful in differentiating these disorders. In this chapter, the different myelomonocytic cutaneous infiltrates including cutaneous extramedullary hematopoiesis, cutaneous myelomonocytic infiltrates in patients with myelodysplastic syndrome (MDS)/myeloproliferative disorders (MPD), myeloid sarcoma, blastic plasmacytoid dendritic cell neoplasm (BPDCN), dendritic cell infiltrates,

and histiocytic infiltrates are reviewed in detail. Table 16.1 highlights the cutaneous findings and epidemiology of the different myelomonocytic subtypes, and Table 16.2 outlines the immunophenotypical findings.

Cutaneous Extramedullary Hematopoiesis

Extramedullary hematopoiesis (EMH) is a common finding among patients with myeloid malignancies and hemoglobinopathies (Korsten et al. 1970; Glew et al. 1973; Rice et al. 1980; Lewkow and Shah 1984; Gowitt and Zaatari 1985; Gumbs et al. 1987; Shih et al. 1988; de Morais et al. 1996; Dibbern et al. 1997) or due to compromise of normal marrow space from foreign cells, cytokine-driven myeloid expansion, or stromal fibrosis (O'Malley 2007).

Definition

Cutaneous extramedullary hematopoiesis (CEMH) is defined as involvement of the skin with precursor hematopoietic tissue, which is normally in the bone marrow. The usual EMH sites include the liver and spleen, but almost all anatomical body locations can be affected including the skin (Koch et al. 2003; Pitcock et al. 1962; Mizoguchi et al. 1990). EMH is essential in fetal life, but after birth it is usually considered an

S. Dalia, MD (✉)
Department of Malignant Hematology, H. Lee Moffitt Cancer Center and Research Institute,
700 S Harbour Island Blvd, Unit 330, Tampa, FL 33602, USA
e-mail: samir.dalia@moffitt.org; sdalia@gmail.com

L. Sokol, MD, PhD
Department of Malignant Hematology, Moffitt Cancer Center, Tampa, FL USA

H.D. Cualing, MD
Department of Hematopathology and Cutaneous Lymphoma, IHCFLOW Diagnostic Laboratory, Lutz, FL, USA

H.D. Cualing et al. (eds.), *Cutaneous Hematopathology*,
DOI 10.1007/978-1-4939-0950-6_16, © Springer Science+Business Media New York 2014

Table 16.1 Cutaneous signs, epidemiological, and pattern of infiltration of cutaneous myelomonocytic infiltrates

Type of infiltrate	Cutaneous findings	Epidemiology	Pattern of infiltration
Extramedullary hematopoiesis	Pink, red, or bluish plaques, papules, or nodules	Most common with myelofibrosis	Perivascular and limited to dermis
Myeloid sarcoma	Papules, plaques, and nodules usually on the upper body	Male predominance, median age of 56 years	Dermis and subcutaneous tissue
Blastic plasmacytoid dendritic cell neoplasm (BPDCN)	Brown to violaceous nodules, plaques, or bruises	Male predominance, mean age of 61 years	Diffuse monomorphous infiltrate of medium-sized blast cells
Interdigitating dendritic cell sarcoma (IDCS)	Asymptomatic nodular lesions	Male predominance, median age 56.5 years	Dermis, spares epidermis
Follicular dendritic cell sarcoma (FDCS)	Subcutaneous nodules, can have paraneoplastic pemphigus	Mean age of 44 years Associated with Castleman disease and EBV	Dermis, can extend to subcutaneous or muscle but spares the epidermis
Langerhans cell histiocytosis (LCH)	Can resemble seborrheic dermatitis. Reddish-brown nodules or papules, rarely tumors	Male predominance	Dermis, often with epidermotropism
Dermal dendrocytic infiltrates	Well-circumscribed atrophic and wrinkled patch on the skin	Usually found in infancy or in childhood	Dermis, has epidermal atrophy
Indeterminate dendritic cell infiltrates	Solitary or multiple maculopapular or papulo-nodular lesions	Associated with low-grade B lymphomas	Dermis and can extend into subcutaneous fat

Table 16.2 Immunophenotypical markers of myelomonocytic cutaneous infiltrates

Marker	Myeloid sarcoma	Blastic plasmacytoid dendritic cell neoplasm	Interdigitating dendritic cell sarcoma	Follicular dendritic cell sarcoma	Langerhans cell histiocytosis	Dermal dendrocytic infiltrates	Indeterminate dendritic cell infiltrates
CD1a	−	−	−	−	++	−	+
CD4	+/−	+	+	+	+	+/−	+
CD21	−	−	−	++	−	−	−
CD34	++	−	−	−	−	++	−
CD35	−	−	−	++	−	−	−
CD45	++/−	+/−	+/−	−/wk+	+	−	+
CD68	+	+	+	+/−	+/−	+/−	+/−
CD123	−	++	−	−	−	−	−
Factor XIIa	−	−	−	−	−	++	−
Fascin	−	−	++	++	+	−	+
Lysozyme	+	−	+/−	−	+/−	−	+
S100	−	−	++	−/+	++	−	++
TCL1	−	++	−	−	−	−	−
Birbeck granules	−	−	−	−	++	−	−

Expression: ++ high, + present, +/− low or varies, − not present

abnormality (Koch et al. 2003). In a series of 510 patients with EMH, there were 27 patients (5.3 %) who were diagnosed with nonhepatosplenic EMH, and out of these, two patients had cutaneous EMH (Koch et al. 2003).

Epidemiology

The most common underlying condition associated with EMH is primary myelofibrosis. Little is known about the exact etiology of CEMH because of its rarity, with most information coming from case reports or small series. Large series from three reports of 220 patients with myelofibrosis reported only one with CEMH (Bouroncle and Doan 1962; Pitcock et al. 1962; Ward and Block 1971). Literature documentation of CEMH comprises a total of about 30 cases and appears to be most frequently associated with myelofibrosis or myeloproliferative disorders (Patel et al. 1995; Revenga et al. 2000; Fernandez Acenero et al. 2003). Increased levels of transforming growth factor-beta appear to be associated with CEMH in patients with idiopathic myelofibrosis (Collie et al. 2013; Corella et al. 2008; Haniffa et al. 2006; Kawakami et al. 2008; Kwon et al. 1999; Lane et al. 2002; Miyata et al. 2008; Mizoguchi et al. 1990; Pagerols et al. 1998; Rodriguez et al. 1991; Rogalski et al. 2002; Ruberto et al. 1995).

Clinical Appearance of Cutaneous Lesions

Lesions presented as firm nodules in dermis and subcutaneous tissue. Pink, reddish, or bluish plaques, papules, or nodules are commonly seen and hemorrhage can develop around the lesion (Mizoguchi et al. 1990).

Pattern of Infiltration

Infiltrates are perivascular and may be limited to the dermis and subcutaneous tissue without epidermotropism.

Cytomorphology

Hematopoietic cells of different lineages and admixture could be seen. These include myeloid precursor cells in several stages of maturation, nucleated erythroid precursors, and mature megakaryocytes (Haniffa et al. 2006) (see Fig. 16.1). The presence of pure myeloid or erythroid precursors is rare, and in those cases with immature cells or blasts, a diagnosis of myeloid sarcoma should be ruled out (Mizoguchi et al. 1990).

Clinical Behavior

The prognosis in patients with nonhepatosplenic EMH is based on the underlying etiology. Hence, finding a cutaneous EMH should prompt a process for finding a systemic cause or even performing a bone marrow biopsy and a hematology consult. As a group, nonhepatosplenic EMH have

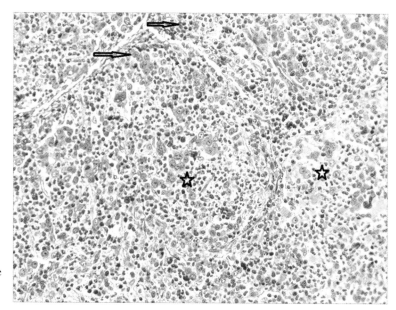

Fig 16.1 Extramedullary myeloid infiltrate in a child post-chemotherapy, (*arrows*) point to immature erythroid precursors and (*stars*) note the multinucleated megakaryocytes

poor outcome with the median survival of 13 months (Koch et al. 2003). Treatment is based on treating the underlying disorder, most commonly primary myelofibrosis.

Differential Diagnosis

CEMH is a type of infiltrative process in the "cutis" and is seen in patients with an underlying marrow disorder or even acute leukemia, and a bone marrow biopsy should be done in patients with isolated CEMH. Myeloid sarcoma with differentiated cells can also mimic CEMH, and immunohistochemistry for myeloid-monocytic markers such as CD43, lysozyme, CD68, and stem cell markers CD34 or CD117 may separate the immature from mature extramedullary hematopoiesis (Porcu et al. 1999). In general, a CD3-negative and CD43-positive immature single-field dermal infiltrate suggests a myeloid sarcoma instead of T-cell lymphoma.

Cutaneous Myelomonocytic Infiltrate in Patients with MDS/MPD

Introduction

Common myelomonocytic infiltrations under the generic nonspecific term "leukemia cutis" and more specifically myeloid sarcoma have been observed in patients with cutaneous lesions (List et al. 1991). Patients with an underlying myeloid disorder can develop specific (clonal, malignant) or nonspecific (reactive, benign) cutaneous lesions (Bluefarb and Webster 1953; Wong et al. 1995). Lesions that are specific are those in which the skin is involved by myelomonocytic leukemic cells and show histological changes compatible with leukemia cutis (LC). Nonspecific lesions include leukemoid reactions that may be due to bacterial, viral, and fungal infections secondary to immunosuppression or a hemorrhagic diathesis resulting in petechiae or purpura (Wong et al. 1995). Another subset of patients can developed

neutrophilic infiltrates of the skin such as seen in pyoderma gangrenosum, bullous pyoderma, and Sweet's syndrome (Burton 1980) (see Chap. 15 *for discussion on pyoderma gangrenosum and Sweet's syndrome*). This chapter focuses the discussion on LC.

Definition

Cutaneous infiltrates that have similar histopathologic findings to the clonal underlying hematopoietic disorder are characterized as leukemia cutis (LC). LC is a clinical term applied to tumors in skin associated with underlying primary bone marrow neoplasms which could include mature and immature leukemia such as chronic lymphocytic leukemia, precursor lymphoblastic/leukemia, and acute to chronic myelomonocytic leukemia (Su 1994; Kumar 1997; Burns et al. 2005; Kaune et al. 2009; Lee et al. 2010; Wagner et al. 2012). LC discussion in this section is limited to those infiltrates that are histopathologically of myelomonocytic in origin.

Epidemiology

LC has been well described in patients with acute myelogenous leukemia but has rarely been associated with MDS or MPD. In one series of 44 cases of LC, 41 cases were related to myeloid leukemia and 2 to MDS, and 1 was related to polycythemia vera (Wong et al. 1995).

Clinical Appearance of Cutaneous Lesions

Lesions can be located anywhere on the body and can appear as either solitary or multiple purpuric papules or plaques. They can also be ulcerated or non-ulcerated nodules or subcutaneous masses. The most common anatomical location is the lower extremities, followed by the upper extremities, back, trunk, and face (Paydas and Zorludemir 2000).

Pattern of Infiltration

Dense and diffuse cellular infiltrate occupying the dermis and extending into the subcutaneous tissue is seen (Wong et al. 1995). In 18 of 44 cases of nonlymphocytic leukemias (mostly acute myeloid leukemia, two MDS, and a polycythemia vera), sparing of the grenz zone was observed. Infiltration of the nerves as well as the hair follicles, sebaceous glands, sweat glands, and vessels with a prominent "Indian filing"; perivascular targetoid pattern; or single-cell filing pattern of immature blast forms was also seen. Some infiltrates also involved exclusively the subcutaneous fat. Less common patterns include kaposiform-like and neutrophilic infiltrates with scattered blasts (8 of 52 cases), and atypical immature myeloid cells with a predominately perivascular pattern with associated MDS (Wong et al. 1995).

Cytomorphology

Morphology is similar to the primary myeloid neoplasm and shows dysplastic cells in those with an underlying myelodysplastic syndrome or myeloproliferative syndrome. At higher power, these cells can show variable cytological differentiation and marked pleomorphism and can stain positive for chloroacetate esterase or Leder stain if myelomonocytic in origin. Periodic acid-Schiff (PAS) stains most lymphoblasts in a dot pattern.

Depending on tumor cell differentiation, a blastic (undifferentiated) or maturing (differentiated) morphology could be seen. Blastic pattern shows monomorphous infiltrate of blasts. Neoplastic, neutrophilic, or eosinophilic precursors could be seen in differentiated forms (see Fig. 16.2a). Round myeloblasts admixed with myelocytes with nuclear folds are the rule in acute myeloid leukemia and in chronic myeloid leukemia (CML) and other myeloproliferative/MDS disorders. The morphologic hallmark is a maturing leukemic cellular pattern of myeloblasts, eosinophilic myelocytes, bands, and neutrophils that mimic the marrow appearance of CML. In acute monocytic leukemia, deeply folded grooved or kidney-shaped vesicular nuclei, positive for nonspecific esterase but negative for Leder stain, are the typical picture.

Immunophenotype

Immunophenotypical markers corresponding to the primary underlying myeloid neoplasm are observed. Most myeloid sarcoma should stain with CD43, lysozyme, and myeloperoxidase (MPO). MPO staining may be absent in monocytic LC (Cho-Vega et al. 2008).

Cytogenetic/Molecular Findings

LC is seen commonly in patients with acute myeloid leukemia with trisomy of chromosome 8 (Sen et al. 2000; Agis et al. 2002; Pileri et al. 2007). Tetrasomy and pentasomy of chromosome 8 have been reported as well (Ferrara et al. 1996; Gould et al. 2000).

Clinical Behavior

Patients with LC follow a clinical course similar to that of the underlying disease.

Differential Diagnosis

Myeloid sarcoma and Langerhans cell histiocytosis should be ruled out in patients with LC. Myeloid sarcoma can present as a type of leukemia cutis but can be differentiated from mature lymphocytic and lymphoblastic forms based on morphology, clinical history, and immunohistochemical profiling (see text on myeloid sarcoma). Most precursor B lymphoblasts should stain with CD79a, TDT, or CD10 with precursor T blast staining with cytoplasmic CD3 instead. Mature lymphocytic leukemia will mark with corresponding markers for chronic lymphocytic leukemia/lymphoma (CLL): CD23, CD5, and CD20 (see Fig. 16.2b).

Fig. 16.2 (**a**) Myeloid sarcoma from a patient with a myeloproliferative neoplasm with eosinophilic differentiation. Note the cytoplasmic eosinophilic granules in some dysplastic eosinophils and immature cells. (**b**) Chronic lymphocytic leukemia/lymphoma involving skin with prolymphocytes (*inset*) CD20 (*inset2*) CD5 and (**c**) CD23 positivity

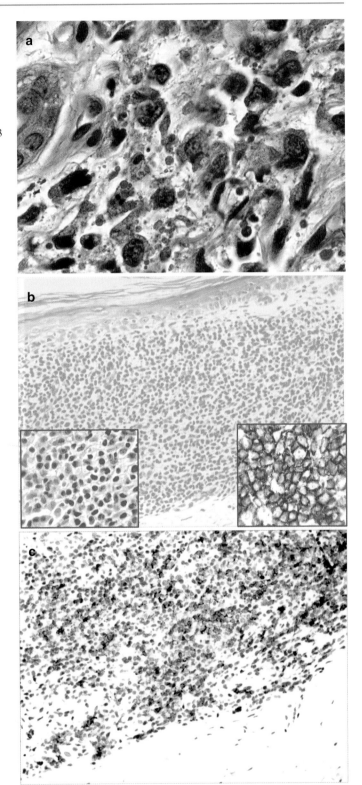

Myeloid or Granulocytic Sarcoma

The skin is one of the most common sites of involvement of myeloid sarcoma (MS). The mechanism by which myeloid blasts migrate to the skin is poorly understood, but it may be due to the expression of chemokine receptors and adhesion molecules by the blasts and the various cell types residing in the skin (Cho-Vega et al. 2008).

Definition

A myeloid sarcoma is by definition a tumor mass that is composed of myeloid blasts with or without maturation occurring at any anatomical site other than the bone marrow and resulting in an effacement of underlying tissue architecture. The lesion was first described by Burns in 1811 (Burns 1811). In 1853 the term "chloroma" was given to the lesion because such tumors often display a greenish color that fades on exposure to air due to the presence of myeloperoxidase (King 1853). MS is also known as a granulocytic sarcoma, chloroma, or extramedullary myeloid cell tumor (Rappaport 1966). MS is included in the 2008 WHO classification of myeloid neoplasm as distinct manifestation of acute myeloid leukemia (Swerdlow et al.2008). Patients with known myeloid leukemia infiltrates of any site of the body by myeloid blasts are not classified as MS unless the tumor effaces the tissue architecture. Skin, lymph node, gastrointestinal tract, bone, soft tissue, and testis are the most frequently affected sites (Falini et al. 2007; Pileri et al. 2007). Rarely, multiple anatomical sites are affected in a single patient.

Epidemiology

MS has been reported in 2.5–9.1 % of patients with AML and can occur concomitantly, following, or prior to systemic bone marrow leukemia (Wiernik and Serpick 1970; Liu et al. 1973; Krause 1979; Neiman et al. 1981). Males are more affected than females with a ratio of 1.2:1. Median age is 56 years but is also seen in older patients (Falini et al. 2007; Pileri et al. 2007; Hurley et al. 2013). In one series of 61 biopsied cases, 13 had skin involvement (Neiman et al. 1981). Incidence of MS after allogeneic hematopoietic cell transplantation has been reported to be 0.2–1.3 % with poor overall survival (Bekassy et al. 1996; Szomor et al. 1997).

Clinical Appearance of Cutaneous Lesions

Multiple skin lesions such as papules, plaques, and/or nodules are commonly described. The torso is more commonly involved, but one study did favor the involvement of the upper body (Hurley et al. 2013).

Pattern of Infiltration

Pleomorphic blasts are seen in the dermis and subcutaneous tissue.

Cytomorphology

Blasts are identifiable by their immature cytomorphology with dispersed nuclear chromatin with nucleoli and abundant mitotic activity with scattered apoptotic cells (Liu et al. 1973; Krause 1979; Neiman et al. 1981; Eshghabadi et al. 1986; Meis et al. 1986). Eosinophilic myelocytes can also been seen (Lin et al. 1990). Myelomonocytic or pure monoblastic morphology can be seen (Falini et al. 2007; Pileri et al. 2007) (see Fig. 16.3).

Immunophenotype

CD68/KP1 is the most commonly expressed marker followed by MPO, CD117, CD99, lysozyme, CD34, TdT, CD56, CD61, CD30, and CD4 (Pileri et al. 2007). In one series lysozyme was positive in all cases, with myeloperoxidase in 56 %, CD68 in 100 %, and CD34 in 19 % of patients (Hurley et al. 2013). Cases can

Fig. 16.3 Myeloid sarcoma without differentiation (blastic form). Note the atypical blasts with open vesicular and dispersed chromatin

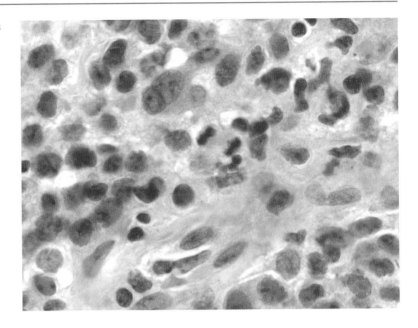

demonstrate aberrant expression of T- or B-cell lineages which can lead to an erroneous diagnosis (Hanson et al. 1993).

Cytogenetic/Molecular Findings

Chromosomal aberrations by FISH or cytogenetics are detectable in 55 % of cases (Pileri et al. 2007). Monosomy 7; *MLL* (myeloid/lymphoid or mixed-lineage leukemia) rearrangement; trisomy 4; monosomy 16, 16q, 5q, and 20q; and trisomy 11 are some of the reported abnormalities (Pileri et al. 2007). Trisomy of chromosome 8 and inversion 16 are more common in MS involving the skin (Dachary et al. 1986; Cronin et al. 2009; Hurley et al. 2013). *NPM1* mutations are seen in 16 % of cases (Falini et al. 2005, 2007).

Clinical Behavior

Prognosis is poor in patients with MS. MS is considered an equivalent of a diagnosis of acute myeloid leukemia and should be treated with induction chemotherapy (Eshghabadi et al. 1986; Lin et al. 1990). Allogeneic hematopoietic cell transplantation carries a higher probability of

prolonged survival or cure (Breccia et al. 2004; Pileri et al. 2007). Radiation therapy can be useful in emergency or palliative settings (Bakst et al. 2012).

Differential Diagnosis

T- and B-cell malignancies especially non-Hodgkin lymphoma can be differentiated by cytomorphology and immunohistochemistry (46 % of cases in one series) (Byrd et al. 1995). Lymphoblastic leukemia, melanoma, Ewing's sarcoma, blastic plasmacytoid dendritic cell neoplasm (see section on BPDCN below), and immature EMH should be considered as well (Ngu et al. 2001).

Blastic Plasmacytoid Dendritic Cell Neoplasm (BPDCN)

Definition

BPDCN is an aggressive tumor derived from the precursors of plasmacytoid dendritic cells. BPDCNs have myeloid ancestors in common with monocytes and are found in the bone marrow and skin (Liu et al. 2009). BPDCN was previously known as blastic NK-cell lymphoma, CD4 + CD56+ hematodermic neoplasm, and plasmacytic dendritic cell leukemia, making it difficult to track historically (Lim et al. 2013). Cutaneous findings are seen universally in BPDCN and 50 % of patients present with isolated cutaneous lesions (Cota et al. 2010).

Epidemiology

BPDCN is a very rare neoplasm representing approximately 0.8 % of the primary cutaneous lymphomas (Petrella and Facchetti 2010). There is a 3.3:1 male/female ratio with most patients being elderly with a mean age at diagnosis of 61 years. Though it usually occurs in the elderly, it can occur in children and has been reported in patients as young as 8 years of age (Lim et al. 2013). There is no increased incidence in any one ethnic group (Feuillard et al. 2002; Jacob et al. 2003; Herling and Jones 2007).

Clinical Appearance of Cutaneous Lesions

Patients usually present with asymptomatic brownish to violaceous nodules, plaques, or bruise-like areas which can be solitary or in multiple locations on the skin (Feuillard et al. 2002; Julia et al. 2013; Lim et al. 2013). In one study 73 % of patients had nodular lesions only and 12 % had bruise-like patches, while 15 % had disseminated and mixed lesions (Julia et al. 2013). Twenty percent of patients will have regional lymphadenopathy (Lim et al. 2013).

Pattern of Infiltration

BPDCN is characterized by a diffuse, monomorphous infiltrate of medium-sized blast cells with irregular nuclei, fine chromatin, and one to several small nucleoli. Tumor cells occupy the dermis and spare the epidermis but will eventually invade the subcutaneous fat (Petrella et al. 1999, 2005; Cota et al. 2010).

Cytomorphology

A plasmacytoid cytological appearance is seen in medium- to high-power view, but these cells usually lack a perinuclear hof of true plasma cells (see Fig. 16.4). The cells are derived from plasmacytoid dendritic cells, an antigen presenting cell, resident in skin and lymph nodes. Cytoplasm is usually scant to moderate, may be eccentric, and appears gray blue and agranular on Giemsa stain. Mitoses are rarely prominent and angioinvasion is rare. BPDCN is negative with nonspecific esterase and myeloperoxidase cytochemical stains.

Immunophenotype

BPDCN cells are positive for CD4, CD56, CD123, and TCL1 (Tecchio et al. 2009; Cota et al. 2010). Rarely CD56 can be negative, but if CD4, CD123, and TCL1 are present, this does not exclude the diagnosis. Occasionally CD7, CD33, CD43, CD45RA, TL1-A, and HLA-DR can be positive. Most tumors lack conventional myeloid and lymphoid T- and B-cell antigens (Petrella et al. 1999, 2002; Herling et al. 2003; Petrella et al. 2004, 2005; Reichard et al. 2005; Willemze et al. 2005; Assaf et al. 2007; Herling and Jones 2007; Pilichowska et al. 2007; Garnache-Ottou et al. 2009). Newer markers that can be diagnostic include CD2AP (Marafioti et al. 2008), BDCA-2 (CD303), and BDCA-4 (CD304) (Garnache-Ottou et al. 2009). CD68 is expressed in 50 % of cases as small cytoplasmic dots (Petrella et al. 2004, 2005).

Cytogenetic/Molecular Findings

Cytogenetic analysis often shows a complex karyotype (Feuillard et al. 2002; Petrella et al. 2005; Herling and Jones 2007; Ascani et al. 2008; Garnache-Ottou et al. 2009) or deletions of tumor suppressor genes in the majority of cases (Jardin et al. 2009). Genomic losses affecting 5q21 or 5q34, 12p13, 13q21, 6q23, 15q, and chromosome 9 have been reported (Petrella et al.

Fig. 16.4 Blastic plasmacytoid dendritic cell leukemia involving the skin. (**a**) Subepidermal plasmacytoid blasts with single-cell pattern. (**b**) Targetoid perivascular pattern

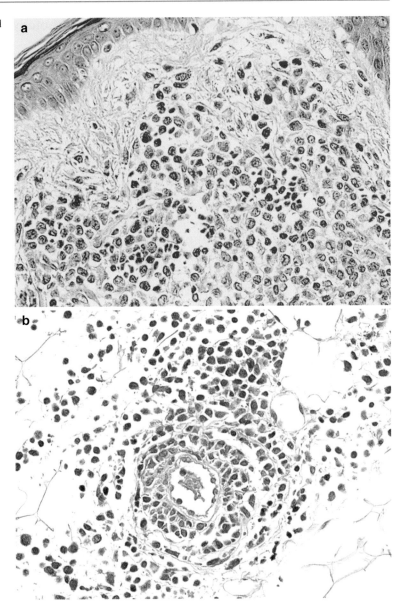

1999; Leroux et al. 2002; Reichard et al. 2005; Guo et al. 2011; Lucioni et al. 2011; Julia et al. 2013). A recent study suggested that a mutation of *CDKN2A/CDKN2B* on chromosome 9 could help identify more aggressive cases (Lucioni et al. 2011). One study showed that IgH and TCR-gamma gene rearrangement analysis done in 34 biopsies from 27 patients showed a polyclonal smear in all cases (Cota et al. 2010).

Clinical Behavior

The majority of patients present with asymptomatic solitary or multiple skin lesions usually with nodules and plaques. Low-level bone marrow involvement is often seen at presentation or soon after (Feuillard et al. 2002; Herling and Jones 2007; Ascani et al. 2008; Garnache-Ottou et al. 2009). Leukemic dissemination is part of the natural progression of the disease and can be present before, at the same time with, or after skin lesions (Julia et al. 2013). In one series 61 % of patients had bone marrow, lymph node, and/or blood involvement (Julia et al. 2013). Lymphadenopathy and/or splenomegaly are common. Overall prognosis is poor with medial overall survival duration of 12–14 months (Feuillard et al. 2002; Lim et al. 2013). Increased age predicts a worse prognosis. Patients with skin involvement only have initially less aggressive course and can benefit from skin-directed therapy or steroids (Pileri et al. 2012). This approach is especially useful in older patients or younger patients with multiple comorbidities who are not eligible for systemic intensive chemotherapy or allogeneic stem cell transplant. Treatment with radiation therapy and chemotherapy has been used with varying success in patients with BPDCN. Radiation therapy can achieve a complete response in 80 % of patients with localized disease but is associated with a short time to relapse, with a mean of 5.5 months (Dalle et al. 2010). Combined chemotherapy regimens have been given with varying success including cyclophosphamide, doxorubicin, vincristine, prednisone (CHOP-like), or cytarabine-based treatments. Complete responses have been documented in 50–75 % of patients, but relapses usually occur within months and chemotherapy resistance develops (Ng et al. 2006; Dalle et al. 2010). Recently, the incorporation of L-asparaginase in chemotherapy regimen showed promising results (Gruson et al. 2013). Skin findings are almost always present at relapse. In elderly patients who are not a candidate for systemic therapy, skin lesions can respond to monotherapy with steroids. Allogeneic stem cell transplantation is the only known curative approach with mean survival of 31 months. It should be considered in younger patients who achieve complete remission with induction chemotherapy (Reimer et al. 2003; Dalle et al. 2010).

Differential Diagnosis

Skin localizations of myelomonocytic disorders and MS would have overlapping immunohisto-

logic findings, but a CD56, CD4, and CD123 positive blastic skin leukemic infiltrate with plasmacytoid cytomorphology would favor a BPDCN. Extranodal natural killer/T-cell nasal-type tumors and PTCL-unspecified and pleomorphic T-cell lymphomas can be ruled out with immunohistochemistry and cytomorphology with EBV + favoring extranodal NK cell and T cells that are CD30- and CD68-negative T-cell infiltrate, favoring the two latter entities (Petrella et al. 2005).

Interdigitating Dendritic Cell Sarcoma (IDCS)

Definition

Interdigitating dendritic cells present antigens to T cells and regulate cellular immune response (Steinman et al. 1997; Imai et al. 1998; Steinman 2003; Chung et al. 2004; Maeda et al. 2005; Saygin et al. 2013). These cells originate from hematopoietic precursors through the conversion of Langerhans cells as they travel to the lymph node and from the differentiation of myeloid and lymphoid precursor cells (Wood et al. 1985; Rosenzweig et al. 1996; Steinman et al. 1997; Wu and Liu 2007; Saygin et al. 2013). IDCS is a malignant disorder of interdigitating dendritic cells.

Epidemiology

IDCS is an extremely rare disease and skin involvement has rarely been reported. In a large pooled analysis of a total of 462 cases of dendritic cell sarcomas, there were 100 cases of IDCS with seven having skin findings (Saygin et al. 2013). Median age at diagnosis in this pooled analysis was 56.5 years (range 21 months to 88 years) with an M/F ratio of 1.38:1 (Saygin et al. 2013). A clonal relationship between IDCS and low-grade B-cell lymphomas has been reported in patients with both diseases (Feldman et al. 2008; Fraser et al. 2009; Shao et al. 2011). IDCS has been reported following the use of calcineurin inhibitors, and this may be due to their effect by dampening the responses of T cells to which IDCs present antigens (Gordon et al. 2007; Wu et al. 2010; Saygin et al. 2013).

Clinical Appearance of Cutaneous Lesions

Most lesions are asymptomatic and are nodular in nature. Nodules can be erythematous or brownish but not ulcerative. These lesions can occur anywhere and can appear in crops (Hui et al. 1987; Lee et al. 2009).

Pattern of Infiltration

IDCS usually is found throughout the dermis but spares the epidermis. The tumor can invade the subcutaneous tissue and can be seen in a fascicular pattern forming intertwining bundles (Hui et al. 1987; Lee et al. 2009).

Cytomorphology

Large spindle to ovoid cells are seen forming whorls. Cells have coarse nuclear chromatin with moderate to abundant cytoplasm resembling histiocytes albeit with indistinct borders (Ylagan et al. 2003). Small lymphocytes intermingling with the large histiocytic cell population is a key diagnostic feature that is less typical of carcinomas and sarcomas (Ylagan et al. 2003). In one series lymphoplasmacytic infiltration was seen in 63 % of tumors and rarely epithelioid cells were seen (7 %) (Saygin et al. 2013).

Immunophenotype

Cells are S100 positive and CD45 positive and have variable CD68 positivity (Gaertner et al.

2001; Pileri et al. 2002). Some IDCS are vimentin, HLA-DR, and fascin positive (Maeda et al. 2005). Lysozyme can also be positive (Gaertner et al. 2001). CD21 and CD35 will be negative (Ylagan et al. 2003). B-cell markers such as CD20 and T-cell markers such as CD3 and CD5 are usually negative. Cytokeratin, myeloperoxidase, CD1a, CD21, CD23, CD30, CD35, CD21, CD34, CD79a, BCL-2, and BCL-6 should all be negative (Gaertner et al. 2001; Pileri et al. 2002, 2007; Jiang et al. 2013). ATPase can be strongly positive in some cases (Turner et al. 1984; Fonseca et al. 1998). Birbeck granules are not seen on ultrastructure examination (Gaertner et al. 2001; Pileri et al. 2002).

Cytogenetic/Molecular Findings

Immunoglobulin and T-cell receptor genes are in a germ line configuration (Weiss et al. 1990).

Clinical Behavior

Prognosis is poor in cases of disseminated disease, and about half the patients will die of their disease. In the pooled analysis of 100 cases of IDCS, the median survival for patients with metastatic disease was 9 months, but cases with local disease did not reach median and 2-year survival rates (Saygin et al. 2013). In patients with localized disease, there was no difference in the overall survival between surgery and nonsurgical modalities such as radiation therapy (Saygin et al. 2013). In the metastatic setting, combined chemotherapy such as CHOP, ICE, and ABVD was most commonly used in patients with IDCS (Saygin et al. 2013). In metastatic IDCS, there was a statistical trend ($P=0.1$) toward improved overall survival in those patients who received surgery, and these authors recommended surgery with adjuvant chemotherapy (Saygin et al. 2013).

Differential Diagnosis

Inflammatory pseudotumors typically show no histological atypia and are seen in patients with fever and other constitutional symptoms. Hodgkin lymphoma, which is remarkably rare in skin, and non-Hodgkin lymphoma may be considered if fibrosis is present inducing a pseudospindle morphology (Jayaram and Abdul Rahman 1997; Fonseca et al. 1998; Mohanty et al. 2003; Pillay et al. 2004). Langerhans cell sarcomas and other sarcomas such as peripheral nerve sheath tumors should be ruled out (Ylagan et al. 2003). Intranodal myofibroblastoma, true histiocytic lymphomas, melanomas, and anaplastic large-cell lymphomas are also considerations if spindle and anaplastic pattern is prominent (Fonseca et al. 1998).

Follicular Dendritic Cell Sarcoma (FDCS)

Definition

Follicular dendritic cells (FDC) present and retain antigens for B cells and stimulate B-cell proliferation and differentiation while having complex interactions with T cells (Tew et al. 1990; Wu et al. 1996; Fonseca et al. 1998). They are of mesenchymal origin. FDCS is a malignant expansion of FDC. FDCS usually presents as lymphadenopathy in the majority of cases but can present in a wide variety of extra nodal sites including the skin. In a large pooled analysis including 462 cases, 343 had FDCS and two of these had skin findings (Saygin et al. 2013).

Epidemiology

There is a wide age range with an adult predominance and a mean age of 44 years (Pileri et al. 2002; Nguyen et al. 2005). There is a female predominance for the inflammatory pseudotumor variant (Cheuk et al. 2001; Pileri et al. 2002; Vargas et al. 2002). FDCS can occur in association with Castleman disease usually in the hyaline vascular type (Chan et al. 1994). The inflammatory pseudotumor-like variant is associated with Epstein-Barr virus (EBV) (Arber et al. 1998). There may be an association between FDCS and autoimmunity with paraneoplastic pemphigus and myasthenia gravis seen in cases of FDCS (Lee et al. 1999; Wang et al. 2005; Meijs et al. 2008; Saygin et al. 2013).

Clinical Appearance of Cutaneous Lesions

Lesions can appear as subcutaneous nodules (Kazakov et al. 2005). In patients with FDCS, a paraneoplastic pemphigus can also occur and resembles ulcerations on the skin or mucosal surfaces, erythematous patches, or lichen planus.

Pattern of Infiltration

FDCS invading the tissue presents as spindle-shaped infiltrates in the dermis that may extend into the subcutaneous or even muscle but spares the epidermis (Kazakov et al. 2005).

Cytomorphology

Spindled to ovoid cells forming fascicles, whorls, diffuse sheets, or nodules are characteristic. Individual cells generally show indistinct cell borders and a moderate amount of eosinophilic cytoplasm. Nuclei are oval or elongated and finely dispersed chromatin. Nuclear pseudo-inclusions are common and binucleated and multinucleated tumor cells are seen (2008). On electron microscopy, the long cytoplasmic projections and desmosomal junctions are seen, while Birbeck granules and numerous lysosomes are not seen (Fonseca et al. 1998).

Fig. 16.5 Follicular dendritic cell sarcoma (FDCS) with CD21 + CD35+ (*inset*) histiocytes

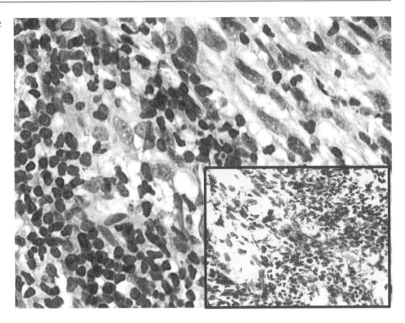

Lymphoplasmacytic infiltration is frequently present in greater than 90 % of cases (Saygin et al. 2013). Rarely, Reed-Sternberg-like cells can lead to a mistaken diagnosis of Hodgkin disease (Mohanty et al. 2003) (see Fig. 16.5).

Immunophenotype

CD21, CD35, R4/23, Ki-FDC1p, and KiM4 are positive in FDCS (Chan et al. 1997; Fonseca et al. 1998; Ylagan et al. 2003). There is variable expression of CD68. Clusterin is strongly positive but is negative or weakly positive in other dendritic cell tumors (Grogg et al. 2004, 2005). Desmoplakin, vimentin, fascin, epidermal growth factor receptor (EGFR), CD45, and HLA-DR can be variable (Chan and Chan 1997; Fonseca et al. 1998; Sun et al. 2003; Ylagan et al. 2003).

Cytogenetic/Molecular Findings

Immunoglobulin and T-cell receptor genes are germ line configuration (Weiss et al. 1990). There is very limited data on genetic changes seen in patients with FDCS (Sander et al. 2007).

Clinical Behavior

Not much is known about skin-specific findings or clinical behavior because of the rarity of this disease in the skin. The most frequent location of lymphadenopathy is cervical and intra-abdominal and about half of patients will present with a local mass (Saygin et al. 2013). FDCS has a fairly benign course with median survival for local disease was 168 months (range 2–360 months). Risk of local recurrence and distant metastasis is around 27–28 % (Saygin et al. 2013). Larger tumor size (≥6 cm), presence of coagulative necrosis, high mitotic count (≥5 per 10 high-power fields), and cytological atypia are associated with poor prognosis (Chan et al. 1997; Shia et al. 2006; Saygin et al. 2013). Surgery is the mainstay of treatment for FDCS. Adjuvant therapy for fully resected patients is unclear. A pooled analysis showed no benefit of adjuvant radiation therapy (Saygin et al. 2013). This analysis did show that in the metastatic setting, treatment with combined adjuvant chemotherapy and radiotherapy ($n=23$) only resulted in two deaths due to disease showing the importance of adjuvant treatment in advanced FDCS. Regimens designed for the management of aggressive lymphomas such as

CHOP (cyclophosphamide, vincristine, doxorubicin, prednisone), ICE (ifosfamide, carboplatin, etoposide), and ABVD (adriamycin, bleomycin, vincristine, dacarbazine) have been tried with variable success (Saygin et al. 2013).

Differential Diagnosis

FDCS has the same differential diagnosis as IDCS. This includes ruling out inflammatory pseudotumors, histiocytic lymphomas, melanomas, Langerhans cell sarcomas, other sarcomas such as peripheral nerve sheath tumors (Ylagan et al. 2003), ALCL, IDCS, Hodgkin disease, intranodal myofibroblastoma, and NHL (Jayaram and Abdul Rahman 1997; Fonseca et al. 1998; Mohanty et al. 2003; Pillay et al. 2004).

Cutaneous Langerhans Cell Histiocytosis

Definition

Langerhans cell histiocytosis (LCH) represents a clonal accumulation of Langerhans cells that are a cutaneous antigen presenting cells (Newman et al. 2007). After being triggered by a new antigen, the LC migrates to the regional lymph nodes and activates antigen-specific T cells that return to the skin (Romani et al. 2003). Cutaneous lesions are present in one third of patients. In the Hashimoto-Pritzker disease, also known as congenital, self-healing reticulohistiocytosis, disease is limited to the skin and resolves rapidly over a period of weeks (Divaris et al. 1991). This is a rare disease and is more commonly seen in children than adults.

Epidemiology

Incidence is 5 per million populations per year with most cases occurring in childhood. There is a predilection for males (Pileri et al. 2002;

Salotti et al. 2009). The WHO states that the disease is more common in northern European descent patients and rare in blacks (2008). LCH usually presents with either unifocal or multifocal bone disease or as a multisystem disease. LCH has been associated with Epstein-Barr virus, malaria, and leukemias (Newman et al. 2007). In a large series of 314 patients diagnosed between 1946 and 1996, the median age at diagnosis was 24.5 years (Howarth et al. 1999). Isolated skin findings were seen in 14 patients of this series. There are disease processes that include LCH. Letterer-Siwe disease usually presents in the first 2 years of life and is the acute disseminated form of LCH (Newman et al. 2007). Hand-Schuller-Christian disease is a chronic multisystem disease seen in older children and consists of the classic triad of bone disease, diabetes insipidus, and exophthalmos (Gianotti and Caputo 1985). Eosinophilic granuloma of bone is a common manifestation of LCH in adults. The most frequent anatomical sites of LCH in adults were the lung (62 %), bone (50 %), and skin (15 %). One-third of patients developed multiple organ involvement (Gotz and Fichter 2004).

In contrast to acute illness observed in children, LCH in adults has usually more chronic course.

Clinical Appearance of Cutaneous Lesions

Patients with Letterer-Siwe disease have extensive cutaneous lesions and classically resemble seborrheic dermatitis with involvement of the scalp, face, trunk, and perineum (Zachary and MacDonald 1983). Hand-Schuller-Christian disease has papulonodular, granulomatous, or seborrheic dermatitis-like lesions (Zachary and MacDonald 1983). In Hashimoto-Pritzker disease, lesions are seen at birth and are widespread reddish-brown nodules that regress (Divaris et al. 1991). LCH can also present with papules, pustules, vesicles, petechiae, or purpura (Zachary and MacDonald 1983; Stein et al. 2001; Park et al. 2012).

Fig. 16.6 Langerhans cell histiocytosis with eosinophilic neoplastic cells, some with grooved nuclei positive for CD1a and S100

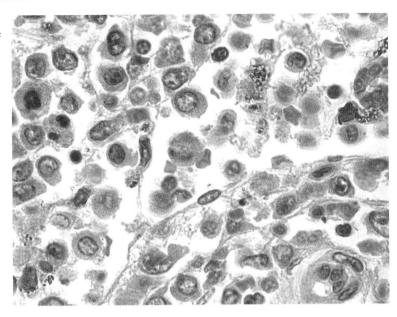

Pattern of Infiltration

Dermal infiltrate of large epithelioid cells with abundant eosinophilic cytoplasm and indented or reniform nuclei (Hashimoto and Pritzker 1973).

Cytomorphology

Oval cells about 10–15 μm in size with grooved, folded, or indented or lobulated nuclei with fine chromatin are seen (2008) (WHO) (see Fig. 16.6). Placental alkaline phosphatase can be used in archival material to evaluate for LCH (Newman et al. 2007). Eosinophils are scattered throughout the infiltrate and the epidermis is free of infiltrating cells (Hashimoto and Pritzker 1973). Letterer-Siwe disease has infiltrates that are composed largely of LCs with scattered lymphocytes, eosinophils, and occasional neutrophils (Wells 1979). In Hand-Schuller-Christian disease, there is a prominent granulomatous reaction made of aggregates of histiocytes and rarely cells with xanthomatous changes (Altman and Winkelmann 1963). In Hand-Schuller-Christian disease, clusters of eosinophils are prominent

and there are occasional multinucleated giant cells (Risdall et al. 1983). Birbeck granules which have a tennis racquet shape and zipper-like appearance are present in 0–40 % of cells by electron microscopy (Zunino-Goutorbe et al. 2008). An ultrastructural finding that has been proposed to be specific for congenital self-healing reticulohistiocytosis (CSHR) is the presence of concentrically laminated dense-core bodies in the same cells that contain Birbeck granules (Hashimoto et al. 1984).

Immunophenotype

LCH stain positive for S-100 protein, CD1a, CD45, and CD101. CD1a staining is specific for LCH (Newman et al. 2007). CD68 staining can be positive (Wheller et al. 2013). Langerin (CD207) is also specific for LCH (Chikwava and Jaffe 2004; Lau et al. 2008). Placental alkaline phosphatase can be used in archival material to evaluate for LCH (Newman et al. 2007). LCH do not express CD34 or MS-1 (a marker for dendritic perivascular macrophages that are found in non-LCD histiocytosis) (Goerdt et al. 1993).

Cytogenetics/Molecular Findings

LCH has been shown to be clonal by X-linked androgen receptor gene assay (HUMARA) (Willman et al. 1994; Yu et al. 1994; Yousem et al. 2001). No consistent molecular genetic defect has been identified (Murakami et al. 2002). Recently, recurrent BRAF V600E somatic mutation was identified in 35 of 61 patients (57 %) with LCH (Badalian-Very et al. 2010).

Clinical Behavior

Self-limited LCH should be distinguished from other forms of LCH because disseminated disease has a worse prognosis and requires an aggressive therapy such as chemotherapy. Thorough investigation and follow-up of patients with LCH should be performed because clinically, histopathologically, and immunohistochemically, one cannot determine those individuals with more aggressive disease (Kapur et al. 2007; Wheller et al. 2013). In self-limited disease, one group suggests a follow-up period of 2 years including laboratory tests and radiographs (abdominal ultrasound and chest x-ray) (Zunino-Goutorbe et al. 2008). LCH can lead to diabetes insipidus due to infiltration and scarring in the hypothalamic pituitary area or due to an autoimmune process with antibodies to vasopressin (Dunger et al. 1989; Grois et al. 1995, 2006). The most important risk factor for developing DI in patients with LCH was multisystem disease (Grois et al. 2006). Self-limited disease of the skin can be treated with topical nitrogen mustard (Wong et al. 1986; Munn and Chu 1998; Stein et al. 2001), psoralen plus ultraviolet A (PUVA) phototherapy (Munn and Chu 1998; Stein et al. 2001), imiquimod (Taverna et al. 2006), excimer laser (Vogel et al. 2008), and radiation therapy (Lichtenwald et al. 1991). Though most patients are initially treated with corticosteroids, thalidomide (Imanaka et al. 2004; Park et al. 2012), and etoposide have the best results for patients with widespread cutaneous disease (Munn and Chu 1998; McClain 2005; McClain and Kozinetz 2007; Gadner et al. 2008; Park et al. 2012).

Agents such as methotrexate, cyclophosphamide, cyclosporine, 6-mercaptopurine, and vinblastine have also been reported to work (McLelland et al. 1990; Munn and Chu 1998; Stockschlaeder and Sucker 2006; Park et al. 2012). Current treatment should be based on the Histiocyte Society evaluation and treatment guidelines with current recommendations for treatment of all categories, excluding single-system disease to be systemic therapy (Minkov et al. 2009; French Histiocytosis Society 1996). Currently, for systemic involvement, prednisone and vinblastine for 12 months are the recommended treatment (Gadner et al. 2008; Minkov et al. 2009; Gadner et al. 2013). One year of therapy was proven to decrease recurrence when compared to six cycles (Gadner et al. 2013). Progressive disease or recurrence should be treated with 2-chlorodeoxyadenosine and cytarabine (Bernard et al. 2005). Stem cell transplantation should be considered in these patients (Steiner et al. 2005). This disease can affect the skin or other organs. Recent case series has suggested that an inhibitor of mutated BRAF (vemurafenib) could be a novel promising targeted therapy for patients with LCH carrying V600E mutation (Haroche et al. 2013).

Differential Diagnosis

LCH can be mistaken for disorders that cause Langerhans cell hyperplasia such as scabies, contact dermatitis, indeterminate dendritic cell infiltrates, pityriasis lichenoides et varioliformis acuta, and different T-cell lymphoproliferative disorders such as lymphomatoid papulosis, mycosis fungoides, parapsoriasis, or cutaneous T-cell hyperplasia (Christie et al. 2006; Pigozzi et al. 2006; Bhattacharjee and Glusac 2007; Drut et al. 2010). Since it can involve the skeleton in adults, it can be confused for multiple myeloma (Malpas 1998).

Dermal Dendrocytic Infiltrates

Definition

Dermal dendrocytes encompass a double population of dermal-resident cells that include

CD34+ cells and factor XIIIa-positive cells. These two cell types have different resident sites and function (Sontheimer et al. 1989; Hoyo et al. 1993; Narvaez et al. 1996; Drut 2007). CD34 also labels dermal dendrocytes, with an overlapping immunoprofile with CD34 expression seen in cellular dermatofibroma. Lesions may harbor some cells expressing the alternative antigen though the majority do not (Goldblum and Tuthill 1997).

Epidemiology

Rare cases often mistaken for neurofibromas. Can present in infant and early childhood as hamartomas.

Clinical Appearance of Cutaneous Lesions

Well-circumscribed atrophic and wrinkled patch on the skin. These can look similar to a congenital melanocytic nevus or skin-colored papules (Cerio et al. 1989; Ohata and Kawahara 2002; Drut 2007).

Pattern of Infiltration

Dermal proliferation of fusiform cells. Epidermal atrophy can be seen.

Cytomorphology

Fusiform or spindle-shaped cells that are seen in the dermis. These can be arranged in several layers and around small vessels (Drut 2007).

Immunophenotype

The tumor cells are positive for CD34+ and factor XIIIa and are usually negative for S100 (Cerio et al. 1989; Hoyo et al. 1993; Narvaez et al. 1996; Goldblum and Tuthill 1997).

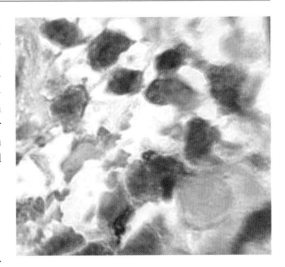

Fig. 16.7 Factor XIIIa positive dendrocytes

Clinical Behavior

These lesions are usually benign and do not require intensive treatment (see Fig. 16.7).

Differential Diagnosis

Neurofibroma, dermatofibrosarcoma protuberans, and giant-cell fibroblastoma should all be considered in the differential. Xanthomas and even indeterminate dendritic neoplasm can stain with Factox XIII and figures in the differential of immunstain results. Staining for factor XIIIa is the most sensitive test for dermal dendrocytic infiltrates (Cerio et al. 1989; Sontheimer et al. 1989; Gray et al. 1990; Hoyo et al. 1993; Narvaez et al. 1996; Goldblum and Tuthill 1997; Ohata and Kawahara 2002; Drut 2007).

Indeterminate Dendritic Cell Infiltrates

Definition

Indeterminate dendritic cell tumor, also known as indeterminate cell histiocytosis (ICH), is a neoplastic proliferation of normal dendritic accessory cells, usually found in the dermis. These cells should lack intracytoplasmic Birbeck granules but share morphologic and immunophenotypical features with Langerhans cells (Ferran et al. 2007). Since Langerhans cells lose their Birbeck granules when cultured and since some indeterminate cells migrate to the epidermis and may become Langerhans cells, some authors speculate that indeterminate cells may represent a mature form of Langerhans cells (Chu et al. 1982; Romani et al. 1989; Teunissen et al. 1990; Weiss et al. 2005).

Epidemiology

Indeterminate dendritic cell tumor is a very rare disorder and may be associated with low-grade B-cell lymphoma (Vasef et al. 1995).

Clinical Appearance of Cutaneous Lesions

Solitary or multiple asymptomatic maculopapular or papulo-nodular lesions (Rosenberg and Morgan 2001; Ferran et al. 2007). Most lesions are located on the trunk, face, neck, or extremities. Rarely, generalized distribution has been reported (Sidoroff et al. 1996).

Pattern of Infiltration

A diffuse infiltrate comprising of cells with irregular nuclear grooves and clefts that resemble Langerhans cells. Infiltration is seen in the dermis but may extend into the subcutaneous fat. The epidermis is spared (Rosenberg and Morgan 2001).

Cytomorphology

Cells resemble Langerhans cells with irregular nuclear grooves and clefts. Cytoplasm is abundant and eosinophilic. Multinucleated

giant cells may be seen and there may be spindling of some cells. Cytoplasm is abundant and is eosinophilic. These cells lack Birbeck granules. Desmosomes are lacking but the cells can have interdigitating cell processes (2008).

Immunophenotype

Indeterminate cells usually express S-100 and CD1a antigens but always lack Birbeck granules on ultrastructural exam (Ferran et al. 2007). Desmosomes are lacking but there can be complex interdigitating cell processes. These cells are negative for specific B- and T-cell markers, CD30, CD163, CD21, CD23, and CD35. There is variable positivity for CD45, CD68, lysozyme, and CD4 (Vener et al. 2007) (see Fig. 16.8).

Cytogenetic/Molecular Findings

One case was shown to be clonal by human androgen receptor gene assay (Vener et al. 2007).

Clinical Behavior

Disease is usually limited to the skin and extra cutaneous lesions and systemic symptoms are rare (Ferran et al. 2007). Etiology of this disorder remains unknown, but it has been postulated that it can represent a reactive disorder secondary to antigenic exposure (Ratzinger et al. 2005). Proliferations of indeterminate cells have been seen in nodular scabies (Hashimoto et al. 2000) and in healed lesions of pityriasis rosea (Wollenberg et al. 2002).

Differential Diagnosis

The differential diagnosis is similar to that for LCH and includes LCH, scabies, pityriasis rosea, and T-cell lymphomas.

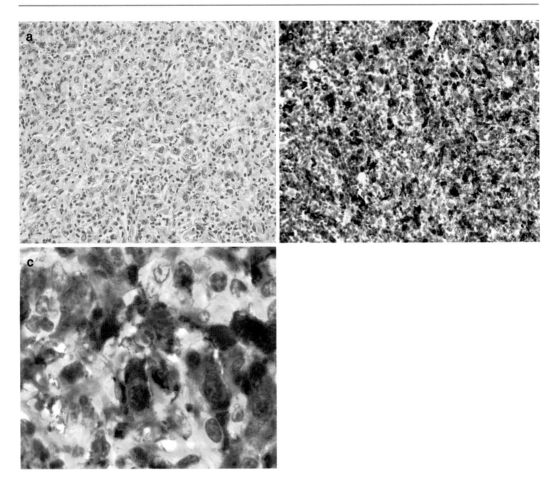

Fig. 16.8 (**a**) Indeterminate dendritic cell sarcoma. (**b**) CD68 stain. (**c**) S100 stain

> **Conclusions**
>
> The different myelomonocytic infiltrates can be associated with underlying systemic disorders such as EMH in patients with primary myelofibrosis or infiltrates related to MDS or AML or can be a primary disorder on their own. The broad differential diagnosis includes being able to differentiate myelomonocytic infiltrates into a specific subtype and also to exclude other similar causes such as precursor lymphoblastic leukemia (see Fig. 16.9) which may present with papulo-nodular tumors as with other myelomonocytic infiltrates but will have a different cytomorphology and immunophenotypical profile (CD10, Pax5, CD22 positive). Table 16.2 summarizes the different immunophenotypical markers that can be used to help differentiate between the different myelomonocytic infiltrates discussed above.
>
> Differentiation of each disease entity relies on the use of clinical findings and careful evaluation of the cytomorphology and immunophenotypical profile including evaluation of atypical cells circulating in the peripheral blood (see Fig. 16.10).
>
> Consensus on the treatment of these disorders continues to be difficult due to the rare nature of many of these diseases. Consortium group recommendations and when possible, clinical trials should be the mainstay of treatment decisions. Prognosis can be variable and further research is needed to use targeted therapy in these rare tumor subtypes.

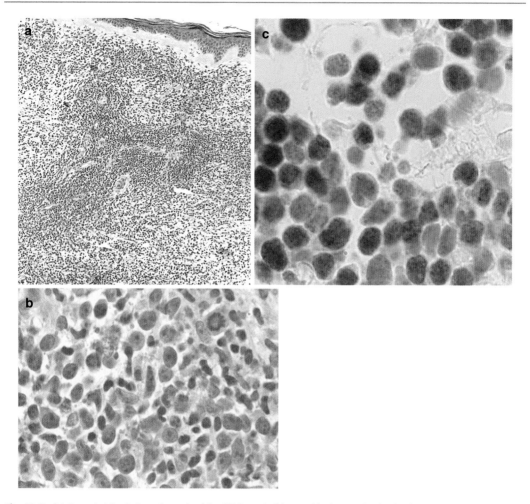

Fig. 16.9 (**a**) Lymphoblastic lymphoma in skin. (**b**) Lymphoblasts with abnormal mitosis, finely dispersed chromatin. (**c**) TdT nuclear-positive lymphoblasts

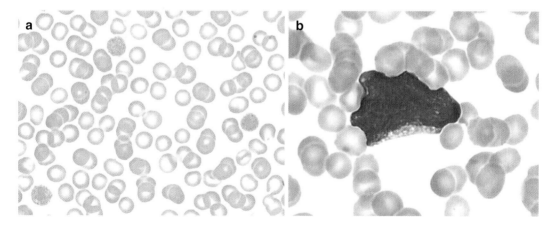

Fig. 16.10 (**a**) Circulating cerebriform lymphocytes and (**b**) circulating blast, in oil magnification, to contrast the nuclear chromatin pattern and contours

References

A multicentre retrospective survey of Langerhans' cell histiocytosis: 348 cases observed between 1983 and 1993. The French Langerhans' Cell Histiocytosis Study Group. Arch Dis Child. 1996;75(1): 17–24.

Swerdlow et al. (eds). WHO classification of tumours of haematopoietic and lymphoid tissues. Lyon: International Agency for Research on Cancer; 2008.

Agis H, Weltermann A, et al. A comparative study on demographic, hematological, and cytogenetic findings and prognosis in acute myeloid leukemia with and without leukemia cutis. Ann Hematol. 2002;81(2):90–5.

Altman J, Winkelmann RK. Xanthomatous cutaneous lesions of histiocytosis X. Arch Dermatol. 1963; 87:164–70.

Arber DA, Weiss LM, et al. Detection of Epstein-Barr virus in inflammatory pseudotumor. Semin Diagn Pathol. 1998;15(2):155–60.

Ascani S, Massone C, et al. CD4-negative variant of CD4+/CD56+ hematodermic neoplasm: description of three cases. J Cutan Pathol. 2008;35(10):911–5.

Assaf C, Gellrich S, et al. CD56-positive haematological neoplasms of the skin: a multicentre study of the Cutaneous Lymphoma Project Group of the European Organisation for Research and Treatment of Cancer. J Clin Pathol. 2007;60(9):981–9.

Badalian-Very G, Vergilio JA, et al. Recurrent BRAF mutations in Langerhans cell histiocytosis. Blood. 2010;116(11):1919–23.

Bakst R, Wolden S, et al. Radiation therapy for chloroma (granulocytic sarcoma). Int J Radiat Oncol Biol Phys. 2012;82(5):1816–22.

Bekassy AN, Hermans J, et al. Granulocytic sarcoma after allogeneic bone marrow transplantation: a retrospective European multicenter survey. Acute and Chronic Leukemia Working Parties of the European Group for Blood and Marrow Transplantation. Bone Marrow Transplant. 1996;17(5):801–8.

Bernard F, Thomas C, et al. Multi-centre pilot study of 2-chlorodeoxyadenosine and cytosine arabinoside combined chemotherapy in refractory Langerhans cell histiocytosis with haematological dysfunction. Eur J Cancer. 2005;41(17):2682–9.

Bhattacharjee P, Glusac EJ. Langerhans cell hyperplasia in scabies: a mimic of Langerhans cell histiocytosis. J Cutan Pathol. 2007;34(9):716–20.

Bluefarb SM, Webster JR. Leukemia cutis simulating venereal disease. Q Bull Northwest Univ Med Sch. 1953;27(1):18–20.

Bouroncle BA, Doan CA. Myelofibrosis. Clinical, hematologic and pathologic study of 110 patients. Am J Med Sci. 1962;243:697–715.

Breccia M, Mandelli F, et al. Clinico-pathological characteristics of myeloid sarcoma at diagnosis and during follow-up: report of 12 cases from a single institution. Leuk Res. 2004;28(11):1165–9.

Burns A. Observations of surgical anatomy, head and neck. Edinburgh: Thomas Royace and Company; 1811. p. 364–6.

Burns CA, Scott GA, et al. Leukemia cutis at the site of trauma in a patient with Burkitt leukemia. Cutis. 2005;75(1):54–6.

Burton JL. Sweet's syndrome, pyoderma gangrenosum and acute leukaemia. Br J Dermatol. 1980;102(2): 239.

Byrd JC, Edenfield WJ, et al. Extramedullary myeloid cell tumors in acute nonlymphocytic leukemia: a clinical review. J Clin Oncol. 1995;13(7):1800–16.

Cerio R, Spaull J, et al. Histiocytoma cutis: a tumour of dermal dendrocytes (dermal dendrocytoma). Br J Dermatol. 1989;120(2):197–206.

Chan J, Chan J. PRoliferative lesions of follicular dendritic cells: an overview, including a detailed account of follicular dendritic cell sarcoma, a neoplasm with many faces and uncommon etiologic associations. Adv Anat Pathol. 1997;4:387–411.

Chan JK, Fletcher CD, et al. Follicular dendritic cell sarcoma. Clinicopathologic analysis of 17 cases suggesting a malignant potential higher than currently recognized. Cancer. 1997;79(2):294–313.

Chan JK, Tsang WY, et al. Follicular dendritic cell tumor and vascular neoplasm complicating hyaline-vascular Castleman's disease. Am J Surg Pathol. 1994;18(5): 517–25.

Cheuk W, Chan JK, et al. Inflammatory pseudotumor-like follicular dendritic cell tumor: a distinctive low-grade malignant intra-abdominal neoplasm with consistent Epstein-Barr virus association. Am J Surg Pathol. 2001;25(6):721–31.

Chikwava K, Jaffe R. Langerin (CD207) staining in normal pediatric tissues, reactive lymph nodes, and childhood histiocytic disorders. Pediatr Dev Pathol. 2004;7(6):607–14.

Cho-Vega JH, Medeiros LJ, et al. Leukemia cutis. Am J Clin Pathol. 2008;129(1):130–42.

Christie LJ, Evans AT, et al. Lesions resembling Langerhans cell histiocytosis in association with other lymphoproliferative disorders: a reactive or neoplastic phenomenon? Hum Pathol. 2006;37(1):32–9.

Chu A, Eisinger M, et al. Immunoelectron microscopic identification of Langerhans cells using a new antigenic marker. J Invest Dermatol. 1982;78(2):177–80.

Chung NP, Chen Y, et al. Dendritic cells: sentinels against pathogens. Histol Histopathol. 2004;19(1):317–24.

Collie AM, Uchin JM, et al. Cutaneous intravascular extramedullary hematopoiesis in a patient with post-polycythemia vera myelofibrosis. J Cutan Pathol 2013;40(7):616–20.

Corella F, Barnadas MA, et al. A case of cutaneous extra-medullary hematopoiesis associated with idiopathic myelofibrosis. Actas Dermosifiliogr 2008;99(4): 297–300.

Cota C, Vale E, et al. Cutaneous manifestations of blastic plasmacytoid dendritic cell neoplasm-morphologic and phenotypic variability in a series of 33 patients. Am J Surg Pathol. 2010;34(1):75–87.

Cronin DM, George TI, et al. An updated approach to the diagnosis of myeloid leukemia cutis. Am J Clin Pathol. 2009;132(1):101–10.

Dachary D, Bernard P, et al. Acute myeloid leukemia with marrow hypereosinophilia and chromosome 16 abnormality. Cancer Genet Cytogenet. 1986;20(3–4):241–6.

Dalle S, Beylot-Barry M, et al. Blastic plasmacytoid dendritic cell neoplasm: is transplantation the treatment of choice? Br J Dermatol. 2010;162(1):74–9.

de Morais JC, Spector N, et al. Spinal cord compression due to extramedullary hematopoiesis in the proliferative phase of polycythemia vera. Acta Haematol. 1996;96(4):242–4.

Dibbern Jr DA, Loevner LA, et al. MR of thoracic cord compression caused by epidural extramedullary hematopoiesis in myelodysplastic syndrome. AJNR Am J Neuroradiol. 1997;18(2):363–6.

Divaris DX, Ling FC, et al. Congenital self-healing histiocytosis. Report of two cases with histochemical and ultrastructural studies. Am J Dermatopathol. 1991;13(5):481–7.

Drut R. Polypoid dermal dendrocytic hamartoma in a giant congenital melanocytic nevus. Int J Surg Pathol. 2007;15(1):73–6.

Drut R, Peral CG, et al. Langerhans cell hyperplasia of the skin mimicking Langerhans cell histiocytosis: a report of two cases in children not associated with scabies. Fetal Pediatr Pathol. 2010;29(4):231–8.

Dunger DB, Broadbent V, et al. The frequency and natural history of diabetes insipidus in children with Langerhans-cell histiocytosis. N Engl J Med. 1989;321(17):1157–62.

Eshghabadi M, Shojania AM, et al. Isolated granulocytic sarcoma: report of a case and review of the literature. J Clin Oncol. 1986;4(6):912–7.

Falini B, Lenze D, et al. Cytoplasmic mutated nucleophosmin (NPM) defines the molecular status of a significant fraction of myeloid sarcomas. Leukemia. 2007;21(7):1566–70.

Falini B, Mecucci C, et al. Cytoplasmic nucleophosmin in acute myelogenous leukemia with a normal karyotype. N Engl J Med. 2005;352(3):254–66.

Feldman AL, Arber DA, et al. Clonally related follicular lymphomas and histiocytic/dendritic cell sarcomas: evidence for transdifferentiation of the follicular lymphoma clone. Blood. 2008;111(12):5433–9.

Fernandez Acenero MJ, Borbujo J, et al. Extramedullary hematopoiesis in an adult. J Am Acad Dermatol. 2003;48(5 Suppl):S62–3.

Ferran M, Toll A, et al. Acquired mucosal indeterminate cell histiocytoma. Pediatr Dermatol. 2007;24(3):253–6.

Ferrara F, Cancemi D, et al. Tetrasomy 8 and t(1;11)(p32;q24) in acute myelo-monocytic leukemia with extensive leukemic cutaneous involvement. Leuk Lymphoma. 1996;20(5–6):513–5.

Feuillard J, Jacob MC, et al. Clinical and biologic features of CD4(+)CD56(+) malignancies. Blood. 2002;99(5):1556–63.

Fonseca R, Yamakawa M, et al. Follicular dendritic cell sarcoma and interdigitating reticulum cell sarcoma: a review. Am J Hematol. 1998;59(2):161–7.

Fraser CR, Wang W, et al. Transformation of chronic lymphocytic leukemia/small lymphocytic lymphoma to interdigitating dendritic cell sarcoma: evidence for transdifferentiation of the lymphoma clone. Am J Clin Pathol. 2009;132(6):928–39.

Gadner H, Grois N, et al. Improved outcome in multisystem Langerhans cell histiocytosis is associated with therapy intensification. Blood. 2008;111(5):2556–62.

Gadner H, Minkov M, et al. Therapy prolongation improves outcome in multisystem Langerhans cell histiocytosis. Blood. 2013;121(25):5006–14.

Gaertner EM, Tsokos M, et al. Interdigitating dendritic cell sarcoma. A report of four cases and review of the literature. Am J Clin Pathol. 2001;115(4):589–97.

Garnache-Ottou F, Feuillard J, et al. Extended diagnostic criteria for plasmacytoid dendritic cell leukaemia. Br J Haematol. 2009;145(5):624–36.

Gianotti F, Caputo R. Histiocytic syndromes: a review. J Am Acad Dermatol. 1985;13(3):383–404.

Glew RH, Haese WH, et al. Myeloid metaplasia with myelofibrosis. The clinical spectrum of extramedullary hematopoiesis and tumor formation. Johns Hopkins Med J. 1973;132(5):253–70.

Goerdt S, Kolde G, et al. Immunohistochemical comparison of cutaneous histiocytoses and related skin disorders: diagnostic and histogenetic relevance of MS-1 high molecular weight protein expression. J Pathol. 1993;170(4):421–7.

Goldblum JR, Tuthill RJ. CD34 and factor-XIIIa immunoreactivity in dermatofibrosarcoma protuberans and dermatofibroma. Am J Dermatopathol. 1997;19(2):147–53.

Gordon MK, Kraus M, et al. Interdigitating dendritic cell tumors in two patients exposed to topical calcineurin inhibitors. Leuk Lymphoma. 2007;48(4):816–8.

Gotz G, Fichter J. Langerhans'-cell histiocytosis in 58 adults. Eur J Med Res. 2004;9(11):510–4.

Gould J, Iqbal A, et al. Pentasomy 8 in acute monoblastic leukemia. Cancer Genet Cytogenet. 2000;117(2):146–8.

Gowitt GT, Zaatari GS. Bronchial extramedullary hematopoiesis preceding chronic myelogenous leukemia. Hum Pathol. 1985;16(10):1069–71.

Gray MH, Smoller BR, et al. Giant dermal dendrocytoma of the face: a distinct clinicopathologic entity. Arch Dermatol. 1990;126(5):689–90.

Grogg KL, Lae ME, et al. Clusterin expression distinguishes follicular dendritic cell tumors from other dendritic cell neoplasms: report of a novel follicular dendritic cell marker and clinicopathologic data on 12 additional follicular dendritic cell tumors and 6 additional interdigitating dendritic cell tumors. Am J Surg Pathol. 2004;28(8):988–98.

Grogg KL, Macon WR, et al. A survey of clusterin and fascin expression in sarcomas and spindle cell neoplasms: strong clusterin immunostaining is highly specific for follicular dendritic cell tumor. Mod Pathol. 2005;18(2):260–6.

Grois N, Flucher-Wolfram B, et al. Diabetes insipidus in Langerhans cell histiocytosis: results from the

DAL-HX 83 study. Med Pediatr Oncol. 1995; 24(4):248–56.

Grois N, Potschger U, et al. Risk factors for diabetes insipidus in Langerhans cell histiocytosis. Pediatr Blood Cancer. 2006;46(2):228–33.

Gruson B, Vaida I, et al. L-asparaginase with methotrexate and dexamethasone is an effective treatment combination in blastic plasmacytoid dendritic cell neoplasm. Br J Haematol. 2013;163:543–5.

Gumbs RV, Higginbotham-Ford EA, et al. Thoracic extramedullary hematopoiesis in sickle-cell disease. AJR Am J Roentgenol. 1987;149(5):889–93.

Guo J, Si L, et al. Phase II, open-label, single-arm trial of imatinib mesylate in patients with metastatic melanoma harboring c-Kit mutation or amplification. J Clin Oncol. 2011;29(21):2904–9.

Haniffa MA, Wilkins BS, et al. Cutaneous extramedullary hemopoiesis in chronic myeloproliferative and myelodysplastic disorders. J Am Acad Dermatol. 2006;55(2 Suppl):S28–31.

Hanson CA, Abaza M, et al. Acute biphenotypic leukaemia: immunophenotypic and cytogenetic analysis. Br J Haematol. 1993;84(1):49–60.

Haroche J, Cohen-Aubart F, et al. Dramatic efficacy of vemurafenib in both multisystemic and refractory Erdheim-Chester disease and Langerhans cell histiocytosis harboring the BRAF V600E mutation. Blood. 2013;121(9):1495–500.

Hashimoto K, Fujiwara K, et al. Post-scabetic nodules: a lymphohistiocytic reaction rich in indeterminate cells. J Dermatol. 2000;27(3):181–94.

Hashimoto K, Pritzker MS. Electron microscopic study of reticulohistiocytoma. An unusual case of congenital, self-healing reticulohistiocytosis. Arch Dermatol. 1973;107(2):263–70.

Hashimoto K, Takahashi S, et al. Congenital self-healing reticulohistiocytosis. Report of the seventh case with histochemical and ultrastructural studies. J Am Acad Dermatol. 1984;11(3):447–54.

Herling M, Jones D. CD4+/CD56+ hematodermic tumor: the features of an evolving entity and its relationship to dendritic cells. Am J Clin Pathol. 2007;127(5):687–700.

Herling M, Teitell MA, et al. TCL1 expression in plasmacytoid dendritic cells (DC2s) and the related CD4+ CD56+ blastic tumors of skin. Blood. 2003; 101(12):5007–9.

Howarth DM, Gilchrist GS, et al. Langerhans cell histiocytosis: diagnosis, natural history, management, and outcome. Cancer. 1999;85(10):2278–90.

Hoyo E, Kanitakis J, et al. The dermal dendrocyte. Pathol Biol (Paris). 1993;41(7):613–8.

Hui PK, Feller AC, et al. Skin tumor of T accessory cells (interdigitating reticulum cells) with high content of T lymphocytes. Am J Dermatopathol. 1987;9(2): 129–37.

Hurley MY, Ghahramani GK, et al. Cutaneous myeloid sarcoma: natural history and biology of an uncommon manifestation of acute myeloid leukemia. Acta Derm Venereol. 2013;93(3):319–24.

Imai Y, Yamakawa M, et al. The lymphocyte-dendritic cell system. Histol Histopathol. 1998;13(2):469–510.

Imanaka A, Tarutani M, et al. Langerhans cell histiocytosis involving the skin of an elderly woman: a satisfactory remission with oral prednisolone alone. J Dermatol. 2004;31(12):1023–6.

Jacob MC, Chaperot L, et al. CD4+ CD56+ lineage negative malignancies: a new entity developed from malignant early plasmacytoid dendritic cells. Haematologica. 2003;88(8):941–55.

Jardin F, Callanan M, et al. Recurrent genomic aberrations combined with deletions of various tumour suppressor genes may deregulate the G1/S transition in CD4+CD56+ haematodermic neoplasms and contribute to the aggressiveness of the disease. Leukemia. 2009;23(4):698–707.

Jayaram G, Abdul Rahman N. Cytology of Ki-1-positive anaplastic large cell lymphoma. A report of two cases. Acta Cytol. 1997;41(4 Suppl):1253–60.

Jiang YZ, Dong NZ, et al. Interdigitating dendritic cell sarcoma presenting simultaneously with acute myelomonocytic leukemia: report of a rare case and literature review. Int J Hematol. 2013;97(5):657–66.

Julia F, Petrella T, et al. Blastic plasmacytoid dendritic cell neoplasm: clinical features in 90 patients. Br J Dermatol. 2013;169:579–86.

Kapur P, Erickson C, et al. Congenital self-healing reticulohistiocytosis (Hashimoto-Pritzker disease): ten-year experience at Dallas Children's Medical Center. J Am Acad Dermatol. 2007;56(2):290–4.

Kaune KM, Baumgart M, et al. Solitary cutaneous nodule of blastic plasmacytoid dendritic cell neoplasm progressing to overt leukemia cutis after chemotherapy: immunohistology and FISH analysis confirmed the diagnosis. Am J Dermatopathol. 2009;31(7):695–701.

Kawakami T, Kimura S, et al. Transforming growth factor-beta overexpression in cutaneous extramedullary hematopoiesis of a patient with myelodysplastic syndrome associated with myelofibrosis. J Am Acad Dermatol 2008;58(4):703–6.

Kazakov DV, Morrisson C, et al. Sarcoma arising in hyaline-vascular castleman disease of skin and subcutis. Am J Dermatopathol. 2005;27(4):327–32.

King A. A case of chloroma. Mon J Med. 1853;17:97.

Koch CA, Li CY, et al. Nonhepatosplenic extramedullary hematopoiesis: associated diseases, pathology, clinical course, and treatment. Mayo Clin Proc. 2003;78(10):1223–33.

Korsten J, Grossman H, et al. Extramedullary hematopoiesis in patients with thalassemia anemia. Radiology. 1970;95(2):257–63.

Krause JR. Granulocytic sarcoma preceding acute leukemia: a report of six cases. Cancer. 1979;44(3): 1017–21.

Kumar PV. Leukemia cutis. Fine needle aspiration findings. Acta Cytol. 1997;41(3):666–71.

Kwon KS, Lee JB, et al. A case of cutaneous extramedullary hematopoiesis in myelofibrosis with a preponderance of eosinophilic precursor cells. J Dermatol 1999;26(6):379–84.

Lane JE, Walker AN, et al. Cutaneous sclerosing extramedullary hematopoietic tumor in chronic myelogenous leukemia. J Cutan Pathol 2002;29(10):608–12.

Lau SK, Chu PG, et al. Immunohistochemical expression of Langerin in Langerhans cell histiocytosis and non-Langerhans cell histiocytic disorders. Am J Surg Pathol. 2008;32(4):615–9.

Lee IJ, Kim SC, et al. Paraneoplastic pemphigus associated with follicular dendritic cell sarcoma arising from Castleman's tumor. J Am Acad Dermatol. 1999;40(2 Pt 2):294–7.

Lee JC, Christensen T, et al. Metastatic interdigitating dendritic cell sarcoma masquerading as a skin primary tumor: a case report and review of the literature. Am J Dermatopathol. 2009;31(1):88–93.

Lee E, Park HJ, et al. Leukemia cutis as early relapse of T-cell acute lymphoblastic leukemia. Int J Dermatol. 2010;49(3):335–7.

Leroux D, Mugneret F, et al. CD4(+), CD56(+) DC2 acute leukemia is characterized by recurrent clonal chromosomal changes affecting 6 major targets: a study of 21 cases by the Groupe Francais de Cytogenetique Hematologique. Blood. 2002;99(11):4154–9.

Lewkow LM, Shah I. Sickle cell anemia and epidural extramedullary hematopoiesis. Am J Med. 1984;76(4):748–51.

Lichtenwald DJ, Jakubovic HR, et al. Primary cutaneous Langerhans cell histiocytosis in an adult. Arch Dermatol. 1991;127(10):1545–8.

Lim D, Goodman H, et al. Blastic plasmacytoid dendritic cell neoplasm. Australas J Dermatol. 2013;54(2):e43–5.

Lin CK, Liang R, et al. Myelodysplastic syndrome presenting with generalized cutaneous granulocytic sarcomas. Acta Haematol. 1990;83(2):89–93.

List AF, Gonzalez-Osete G, et al. Granulocytic sarcoma in myelodysplastic syndromes: clinical marker of disease acceleration. Am J Med. 1991;90(2):274–6.

Liu PI, Ishimaru T, et al. Autopsy study of granulocytic sarcoma (chloroma) in patients with myelogenous leukemia, Hiroshima-Nagasaki 1949–1969. Cancer. 1973;31(4):948–55.

Liu K, Victora GD, et al. In vivo analysis of dendritic cell development and homeostasis. Science. 2009;324(5925):392–7.

Lucioni M, Novara F, et al. Twenty-one cases of blastic plasmacytoid dendritic cell neoplasm: focus on biallelic locus 9p21.3 deletion. Blood. 2011;118(17):4591–4.

Maeda K, Takahashi T, et al. Interdigitating cell sarcoma: a report of an autopsy case and literature review. J Clin Exp Hematopathol. 2005;45:37–44.

Malpas JS. Langerhans cell histiocytosis in adults. Hematol Oncol Clin N Am. 1998;12(2):259–68.

Marafioti T, Paterson JC, et al. Novel markers of normal and neoplastic human plasmacytoid dendritic cells. Blood. 2008;111(7):3778–92.

McClain KL. Drug therapy for the treatment of Langerhans cell histiocytosis. Expert Opin Pharmacother. 2005;6(14):2435–41.

McClain KL, Kozinetz CA. A phase II trial using thalidomide for Langerhans cell histiocytosis. Pediatr Blood Cancer. 2007;48(1):44–9.

McLelland J, Broadbent V, et al. Langerhans cell histiocytosis: the case for conservative treatment. Arch Dis Child. 1990;65(3):301–3.

Meijs M, Mekkes J, et al. Paraneoplastic pemphigus associated with follicular dendritic cell sarcoma without Castleman's disease; treatment with rituximab. Int J Dermatol. 2008;47(6):632–4.

Meis JM, Butler JJ, et al. Granulocytic sarcoma in nonleukemic patients. Cancer. 1986;58(12):2697–709.

Minkov M, Grois N, et al. Langerhans cell histiocytosis: histiocyte society evaluation and treatment guidelines. 2009. Retrieved from https://www.histiocytesociety.org/document.doc?id=290. Accessed 23 June 2013.

Miyata T, Masuzawa M, et al. Cutaneous extramedullary hematopoiesis in a patient with idiopathic myelofibrosis. J Dermatol 2008;35(7):456–61.

Mizoguchi M, Kawa Y, et al. Cutaneous extramedullary hematopoiesis in myelofibrosis. J Am Acad Dermatol. 1990;22(2 Pt 2):351–5.

Mohanty SK, Dey P, et al. Cytologic diagnosis of follicular dendritic cell tumor: a diagnostic dilemma. Diagn Cytopathol. 2003;29(6):368–9.

Munn S, Chu AC. Langerhans cell histiocytosis of the skin. Hematol Oncol Clin N Am. 1998;12(2):269–86.

Murakami I, Gogusev J, et al. Detection of molecular cytogenetic aberrations in Langerhans cell histiocytosis of bone. Hum Pathol. 2002;33(5):555–60.

Narvaez D, Kanitakis J, et al. Immunohistochemical study of CD34-positive dendritic cells of human dermis. Am J Dermatopathol. 1996;18(3):283–8.

Neiman RS, Barcos M, et al. Granulocytic sarcoma: a clinicopathologic study of 61 biopsied cases. Cancer. 1981;48(6):1426–37.

Newman B, Hu W, et al. Aggressive histiocytic disorders that can involve the skin. J Am Acad Dermatol. 2007;56(2):302–16.

Ng AP, Lade S, et al. Primary cutaneous CD4+/CD56+ hematodermic neoplasm (blastic NK-cell lymphoma): a report of five cases. Haematologica. 2006;91(1):143–4.

Ngu IW, Sinclair EC, et al. Unusual presentation of granulocytic sarcoma in the breast: a case report and review of the literature. Diagn Cytopathol. 2001;24(1):53–7.

Nguyen TT, Schwartz EJ, et al. Expression of CD163 (hemoglobin scavenger receptor) in normal tissues, lymphomas, carcinomas, and sarcomas is largely restricted to the monocyte/macrophage lineage. Am J Surg Pathol. 2005;29(5):617–24.

O'Malley DP. Benign extramedullary myeloid proliferations. Mod Pathol. 2007;20(4):405–15.

Ohata C, Kawahara K. CD34-reactive myxoid dermal dendrocytoma. Am J Dermatopathol. 2002;24(1):50–3.

Pagerols X, Curc N, et al. Cutaneous extramedullary haematopoiesis associated with blast crisis in myelofibrosis. Clin Exp Dermatol 1998;23(6):296–97.

Park L, Schiltz C, et al. Langerhans cell histiocytosis. J Cutan Med Surg. 2012;16(1):45–9.

Patel BM, Su WP, et al. Cutaneous extramedullary hematopoiesis. J Am Acad Dermatol. 1995;32(5 Pt 1): 805–7.

Paydas S, Zorludemir S. Leukaemia cutis and leukaemic vasculitis. Br J Dermatol. 2000;143(4):773–9.

Petrella T, Facchetti F. Tumoral aspects of plasmacytoid dendritic cells: what do we know in 2009? Autoimmunity. 2010;43(3):210–4.

Petrella T, Dalac S, et al. CD4+ CD56+ cutaneous neoplasms: a distinct hematological entity? Groupe Francais d'Etude des Lymphomes Cutanes (GFELC). Am J Surg Pathol. 1999;23(2):137–46.

Petrella T, Comeau MR, et al. 'Agranular CD4+ CD56+ hematodermic neoplasm' (blastic NK-cell lymphoma) originates from a population of CD56+ precursor cells related to plasmacytoid monocytes. Am J Surg Pathol. 2002;26(7):852–62.

Petrella T, Meijer CJ, et al. TCL1 and CLA expression in agranular CD4/CD56 hematodermic neoplasms (blastic NK-cell lymphomas) and leukemia cutis. Am J Clin Pathol. 2004;122(2):307–13.

Petrella T, Bagot M, et al. Blastic NK-cell lymphomas (agranular CD4+CD56+ hematodermic neoplasms): a review. Am J Clin Pathol. 2005;123(5):662–75.

Pigozzi B, Bordignon M, et al. Expression of the CD1a molecule in B- and T-lymphoproliferative skin conditions. Oncol Rep. 2006;15(2):347–51.

Pileri SA, Grogan TM, et al. Tumours of histiocytes and accessory dendritic cells: an immunohistochemical approach to classification from the International Lymphoma Study Group based on 61 cases. Histopathology. 2002;41(1):1–29.

Pileri SA, Ascani S, et al. Myeloid sarcoma: clinicopathologic, phenotypic and cytogenetic analysis of 92 adult patients. Leukemia. 2007;21(2):340–50.

Pileri A, Delfino C, et al. Blastic plasmacytoid dendritic cell neoplasm (BPDCN): the cutaneous sanctuary. G Ital Dermatol Venereol. 2012;147(6):603–8.

Pilichowska ME, Fleming MD, et al. CD4+/CD56+ hematodermic neoplasm ("blastic natural killer cell lymphoma"): neoplastic cells express the immature dendritic cell marker BDCA-2 and produce interferon. Am J Clin Pathol. 2007;128(3):445–53.

Pillay K, Solomon R, et al. Interdigitating dendritic cell sarcoma: a report of four paediatric cases and review of the literature. Histopathology. 2004;44(3):283–91.

Pitcock JA, Reinhard EH, et al. A clinical and pathological study of seventy cases of myelofibrosis. Ann Intern Med. 1962;57:73–84.

Porcu P, Neiman RS, et al. Splenectomy in agnogenic myeloid metaplasia. Blood. 1999;93(6):2132–4.

Rappaport H. Tumors of the hematopoietic system, atlas of tumor pathology, section III, fascicle 8. Washington, DC: Armed Forces Institute of Pathology; 1966. p. 241–3.

Ratzinger G, Burgdorf WH, et al. Indeterminate cell histiocytosis: fact or fiction? J Cutan Pathol. 2005; 32(8):552–60.

Reichard KK, Burks EJ, et al. CD4(+) CD56(+) lineage-negative malignancies are rare tumors of plasmacytoid dendritic cells. Am J Surg Pathol. 2005;29(10):1274–83.

Reimer P, Rudiger T, et al. What is CD4+CD56+ malignancy and how should it be treated? Bone Marrow Transplant. 2003;32(7):637–46.

Revenga F, Horndler C, et al. Cutaneous extramedullary hematopoiesis. Int J Dermatol. 2000;39(12):957–8.

Rice GP, Assis LJ, et al. Extramedullary hematopoiesis and spinal cord compression complicating polycythemia rubra vera. Ann Neurol. 1980;7(1):81–4.

Risdall RJ, Dehner LP, et al. Histiocytosis X (Langerhans' cell histiocytosis). Prognostic role of histopathology. Arch Pathol Lab Med. 1983;107(2):59–63.

Rodriguez Ramirez J, Redondo Martinez E, et al. Idiopathic myelofibrosis with cutaneous extramedullary hematopoiesis. Med Clin (Barc) 1991;97(1):24–6.

Rogalski C, Paasch U, et al. Cutaneous extramedullary hematopoiesis in idiopathic myelofibrosis. Int J Dermatol 2002;41(12):883–84.

Romani N, Lenz A, et al. Cultured human Langerhans cells resemble lymphoid dendritic cells in phenotype and function. J Invest Dermatol. 1989;93(5):600–9.

Romani N, Holzmann S, et al. Langerhans cells – dendritic cells of the epidermis. APMIS. 2003;111(7–8):725–40.

Rosenberg AS, Morgan MB. Cutaneous indeterminate cell histiocytosis: a new spindle cell variant resembling dendritic cell sarcoma. J Cutan Pathol. 2001; 28(10):531–7.

Rosenzweig M, Canque B, et al. Human dendritic cell differentiation pathway from CD34+ hematopoietic precursor cells. Blood. 1996;87:535–44.

Ruberto E, Espinola R, et al. Idiopathic myelofibrosis with extramedullary hematopoiesis foci in the skin and testicles. Report of a case. Sangre (Barc) 1995; 40(2):157–160.

Salotti JA, Nanduri V, et al. Incidence and clinical features of Langerhans cell histiocytosis in the UK and Ireland. Arch Dis Child. 2009;94(5):376–80.

Sander B, Middel P, et al. Follicular dendritic cell sarcoma of the spleen. Hum Pathol. 2007;38(4):668–72.

Saygin C, Uzunaslan D, et al. Dendritic cell sarcoma: a pooled analysis including 462 cases with presentation of our case series. Crit Rev Oncol Hematol. 2013;88:253–71.

Sen F, Zhang XX, et al. Increased incidence of trisomy 8 in acute myeloid leukemia with skin infiltration (leukemia cutis). Diagn Mol Pathol. 2000;9(4):190–4.

Shao H, Xi L, et al. Clonally related histiocytic/dendritic cell sarcoma and chronic lymphocytic leukemia/small lymphocytic lymphoma: a study of seven cases. Mod Pathol. 2011;24(11):1421–32.

Shia J, Chen W, et al. Extranodal follicular dendritic cell sarcoma: clinical, pathologic, and histogenetic characteristics of an underrecognized disease entity. Virchows Arch. 2006;449(2):148–58.

Shih LY, Lin FC, et al. Cutaneous and pericardial extramedullary hematopoiesis with cardiac tamponade in chronic myeloid leukemia. Am J Clin Pathol. 1988;89(5):693–7.

Sidoroff A, Zelger B, et al. Indeterminate cell histiocytosis–a clinicopathological entity with features of both X- and non-X histiocytosis. Br J Dermatol. 1996;134(3):525–32.

Sontheimer RD, Matsubara T, et al. A macrophage phenotype for a constitutive, class II antigen-expressing, human dermal perivascular dendritic cell. J Invest Dermatol. 1989;93(1):154–9.

Stein SL, Paller AS, et al. Langerhans cell histiocytosis presenting in the neonatal period: a retrospective case series. Arch Pediatr Adolesc Med. 2001;155(7):778–83.

Steiner M, Matthes-Martin S, et al. Improved outcome of treatment-resistant high-risk Langerhans cell histiocytosis after allogeneic stem cell transplantation with reduced-intensity conditioning. Bone Marrow Transplant. 2005;36(3):215–25.

Steinman RM. Some interfaces of dendritic cell biology. APMIS. 2003;111(7–8):675–97.

Steinman RM, Pack M, et al. Dendritic cells in the T-cell areas of lymphoid organs. Immunol Rev. 1997;156:25–37.

Stockschlaeder M, Sucker C. Adult Langerhans cell histiocytosis. Eur J Haematol. 2006;76(5):363–8.

Su WP. Clinical, histopathologic, and immunohistochemical correlations in leukemia cutis. Semin Dermatol. 1994;13(3):223–30.

Sun X, Chang KC, et al. Epidermal growth factor receptor expression in follicular dendritic cells: a shared feature of follicular dendritic cell sarcoma and Castleman's disease. Hum Pathol. 2003;34(9):835–40.

Szomor A, Passweg JR, et al. Myeloid leukemia and myelodysplastic syndrome relapsing as granulocytic sarcoma (chloroma) after allogeneic bone marrow transplantation. Ann Hematol. 1997;75(5–6):239–41.

Taverna JA, Stefanato CM, et al. Adult cutaneous Langerhans cell histiocytosis responsive to topical imiquimod. J Am Acad Dermatol. 2006;54(5):911–3.

Tecchio C, Colato C, et al. Plasmacytoid dendritic cell leukemia: a rapidly evolving disease presenting with skin lesions sensitive to radiotherapy plus hyperthermia. Oncologist. 2009;14(12):1205–8.

Teunissen MB, Wormmeester J, et al. Human epidermal Langerhans cells undergo profound morphologic and phenotypical changes during in vitro culture. J Invest Dermatol. 1990;94(2):166–73.

Tew JG, Kosco MH, et al. Follicular dendritic cells as accessory cells. Immunol Rev. 1990;117:185–211.

Turner RR, Wood GS, et al. Histiocytic malignancies. Morphologic, immunologic, and enzymatic heterogeneity. Am J Surg Pathol. 1984;8(7):485–500.

Vargas H, Mouzakes J, et al. Follicular dendritic cell tumor: an aggressive head and neck tumor. Am J Otolaryngol. 2002;23(2):93–8.

Vasef MA, Zaatari GS, et al. Dendritic cell tumors associated with low-grade B-cell malignancies. Report of three cases. Am J Clin Pathol. 1995;104(6):696–701.

Vener C, Soligo D, et al. Indeterminate cell histiocytosis in association with later occurrence of acute myeloblastic leukaemia. Br J Dermatol. 2007;156(6):1357–61.

Vogel CA, Aughenbaugh W, et al. Excimer laser as adjuvant therapy for adult cutaneous Langerhans cell histiocytosis. Arch Dermatol. 2008;144(10):1287–90.

Wagner G, Fenchel K, et al. Leukemia cutis – epidemiology, clinical presentation, and differential diagnoses. J Dtsch Dermatol Ges. 2012;10(1):27–36.

Wang J, Bu DF, et al. Autoantibody production from a thymoma and a follicular dendritic cell sarcoma associated with paraneoplastic pemphigus. Br J Dermatol. 2005;153(3):558–64.

Ward HP, Block MH. The natural history of agnogenic myeloid metaplasia (AMM) and a critical evaluation of its relationship with the myeloproliferative syndrome. Medicine (Baltimore). 1971;50(5):357–420.

Weiss LM, Berry GJ, et al. Spindle cell neoplasms of lymph nodes of probable reticulum cell lineage. True reticulum cell sarcoma? Am J Surg Pathol. 1990;14(5):405–14.

Weiss T, Weber L, et al. Solitary cutaneous dendritic cell tumor in a child: role of dendritic cell markers for the diagnosis of skin Langerhans cell histiocytosis. J Am Acad Dermatol. 2005;53(5):838–44.

Wells GC. The pathology of adult type Letterer-Siwe disease. Clin Exp Dermatol. 1979;4(4):407–12.

Wheller L, Carman N, et al. Unilesional self-limited Langerhans cell histiocytosis: a case report and review of the literature. J Cutan Pathol. 2013;40(6):595–9.

Wiernik PH, Serpick AA. Granulocytic sarcoma (chloroma). Blood. 1970;35(3):361–9.

Willemze R, Jaffe ES, et al. WHO-EORTC classification for cutaneous lymphomas. Blood. 2005;105(10):3768–85.

Willman CL, Busque L, et al. Langerhans'-cell histiocytosis (histiocytosis X) – a clonal proliferative disease. N Engl J Med. 1994;331(3):154–60.

Wollenberg A, Burgdorf WH, et al. Long-lasting "christmas tree rash" in an adolescent: isotopic response of indeterminate cell histiocytosis in pityriasis rosea? Acta Derm Venereol. 2002;82(4):288–91.

Wong E, Holden CA, et al. Histiocytosis X presenting as intertrigo and responding to topical nitrogen mustard. Clin Exp Dermatol. 1986;11(2):183–7.

Wong TY, Suster S, et al. Histologic spectrum of cutaneous involvement in patients with myelogenous leukemia including the neutrophilic dermatoses. Int J Dermatol. 1995;34(5):323–9.

Wood GS, Turner RR, et al. Human dendritic cells and macrophages. In situ immunophenotypic definition of subsets that exhibit specific morphologic and microenvironmental characteristics. Am J Pathol. 1985;119(1):73–82.

Wu L, Liu YJ. Development of dendritic-cell lineages. Immunity. 2007;26(6):741–50.

Wu J, Qin D, et al. Follicular dendritic cell-derived antigen and accessory activity in initiation of memory IgG responses in vitro. J Immunol. 1996;157(8):3404–11.

Wu Q, Liu C, et al. Interdigitating dendritic cell sarcoma involving bone marrow in a liver transplant recipient. Transplant Proc. 2010;42(5):1963–6.

Ylagan LR, Bartlett NL, et al. Interdigitating dendritic reticulum cell tumor of lymph nodes: case report with differential diagnostic considerations. Diagn Cytopathol. 2003;28(5):278–81.

Yousem SA, Colby TV, et al. Pulmonary Langerhans' cell histiocytosis: molecular analysis of clonality. Am J Surg Pathol. 2001;25(5):630–6.

Yu RC, Chu C, et al. Clonal proliferation of Langerhans cells in Langerhans cell histiocytosis. Lancet. 1994;343(8900):767–8.

Zachary CB, MacDonald DM. Hand-Schuller-Christian disease with secondary cutaneous involvement. Clin Exp Dermatol. 1983;8(2):177–83.

Zunino-Goutorbe C, Eschard C, et al. Congenital solitary histiocytoma: a variant of Hashimoto-Pritzker histiocytosis. A retrospective study of 8 cases. Dermatology. 2008;216(2):118–24.

Cutaneous Intravascular Conditions

17

Vincent Liu

Intravascular Large B-Cell Lymphoma

Introduction

Since its first description in 1959 (Pfleger and Tappeiner 1959), establishment of intravascular large B-cell lymphoma as a distinct clinicopathologic entity arose from the recognition that the observed atypical cells within blood vessels were in fact lymphoid in nature (Bhawan et al. 1985; Mori et al. 1985; Sheibani et al. 1986; Wick et al. 1986; Wrotnowski et al. 1985), rather than endothelial ("angioendotheliomatosis proliferans systemica," "malignant angioendotheliomatosis"), as originally suspected. With this more accurate characterization of the tumor cells, intravascular large B-cell lymphoma was accepted by the WHO (World Health Organization) classification of hematolymphoid tumors (Nakamura et al. 2008) as a subtype of extranodal large B-cell lymphoma and was similarly adopted as a subtype of large B-cell lymphoma by the WHO-EORTC (World Health Organization-European Organization for Research and Treatment of Cancer) classification of primary cutaneous lymphomas (Willemze et al. 2005). This current category captures conditions variably termed in the past (e.g., "angiotropic lymphoma," "intravascular lymphomatosis," "angioendotheliotropic (intravascular) lymphomatosis," [Kiel] "angiotropic large-cell lymphoma" [Lukes-Collins]) (Domizio et al. 1989; Fredericks et al. 1991), which all share reference to atypical lymphoid forms honing to the intravascular space (Zuckerman et al. 2006), possibly prevented from vessel escape due to altered surface ligand expression by tumor cells (Ponzoni et al. 2000). Cumulative experience with this rare condition, collected largely from case reports, case series, and reviews, documents common themes of cutaneous, neurologic, and other systemic involvement, although much more remains to be learned with respect to pathophysiology, prognosis, and treatment.

Definition

Intravascular large B-cell lymphoma may be defined as an intravascular malignant proliferation of B-lymphocytes, characterized by cutaneous, neurologic, and other systemic manifestations, typically with aggressive behavior, and lacking a significant extravascular lymphoma component including frequent sparing of the reticuloendothelial system (Nakamura et al. 2008) (Table 17.1). Whether reports of intravascular large B-cell lymphoma occurring in the setting of a prior or concomitant other lymphoma (Asagoe et al. 2003;

V. Liu, MD
Department of Dermatology and Pathology,
University of Iowa Hospitals and Clinics,
200 Hawkins Drive, 40035 PFP, Iowa City, IA
52242-1090, USA
e-mail: vincent-liu@uiowa.edu

H.D. Cualing et al. (eds.), *Cutaneous Hematopathology*,
DOI 10.1007/978-1-4939-0950-6_17, © Springer Science+Business Media New York 2014

Table 17.1 Intravascular large B-cell lymphoma synopsis

Clinical	Cutaneous	Indurated plaques, telangiectatic erythema; trunk predilection
	Extracutaneous	Neurologic complications
	Course	Aggressive
Pathologic	Pattern	Occupies vascular lumina of superficial to deep dermis, panniculus
	Cytology	Atypical, large lymphoid forms
	Immunophenotype	CD20+, CD79a+, Bcl-2+, MUM-1+
	Molecular	IgJ clonality (fresh tissue)

Carter et al. 1996; Kamath et al. 2001; Zhao et al. 2005) represent true intravascular large B-cell lymphoma or intravascular involvement/recurrence of the original lymphoma has been questioned (Cerroni et al. 2009). This rare condition is estimated to represent less than 1 % of all cutaneous lymphomas (Willemze et al. 2005) and to affect less than 1 person per million per year (Zuckerman et al. 2006).

Clinical Appearance of Lesions

A rare malignancy, intravascular B-cell lymphoma, affects older adults of either gender, commonly in the sixth to seventh decades, although younger adults in their 30s have been reported. Clinical manifestations largely reflect end-organ effects from vascular compromise. Skin and central nervous system highlight the organ systems involved, although virtually any organ, including the lungs (Aouba et al. 2005; Martusewicz-Boros et al. 2007; Walls et al. 1999), kidneys (Cossu et al. 2004), heart (Bauer et al. 2005), adrenals (Fukushima et al. 2003), joints (Estalilla et al. 1999; von Kempis et al. 1998), and bone marrow, may be affected (Ferreri et al. 2004).

Cutaneous manifestations of intravascular lymphoma, presenting in approximately 39 % of cases in a large series (Ferreri et al. 2004), are not entirely specific, appearing variably as solitary or multiple, indurated violaceous patches, plaques, and nodules and/or as patchy, variably telangiectatic, violaceous erythema (Fig. 17.1); however, an impressive spectrum of morphologies ("maculopapular" eruptions, hyperpigmented patches, palpable purpura, or ulcers) is recorded in the literature (Chang et al. 1998; Digiuseppe

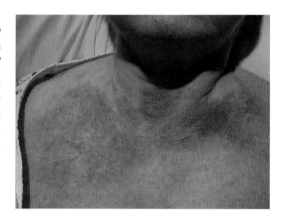

Fig. 17.1 Telangiectatic erythema of the chest in a woman with intravascular large B-cell lymphoma (Reprinted from Brinster et al. (2011). With permission from Elsevier)

et al. 1994; Kiyohara et al. 2000; Ozguroglu et al. 1997; Stroup et al. 1990; Yegappan et al. 2001; Sukpanichnant and Visuthisakchai 2006). Similarly, presenting in approximately 34 % of cases (Ferreri et al. 2004), a range of neurologic sequelae can occur, including focal sensory or motor deficits, seizures, dysarthria, and progressive dementia, among other abnormalities (Calamia et al. 1999; Glass et al. 1993; Hsu et al. 2005; Legerton and Sergent 1993; Nakahara et al. 1999; Vieren et al. 1999; Debiais et al. 2004). Constitutional symptoms commonly accompany these organ-specific manifestations, with fever, night sweats, and/or weight loss occurring in the majority of individuals; in fact, fever of unknown origin may be the primary presenting symptom in some patients (Zuckerman et al. 2006; Hoshino et al. 2004; Kidson-Gerber et al. 2005). Associated elevated serum lactate dehydrogenase (LDH), elevated erythrocyte sedimentation rate (ESR), and anemia are commonly seen.

Table 17.2 Proposed clinical forms of intravascular large B-cell lymphoma

	Non-hemophagocytosis-associated ("classical") form	Hemophagocytosis-associated form
Demographics	Western countries	Asian countries (esp. Japan)
Skin manifestations	Common	Rare
Neurologic manifestations	Common	Uncommon
Hematolymphoid involvement	Uncommon	Nearly always
Hemophagocytosis	Absent	Present

The tremendous variations from patient to patient of intravascular large B-cell lymphoma notwithstanding two general clinicopathologic patterns seem to emerge from review of the international experience (Ferreri et al. 2004): a "classical," non-hemophagocytosis (HPC) variant emphasizing cutaneous and neurologic features and arising usually in Western nations and a variant featuring hemophagocytosis, occurring usually in Asian countries (Kuratsune et al. 1988; Murase et al. 2000) (Table 17.2). In contrast to the prominent neurocutaneous hallmarks of the "classical" form, skin and neurologic manifestations are not typically seen in the HPC-associated form preferentially reported in Asian patients, in whom fever, anemia, thrombocytopenia, and hepatosplenomegaly dominate. At the other end of the spectrum, individuals with only skin involvement have been documented, suggesting the possibility of a "cutaneous-only" variant with good prognosis (Ferreri et al. 2004).

This ability of intravascular large B-cell lymphoma to present with a spectrum of protean and often nonspecific clinical features often delays correct diagnosis (Detsky et al. 2006), and often the discovery of intravascular large B-cell lymphoma is made only in retrospect at autopsy (Narimatsu et al. 2004).

Pattern of Infiltration

Tumor cells occupy the intravascular space, typically of distended capillaries and small venules, within the dermis and occasionally the subcutis (Fig. 17.2). Similar vascular congestion by atypical lymphocytes is observed in the other organ systems affected (Fig. 17.3). Intraluminal tumor cells may be arranged in aggregated clusters with obvious adherence to the vessel wall or may appear to "float" freely. The relative sparing of the surrounding tissue is remarkable, although comparatively minor component of extravascular lymphomatous involvement can be present (Ponzoni et al. 2000). In addition, scattered perivascular mixed inflammatory cells may be observed. Of note, intravascular lymphoma occurring within vascular proliferations such as cherry angiomas has been reported in multiple cases, including cases lacking evidence of other involvement, raising suspicion that tumor cells may exhibit tropism for vascular lesions (Cerroni et al. 2004; Kobayashi et al. 2000; Nixon et al. 2005; Rubin et al. 1997; Satoh et al. 2003).

Cytomorphology

Malignant lymphocytes exhibit predominantly large cytomorphology, with pleomorphic, enlarged, vesicular nuclei, nuclear contour irregularity, and one to several nucleoli, frequently resembling immunoblasts (Fig. 17.4). Over time, diagnostic criteria have expanded to include lymphocytes of smaller size (Ponzoni et al. 2007).

Immunophenotype

Tumor cells express B-lymphocyte-associated antigens (CD19, CD20, CD22, CD79a), as well as antigens which typically characterize diffuse large B-cell lymphoma (Bcl-2, MUM-1) (Fig. 17.5). CD5 expression by tumor cells is

Fig. 17.2 Histopathology of intravascular large B-cell lymphoma of the skin. (**a**) Dilated, thin-walled, dermal blood vessels congested with large, atypical lymphoid forms [H&E; 200×]. (**b**) Tumor cells may appear to float freely within the vascular space [H&E; 400×]

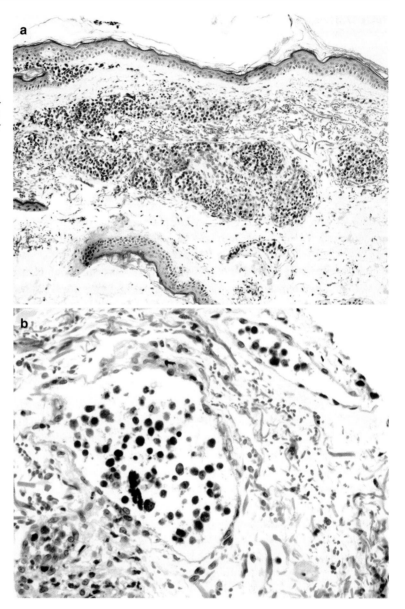

variable (Murase et al. 2007; Khalidi et al. 1998). Immunoglobulin light chain restriction is typically present, although usually only detectable on frozen tissue (Cerroni et al. 2009). On the other hand, tumor cells typically stain negatively for antibodies directed against CD3, cyclin D1, and CD56. In a minority of cases, positive staining for Bcl-6 and/or CD10 is observed. In addition, positive staining for prostate acid phosphatase has been reported in one small series (Seki et al. 2004). Assays for Epstein-Barr virus (EBV) are usually negative, although EBV has been detected in a handful of cases (Hsiao et al. 1999; Tranchida et al. 2003; Yamada et al. 2005). Negative staining for vascular endothelial markers (e.g., CD31, CD34) helps highlight the distinction of the tumor cells from the surrounding vascular lining. Occasional positive staining for Factor VIII has been interpreted as staining of adsorbed antigen by the tumor cells (Mori et al. 1985; Wrotnowski et al. 1985).

Immunophenotyping has further offered potential insight into why tumor cells are uniquely trapped within small blood vessels.

Fig. 17.3 Histopathology of intravascular large B-cell lymphoma of internal organs. (**a**) Intravascular B-cell lymphoma involving the kidney [H&E; 200×] (Courtesy of Dr. Sergei Syrbu, University of Iowa). (**b**) Intravascular B-cell lymphoma involving the lung [H&E; 200×] (Courtesy of Dr. Sergei Syrbu, University of Iowa)

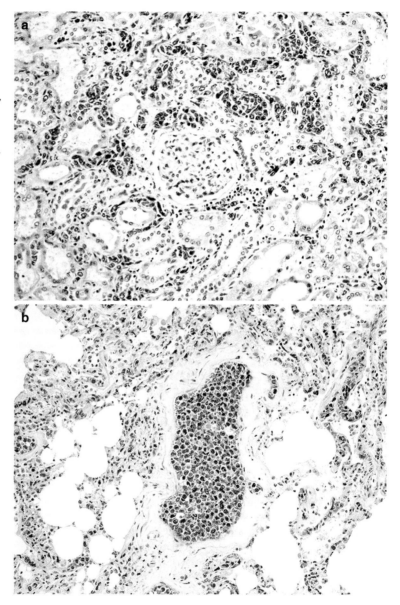

Abnormal expression of cell surface markers on tumor cells has been detected, including aberrant expression of CD11a and CD49d (Kanda et al. 1999), deficiency in the Hermes-3-defined homing receptor antigen (Ferry et al. 1988), the absence of the receptor for peanut agglutinin (Jalkanen et al. 1989), and most intriguingly the loss of CD29 (β1 integrin) and CD54 (ICAM-1) (Ponzoni et al. 2000), suggesting that altered tumor cell surface-endothelial interaction may account, at least in part, for the peculiar intravascular predilection of this lymphoma.

Cytogenetics and Molecular Findings

Although occasional chromosomal abnormalities have been reported (Khoury et al. 2003; Tsukadaira et al. 2002), including detection of t(14;18) translocation (Vieites et al. 2005), reliably consistent cytogenetic findings have not yet been identified. IgJ heavy chain clonality has been reported in fresh frozen tissue samples, although not routinely in formalin-fixed, paraffin-embedded specimens (Cerroni et al. 2009; Baehring et al. 2003; Kojima et al. 2002).

Fig. 17.4 Atypical, large, lymphocytes exhibiting nuclear enlargement, nuclear contour irregularity, and nucleoli [H&E; 600×]

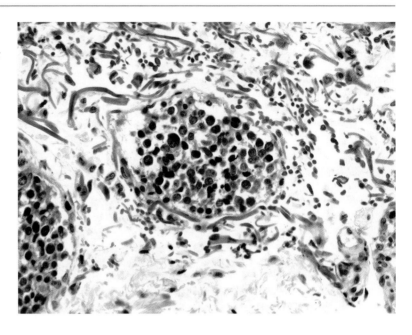

Clinical Behavior

Intravascular large B-cell lymphoma generally exhibits aggressive behavior, with overall poor prognosis. Five-year survival rate is estimated to be 65 % (Willemze et al. 2005), with most patients eventually succumbing to complications of progressive disease. Recognition of "classical" (Western) and "Asian" variants (Ferreri et al. 2004) offers clues on patterns of presentation but does not stratify reliably with regard to prognosis, with the notable exception of the cutaneous form of intravascular large B-cell lymphoma, which does appear to benefit from an indolent course (Ferreri et al. 2004). Laboratory parameters, such as frequently encountered elevated serum LDH (lactate dehydrogenase), have not been demonstrated to represent independent prognostic variables.

The overall aggressive nature of the noncutaneous form of intravascular large B-cell lymphoma warrants correspondingly aggressive systemic therapy (Digiuseppe et al. 1994). Typically, anthracycline-based multi-agent chemotherapy (e.g., CHOP: cyclophosphamide, doxorubicin, vincristine, and prednisone) is initially administered (Ferreri et al. 2004; Bouzani

et al. 2006; Feugier et al. 2005; Shimada et al. 2008), often with rituximab (R-CHOP) (Ferreri et al. 2008; Bazhenova et al. 2006; Cartron et al. 2002; Ganguly 2007). Special attention is given to any central nervous system involvement (Baehring et al. 2003; Harris et al. 1994; Sawamoto et al. 2006; Yamaguchi et al. 2001). For refractory cases, stem cell transplantation may be indicated (Ferreri et al. 2004; Koizumi et al. 2001). Positron emission tomography has been used to assess treatment response (Juweid et al. 2007).

Differential Diagnosis

Labeled a "great imitator" (Zuckerman et al. 2006), intravascular B-cell lymphoma can mimic a number of other conditions, both clinically and pathologically. From a clinical perspective, the variably livedoid erythema can generate differential considerations for vasculopathic states or reactive erythemas (Ferreri et al. 2004; Ponzoni et al. 2007). The indurated plaques and nodules can be confused with panniculitis (Kiyohara et al. 2000) or with other neoplasms. The polymorphous cutaneous presentations of

Fig. 17.5 Typical immunophenotypic profile of
intravascular large B-cell
lymphoma involving the lung:
(**a**) CD20-positive staining
[CD20; 200×]. (**b**) Contrasting
CD31-positive staining of
surrounding endothelial cells
[CD31; 200×]

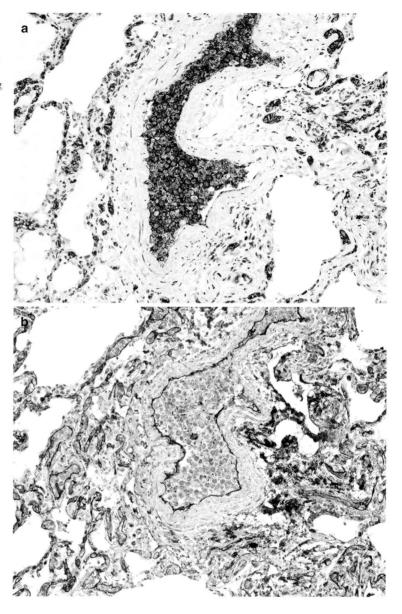

intravascular lymphoma have led to varied clinical impressions ranging from cellulitis (Roglin
and Boer 2007) to vasculitis to vascular tumors
(e.g., Kaposi's sarcoma) (Demirer et al. 1994) to
keratinocytic tumors (e.g., squamous cell carcinoma) (Stroup et al. 1990).

From a pathologic standpoint, the main differential diagnosis includes other lymphomas/
leukemias, metastatic disease (Fig. 17.6), reactive

intravascular conditions (reactive angioendotheliomatosis), and intravascular histiocytosis. With
regard to pathologic mimics for intravascular lymphoma featuring atypical lymphoid forms within
vessels, chronic lymphocytic leukemia, mantle
zone lymphoma, and splenic marginal zone
lymphoma in particular need to be considered,
although even infectious mononucleosis may
also demonstrate atypical intravascular lymphoid

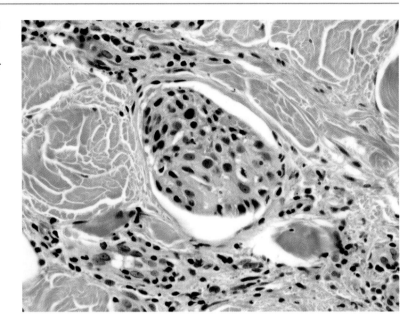

Fig. 17.6 Lymphovascular invasion by squamous cell carcinoma as a histopathologic mimic of intravascular lymphoma

forms, causing confusion with intravascular lymphoma (Ponzoni et al. 2007). Appropriate immunohistochemical studies and the relative absence of extravascular infiltration of malignant cells into surrounding tissue can aid in distinction from other lymphomas. Of note, biopsies of apparently non-lesional skin have been shown to be pathologically diagnostic of intravascular large B-cell lymphoma (Asada et al. 2007; Gill et al. 2003; Le et al. 2008).

Intravascular Large NK-/T-Cell Lymphoma

Introduction

Not officially recognized by the WHO or the WHO-EORTC as its own distinct lymphoma entity, intravascular large NK-/T-cell lymphoma represents the NK-/T-cell counterpart to the rare but more common and officially recognized intravascular large B-cell lymphoma (Ferreri et al. 2004; Cerroni et al. 2008; Song et al. 2007). Characterization of this very rare T- or NK-cell phenotypic variant of intravascular lymphoma is

limited by small numbers of cases (total less than 100) which have reported variably thorough immunophenotypic evaluations. Nonetheless, the overall clinical behavior of intravascular large NK-/T-cell lymphoma appears similar to intravascular large B-cell lymphoma, suggesting the cell of origin to be of lesser importance than histomorphology, a feature unique among lymphoma entities (Cerroni et al. 2008). Due to the overlapping immunophenotypic markers between T-lymphocytes and NK-cells, they have conventionally been grouped together in the context of intravascular lymphoma. Included in this discussion of intravascular large NK-/T-cell lymphoma are exceptional cases expressing the CD30 antigen.

Definition

Intravascular large NK-/T-cell lymphoma represents an intravascular malignant T-lymphocytic or NK-cell proliferation generally lacking a significant extravascular lymphoma component, characterized most commonly by cutaneous and neurologic manifestations and by aggressive behavior (Table 17.3).

Table 17.3 Intravascular large NK-/T-cell lymphoma synopsis

Clinical	Cutaneous	Solitary or multiple, erythematous-violaceous patches, indurated plaques, often with associated livedoid erythema
	Extracutaneous	Neurologic most frequent
	Course	Aggressive
Pathologic	Morphology	Tumor aggregates with distended vascular lumina
	Cytology	Large, atypical, lymphoid appearance
	Immunophenotype	CD2+, CD3+, CD5−, CD56+, EBER often positive; CD30+ in very rare intravascular anaplastic large-cell lymphoma subset
	Molecular	Monoclonal TCR gene rearrangements may be detected

Clinical Appearance of Lesions

Overall, the clinical features of intravascular large NK-/T-cell lymphoma appear similar to intravascular large B-cell lymphoma, with the exception that intravascular T-cell lymphoma appears more commonly associated with EBV (Cerroni et al. 2009; Nakamichi et al. 2008). While a congenital case has been reported (Tateyama et al. 1991), intravascular large NK-/T-cell lymphoma typically affects middle to older age adults and characteristically demonstrates cutaneous and neurologic features, resembling intravascular B-cell lymphoma. The heterogeneous skin lesions range from indurated plaques and nodules to patchy, variably livedoid erythema. The spectrum of neurologic complications encompasses focal sensory/motor as well as global neurologic deficits. Like intravascular large B-cell lymphoma, virtually any organ system (including the kidney, liver, lung, adrenal, bone marrow, spleen, pituitary gland, ovary, cervix, ileum) may be involved (Cerroni et al. 2009; Williams et al. 2005; Wu et al. 2005).

Pattern of Infiltration

Identical to intravascular large B-cell lymphoma, small blood vessels (typically capillaries and small venules) are variably filled and distended by tumor cells within the dermis and subcutis. Perivascular scattered mixed inflammatory cells may be seen, although significant extravascular lymphoma is not expected.

Cytomorphology

Malignant lymphocytes exhibit predominantly medium to large cytomorphology, with pleomorphic, enlarged, vesicular nuclei, with nuclear contour irregularity.

Immunophenotype

As expected by lineage, tumor cells of intravascular large NK-/T-cell lymphoma express CD2 and CD3, although usually not CD5. As most cases exhibit an NK-/T-cell cytotoxic phenotype reminiscent of extranodal NK-/T-cell lymphoma, tumor cells of intravascular large NK-/T-cell lymphoma usually also express cytotoxic proteins such as TIA-1 and granzyme B and frequently express CD56 and EBER-1 (Cerroni et al. 2008). In fact, the intravascular large NK-/T-cell lymphoma appears associated with EBV more frequently than is its B-cell counterpart (Au et al. 1997). Notably, the beta-F1 marker of alpha/beta T-lymphocytes is not detected.

Exceptional reports of the so-called intravascular anaplastic large-cell lymphoma have documented the tumor cells in a subset of intravascular NK-/T-cell lymphoma cases as prominently expressing CD30, associated with a general tendency toward relapse and frequently a rapidly fatal course (Ko et al. 1997; Takahashi et al. 2005; Wang et al. 2011; Zizi-Sermpetzoglou et al. 2009).

Cytogenetics and Molecular Findings

Monoclonal rearrangements of the T-cell receptor-gamma gene may be detected in a minority (approximately one-third) of cases, with the remainder possibly representing those of true NK-cell lineage (Cerroni et al. 2009).

Clinical Behavior

Intravascular large NK-/T-cell lymphoma overall exhibits aggressive behavior and poor prognosis, generally comparable to that of intravascular large B-cell lymphoma. Accordingly, treatment with multi-agent chemotherapy is typically administered for these patients. Stratification of intravascular large NK-/T-cell lymphoma into reliably predictive, sharply defined subsets is precluded by the rarity of the disease, but the overall tendency appears that more limited organ (e.g., skin) involvement portends better prognosis. Patients with CD30-positive, intravascular anaplastic large-cell lymphoma appear to similarly suffer poor outcomes, with many experiencing rapid deterioration and death from disease (Takahashi et al. 2005), although if disease is limited to the skin, the course may be more indolent (Wang et al. 2011).

Differential Diagnosis

As with its immunophenotypic cousin intravascular large B-cell lymphoma, intravascular large NK-/T-cell lymphoma can wear a variety of clinical costumes, allowing it to masquerade both as inflammatory conditions and as other neoplasms. Presentation by intravascular NK-/T-cell lymphoma as erythematous to violaceous patches variably exhibiting a livedo racemosa pattern can raise suspicion for varied vasculopathic states, while indurated plaques and nodules can be confused with infiltrative processes, cellulitis, panniculitis, or possibly vascular tumors (Krishnan et al. 2009).

Primary pathologic differential considerations cover other malignancies, including metastatic tumors (e.g., carcinomas, melanoma) and vascular proliferations, as well as intravascular reactive conditions (Bryant et al. 2007), including intravascular histiocytosis. With respect to intravascular ALCL in particular, pathologic simulants exhibiting CD30-positive atypical, large blast-like forms have been observed in apparently benign settings (Fig. 17.7) (Baum et al. 2009; Riveiro-Falkenbach et al. 2013).

Intralymphatic Histiocytosis

Introduction

Histiocytes, rather than lymphocytes or endothelial cells, can occupy the lumina of vessels in certain states, collectively termed "intralymphatic histiocytosis." Understanding of intralymphatic histiocytosis has evolved over its brief history, beginning with identification of the intravascular occupants as of macrophagic-histiocytic lineage, followed by recognition of the lymphatic nature of the involved vessels, and continuing to the present day with ongoing debate over the condition's possible relationship with benign reactive angioendotheliomatosis. The various terms used to describe this entity ("intravascular histiocytosis," "rheumatoid intravascular or intralymphatic histiocytosis of the skin," "cutaneous histiocytic lymphangitis," "rheumatoid arthritis-associated intravascular histiocytopathy," "intralymphatic histiocytosis") reflect its evolving conceptualization.

"Intravascular histiocytosis" was first coined by O'Grady et al. two decades ago in reference to their description of a 77-year-old woman with plaques on her left lower leg which histopathologically revealed immunohistochemically confirmed macrophagic histiocytes distending small dermal vessels (O'Grady and Shahidullah 1994), and the authors specifically contrasted their case with intravascular lymphoma. The resemblance of intravascular histiocytosis to benign reactive angioendotheliomatosis was highlighted by Rieger et al. 5 years later, in their discussion of two additional patients, with the authors postulating that conditions beginning as intravascular histiocytosis subsequently become associated with

Fig. 17.7 Reactive CD30-positive intravascular condition of the skin. (**a**) Irregularly contoured lymphocytes within cutaneous dermal vessels [H&E; 400×]. (**b**) CD3-positive staining of intravascular lymphocytic population [CD3; 400×]. (**c**) Larger atypical lymphoid forms stain express CD30 [CD30; 400×]

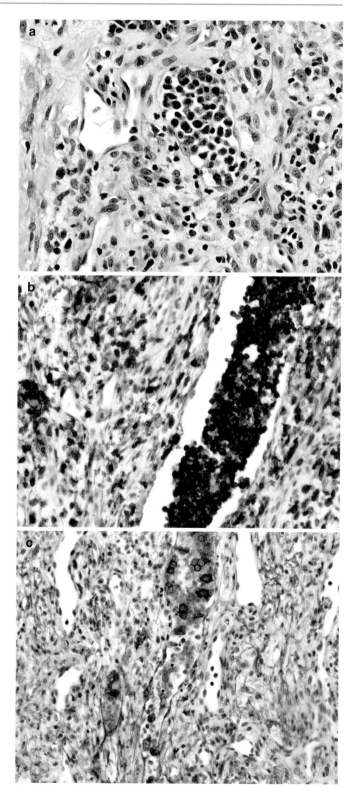

intravascular thrombi, which in turn results in endothelial proliferation recognized as angioendotheliomatosis (Rieger et al. 1999). The frequent association between intravascular histiocytosis and rheumatoid arthritis was demonstrated by subsequent reports (Magro and Crowson 2003; Takiwaki et al. 2004; Catalina-Fernandez et al. 2007). Takiwaki et al. further acknowledged that the nature of the vessels housing the histiocytic infiltrates was uncertain, entertaining the possibility that they could be lymphatic. The lymphatic identity of the involved vessels was confirmed the following year, as Okazaki et al. discovered vessel expression of the lymphatic marker podoplanin (Okazaki et al. 2005). In the largest series to date of 16 patients, Requena et al. expanded on the clinicopathologic spectrum of the condition and corroborated the lymphatic nature of the involved vessels. Indeed, based upon the lymphatic predilection for this condition rather than blood vessels involved in reactive angioendotheliomatosis, Requena et al. favored intravascular histiocytosis and reactive angioendotheliomatosis to be separate and distinct entities, contrasting with the Rieger's hypothesis a decade earlier proposing a link between the two conditions (Requena et al. 2009).

Definition

Intralymphatic histiocytosis refers to the group of reactive conditions characterized by the phenomenon of lymphatic vessels containing histiocytes (Table 17.4).

Clinical Appearance of Lesions

Intravascular histiocytosis typically occurs in middle-aged to elderly individuals, affecting both men and women, although a report of intravascular histiocytosis arising in a teenager has been reported (Asagoe et al. 2006). Associated systemic disease is frequent, with rheumatoid arthritis present in approximately half of cases. Ill-defined erythematous to violaceous patches and plaques, frequently featuring livedo reticularis-like morphology, usually distributed on the proximal extremities but also on the trunk, represent the most common cutaneous manifestations of intravascular histiocytosis. Predilection for cutaneous lesions to be located over or around joints has been noted. The constituent papules and plaques characteristically exhibit a wavy or branching arrangement suggestive of a vascular pattern. Associated edema within the plaques may be appreciated. A report of intravascular histiocytosis manifesting as vulvar necrosis has been described (Pouryazdanparast et al. 2009).

Pattern of Infiltration

Variably cohesive histiocytic aggregates are featured within distended lymphatics of the reticular dermis. Surrounding patchy mixed inflammation including small lymphocytes, histiocytes, and plasma cells may be seen, in some cases forming lymphoid aggregates protruding into the vessel lumen (Requena et al. 2009).

Table 17.4 Intralymphatic histiocytosis synopsis

Clinical	Cutaneous	Livedoid erythematous patches of proximal extremities, trunk
	Extracutaneous	Associated with rheumatoid arthritis (common)
	Course	Indolent
Pathologic	Morphology	Reticular dermal lymphatic vessels
	Cytology	Epithelioid histiocytes
	Immunophenotype	Monocyte/histiocyte markers positive (CD68); lymphatic vascular markers (e.g., CD31; CD34; Lyve-1; podoplanin; D2-40)
	Molecular	No aberrations detected

Cytomorphology

Lesional histiocytes typically exhibit epithelioid mononuclear cytomorphology, demonstrating round to oval, vesicular, uniform nuclei surrounded by ample, eosinophilic, finely granular cytoplasm. Admixed neutrophils and small lymphocytes also may be seen within the vascular space.

Immunophenotype

Intravascular lesional cells express CD68 and other macrophagic-histiocytic markers. The lymphatic nature of the containing vessels is confirmed by positive staining not only for CD31 and CD34 but also for podoplanin, Lyve-1, Prox-1, and D2-40.

Cytogenetics and Molecular Findings

No reproducible cytogenetic abnormalities or clonality is detected in intravascular histiocytosis, consistent with its reactive nature.

Clinical Behavior

As a reactive condition, intravascular histiocytosis generally follows an indolent, waxing-waning, but often chronic course; no malignant transformation has yet been reported. Frequent association with underlying inflammatory disease, usually rheumatoid arthritis, is characteristic of the condition, although the cutaneous lesions do not reliably reflect the underlying disease activity. In addition to therapy administered for any underlying disease, a variety of skin-directed therapies (including topical corticosteroids, pressure bandage (Washio et al. 2011), cyclophosphamide, pentoxifylline, amoxicillin + acetylsalicylic acid) have been attempted with variable response.

Differential Diagnosis

Clinically, the erythematous indurated patches and plaques of intralymphatic histiocytosis may resemble infections (e.g., cellulitis, herpetic infections), allergic contact dermatitis, or infiltrative conditions (e.g., granuloma annulare, mycosis fungoides), while cases featuring a livedo reticularis pattern may evoke consideration for other vasculopathic states. From a pathologic standpoint, the main differential diagnosis includes intravascular lymphoma, lymphovascular invasion by carcinoma, or reactive angioendotheliomatosis. The conceptual evolution of "angioendotheliomatosis," with its separation into malignant and benign forms, eventuating into our modern diagnoses of intravascular lymphoma and reactive angioendotheliomatosis, respectively, highlights the diagnostic challenge of intravascular histiocytosis. As mentioned previously, the relationship between intralymphatic histiocytosis and reactive angioendotheliomatosis has been debated (Requena et al. 2009). Of note, a patient was recently reported who had a cutaneous angioma featuring intralymphatic atypical T-cells (Ardighieri et al. 2010). Immunohistochemical demonstration of positive staining for lymphatic markers (e.g., podoplanin, see Table 17.4 for other markers.) by the affected vessels with concurrent positive staining for macrophagic-histiocytic markers (e.g., CD68) by the intravascular population helps confirm the diagnosis of intralymphatic histiocytosis.

References

Aouba A, Diop S, Saadoun D, Trebbia G, Vilde F, Patri B, et al. Severe pulmonary arterial hypertension as initial manifestation of intravascular lymphoma: case report. Am J Hematol. 2005;79(1):46–9. PubMed PMID: WOS:000228843000008. English.

Ardighieri L, Lonardi S, Vermi W, Medicina D, Cerroni L, Facchetti F. Intralymphatic atypical T-cell proliferation in a cutaneous hemangioma. J Cutan Pathol. 2010;37(4):497–503. PubMed PMID: WOS: 000274451700017. English.

Asada N, Odawara J, Kimura SI, Aoki T, Yamakura M, Takeuchi M, et al. Use of random skin biopsy for diagnosis of intravascular large B-Cell lymphoma. Mayo Clin Proc. 2007;82(12):1525–7. PubMed PMID: WOS:000251384300013. English.

Asagoe K, Fujimoto W, Yoshino T, Mannami T, Liu YX, Kanzaki H, et al. Intravascular lymphomatosis of the skin as a manifestation of recurrent B-cell lymphoma. J Am Acad Dermatol. 2003;48(2):S1–4. PubMed PMID: WOS:000181166900001. English.

Asagoe K, Torigoe R, Ofuji R, Iwatsuki K. Reactive intravascular histiocytosis associated with tonsillitis. Brit J Dermatol. 2006;154(3):560–3. PubMed PMID: WOS:000234918900032. English.

Au WY, Shek WH, Nicholls J, Tse KM, Todd D, Kwong YL. T-cell intravascular lymphomatosis (angiotropic large cell lymphoma): association with Epstein-Barr viral infection. Histopathology. 1997;31(6):563–7. PubMed PMID: WOS:000071222800010. English.

Baehring JM, Longtine J, Hochberg FH. A new approach to the diagnosis and treatment of intravascular lymphoma. J Neuro Oncol. 2003;61(3):237–48. PubMed PMID: WOS:000181204400008. English.

Bauer A, Perras B, Sufke S, Horny HP, Kreft B. Myocardial infarction as an uncommon clinical manifestation of intravascular large cell lymphoma. Acta Cardiol. 2005;60(5):551–5. PubMed PMID: WOS:000232558700016. English.

Baum CL, Stone MS, Liu V. Atypical intravascular CD30 + T-cell proliferation following trauma in a healthy 17-year-old male: first reported case of a potential diagnostic pitfall and literature review. J Cutan Pathol. 2009;36(3):350–4. PubMed PMID: WOS:000262879800011. English.

Bazhenova L, Higginbottom P, Mason J. Intravascular lymphoma: a role for single-agent rituximab. Leuk Lymphoma. 2006;47(2):337–41. PubMed PMID: WOS:000233641400021. English.

Bhawan J, Wolff SM, Ucci AA, Bhan AK. Malignant-lymphoma and malignant angioendotheliomatosis – one disease. Cancer. 1985;55(3):570–6. PubMed PMID: WOS:A1985ABC5600015. English.

Bouzani M, Karmiris T, Rontogianni D, Delimpassi S, Apostolidis J, Mpakiri M, et al. Disseminated intravascular B-cell lymphoma: clinicopathological features and outcome of three cases treated with anthracycline-based immunochemotherapy. Oncologist. 2006;11(8):923–8. PubMed PMID: WOS: 000240627900008. English.

Brinster NK, Liu V, Diwan H, McKee PH. High yield pathology: dermatopathology. Philadelphia: Elsevier; 2011.

Bryant A, Lawton H, Al-Talib R, Wright DH, Theaker JM. Intravascular proliferation of reactive lymphoid blasts mimicking intravascular lymphoma – a diagnostic pitfall. Histopathology. 2007;51(3):401–2. PubMed PMID: WOS:000249528900012. English.

Calamia KT, Miller A, Shuster EA, Perniciaro C, Menke DM. Intravascular lymphomatosis. A report of ten patients with central nervous system involvement and a review of the disease process. Advances in experimental medicine and biology. Adv Exp Med Biol. 1999;455:249–65. PubMed PMID: 10599352.

Carter DK, Batts KP, de Groen PC, Kurtin PJ. Angiotropic large cell lymphoma (intravascular lymphomatosis) occurring after follicular small cleaved cell lymphoma. Mayo Clin Proc. 1996;71(9):869–73. PubMed PMID: WOS:A1996VF67100008. English.

Cartron G, Dacheux L, Salles G, Solal-Celigny P, Bardos P, Colombat P, et al. Therapeutic activity of humanized anti-CD20 monoclonal antibody and polymorphism in IgG Fc receptor Fc gamma RIIIa gene. Blood. 2002;99(3):754–8. PubMed PMID: WOS:000173527000007. English.

Catalina-Fernandez I, Alvarez AC, Martin FC, Fernandez-Mera JJ, Saenz-Santamaria J. Cutaneous intralymphatic histiocytosis associated with rheumatoid arthritis: report of a case and review of the literature. Am J Dermatopathol. 2007;29(2):165–8. PubMed PMID: WOS:000246792300009. English.

Cerroni L, Zalaudek I, Kerl H. Intravascular large B-cell lymphoma colonizing cutaneous hemangiomas. Dermatology. 2004;209(2):132–4. PubMed PMID: WOS:000223490400011. English.

Cerroni L, Massone C, Kutzner H, Mentzel T, Umbert P, Kerl H. Intravascular large T-cell or NK-cell lymphoma – a rare variant of intravascular large cell lymphoma with frequent cytotoxic phenotype and association with epstein-barr virus infection. Am J Surg Pathol. 2008;32A(6):891–8. PubMed PMID: WOS:000256553000011. English.

Cerroni L, Gatter K, Kerl H. Skin lymphoma. 3rd ed. West Sussex: Wiley-Blackwell; 2009.

Chang A, Zic JA, Boyd AS. Intravascular large cell lymphoma: a patient with asymptomatic purpuric patches and a chronic clinical course. J Am Acad Dermatol. 1998;39(2):318–21. PubMed PMID: WOS:000075182200005. English.

Cossu A, Deiana A, Lissia A, Satta A, Cossu M, Dedola MF, et al. Nephrotic syndrome and angiotropic lymphoma report of a case. Tumori. 2004;90(5):510–3. PubMed PMID: 15656340.

Debiais S, Bonnaud I, Cottier JP, Destrieux C, Saudeau D, de Toffol B, et al. A spinal cord intravascular lymphomatosis with exceptionally good outcome. Neurology. 2004;63(7):1329–30. PubMed PMID: 15477571.

Demirer T, Dail DH, Aboulafia DM. Four varied cases of intravascular lymphomatosis and a literature review. Cancer. 1994;73(6):1738–45. PubMed PMID: 8156502.

Detsky ME, Chiu L, Shandling MR, Sproule ME, Ursell MR. Clinical problem-solving. Heading down the wrong path. N Engl J Med. 2006;355(1):67–74. PubMed PMID: 16822998.

Digiuseppe JA, Nelson WG, Seifter EJ, Boitnott JK, Mann RB. Intravascular lymphomatosis – a clinicopathological study of 10 cases and assessment of response to chemotherapy. J Clin Oncol. 1994;12(12):2573–9. PubMed PMID: WOS:A1994PV81100009. English.

Domizio P, Hall PA, Cotter F, Amiel S, Tucker J, Besser GM, et al. Angiotropic large cell lymphoma (ALCL): morphological, immunohistochemical and genotypic studies with analysis of previous reports. Hematol Oncol. 1989;7(3):195–206. PubMed PMID: 2651272.

Estalilla OC, Koo CH, Brynes RK, Medeiros LJ. Intravascular large B-cell lymphoma – a report of five cases initially diagnosed by bone marrow biopsy. Am J Clin Pathol. 1999;112(2):248–55. PubMed PMID: WOS:000081664800013. English.

Ferreri AJM, Campo E, Seymour JF, Willemze R, Ilariucci F, Ambrosetti A, et al. Intravascular lymphoma:

clinical presentation, natural history, management and prognostic factors in a series of 38 cases, with special emphasis on the 'cutaneous variant'. Brit J Haematol. 2004;127(2):173–83. PubMed PMID: WOS:000224283700006. English.

Ferreri AJM, Dognini GP, Govi S, Crocchiolo R, Bouzani M, Bollinger CR, et al. Can rituximab change the usually dismal prognosis of patients with intravascular large B-cell lymphoma? J Clin Oncol. 2008;26(31):5134–6. PubMed PMID: WOS:000260537600029. English.

Ferry JA, Harris NL, Picker LJ, Weinberg DS, Rosales RK, Tapia J, et al. Intravascular lymphomatosis (Malignant Angioendotheliomatosis) – a B-cell neoplasm expressing surface homing receptors. Modern Pathol. 1988;1(6):444–52. PubMed PMID: WOS:A1988R208300007. English.

Feugier P, Van Hoof A, Sebban C, Solal-Celigny P, Bouabdallah R, Ferme C, et al. Long-term results of the R-CHOP study in the treatment of elderly patients with diffuse large B-cell lymphoma: a study by the groupe d'Etude des lymphomes de l'adulte. J Clin Oncol. 2005;23(18):4117–26. PubMed PMID: WOS:000229886700016. English.

Fredericks RK, Walker FO, Elster A, Challa V. Angiotropic intravascular large-cell lymphoma (Malignant Angioendotheliomatosis) – report of a case and review of the literature. Surg Neurol. 1991;35(3):218–23. PubMed PMID: WOS:A1991EZ63400008. English.

Fukushima A, Okada Y, Tanikawa T, Onaka T, Tanaka A, Higashi T, et al. Primary bilateral adrenal intravascular large B-cell lymphoma associated with adrenal failure. Intern Med. 2003;42(7):609–14. PubMed PMID: 12879956.

Ganguly S. Acute intracerebral hemorrhage in intravascular lymphoma: a serious infusion related adverse event of rituximab. Am J Clin Oncol. 2007;30(2):211–2. PubMed PMID: 17414473.

Gill S, Melosky B, Haley L, ChanYan C. Use of random skin biopsy to diagnose intravascular lymphoma presenting as fever of unknown origin. Am J Med. 2003;114(1):56–8. PubMed PMID: WOS:000180579400011. English.

Glass J, Hochberg FH, Miller DC. Intravascular lymphomatosis. A systemic disease with neurologic manifestations. Cancer. 1993;71(10):3156–64. PubMed PMID: 8490846.

Harris CP, Sigman JD, Jaeckle KA. Intravascular malignant lymphomatosis: amelioration of neurological symptoms with plasmapheresis. Ann Neurol. 1994;35(3):357–9. PubMed PMID: 8122888.

Hoshino A, Kawada E, Ukita T, Itoh K, Sakamoto H, Fujita K, et al. Usefulness of FDG-PET to diagnose intravascular lymphomatosis presenting as fever of unknown origin. Am J Hematol. 2004;76(3):236–9. PubMed PMID: 15224358.

Hsiao CH, Su IJ, Hsieh SW, Huang SF, Tsai TF, Chen MY, et al. Epstein-Barr virus-associated intravascular lymphomatosis within Kaposi's sarcoma in an AIDS patient. Am J Surg Pathol. 1999;23(4):482–7. PubMed PMID: 10199480.

Hsu YH, Tseng BY, Shyu WC, Yen PS. Intravascular lymphomatosis mimicking acute disseminated encephalomyelitis: a case report. Kaohsiung J Med Sci. 2005;21(2):93–7. PubMed PMID: 15825696.

Jalkanen S, Aho R, Kallajoki M, Ekfors T, Nortamo P, Gahmberg C, et al. Lymphocyte homing receptors and adhesion molecules in intravascular malignant lymphomatosis. Int J Cancer. 1989;44(5):777–82. PubMed PMID: WOS:A1989CB05400003. English.

Juweid ME, Stroobants S, Hoekstra OS, Mottaghy FM, Dietlein M, Guermazi A, et al. Use of positron emission tomography for response assessment of lymphoma: consensus of the imaging subcommittee of international harmonization project in lymphoma. J Clin Oncol. 2007;25(5):571–8. PubMed PMID: WOS:000244176000017. English.

Kamath NV, Gilliam AC, Nihal M, Spiro TP, Wood GS. Primary cutaneous large B-cell lymphoma of the leg relapsing as cutaneous intravascular large B-cell lymphoma. Arch Dermatol. 2001;137(12):1657–8. PubMed PMID: WOS:000172792700022. English.

Kanda M, Suzumiya J, Ohshima K, Tamura K, Kikuchi M. Intravascular large cell lymphoma: clinicopathological, immuno-histochemical and molecular genetic studies. Leuk Lymphoma. 1999;34(5–6):569. PubMed PMID: WOS:000082619100017. English.

Khalidi HS, Brynes RK, Browne P, Koo CH, Battifora H, Medeiros LJ. Intravascular large B-cell lymphoma: the CD5 antigen is expressed by a subset of cases. Modern Pathol. 1998;11(10):983–8. PubMed PMID: WOS:000076505600012. English.

Khoury H, Lestou VS, Gascoyne RD, Bruyere H, Li CH, Nantel SH, et al. Multicolor karyotyping and clinico-pathological analysis of three intravascular lymphoma cases. Modern Pathol. 2003;16(7):716–24. PubMed PMID: WOS:000184284000014. English.

Kidson-Gerber G, Bosco A, MacCallum S, Dunkley S. Two cases of intravascular lymphoma: highlighting the diagnostic difficulties in pyrexia of unknown origin. Intern Med J. 2005;35(9):569–70. PubMed PMID: WOS:000231147300014. English.

Kiyohara T, Kumakiri M, Kobayashi H, Shimizu T, Ohkawara A, Ohnuki M. A case of intravascular large B-cell lymphoma mimicking erythema nodosum: the importance of multiple skin biopsies. J Cutan Pathol. 2000;27(8):413–8. PubMed PMID: WOS:000088444100007. English.

Ko YH, Han JH, Go JH, Kim DS, Kwon OJ, Yang WI, et al. Intravascular lymphomatosis: a clinicopathological study of two cases presenting as an interstitial lung disease. Histopathology. 1997;31(6):555–62. PubMed PMID: WOS:000071222800009. English.

Kobayashi T, Munakata S, Sugiura H, Koizumi M, Sumida M, Murata K, et al. Angiotropic lymphoma: proliferation of B cells in the capillaries of cutaneous angiomas. Brit J Dermatol. 2000;143(1):162–4. PubMed PMID: WOS:000088012700027. English.

Koizumi M, Nishimura M, Yokota A, Munekata S, Kobayashi T, Saito Y. Case report – successful treatment of intravascular malignant lymphomatosis with high-dose chemotherapy and autologous peripheral blood stem cell transplantation. Bone Marrow Transpl. 2001;27(10):1101–3. PubMed PMID: WOS:000169416400015. English.

Kojima K, Kaneda K, Yasukawa M, Tanaka K, Inoue T, Yamashita T, et al. Specificity of polymerase chain reaction-based clonality analysis of immunoglobulin heavy chain gene rearrangement for the detection of bone marrow infiltrate in B-cell lymphoma-associated haemophagocytic syndrome. Brit J Haematol. 2002;119(3):616–21. PubMed PMID: WOS:000179283600006. English.

Krishnan C, Moline S, Anders K, Warnke RA. Intravascular ALK-positive anaplastic large-cell lymphoma mimicking inflammatory breast carcinoma. J Clin Oncol. 2009;27(15):2563–5. PubMed PMID: WOS:000266195400024. English.

Kuratsune H, Machii T, Aozasa K, Ueda E, Tokumine Y, Morita T, et al. B-cell lymphoma showing clinicopathological features of malignant histiocytosis. Acta Haematol-Basel. 1988;79(2):94–8. PubMed PMID: WOS:A1988M292800009. English.

Le EN, Gerstenblith MR, Gelber AC, Manno RL, Ranasinghe PD, Sweren RJ, et al. The use of blind skin biopsy in the diagnosis of intravascular B-cell lymphoma. J Am Acad Dermatol. 2008;59(1):148–51. PubMed PMID: WOS:000257118300021. English.

Legerton CW, Sergent JS. Intravascular malignant-lymphoma mimicking central-nervous-system lupus. Arthritis Rheum. 1993;36(1):135. PubMed PMID: WOS:A1993KK74600022. English.

Magro CM, Crowson AN. The spectrum of cutaneous lesions in rheumatoid arthritis: a clinical and pathological study of 43 patients. J Cutan Pathol. 2003;30(1):1–10. PubMed PMID: WOS:000180529300001. English.

Martusewicz-Boros M, Wiatr E, Radzikowska E, Roszkowski-Sliz K, Langfort R. Pulmonary intravascular large B-cell lymphoma as a cause of severe hypoxemia. J Clin Oncol. 2007;25(15):2137–9. PubMed PMID: WOS:000246804200032. English.

Mori S, Itoyama S, Mohri N, Shibuya A, Hirose T, Takanashi R, et al. Cellular characteristics of neoplastic angioendotheliosis – an immunohistological marker study of 6 cases. Virchows Arch A. 1985;407(2):167–75. PubMed PMID: WOS:A1985AMQ8400004. English.

Murase T, Nakamura S, Kawauchi K, Matsuzaki H, Sakai C, Inaba T, et al. An Asian variant of intravascular large B-cell lymphoma: clinical, pathological and cytogenetic approaches to diffuse large B-cell lymphoma associated with haemophagocytic syndrome. Brit J Haematol. 2000;111(3):826–34. PubMed PMID: WOS:000165938900017. English.

Murase T, Yamaguchi M, Suzuki R, Okamoto M, Sato Y, Tamaru JI, et al. Intravascular large B-cell lymphoma (IVLBCL): a clinicopathologic study of 96 cases with special reference to the immunophenotypic heterogeneity of CD5. Blood. 2007;109(2):478–85. PubMed PMID: WOS:000243416600018. English.

Nakahara T, Saito T, Muroi A, Sugiura Y, Ogata M, Sugiyama Y, et al. Intravascular lymphomatosis presenting as an ascending cauda equina: conus medullaris syndrome: remission after biweekly CHOP therapy. J Neurol Neurosurg Psychiatry. 1999;67(3):403–6. PubMed PMID: 10449569. Pubmed Central PMCID: 1736537.

Nakamichi N, Fukuhara S, Aozasa K, Morii E. NK-cell intravascular lymphomatosis–a mini-review. Eur J Haematol. 2008;81(1):1–7. PubMed PMID: 18462254.

Nakamura S, Ponzoni M, Campo E. Intravascular large B-cell lymphoma. In: Swerdlow SH, Campo E, Harris NL, et al., editors. WHO classification of tumours of haematopoietic and lymphoid tissues. 4th ed. Lyon: IARC Press; 2008.

Narimatsu H, Morishita Y, Saito S, Shimada K, Ozeki K, Kohno A, et al. Usefulness of bone marrow aspiration for definite diagnosis of Asian variant of intravascular lymphoma: four autopsied cases. Leuk Lymphoma. 2004;45(8):1611–6. PubMed PMID: 15370213.

Nixon BK, Kussick SJ, Carlon MJ, Rubin BP. Intravascular large B-cell lymphoma involving hemangiomas: an unusual presentation of a rare neoplasm. Mod Pathol: Off J U S Can Acad Pathol Inc. 2005;18(8):1121–6. PubMed PMID: 15803190.

O'Grady JT, Shahidullah H, Doherty VR, al-Nafussi A. Intravascular histiocytosis. Histopathology. 1994;24(3):265–8. PubMed PMID: 8200627.

Okazaki A, Asada H, Niizeki H, Nonomura A, Miyagawa S. Intravascular histiocytosis associated with rheumatoid arthritis: report of a case with lymphatic endothelial proliferation. Br J Dermatol. 2005;152(6):1385–7. PubMed PMID: 15949027.

Ozguroglu E, Buyulbabani N, Ozguroglu M, Baykal C. Generalized telangiectasia as the major manifestation of angiotropic (intravascular) lymphoma. Br J Dermatol. 1997;137(3):422–5. PubMed PMID: 9349342.

Pfleger L, Tappeiner J. On the recognition of systematized endotheliomatosis of the cutaneous blood vessels (reticuloendotheliosis)? Der Hautarzt Zeitschrift Dermatologie Venerologie verwandte Gebiete. 1959;10:359–63. PubMed PMID: 14432547.

Ponzoni M, Arrigoni G, Gould VE, Del Curto B, Maggioni M, Scapinello A, et al. Lack of CD 29 (beta 1 integrin) and CD 54 (ICAM-1) adhesion molecules in intravascular lymphomatosis. Hum Pathol. 2000;31(2):220–6. PubMed PMID: WOS:000085237900011. English.

Ponzoni M, Ferreri AJM, Campo E, Facchetti F, Mazzucchelli L, Yoshino T, et al. Definition, diagnosis, and management of intravascular large B-Cell lymphoma: proposals and perspectives from an international consensus meeting. J Clin Oncol. 2007;25(21):3168–73. PubMed PMID: WOS:000248743800028. English.

Pouryazdanparast P, Cho K, Fullen D, Yu L, Dalton V, Haefner H. Intravascular histiocytosis presenting with extensive vulvar necrosis. J Cutan Pathol. 2009;36(1):105. PubMed PMID: WOS:000262129600023. English.

Requena L, El-Shabrawi-Caelen L, Walsh SN, Segura S, Ziemer M, Hurt MA, et al. Intralymphatic histiocytosis. A clinicopathologic study of 16 cases. Am J Dermatopathol. 2009;31(2):140–51. PubMed PMID: WOS:000264558100005. English.

Rieger E, Soyer HP, Leboit PE, Metze D, Slovak R, Kerl H. Reactive angioendotheliomatosis or intravascular histiocytosis? An immunohistochemical and ultrastructural study in two cases of intravascular histiocytic cell proliferation. Br J Dermatol. 1999;140(3):497–504. PubMed PMID: WOS:000079498800021. English.

Riveiro-Falkenbach E, Fernandez-Figueras MT, Rodriguez-Peralto JL. Benign atypical intravascular CD30(+) T-cell proliferation: a reactive condition mimicking intravascular lymphoma. Am J Dermatopathol. 2013;35(2):143–50. PubMed PMID: WOS:000316941200005. English.

Roglin J, Boer A. Skin manifestations of intravascular lymphoma mimic inflammatory diseases of the skin. Brit J Dermatol. 2007;157(1):16–25. PubMed PMID: WOS:000247318900003. English.

Rubin MA, Cossman J, Freter CE, Azumi N. Intravascular large cell lymphoma coexisting within hemangiomas of the skin. Am J Surg Pathol. 1997;21(7):860–4. PubMed PMID: WOS:A1997XW92300016. English.

Satoh S, Yamazaki M, Yahikozawa H, Ichikawa N, Saito H, Hanyuu N, et al. Intravascular large B cell lymphoma diagnosed by senile angioma biopsy. Internal Med. 2003;42(1):117–20. PubMed PMID: WOS:000180716100024. English.

Sawamoto A, Narimatsu H, Suzuki T, Kurahashi S, Sugimoto T, Sugiura I. Long-term remission after autologous peripheral blood stem cell transplantation for relapsed intravascular lymphoma. Bone Marrow Transpl. 2006;37(2):233–4. PubMed PMID: WOS:000234554900018. English.

Seki K, Miyakoshi S, Lee GH, Matsushita H, Mutoh Y, Nakase K, et al. Prostatic acid phosphatase is a possible tumor marker for intravascular large B-cell lymphoma. Am J Surg Pathol. 2004;28(10):1384–8. PubMed PMID: WOS:000224109400016. English.

Sheibani K, Battifora H, Winberg CD, Burke JS, Benezra J, Ellinger GM, et al. Further evidence that malignant angioendotheliomatosis is an angiotropic large-cell lymphoma. New Engl J Med. 1986;314(15):943–8. PubMed PMID: WOS:A1986A741400002. English.

Shimada K, Matsue K, Yamamoto K, Murase T, Ichikawa N, Okamoto M, et al. Retrospective analysis of intravascular large B-cell lymphoma treated with rituximab-containing chemotherapy as reported by the IVL study group in Japan. J Clin Oncol. 2008;26(19):3189–95. PubMed PMID: WOS:000257416400015. English.

Song DE, Lee MW, Ryu MH, Kang DW, Kim SJ, Huh J. Intravascular large cell lymphoma of the natural killer cell type. J Clin Oncol. 2007;25(10):1279–82. PubMed PMID: WOS:000245677300020. English.

Stroup RM, Sheibani K, Moncada A, Purdy LJ, Battifora H. Angiotropic (Intravascular) large cell lymphoma – a clinicopathological study of 7 cases with unique clinical presentations. Cancer. 1990;66(8):1781–8. PubMed PMID: WOS:A1990EE78300022. English.

Sukpanichnant S, Visuthisakchai S. Intravascular lymphomatosis: a study of 20 cases in Thailand and a review of the literature. Clin Lymphoma Myelom. 2006;6(4):319–28. PubMed PMID: WOS:000237846400011. English.

Takahashi E, Kajimoto K, Fukatsu T, Yoshida M, Eimoto T, Nakamura S. Intravascular large T-cell lymphoma: a case report of CD30-positive and ALK-negative anaplastic type with cytotoxic molecule expression. Virchows Arch. 2005;447(6):1000–6. PubMed PMID: WOS:000233526900013. English.

Takiwaki H, Adachi A, Kohno H, Ogawa Y. Intravascular or intralymphatic histiocytosis associated with rheumatoid arthritis: a report of 4 cases. J Am Acad Dermatol. 2004;50(4):585–90. PubMed PMID: WOS:000220548000008. English.

Tateyama H, Eimoto T, Tada T, Kamiya M, Fujiyoshi Y, Kajiura S. Congenital angiotropic lymphoma (Intravascular Lymphomatosis) of the T-Cell type. Cancer. 1991;67(8):2131–6. PubMed PMID: WOS:A1991FE03200020. English.

Tranchida P, Bayerl M, Voelpel MJ, Palutke M. Testicular ischemia due to intravascular large B-cell lymphoma: a novel presentation in an immunosuppressed individual. Int J Surg Pathol. 2003;11(4):319–24. PubMed PMID: WOS:000186571500014. English.

Tsukadaira A, Okubo Y, Ogasawara H, Urushibata K, Honda T, Miura I, et al. Chromosomal aberrations in intravascular lymphomatosis. Am J Clin Oncol-Canc. 2002;25(2):178–81. PubMed PMID: WOS:000174906300015. English.

Vieites B, Fraga M, Lopez-Presas E, Pintos E, Garcia-Rivero A, Forteza J. Detection of t(14;18) translocation in a case of intravascular large B-cell lymphoma: a germinal centre cell origin in a subset of these lymphomas? Histopathology. 2005;46(4):466–8. PubMed PMID: WOS:000227899700014. English.

Vieren M, Sciot R, Robberecht W. Intravascular lymphomatosis of the brain: a diagnostic problem. Clin Neurol Neurosurg. 1999;101(1):33–6. PubMed PMID: WOS:000080135500009. English.

von Kempis J, Kohler G, Herbst EW, Peter HH. Intravascular lymphoma presenting as symmetric polyarthritis. Arthritis Rheum. 1998;41(6):1126–30. PubMed PMID: WOS:000074023700020. English.

Walls JG, Hong G, Cox JE, McCabe KM, O'Brien KE, Allerton JP, et al. Pulmonary intravascular – lymphomatosis presentation with dyspnea and air trapping. Chest. 1999;115(4):1207–10. PubMed PMID: WOS:000079655900055. English.

Wang L, Li CX, Gao TW. Cutaneous intravascular anaplastic large cell lymphoma. J Cutan Pathol. 2011;38(2):221–6. PubMed PMID: WOS:000285754200010. English.

Washio K, Nakata K, Nakamura A, Horikawa T. Pressure bandage as an effective treatment for intralymphatic histiocytosis associated with rheumatoid arthritis.

Dermatology. 2011;223(1):20–4. PubMed PMID: WOS:000295798100005. English.

Wick MR, Mills SE, Scheithauer BW, Cooper PH, Davitz MA, Parkinson K. Reassessment of malignant angio-endotheliomatosis – evidence in favor of its reclas-sification as intravascular lymphomatosis. Am J Surg Pathol. 1986;10(2):112–23. PubMed PMID: WOS:A1986A258400004. English.

Willemze R, Jaffe ES, Burg G, Cerroni L, Berti E, Swerdlow SH, et al. WHO-EORTC classification for cutaneous lymphomas. Blood. 2005;105(10):3768–85. PubMed PMID: WOS:000229009000013. English.

Williams G, Foyle A, White D, Greer W, Burrell S, Couban S. Intravascular T-cell lymphoma with bowel involvement: case report and literature review. Am J Hematol. 2005;78(3):207–11. PubMed PMID: WOS:000227412900008. English.

Wrotnowski U, Mills SE, Cooper PH. Malignant angio-endotheliomatosis – an angiotropic lymphoma. Am J Clin Pathol. 1985;83(2):244–8. PubMed PMID: WOS:A1985ABR8000020. English.

Wu HQ, Said JW, Ames ED, Chen C, McWhorter V, Chen P, et al. First reported cases of intravascular large cell lymphoma of the NK cell type – clinical, histologic, immunophenotypic, and molecular features. Am J Clin Pathol. 2005;123(4):603–11. PubMed PMID: WOS:000227966300016. English.

Yamada N, Uchida R, Fuchida S, Okano A, Okamoto M, Ochiai N, et al. CD5+ Epstein-Barr virus-positive intravascular large B-cell lymphoma in the uterus co-existing with huge myoma. Am J Hematol. 2005;78(3):221–4. PubMed PMID: 15726593.

Yamaguchi M, Kimura M, Watanabe Y, Taniguchi M, Masuya M, Kageyama S, et al. Successful autolo-gous peripheral blood stem cell transplantation for relapsed intravascular lymphomatosis. Bone Marrow Transpl. 2001;27(1):89–91. PubMed PMID: WOS:000166676700013. English.

Yegappan S, Coupland R, Arber DA, Wang N, Miocinovic R, Tubbs RR, et al. Angiotropic lymphoma: an immunophenotypically and clinically heterogeneous lymphoma. Modern Pathol. 2001;14(11):1147–56. PubMed PMID: WOS:000172160400012. English.

Zhao XF, Sands AM, Ostrow PT, Halbiger R, Conway JT, Bagg A. Recurrence of nodal diffuse large B-cell lymphoma as intravascular large B-cell lymphoma – is an intravascular component at initial diagnosis pre-dictive? Arch Pathol Lab Med. 2005;129(3):391–4. PubMed PMID: WOS:000227445800020. English.

Zizi-Sermpetzoglou A, Petrakopoulou N, Tepelenis N, Savvaidou V, Vasilakaki T. Intravascular T-cell lym-phoma of the vulva, CD30 positive: a case report. Eur J Gynaecol Oncol. 2009;30(5):586–8. PubMed PMID: WOS:000270030600030. English.

Zuckerman D, Seliem R, Hochberg E. Intravascular lymphoma: the oncologist's "great imitator". Oncologist. 2006;11(5):496–502. PubMed PMID: WOS:000240627300009. English.

Nonlymphoid Tumors Mimicking Lymphoma

Alicia Schnebelen, Jennifer R. Kaley, and Sara C. Shalin

Introduction

No book on cutaneous hematopathology would be complete without a chapter dedicated to non-hematolymphoid tumors that routinely or on occasion masquerade as hematologic malignancies. Mimickers of lymphoma or other hematopoietic infiltrates in the skin are not uncommon and have the potential to pose a major diagnostic challenge to the pathologists. Cutaneous lymphoma mimics include benign entities such as infection, hypersensitivity reactions, drug reactions, and inflammatory dermatoses, as well as neoplasms, including melanoma, sarcoma, and undifferentiated carcinomas. Many of the inflammatory dermatoses that can be histologically confused with a malignant hematolymphoid proliferation have been discussed elsewhere in this book (see Chaps. 5, 7, and 8); this chapter will therefore concentrate on the neoplasms that can mimic hematopoietic malignancies.

Undifferentiated neoplasms in the skin require a broad differential diagnosis. Clinical characteristics of the lesion and pertinent history are help-ful but not always available. When confronted with a cutaneous lesion with ambiguous morphologic characteristics, immunohistochemistry is often necessary to arrive at a final diagnosis, although histologic clues to a non-hematopoietic etiology may usually be detected with careful examination. As a rule, histologic findings should be evaluated in the context of clinical information in order to carefully select a panel of stains that will aid in the accurate diagnosis of a tumor. Cutaneous infiltrates can be broadly generalized into categories based on morphology; a few pertinent examples of such categories include small round cell, spindle cell, epithelioid, and pleomorphic neoplasms (Wick 2008). As cutaneous hematolymphoid neoplasms can fall within many of these morphologic categories, these should not be neglected when forming a differential diagnosis. A strategically selected panel of immunohistochemical stains can then be utilized to support a suspected diagnosis or at the least to narrow the differential diagnosis. In general, molecular testing is secondary to immunohistochemistry, and its use is left to the discretion of the pathologist (Wick 2008). This chapter will focus on entities that may be histologically confused with hematopoietic neoplasms. Each entity will be briefly discussed with a particular concentration on patterns that overlap with cutaneous hematolymphoid infiltrates and the valuable ancillary techniques to distinguish them.

A. Schnebelen, MD • J.R. Kaley, MD
S.C. Shalin, MD, PhD (✉)
Department of Pathology, University of Arkansas for Medical Sciences, 4301 West Markham #517, Little Rock, AR, USA
e-mail: sshalin@uams.edu

Table 18.1 Melanoma incidence by race and gender

Race/ethnicity	Male (per 100,000)	Female (per 100,000)
All races	27.4	16.7
White	31.9	20.0
Black	1.1	1.0
Asian/Pacific Islander	1.6	1.1
American Indian/native Alaskan	4.1	3.5
Hispanic	4.7	4.4

Adapted from the National Cancer Institute Surveillance Epidemiology and End Results.
Rates based on cases diagnosed in 2006–2010 from 18 SEER geographic areas.

Melanoma

Epidemiology

Melanoma is one of the deadliest cutaneous malignancies, with an age-adjusted incidence rate of 21.1 per 100,000 persons per year and an age-adjusted death rate of 2.7 persons per 100,000 per year. The lifetime risk of developing melanoma for Americans is estimated at 2 %, and males are affected slightly more than females (SEER 2012). The average age of presentation is 61 years, although the range of those affected by melanoma is broad and encompasses all ages. Melanoma is extremely rare in infants and young children, although such cases have been reported (Marghoob et al. 1996; Richardson et al. 2002). As with other cutaneous malignancies, Caucasians and fair-skinned individuals have a higher incidence of disease than those of darker pigmentation, a statistic which reflects the significance of ultraviolet (UV) radiation as a contributing factor to the development of melanoma (Table 18.1).

Clinical Features

Classically, melanoma presents as a new or changing darkly pigmented macule, papule, or nodule. Lesions may arise on sun-exposed or sun-protected skin, as well as mucosal sites. Characteristics of concern include large size, asymmetry or irregular borders of the lesion, and uneven or multiple variations in color. Ulceration may or may not be present. Biopsies of clinically concerning lesions should attempt to sample the entire lesion by way of primary excision or deep shave biopsy. Alternatively, a partial biopsy, especially when the lesion is large, generally gives accurate staging information and carries no increased risk of local recurrence, nodal metastasis, or death from disease (Bagley et al. 1981).

Histology and Differential Diagnosis

Different subtypes of melanoma, although not useful as a prognostic indicator of disease, do offer a scaffold by which to conceptualize clinical presentations and classic histologic findings. Melanocytic lesions, not unlike lymphoma, are notorious for their heterogeneity, and indeed, melanoma has been termed "the great mimicker," which derives from its range of histologic patterns and cytologic features. On occasion, the conventional histologic clues that point toward melanoma as a diagnosis, such as melanin production or an intraepidermal component, are absent. For this reason, melanoma should remain on the differential diagnosis of almost any undifferentiated tumor encountered by the pathologist. While a detailed discussion of all of the encountered histologic patterns is beyond the scope of this book, the following section will focus on histologic variants of melanoma that are most likely to demonstrate overlap with hematolymphoid tumors.

Amelanotic Melanoma

While pigmented melanocytic lesions often lead to a clinical differential diagnosis encompassing benign and malignant melanocytic entities, non-pigmented melanomas can be readily mistaken for benign dermatitis or a non-melanocytic neoplasm, including solitary lymphoproliferative processes. Amelanotic melanoma, as the name implies, is a melanoma lacking melanin pigment (Fig. 18.1). The majority of these tumors have been shown to exhibit epithelioid morphology (72 %), with a minority exhibiting spindle cell (18.7 %), desmoplastic (5.3 %), or rhabdoid

Fig. 18.1 Amelanotic melanoma. This nodular tumor extends deeply into the dermis and does not have a classic melanoma in situ component. Higher power (*inset*) shows focal clustering of tumor cells, but pigment production is lacking. Tumor cells expressed S100 protein and MART-1

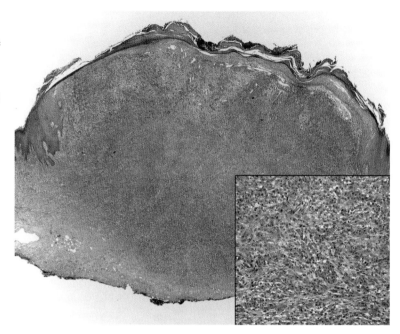

morphologies (4 %) (Cheung et al. 2012). Lesions with epithelioid cytomorphology are more likely to display other unusual features, such as signet ring cells, multinucleated giant cells, or monster cells. When such a variety of atypical cells are present, especially in the absence of melanin pigment or an in situ component in the epidermis, a diagnosis of melanoma is not entirely straightforward; in particular, these tumors may mimic large cell lymphomas, such as anaplastic large cell lymphoma or diffuse large B-cell lymphoma. Fortunately, the absence of melanin pigment does not appear to correlate with expression of melanocytic markers, and examined cases of amelanotic melanoma have reliably retained expression of such markers by immunohistochemistry. This preserved antigenicity also argues the case that amelanotic melanoma is a subtype of melanoma with phenotypic variation rather than a dedifferentiated melanoma (Cheung et al. 2012).

Melanoma with Small Cell Morphology

Small cell melanoma is an uncommon variant of nevoid melanoma with a differential diagnosis encompassing a spectrum of benign and malignant melanocytic lesions as well as nonmelanocytic tumors. The constituent tumor cells resemble those that would typically be seen at the base of an otherwise conventional melanoma. The tumor cells are small with a high nuclear to cytoplasmic ratio, nuclear atypia, hyperchromasia, and prominent nucleoli (Fig. 18.2) (Blessing et al. 2000). In this regard, clusters of small tumor cells on scanning power may mimic small round blue cell tumors, Merkel cell carcinoma, and hematolymphoid neoplasms such as non-Hodgkin lymphoma. Overlying nests of in situ melanoma cells and melanin pigment are useful clues to the diagnosis, but are not always present. The diagnosis is made more challenging in cases of metastases of unknown primary origin, in which pathologists may not consider melanoma within the initial differential diagnosis given the small size and scant cytoplasm of tumor cells (Hanson et al. 2002). Features which help distinguish small cell melanoma from a benign nevus include expansile and often asymmetric growth, deep dermal extension, disorganized growth pattern, monotony without evidence of maturation, and readily identifiable dermal mitoses (Fig. 18.3) (Hanson et al. 2002). Small cell melanomas

Fig. 18.2 Small cell melanoma. Dispersed tumor cells show a high nuclear to cytoplasm ratio and are relatively small (compare to erythrocytes). Individual cell necrosis and mitotic figures are seen, and some of the tumor cells contain pigment

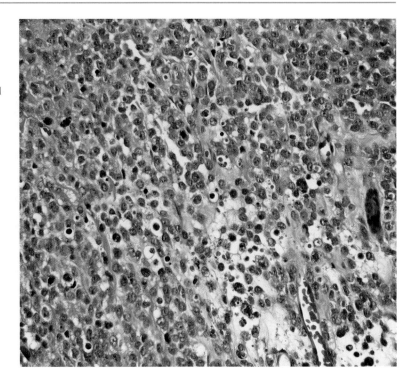

Fig. 18.3 Small cell melanoma. In this case, despite the small cell size and pseudomaturation of melanocytic nests, deep dermal mitoses were evident (*bottom left*), and focally there was sheetlike architecture

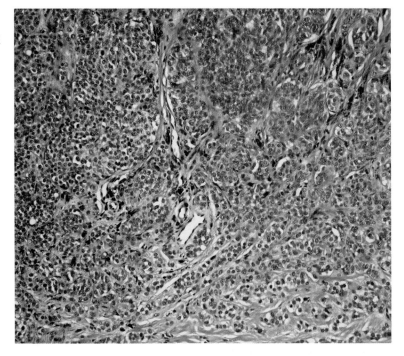

typically maintain expression of melanocytic markers and lack expression of traditional lymphoid markers such as CD45/LCA, so the derivation of the tumor becomes apparent as soon as appropriate immunohistochemical staining is utilized.

Fig. 18.4 Regressing melanoma. Epidermal hyperplasia and a dense lichenoid infiltrate obscure scattered tumor cells (*upper left*). The melanophages are a clue to the regression taking place

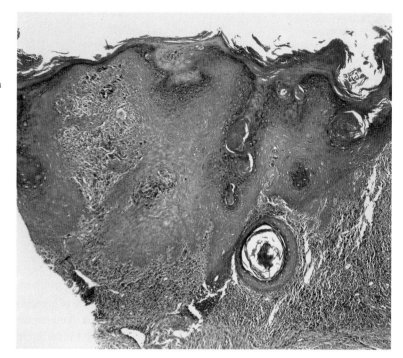

Melanoma with Regression

Active regression of melanoma is thought to represent a host immune response leading to the loss or degeneration of tumor cells. This host response is reflected by a prominent lymphocytic infiltrate (McGovern 1975), whereby tumor cells are likely removed by lymphocyte-mediated apoptosis. Established regression is characterized by a mixed lymphocytic population, vascular fibrosis, and often associated melanophages (Weedon 2010). On occasion, the dense lymphocytic infiltrate of active regression can mask remaining tumor cells and be confused with a reactive or neoplastic hematolymphoid infiltrate, as lymphocytes involved in regression may show nuclear irregularity and epidermotropism (Fig. 18.4). Regressing melanoma has been reported to mimic both mycosis fungoides and cutaneous nodular sclerosing Hodgkin lymphoma. Regressing melanoma can simulate the epidermotropism and Pautrier microabscesses of mycosis fungoides, and residual melanoma cells admixed in a sea of inflammation can mimic the binucleated Reed-Sternberg cells

of Hodgkin lymphoma (Menasce et al. 2005). In fact, Reed-Sternberg-like cells are not unique to Hodgkin lymphoma and are not infrequently reported in melanomas and a variety of other tumors (Strum et al. 1970). In general, regressing melanoma will demonstrate a lymphoid infiltrate primarily composed of CD8-positive cytotoxic T cells, and T-cell gene rearrangement will fail to demonstrate monoclonality. Any remaining atypical dermal cells will prove to be of melanocytic derivation (Menasce et al. 2005).

As an incidental note, it should be remembered that benign nevi can also undergo spontaneous regression. This correlates clinically with a "halo" phenomenon, whereby a pale rim (or halo) surrounds the involuting pigmented lesion. Microscopically, the melanocytic proliferation is engulfed in a dense inflammatory infiltrate which, as in regressing melanoma, can occasionally obscure melanocytes (Fig. 18.5). As in melanoma with regression, the lymphocytic infiltrate associated with a benign nevus undergoing regression is predominantly CD8 positive (Musette et al. 1999; Tokura et al. 1994).

Fig. 18.5 Halo nevus. A brisk lymphocytic infiltrate obscures the dermal component of this nevus from a 15-year-old female. Clinically, the lesion displayed a "halo"

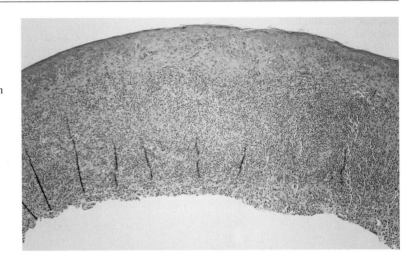

Melanoma on Cytologic Preparations

When applicable, fine-needle aspirate (FNA) is a rapid, minimally invasive technique for diagnosis. Although FNA is considered a procedure with high diagnostic accuracy for melanoma (published sensitivity and specificity values for FNA in metastatic melanoma have ranged between 86.5 % and 100 %), accurate diagnosis of melanoma can be challenging due to the varied morphologic appearances of this disease in cytologic preparations (Basler et al. 1997; Cangiarella et al. 2000; Hafstrom et al. 1980; Murali et al. 2007; Perry et al. 1986b; Rodrigues et al. 2000; Voit et al. 2000). In the absence of tissue architecture, the cytologic features of melanoma cells may be confused with atypical lymphocytes, particularly when the lymph nodes are aspirated with concern for unexplained lymphadenopathy. Care should be taken not to mistake these cells for unusual plasma cells or atypical lymphocyte forms as would be encountered in anaplastic large cell lymphoma or diffuse large B-cell lymphoma (Fig. 18.6). In aspiration smears, melanoma cells are often plasmacytoid and relatively discohesive; upon further investigation, however, foci of more cohesive cell clusters are usually identified, distinguishing melanoma from lymphoma, in which the tumor cells are highly dissociated (Murali et al. 2007). Additional hints that suggest a

diagnosis of melanoma are binucleation and the lack of lymphoglandular bodies (Perry et al. 1986a). Interestingly, the presence of pigment is identified in only one-quarter of melanoma aspirates (Murali et al. 2007). If there is doubt as to the diagnosis, creation of a cell block with subsequent immunohistochemical stains should resolve the dilemma (see immunohistochemistry section discussed below).

Metastatic Melanoma

Clinical history often guides the approach to working up an undifferentiated cutaneous neoplasm and is particularly important in a patient with a history of invasive melanoma. Cutaneous metastasis of melanoma is not uncommon and can be diagnostically challenging, as tumor cells may become undifferentiated, may lose expression of melanocytic markers, and may even acquire aberrant expression of other antigens. If available, review of slides from the original biopsy of the primary tumor can be useful. In some cases, however, an extensive immunohistochemical panel may prove necessary.

Pleomorphic and epithelioid melanoma cells can mimic either Reed-Sternberg cells, as previously discussed, or tumor cells of anaplastic large cell lymphoma. The reverse is also true: primary

Fig. 18.6 Melanoma with plasmacytoid features. This high-power micrograph demonstrates melanoma tumor cells with plasmacytoid morphology, including eccentrically placed nuclei, occasional perinuclear clearing, and prominent nucleoli

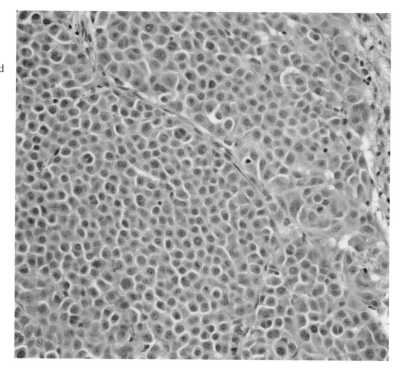

cutaneous anaplastic large cell lymphoma (cALCL) has been reported as a morphologic mimic of metastatic melanoma. In a case report, a man with a remote history of melanoma presented with a new lesion presumed clinically and, at first glance, histologically, to be metastatic melanoma. The absence of expression of melanocytic markers led to an expanded immunohistochemical panel and ultimately a diagnosis of primary cutaneous anaplastic lymphoma, illustrating a pitfall in evaluating poorly differentiated tumors in patients with a known history of melanoma (Pulitzer et al. 2013). Both types of tumors may have a nodular configuration on low-power microscopic examination. Additional overlapping cytologic features of cALCL and metastatic melanoma include abundant cytoplasm, bizarre nuclei, and angulated basophilic nucleoli (Fig. 18.7). However, in cALCL, lymphocytes are more likely to aggregate around the small vessels and to demonstrate classic wreath-shaped "hallmark cells." Although melanoma may lose expression of melanocytic markers and gain anomalous expression of other antigens, it typically remains negative for CD45/LCA, which makes this stain a fairly reliable screening tool to differentiate hematopoietic from melanocytic lineages (Pulitzer et al. 2013). As a subset of anaplastic large cell lymphomas will lack CD45 expression, the addition of CD30 immunohistochemical staining is worthwhile if this entity is within your differential diagnosis (Falini et al. 1990).

In addition to cutaneous metastases, metastatic melanoma within lymph nodes may be challenging to detect. Lymph node metastasis of melanoma, especially when consisting of only a small focus or single cells, may be mistaken for subcapsular/sinusoidal histiocytes. The mitotically active, enlarged lymphocytes comprising germinal centers of lymph nodes may also be a source of diagnostic confusion, especially for those with limited knowledge about normal lymph node architecture (Fig. 18.8). For this reason, the use of immunohistochemistry in the evaluation of sentinel lymph node biopsies has become commonplace and has been shown to be essential in the detection of metastatic disease (Fig. 18.9) (Lobo et al. 2012).

Fig. 18.7 Melanoma. This melanoma demonstrates sheetlike architecture and large pleomorphic tumor cells with admixed inflammatory cells. The lack of clear differentiation and the lack of pigment in this tumor raise a broad differential diagnosis, including anaplastic large cell lymphoma. In this case, tumor cells expressed melanocytic markers

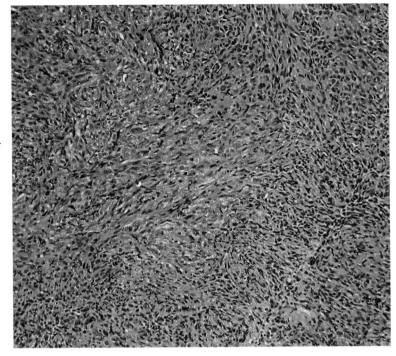

Fig. 18.8 Melanoma metastatic to a sentinel lymph node. Lymph node involvement by melanoma is often subtle. Tumor cells can be seen infiltrating the sinusoidal space adjacent to a lymphoid follicle with germinal center

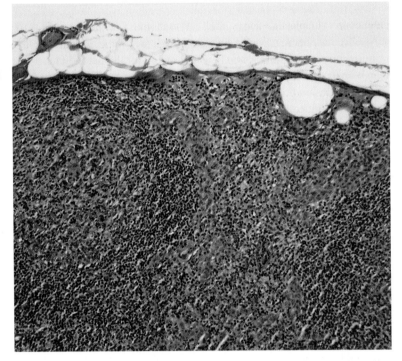

Immunohistochemistry

Evaluation of melanocytic neoplasms may require the use of immunohistochemical stains. The most commonly used antibodies include MART-1/MelanA, HMB-45, S100, and MiTF. MART-1 (melanoma antigen recognized by T cells 1) and MelanA are two separate names for the protein

Fig. 18.9 Melanoma metastatic to a sentinel lymph node. MART-1 immunoreactivity of melanoma tumor cells can assist in confirming or detecting small metastatic deposits

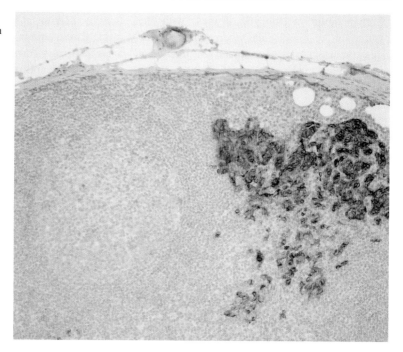

encoded by the human *MLANA* gene and represent a highly specific melanocytic marker. HMB-45, or anti-gp100, is a monoclonal antibody that identifies immature melanosomes and is, therefore, frequently expressed in melanomas that maintain pigment production. S100 protein remains a highly sensitive, albeit not entirely specific, marker of melanocytes. It is particularly useful in the diagnosis of spindle cell or desmoplastic melanomas, as this subtype of melanoma is less likely to express the more specific melanocytic markers. However, S100 is positive in a wide variety of non-melanocytic cell types, including neural-derived cells, adipocytes, chondrocytes, and myoepithelial cells, thereby limiting its specificity. MiTF (microphthalmia transcription factor) is directed against the transcription factor involved in melanocytic development and, as such, represents a nuclear stain for melanocytes. Additional markers for melanocytic neoplasms include tyrosinase, which lacks specificity, and Sox10, a transcription factor and relatively novel nuclear stain which shows promise in providing a more specific marker for the diagnosis of desmoplastic melanoma (Mohamed et al. 2012; Ramos-Herberth et al. 2010). Ki-67 and phosphohistone H3 are markers that serve as surrogates for cell cycle engagement

and mitotic activity and are sometimes useful in determining the proliferative index of a melanocytic lesion. While typically not useful in thin lesions, these markers may be of assistance when encountering a thick melanocytic tumor in which considerations include (benign) nevus versus nevoid melanoma.

Electron Microscopy

Ultrastructural analysis of melanocytic tumors will demonstrate the presence of melanosomes and premelanosomes. Due to the widespread availability and use of immunohistochemical stains, electron microscopy no longer plays a major role in routine diagnosis, although it may be useful in the rare setting of an undifferentiated neoplasm.

Molecular/Genetics

Routine use of molecular studies is not necessary for the diagnosis of straightforward melanocytic lesions. However, molecular techniques are increasingly being employed to aid in the diagnosis of challenging melanocytic lesions, with the assumption that molecular aberrations will be more prevalent and widespread in malignant tumors than in benign ones. Specifically, a 4-probe fluorescent in situ hybridization (FISH) panel (targeting regions on chromosomes 6 and 11) has been designed to detect chromosomal amplifications and deletions of loci that are often mutated in melanoma but are unaltered in benign nevi. This technique was shown to classify melanoma with 86.7 % sensitivity and 95.4 % specificity in initial validation studies (Gerami et al. 2009). Array comparative genome hybridization (aCGH) is another technique by which the entire genome of a tumor is examined for widespread chromosomal gains or losses, with melanomas characteristically demonstrating more aberrations than benign tumors (Bauer and Bastian 2006). Using aCGH performed on human cell lines derived from metastatic melanoma, many genetic alterations specific to melanoma have been identified, including deletions of the *CDKN2A* and *PTEN* loci and amplifications of loci encoding genes previously implicated in melanoma such as *BRAF, NRAS, EGFR, MITF, NOTCH2, CCND1, MDM2, CCNE1,* and *CDK4* (Gast et al. 2010). In addition, mass spectroscopy represents a novel field whereby the specific protein expression within a lesion gives clues to its biological potential. For instance, imaging mass spectrometry has been reported to correctly differentiate Spitz nevus from Spitzoid melanoma with 97 % sensitivity and 90 % specificity (Lazova et al. 2012).

A thorough discussion of all of the specific genetic mutations associated with melanoma is beyond the scope of this chapter, and the reader is referred to one of many excellent reviews on the subject (Nelson and Tsao 2009). However, special mention to the *BRAF* mutation seems warranted, as the presence of this mutation in metastatic lesions confers eligibility for treatment with the recently FDA-approved BRAF inhibitor. Approximately 40–60 % of melanomas exhibit a point mutation in BRAF kinase, in which glutamic acid (most commonly) is substituted for a valine at amino acid position 600 (V600E) on chromosome 7, leading to increased kinase activity of the protein and

thereby driving malignancy (Chapman et al. 2011, Rubinstein et al. 2010). BRAF inhibitors are specifically formulated against the mutated BRAF kinase and represent targeted drug therapy that has been associated with relatively prolonged survival in patients with metastatic melanoma, compared to prior treatment regimens (Chapman et al. 2011).

Prognosis/Course

In the absence of identifiable regional or distant metastases, the prognosis of patients with melanoma depends predominantly on the depth (Breslow's measurement) of the primary tumor. Additional features that inversely correlate with prognosis include ulceration of the primary tumor, increased mitotic activity (measured per millimeter squared), and extensive regression (Edge et al. 2010). Thin melanomas, generally considered to be less than 1 mm in Breslow's depth, have an overall favorable prognosis and are treated surgically with wide local excision. Thicker tumors are treated with wide local excision with generous (1–2 cm) margins, as well as sentinel lymph node sampling, which is usually followed by completion lymphadenectomy if metastatic deposits are identified within the sentinel node. The medical benefit of these procedures remains debated in the literature, and clinical studies are ongoing (Essner 2010; van Akkooi et al. 2010). Chemotherapy, immunomodulatory therapy, and targeted drug therapies, as described above, are utilized in metastatic disease.

Most recurrences from primary cutaneous melanoma occur within 10 years of initial diagnosis, and the majority of these occur within 3 years. However, patients require lifelong surveillance as second primary melanomas and late-occurring metastases can occur. Colloquial terms to describe delayed metastases include "late" metastases that occur 10 years following diagnosis and "ultralate" metastases that occur 15 years following diagnosis. As such, the pathologist should maintain a degree of suspicion for metastatic melanoma in any biopsy from a patient with a clinical history of melanoma.

Merkel Cell Carcinoma

Epidemiology

Merkel cell carcinoma (MCC), or primary cutaneous neuroendocrine carcinoma, is an uncommon, albeit not rare, cutaneous neoplasm that occurs primarily on sun-exposed skin. Caucasians comprise approximately 95 % of all cases of MCC, with a mean age at diagnosis of 76.2 years for women and 73.6 years for men (Penn and First 1999). In addition to ultraviolet radiation exposure, risk factors for the development of MCC include immunosuppression (Penn and First 1999; Samarendra et al. 2000; Ziprin et al. 2000) and infection with the recently discovered Merkel cell polyomavirus (Feng et al. 2008). The role of the Merkel cell polyomavirus as an independent prognostic factor in MCC has been widely debated and remains unclear (Hall et al. 2012, Higaki-Mori et al. 2012; Sihto et al. 2009).

Clinical Features

Merkel cell carcinoma most often presents as a firm, painless, and rapidly enlarging red to violaceous nodule on the face (27 %), upper extremities (22 %), lower extremities (15 %), or scalp and neck (9 %) (Penn and First 1999). The lesion may ulcerate and may have a more plaque-like, rather than nodular, appearance (Goessling et al. 2002). Most patients present with localized skin involvement; however, some patients have regional lymph node metastases at the time of initial presentation, and a few patients diagnosed with MCC present with distant metastatic disease (Calder and Smoller 2010; Goessling et al. 2002). The diagnosis of MCC is rarely made by clinical account alone, as it may be mistaken for angiosarcoma, basal cell carcinoma, melanoma, or cutaneous lymphoma (Calder and Smoller 2010).

Histology and Differential Diagnosis

Despite the early theory that MCC arose from Merkel cells, slow-acting cutaneous mechanoreceptors (and thus, where it derived its namesake),

MCC is now thought to originate from a totipotent stem cell capable of heterogeneic differentiation, most notably neuroendocrine and epithelial differentiation (Calder and Smoller 2010; Smith and Patterson 2001; Tilling and Moll 2012). As such, MCC displays histologic and immunophenotypic features characteristic of both neuroendocrine and epithelial lineages. Similar to other small round blue cell tumors of the dermis and hematolymphoid neoplasms, MCC is composed of monotonous, round to ovoid basophilic cells with sparse cytoplasm (Fig. 18.10). Epidermotropism is not an uncommon finding in MCC; it is estimated that 10–30 % of MCC cases demonstrate epidermal infiltration by tumor cells (D'Agostino et al. 2010; Kanitakis et al. 2006). Furthermore, the pattern of epidermal infiltration may occasionally assume a Pagetoid configuration or may even resemble the Pautrier microabscesses of mycosis fungoides (D'Agostino et al. 2010; Donner et al. 1992; Hashimoto et al. 1998; Kanitakis et al. 2006; LeBoit et al. 1992; Rocamora et al. 1987). Unlike lymphoma cells, MCC tumor nuclei have finely dispersed chromatin typical of neuroendocrine cells, also known as a vesicular or "salt and pepper" chromatin, and prominent nucleoli are absent (Fig. 18.11). MCC may display other neuroendocrine features such as molding, crush artifact, and pseudorosette formation. Molding is particularly useful in distinguishing MCC, as it gives a clue to the cohesive nature of the cells, in comparison to hematopoietic tumor cells, which are discohesive; these features are likely the result of the presence (in MCC) or lack of (in lymphoid cells) cell surface adhesion molecules. Apoptotic debris and mitotic figures are often plentiful in MCC (Pulitzer et al. 2009). Architecturally, MCC cells may be arranged in the dermis as trabeculae, sheets, or ribbons or may be scattered as single diffuse cells. Again, these patterns usually hint at the epithelial nature of the tumor (Calder and Smoller 2010; Pulitzer et al. 2009). Giant tumor cell aggregates have been reported in one case of MCC, a finding that was described as a potential mimic of diffuse large B-cell lymphoma (Smith and Patterson 2001). However, with closer examination, the giant tumor cells in MCC displayed identical nuclear features and an immunohistochemical

Fig. 18.10 Merkel cell carcinoma. The superficial and deep dermis is involved by sheets, nests, and focally trabeculae of monotonous blue cells

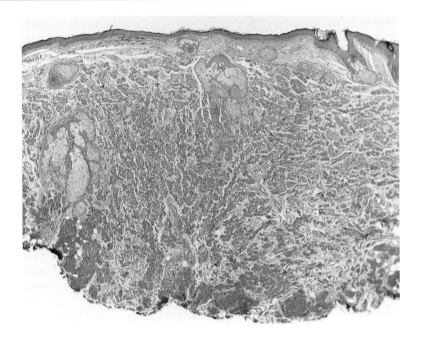

Fig. 18.11 Merkel cell carcinoma. High-power examination of tumor cells reveals nuclei with finely dispersed, "salt and pepper" chromatin and scant cytoplasm. As in other neuroendocrine tumors, nuclear molding is character-istic. Abundant apoptotic debris and frequent mitotic figures are also commonly encountered

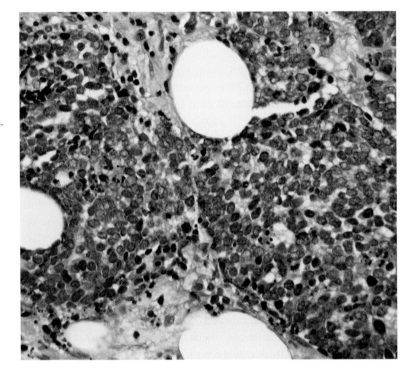

staining pattern belonging to conventional MCC tumor cells. Squamous, adnexal, and sarcoma-tous differentiation have been observed within MCC, prompting the idea of phenotypic trans-formation and further supporting the theory that MCC derives from a totipotent stem cell (Calder

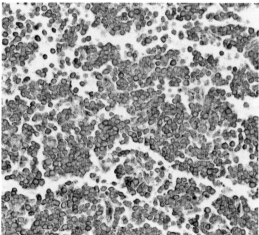

Fig. 18.12 Merkel cell carcinoma. Cytokeratin 20 staining in Merkel cell carcinoma classically highlights malignant cells in a perinuclear "dot-like" pattern (*left image*). Other times, cytokeratin 20 staining can be more diffuse throughout the cytoplasm (*right image*)

Immunohistochemistry

The use of immunohistochemistry can assist in distinguishing MCC from hematolymphoid malignancies and other small round blue cell tumors. Epithelial markers that are expressed in MCC include the low-molecular-weight cytokeratins CK8/CK18 (CAM 5.2), CK19, CK20, MNF116, and epithelial membrane antigen (EMA). The pattern of CK20 staining (often also mirrored in pancytokeratin stains) is particularly useful in identifying MCC. Thought to highlight the perinuclear intermediate filaments seen on electron microscopy, CK20 classically (but not always!) displays a perinuclear dot-like positivity in tumor cells (Fig. 18.12). Additionally, although a minority of MCC will express CK7, cytokeratins CK5/CK6 and CK17 are invariably negative. Neuroendocrine markers that are positive in MCC include neuron-specific enolase (NSE), CD56, synaptophysin, and chromogranin. Tumor cells may also show positivity for vasoactive intestinal peptide (VIP), calcitonin, and somatostatin (Smith and Patterson 2001). Importantly, unlike lymphoma tumor cells, MCC tumor cells do not express leukocyte common antigen (LCA/CD45). MCC is also negative for S100 protein, distinguishing it from melanoma, and while a subset may be positive for CK7, there should be absence of thyroid transcription factor (TTF)-1 expression, distinguishing MCC from metastatic small cell carcinoma of the lung. Interestingly, there are recent reports regarding a subset of MCCs that express terminal deoxynucleotidyl transferase (TdT), PAX5, and anaplastic lymphoma kinase (ALK), markers that have been traditionally described in lymphoblastic lymphomas. These findings potentially induce diagnostic confusion and add to the debate regarding the origin of MCC (Buresh et al. 2008; Filtenborg-Barnkob and Bzorek 2013; Kolhe et al. 2013; Zur Hausen et al. 2013). Moreover, owing to the expression of CD56 in both neuroendocrine tumors and natural killer (NK) cell lymphoma, one may be mistaken for the other, particularly in biopsies with prominent crush artifact or inflammation. CD56 appears to be expressed more strongly in MCC than in NK cell lymphoma, though this

and Smoller 2010; Pulitzer et al. 2009; Smith and Patterson 2001). Moreover, lymphocytic aggregates may surround and/or infiltrate a focus of MCC, thereby further obscuring the diagnosis.

finding is subjective and requires a reference threshold (McNiff et al. 2005). Other more reliable histologic features for distinguishing NK cell lymphoma from MCC include the lack of expression of epithelial markers with concurrent expression of CD2 and CD7 surface antigens, along with cytoplasmic – but not surface – CD3 expression. Reactive lymphocytes in MCC demonstrate a mixed phenotype, with both surface CD3- and CD20-positive cells identified. In addition, NK cell lymphomas will often display angiocentricity and angiodestruction, along with significant eccrine infiltration and/or destruction, features which are typically lacking in MCC (Ansai et al. 1997; McNiff et al. 2005).

Electron Microscopy

Ultrastructural studies reveal characteristic membrane-bound electron-dense core granules and perinuclear intermediate filament aggregates; however, the widespread availability of immunohistochemical staining generally supersedes the use of electron microscopy in aiding in the diagnosis of MCC (Pulitzer et al. 2009; Smith and Patterson 2001).

Molecular/Genetics

Multiple cytogenetic abnormalities have been identified in MCC, particularly within chromo-

somes 1, 11, and 13. These aberrations include gains and losses of genetic material, as well as chromosomal rearrangements. In fact, several mutations identified in MCC have also been detected in small cell carcinoma of the lung. This finding, along with the presence of multiple and diverse genetic abnormalities in MCC, currently does not support the use of cytogenetics studies as an ancillary diagnostic tool for MCC.

Prognosis/Course

A particularly aggressive tumor, MCC has a propensity for rapid enlargement, local recurrence, and early regional lymph node involvement, as well as distant metastatic potential (Goessling et al. 2002; Smith and Patterson 2001). The presence of nodal involvement at the time of presentation, along with immunocompromised status, correlates with poor clinical outcomes, including decreased survival rates and increased risk for the development of distant metastatic disease (Tarantola et al. 2013). Histologic prognostic indicators in MCC have been widely debated and remain somewhat controversial, although features such as size of the primary tumor, depth of tumor invasion, and degree of inflammation are thought to correlate with clinical outcome (Mott et al. 2004; Tarantola et al. 2013). The presence of bcl-2 expression in tumor cells is reported to convey a better clinical prognosis, while p63 expression in tumor cells is thought to correlate

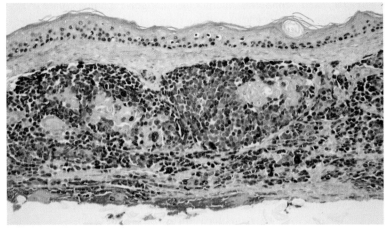

Fig. 18.13 Merkel cell carcinoma. P63 expression in Merkel cell carcinoma has been associated with a more aggressive clinical course and worse prognosis. This Merkel cell carcinoma shows diffuse nuclear immunoreactivity for p63

with adverse outcome (Fig. 18.13) (Hall et al. 2012; Sahi et al. 2012). Current treatment recommendations include wide local excision with sentinel lymph node biopsy, followed by adjuvant radiotherapy of the tumor bed and regional lymph nodes. Systemic chemotherapy is typically reserved for stage 4 metastatic disease, though its use is controversial in localized disease (NCCN 2013, Poulsen et al. 2006; Tai et al. 2000a, b).

Carcinomas

Primary and Metastatic Lymphoepithelioma-Like Carcinoma

Epidemiology

Cutaneous lymphoepithelioma-like carcinoma (LELC) is a remarkably rare dermal neoplasm. Lymphoepithelioma-like carcinoma is a histologically undifferentiated carcinoma that is not unique to the skin; in fact, LELC has been described in nearly every organ, particularly within the head and neck region. The World Health Organization's preferred terminology for tumors with this histologic appearance is "lymphoepithelial carcinoma" (Barnes et al. 2007); however to date, the majority of tumors originating in the skin have been reported in the literature as "lymphoepithelioma-like carcinoma." Unlike its extracutaneous counterparts and sinonasal lymphoepithelial carcinoma, however, lymphoepithelioma-like carcinoma of the skin has not shown an association with Epstein-Barr virus (EBV) (Arsenovic 2008; Carr et al. 1992; Gillum et al. 1996; Weiss et al. 1989) with the exception of one rare case (Aoki et al. 2010). Although its exact histogenesis remains unclear, the tumor is likely derived from epithelial or adnexal origin (Arsenovic 2008; Lopez et al. 2011; Wick et al. 1991).

Clinical Features

Clinically, LELC presents as a slow-growing, flesh-colored or red plaque or nodule arising on the head or neck of middle-aged to elderly patients; there is no gender predilection. It may be clinically mistaken for a basal cell carcinoma or Merkel cell carcinoma, and, in some cases

with epidermal ulceration, it has been mistaken for squamous cell carcinoma (Lopez et al. 2011).

Histology

Histologically, LELC is composed of large, cohesive, epithelioid cells arranged singly or in well-delineated dermal lobules or small nests and surrounded and infiltrated by a mixed population of reactive T and B lymphocytes (Fig. 18.14). The neoplastic cells contain large nuclei with a vesicular chromatin pattern and prominent nucleoli; mitotic activity may be abundant (Fig. 18.15). In cases with a florid lymphocytic infiltrate, the epithelioid component of the tumor may become obscured, making diagnosis particularly more challenging. They key to diagnosis is, therefore, to recognize the neoplastic cells amidst the associated inflammatory infiltrate and to correctly identify them as epithelial in origin (Fig. 18.16).

Immunohistochemistry

Epithelial markers, including cytokeratins, p63, and epithelial membrane antigen (EMA), will highlight inconspicuous epithelioid tumor cells (Fig. 18.17). Primary LELC can be differentiated from metastatic lymphoepithelial carcinoma from other organs by the absence of detection of EBV by either in situ hybridization studies (EBV-encoded RNA, or EBER) or polymerase chain reaction (PCR) on fixed tissues (Gillum et al. 1996). Furthermore, the absence of a separate primary tumor following thorough clinical examination negates the possibility of metastasis.

Differential Diagnosis

Within the differential diagnosis of LELC are squamous cell carcinoma with florid lymphocytic reactivity, Merkel cell carcinoma, poorly differentiated melanoma, and cutaneous lymphoma. Squamous cell carcinoma with reactive lymphocytic infiltrate often reveals a connection to the epidermal surface, and/or epidermal dysplasia. LELC lacks the characteristic CK20 staining pattern and neuroendocrine differentiation of Merkel cell carcinoma, and LELC is negative for melanocytic markers, distinguishing this entity from melanoma. To differentiate LELC from lymphoid malignancies, the polyclonal nature of the

Fig. 18.14
Lymphoepithelioma-like
carcinoma. On low-power
examination, dermal lobules
of tumor cells are obscured by
a dense lymphocytic infiltrate,
almost simulating the
formation of lymphoid
follicles

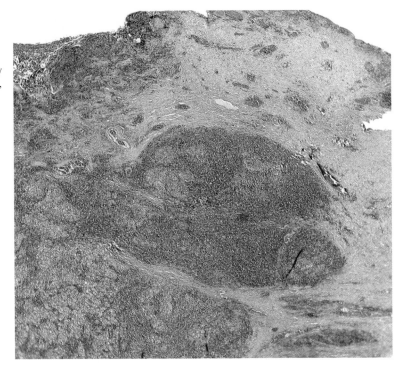

Fig. 18.15
Lymphoepithelioma-like
carcinoma. On high power,
large epithelioid tumor cells
with abundant cytoplasm,
vesicular nuclei, and
prominent nuclei are
appreciated within the
background of small round
lymphocytes and plasma cells

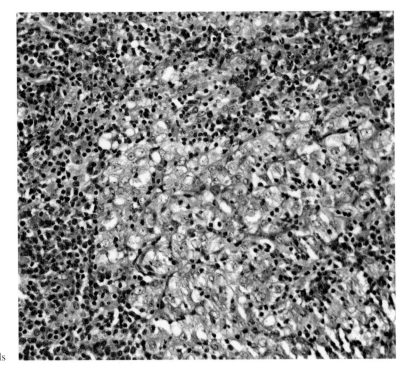

Fig. 18.16
Lymphoepithelioma-like
carcinoma. Focal nesting of
the neoplastic cells provides a
clue to the epithelial nature of
their origin

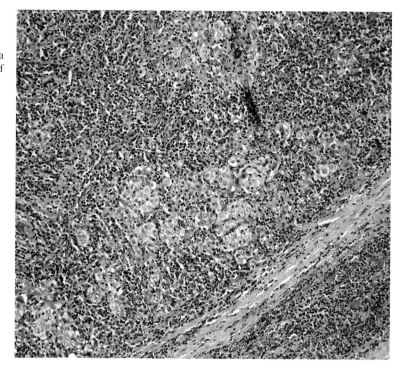

Fig. 18.17
Lymphoepithelioma-like
carcinoma.
Immunohistochemical
staining of the tumor reveals
strong diffuse nuclear p63
immunoreactivity in the
neoplastic cells.
Pancytokeratin stain (not
shown) was also positive in
the tumor cells

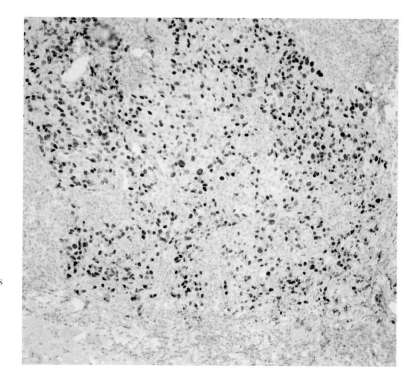

Fig. 18.18 Cutaneous anaplastic large cell lymphoma with pseudoepitheliomatous hyperplasia. On occasion, epithelial changes can overshadow the atypical dermal infiltrate and be mistaken for a squamous cell carcinoma (Slide for photography provided by Dr. Richard Cheney, Roswell Park Hospital, Buffalo, NY)

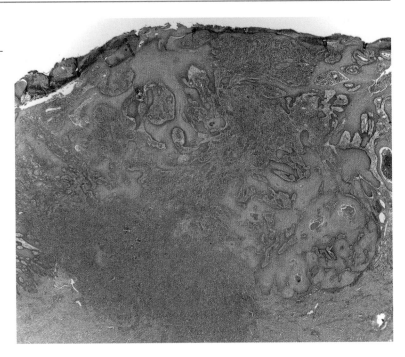

lymphocytic infiltrate can be confirmed by demonstrating a mixed population of CD20- and CD3-positive lymphocytes with mixed kappa and lambda light chain expression of B cells. Any gene rearrangement studies would also be expected to be negative.

As a side remark regarding the capacity of carcinomas and lymphoma to mimic one another, it should also be noted that pseudo-epitheliomatous hyperplasia (epidermal hyperplasia resembling squamous cell carcinoma) has been reported overlying cases of cutaneous anaplastic large cell lymphoma (Biswas et al. 2008). Pseudoepitheliomatous hyperplasia is not associated with LELC; however, the presence of florid pseudoepitheliomatous hyperplasia combined with atypical epithelioid cells in the dermis and an inflammatory infiltrate can easily be misinterpreted as an invasive, poorly differentiated squamous cell carcinoma (Figs. 18.18 and 18.19). Alternatively, lesional cells may be completely overlooked as they are overshadowed by the epidermal proliferation (Biswas et al. 2008). In such cases, dermal epithelioid cells can be evaluated for pancytokeratin and/or p63 (positive in carcinoma) and

CD30 expression (positive in at least 75 % of cells in a membranous and perinuclear pattern in cALCL) to determine the cellular lineage. Conversely, poorly differentiated squamous cell carcinoma consisting of pleomorphic, discohesive dermal cells without obvious epidermal connection or clear keratinocytic atypia may simulate cALCL (Figs. 18.20 and 18.21). Once again, immunohistochemistry easily distinguishes these two entities.

Molecular/Genetics

Routine use of molecular testing is not necessary in cases of LELC. For cases in which lymphoma is considered within the differential diagnosis, T-cell or B-cell clonality studies for gene rearrangement will be negative.

Prognosis/Course

Cutaneous LELC has a tendency for local recurrence when not completely excised (Hall et al. 2006; Lopez et al. 2011). While not often widely metastatic, some case reports document regional lymph node involvement and perineural invasion (Hall et al. 2006; Robins and Perez 1995). Only one death has been reported, which occurred

Fig. 18.19 Cutaneous anaplastic large cell lymphoma with pseudoepitheliomatous hyperplasia. On higher power, pleomorphic, atypical cells are seen within the dermis. The tumor cells expressed CD30 and were negative for pancytokeratin (Slide for photography provided by Dr. Richard Cheney, Roswell Park Hospital, Buffalo, NY)

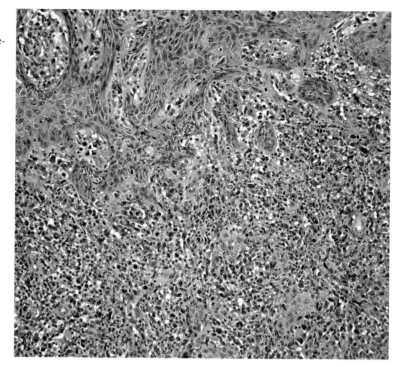

Fig. 18.20 Poorly differentiated squamous cell carcinoma. This case shows a dermal infiltrate of singly dispersed, pleomorphic cells without connection to the overlying epidermis. There is an associated inflammatory infiltrate including eosinophils. Basilar squamous atypia gives a clue to the epithelial nature of the dermal cells

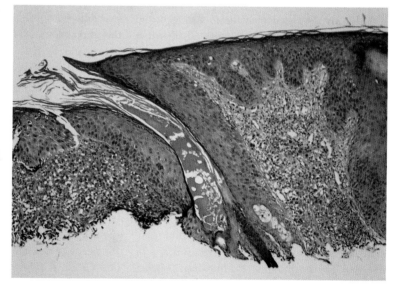

57 months following diagnosis (Swanson et al. 1988). Current treatment strategies include wide local excision or Mohs micrographic surgery (Jimenez et al. 1995; Lopez et al. 2011; Robins and Perez 1995).

Metastatic Carcinoma

Epidemiology

Overall, the skin is an uncommon site for visceral carcinomatous metastasis. When cutaneous

Fig. 18.21 Poorly differentiated squamous cell carcinoma. Pancytokeratin highlights the individual tumor cells in the dermis

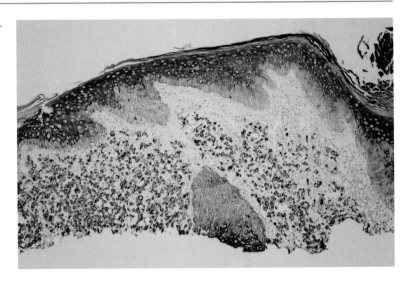

metastasis does occur, it is secondary to hematogenous or lymphatic spread from the primary site, direct extension by an underlying tumor, or iatrogenic deposition following a surgical procedure. A seminal study in the 1970s determined that cutaneous metastases most commonly originated from the lung and colon in males and from the breast, colon, and ovary in females (Brownstein and Helwig 1972). More recent studies have reaffirmed that lung carcinoma remains overall the most common source of cutaneous metastatic carcinoma (Rosen 1980; Saeed et al. 2004). Rarely, a cutaneous metastasis may be the presenting sign of malignancy, with lung, kidney, and ovarian carcinomas being the most commonly reported (Brownstein and Helwig 1972).

Clinical Features

Cutaneous carcinomat metastases typically present as painless, firm, flesh-colored to pink papules or nodules. Lesions may be solitary or multiple and may mimic benign dermal-based skin lesions. Heavily vascularized tumors, such as renal cell carcinoma, may masquerade as vascular tumors clinically. Anatomic location is an important clue to the origin of the neoplasm, as tumors tend to metastasize in the vicinity of the primary tumor. For example, breast and lung cancers have a propensity to metastasize to the chest

wall, while cancers of the colon, ovary, kidney, and bladder often metastasize to the abdomen (Gul et al. 2007).

Histology and Immunohistochemistry

Clinical correlation with a history of malignancy is essential in the evaluation of skin metastases. Often the morphology of the cutaneous metastasis will correspond to the morphology of the primary tumor, and, therefore, review of the original case is elemental to the metastatic work-up. For instance, the presence of glandular structures points to an adenocarcinoma (Fig. 18.22). Particular variants of metastatic carcinoma may impart a histologic appearance that mimic lymphomatoid or leukemic infiltrates; these are given specific mention with their immunophenotypes below.

In general, identifying carcinoma in the dermis in the absence of a clinical history of malignancy requires a panel of immunohistochemical stains for accurate diagnosis. Some authors cite CK7 and CK20 as the most helpful initial screening immunostains (Chu et al. 2000). In another study of 44 cases of skin metastases from unknown origin, CK20, estrogen receptor (ER), and progesterone receptor (PR) were found to be the useful first-line markers in determining primary tumor site by identifying tumors of colorectal and breast origin, respectively (Azoulay et al. 2005).

Fig. 18.22 Metastatic adenocarcinoma. Irregularly shaped glands, some with central necrosis, are deposited in the dermis. In this case, the primary tumor was from the breast

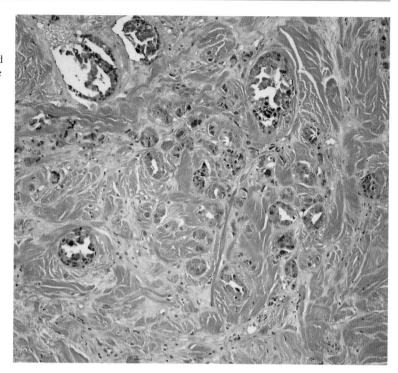

Table 18.2 Immunohistochemical profile of metastatic carcinoma

	CK7	CK20	TTF-1	CDX2	GCDFP15	ER/PR	PAX8
Breast	+	−	−	−	+	+	−
Lung (adenocarcinoma)	++	−/+	+	−	−	−	−
Lung (small cell carcinoma)	+/−	−	+	−	−	+/−	−
Colorectal	−/+	++	−	++	N/A	−	−
Renal	−/+[a]	−	−	−	N/A	−	++
Ovarian	++	+/−	−	−	−	−	++

Note: Exceptions for staining patterns in each of these entities do exist, and this table represents the most commonly observed patterns of staining (Chu et al. 2000; Jagirdar 2008; Nonaka et al. 2008; Park et al. 2007; Saad et al. 2011; Saeed et al. 2004)

++ (almost always positive), + (usually positive), +/− (often positive), −/+ (usually negative)

CK cytokeratin, *TTF* thyroid transcription factor, *GCDFP* gross cystic disease fluid protein, *ER* estrogen receptor, *PR* progesterone receptor, *PAX8* paired box gene 8

[a]CK7 positivity depends on subtype (clear cell RCC is classically CK7 negative; papillary, chromophobe, and collecting duct RCCs are typically CK7 positive)

The addition of S100 can detect melanoma as well (Saeed et al. 2004). Supplementary immunohistochemical stains that are valuable in the investigation of metastatic cutaneous carcinomas are summarized in Table 18.2. This table may be used as a guide; however, as can be expected, many exceptions for staining patterns in each of these entities do exist.

Metastatic Breast Carcinoma

Tumors originating from the breast may metastasize with many different patterns, several of which may be confused with hematolymphoid infiltrates. An undifferentiated, sheetlike pattern is not uncommon (Weedon 2010) and may be readily confused with cutaneous lymphoma.

Fig. 18.23 Metastatic breast cancer. Metastatic breast cancer cells are seen throughout the dermis, dispersed in a single-file pattern. Leukemia cutis can also infiltrate through the dermis in this pattern

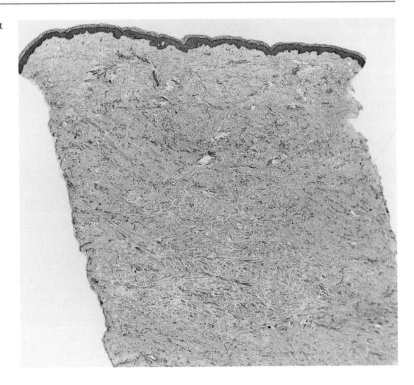

Moreover, metastatic breast carcinoma (particularly of the lobular variant) classically infiltrates in a linear pattern through sclerotic collagen bundles in the dermis (Fig. 18.23). This pattern of infiltration can be similar to the pattern of leukemia cutis, whereby immature myeloid cells infiltrate the skin as sheets, cords, or linear arrays. Additionally, both entities tend to display a Grenz zone, an area of the papillary dermis that is spared from tumor involvement. The presence of intracytoplasmic vacuoles, glandular formation, and lymphatic permeation are helpful clues to the diagnosis of mammary adenocarcinoma (Fig. 18.24), while perivascular and periappendageal "layering" of cells favors a leukemic infiltrate (Weedon 2010). On occasion, metastatic breast cancer may permeate the dermis as individual single cells and may be mistaken for a (nonneoplastic) inflammatory infiltrate (Weedon 2010). Primary lymphoma of the breast, a rare entity, has been described as presenting clinically as inflammatory breast carcinoma, an entity constituting 0.04–0.5 % of breast neoplasms and characterized by plugging of dermal lymphatics

by a poorly differentiated ductal carcinoma with an associated mixed population of inflammatory cells (Anne and Pallapothu 2011).

Differentiating metastatic breast carcinoma from leukemia cutis often necessitates the use of immunohistochemistry. Cytokeratin 7 is expressed by breast metastases in the majority (approximately 2/3) of cases, while estrogen and progesterone receptor positivity, although less sensitive, offer greater specificity to the diagnosis (Azoulay et al. 2005). Gross cystic disease fluid protein-15 (GCDFP15) and mammaglobin are also potential markers of metastatic breast carcinoma, the former of which demonstrates greater specificity and the latter of which confers greater sensitivity (Ormsby et al. 1995). Because the breast is a modified apocrine gland, it is no surprise that primary adnexal neoplasms of the skin and benign adnexal glands also stain with the markers mentioned above, so caution is necessary if such neoplasms are also within the differential diagnosis (Wallace et al. 1995). Additionally, GATA3 is a new and potentially useful marker for metastatic breast carcinoma

Fig. 18.24 Metastatic breast cancer. On higher power examination, the tumor cells are hyperchromatic, atypical, and relatively cohesive. There is focal abortive glandular formation and rare intracytoplasmic vacuoles

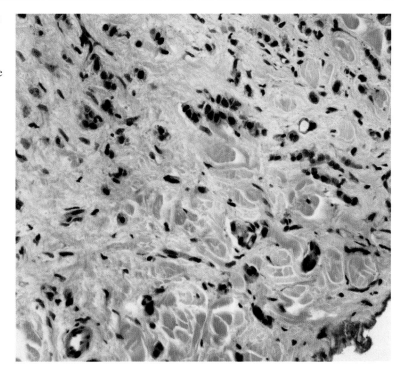

(Cimino-Mathews et al. 2013). The immunophenotype of leukemia cutis varies depending on the degree of cytologic differentiation and cytogenetic abnormalities; CD68 and lysozyme are reported to have the highest sensitivity in the detection of myeloid leukemia cutis, regardless of subtype. Myeloperoxidase is also frequently useful but is less commonly positive in cases of leukemia cutis with monocytic differentiation, which is the most common subtype leukemia involving the skin (Cibull et al. 2008). B- and T-cell specific markers will be useful in confirming a diagnosis of primary breast lymphoma.

Metastatic Small Cell Lung Cancer

Small cell lung cancer is a neuroendocrine carcinoma that only rarely metastasizes to cutaneous sites (Marcoval et al. 2012; Terashima and Kanazawa 1994). Given its neuroendocrine differentiation, it shares histologic similarity to the previously discussed Merkel cell carcinoma. Architecturally, tumor cells invade the dermis in trabeculae, sheets, or ribbons or as single,

diffusely scattered cells (Fig. 18.25). Features typical of neuroendocrine tumors include molding and pseudorosette formation, both of which may hint at the epithelial derivation of the tumor. Tumor nuclei display a vesicular, finely dispersed chromatin pattern, and nucleoli are inconspicuous (Fig. 18.26). As in MCC and aggressive hematolymphoid infiltrates, apoptotic debris, crush artifact, and brisk mitotic activity are often plentiful in small cell carcinoma.

The classic immunophenotype of small cell lung carcinoma is CK7 positive, CK20 negative, and TTF-1 positive (Figs. 18.27 and 18.28). In contrast, although a minority of MCC expresses CK7, MCC is invariably negative for TTF-1 and usually positive for CK20. Similar to MCC, small cell carcinoma can express neuroendocrine markers including synaptophysin, chromogranin, neuron-specific enolase, and CD56. Furthermore, as in MCC, expression of TdT in a subset of small cell lung carcinomas has been identified, leading to a potential for diagnostic confusion with lymphoblastic lymphoma (Kolhe et al. 2013). CD45/LCA is uniformly negative in these tumors, however, and represents a sensitive

Fig. 18.25 Metastatic small cell lung carcinoma. Nodular deposits of blue tumor cells with a nested to sheetlike pattern is present in the dermis

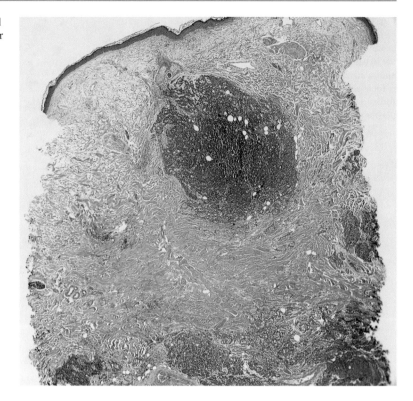

Fig. 18.26 Metastatic small cell lung carcinoma. The tumor cells demonstrate a high nuclear to cytoplasmic ratio and molding. The cells show scant eosinophilic cytoplasm, neuroendocrine-type chromatin, and readily identifiable mitotic figures

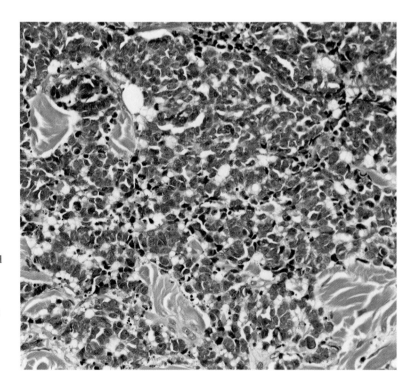

Fig. 18.27 Metastatic small cell lung carcinoma. In metastatic small cell lung carcinoma, tumor cells express cytokeratin 7

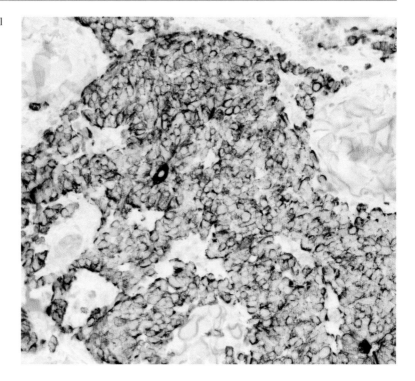

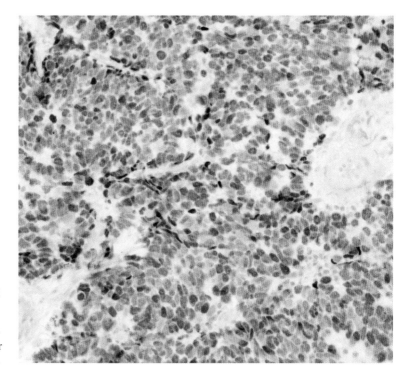

Fig. 18.28 Metastatic small cell lung carcinoma. In metastatic small cell lung carcinoma, tumor cells show nuclear immunoreactivity for thyroid transcription factor-1

stain to distinguish small cell carcinoma from a malignant lymphoid infiltrate.

Molecular/Genetics

Molecular and genetic studies are typically not useful in the evaluation of cutaneous metastases.

Prognosis/Course

Cutaneous metastases typically arise late in disease progression and signify advanced disease with a poor outcome. Survival following the detection of cutaneous carcinoma metastases has been estimated between 5 and 7.5 months (Saeed et al. 2004; Sariya et al. 2007). Metastatic disease can be treated with a combination of surgery, radiation, and/or chemotherapy.

Sarcomas/Other

Like Merkel cell carcinoma and the variants of melanoma and carcinomas described above, some sarcomas and other malignancies can occasionally be mistaken for hematolymphoid neoplasms. Most of these tumor types include those that fall within the "small round blue cell" differential. They may arise either as primary dermal neoplasms or as metastases from non-cutaneous sites. Key histologic and clinical features, as well as immunohistochemical profiles, are useful in distinguishing these entities from cutaneous lymphoma or leukemia.

Primary Cutaneous Ewing Sarcoma/ PNET

Epidemiology

Primary Ewing sarcoma (EWS) of the skin is a remarkably rare neoplasm that was first described in 1975 by Angervall and Enzinger (1975). Like conventional Ewing sarcoma, cutaneous Ewing sarcoma most often affects teenagers and young adults (Boland and Folpe 2013). Whereas mesenchymal Ewing sarcomas display a clear male predominance, the cutaneous variant is identified twice as frequently in women than in men (Ehrig et al. 2007).

Clinical Features

Primary cutaneous EWS often presents as a painless superficial nodule. It is most frequently encountered on the extremities, followed by the trunk and the head and neck (Boland and Folpe 2013; Collier et al. 2011). Cutaneous metastases from deep-seated Ewing sarcoma are rare but have been described (Izquierdo et al. 2002).

Histology, Immunohistochemistry, and Differential Diagnosis

Histologically, the features of cutaneous Ewing sarcoma are identical to its skeletal and deep soft tissue equivalents. The tumors are composed of dense sheets or nests of monomorphic cells containing scant clear to eosinophilic cytoplasm and round nuclei with fine, open chromatin (Fig. 18.29) (Hasegawa et al. 1998). There may be hemorrhagic or necrotic foci within the tumor, and mitotic figures are often easily identified (Collier et al. 2011, Hasegawa et al. 1998). The strong membranous expression of CD99 (MIC2) that is characteristic of extracutaneous Ewing sarcoma is also present in cutaneous EWS tumor cells (Hasegawa et al. 1998; Terrier-Lacombe et al. 2009). A pitfall of CD99, however, is that its expression is not entirely specific for Ewing sarcoma; not only may it be present in other non-Ewing sarcomas, but it is invariably and diffusely expressed in lymphoblastic lymphomas. To further complicate the diagnosis, lymphoblastic lymphomas are frequently negative for CD45, and sometimes negative for CD10, CD20, and CD3 (Boland and Folpe 2013; Hsiao and Su 2003). In these cases, the presence of terminal deoxynucleotidyl transferase (TdT) and CD43 expression may be the most useful antibodies to correctly identify lymphoblastic lymphoma and to distinguish it from other CD99-positive entities (Hsiao and Su 2003). Approximately 25 % of cutaneous EWS demonstrate positivity for the low-molecular-weight cytokeratins (Boland and Folpe 2013).

Molecular/Genetics

Like its deep-seated counterparts, cutaneous EWS derives from a chimeric fusion of the *EWSR1* gene located on chromosome 22q12

Fig. 18.29 Ewing sarcoma. On scanning magnification, the tumor is composed of sheets and nests of small round blue cells. On higher power, the tumor cells are monomorphic, with round nuclei and open chromatin (*inset*)

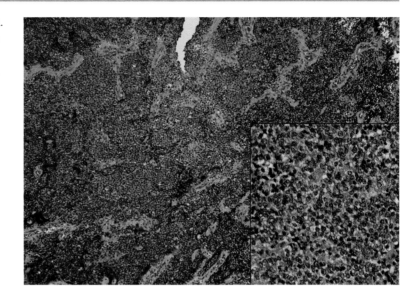

with a member of the E 26 (ETS) family of transcription factors that include *FLI-1* (chromosome 11q24), *ERG* (chromosome 21q22), *ETV1* (chromosome 7p22), *ETV4* (chromosome 17q21), and *FEV* (chromosome 2q36) (Boland and Folpe 2013; Terrier-Lacombe et al. 2009). Immunohistochemical stains for FLI-1 and ERG are commercially available and may be useful in the microscopic work-up of this tumor (Folpe et al. 2000). Additionally, the fusion gene transcripts can be demonstrated via tumor cytogenetics, fluorescence in situ hybridization (FISH), or reverse transcriptase-polymerase chain reaction (RT-PCR). The advantage of performing FISH using break-apart EWSR1 probes is that it is easily carried out on archival, paraffin-embedded tissues and is sensitive, although not specific, in detecting any EWSR1 rearrangement. RT-PCR is particularly helpful in distinguishing cutaneous EWS from other sarcomas that also demonstrate EWSR1 translocations, including clear cell sarcoma, myoepithelioma, and angiomatoid fibrous histiocytoma. Currently, however, RT-PCR can only detect the EWSR1-FLI-1 and EWSR1-ERG fusion products (Boland and Folpe 2013).

Prognosis/Course

Cutaneous EWS carries a better overall prognosis when compared to its osseous and soft tissue counterparts, with less likelihood to locally recur

or metastasize. It is therefore thought to represent a more favorable subtype of Ewing sarcoma (Boland and Folpe 2013; Collier et al. 2011; Delaplace et al. 2012; Ehrig et al. 2007; Hasegawa et al. 1998; Terrier-Lacombe et al. 2009).

Cutaneous Rhabdomyosarcoma

Epidemiology

Rhabdomyosarcoma (RMS) is a malignant small round blue cell tumor with skeletal muscle differentiation and is the most common soft tissue tumor of childhood. While the majority of RMS found in the skin represents metastatic deposits or dermal extension of tumors arising from the deep soft tissues, primary cutaneous RMS has been documented, with the largest series in the literature comprising 11 cases (Brecher et al. 2003; Cobanoglu et al. 2009; Lima et al. 2011; Marburger et al. 2012; Scatena et al. 2012). Both primary and metastatic RMS of the skin demonstrate a bimodal age distribution, and gender predilection is controversial (Marburger et al. 2012; Scatena et al. 2012).

Clinical Features

Three unique subtypes of rhabdomyosarcoma exist: alveolar RMS, embryonal RMS (further divided into botryoid and spindle cell subtypes),

Fig. 18.30 Cutaneous rhabdomyosarcoma. Sheets of monomorphic blue cells fill the dermis. This was classified as alveolar type and may be the most common type to see in the skin

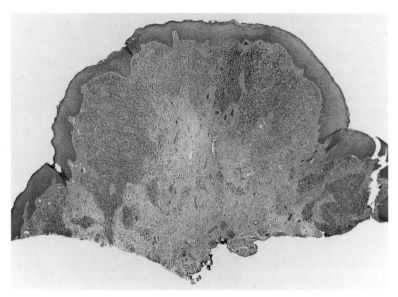

and pleomorphic RMS. With regard to extracutaneous disease, alveolar and embryonal rhabdomyosarcoma subtypes predominate in the pediatric population, the former of which has a proclivity for the extremities and the latter of which involves either the head and neck region or the genitourinary organs. The pleomorphic type arises almost exclusively in adults, which, like alveolar RMS, has a predilection for the extremities. Overall, embryonal RMS is the most common extracutaneous subtype, but alveolar RMS may be the most common subtype to arise in the skin (Setterfield et al. 2002). Primary cutaneous RMS appears to parallel the clinical patterns of its deep-seated counterpart, with alveolar and embryonal RMS being observed in the younger population and pleomorphic RMS occurring in older adults (Marburger et al. 2012). Neonatal alveolar RMS with cutaneous metastases has been reported in association with Beckwith-Wiedemann syndrome (Kuroiwa et al. 2009).

Histology

Histologically, RMS varies broadly in architectural and cytologic appearance depending on the subtype. Alveolar rhabdomyosarcomas are composed of classic small round blue cells with scant cytoplasm and monotonous, hyperchromatic, round to ovoid nuclei (Fig. 18.30). The tumor cells are aggregated between dense fibrous septa with fibrovascular cores. They often become discohesive, creating central, acellular spaces and resembling pulmonary alveoli (Fig. 18.31). The solid variant of alveolar rhabdomyosarcoma poses a particular challenge, as this variant lacks the characteristic fibrous septa and cellular discohesion seen in conventional alveolar RMS and may be confused with cutaneous lymphoma (Fig. 18.32) (Marburger et al. 2012). The tumor cells of embryonal RMS display varying degrees of myogenic differentiation, ranging from small round blue cells like those seen in alveolar RMS to more differentiated "strap cells," which are larger and oblong in shape and contain brightly eosinophilic cytoplasm. Striations, when present, are helpful clues to the diagnosis. Architecturally, embryonal-type RMS is composed of hypercellular areas alternating with hypocellular, myxoid areas (Cobanoglu et al. 2009). Pleomorphic rhabdomyosarcoma, in contrast to the other two subtypes, is composed of cells with varying morphologies, overall with more prominent cytoplasm, eccentrically placed nuclei, and large, conspicuous nucleoli (Fig. 18.33) (Marburger et al. 2012). Given the

Fig. 18.31
Rhabdomyosarcoma, alveolar pattern. This example of alveolar rhabdomyosarcoma demonstrates hyperchromatic tumor cells cling to vascular cores, resulting in central discohesion and resembling pulmonary alveoli

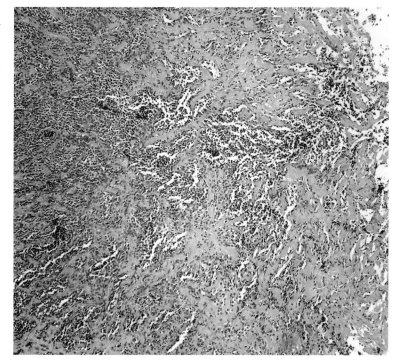

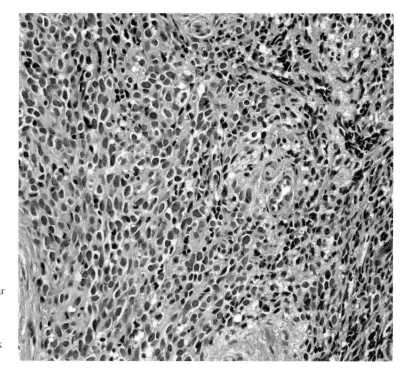

Fig. 18.32
Rhabdomyosarcoma, alveolar type with solid pattern. The tumor cells are enlarged and hyperchromatic and show brisk mitotic activity but lack clear differentiation

Fig. 18.33
Rhabdomyosarcoma,
pleomorphic type with
striations. The tumor cells are
large and atypical, containing
abundant eosinophilic
cytoplasm and displaying
prominent eosinophilic
nucleoli. These large cells are
admixed with small, primitive
cells and spindle cells

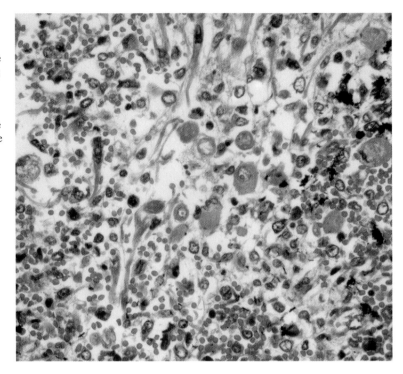

eccentrically located nuclei, the pleomorphic type may be mistaken for plasma cell myeloma or plasmacytoma.

Immunohistochemistry and Differential Diagnosis

Regardless of subtype, rhabdomyosarcoma tumor cells express markers of skeletal muscle differentiation. These markers include desmin, muscle-specific actin (MSA), myogenin, and MYOD1. Marburger and colleagues recommend employing a battery of stains, including desmin, myogenin, and MYOD1, in the work-up of RMS, as single cases may lack expression of one or more markers (Marburger et al. 2012). Myogenin and MYOD1 are nuclear stains, and it should be remembered that even patchy focal nuclear staining (a pattern frequently observed in embryonal-type RMS) should still be interpreted as positive staining (Fig. 18.34). It is not uncommon to observe anomalous expression of cytokeratin, CD56, and NSE in RMS (Marburger et al. 2012; Scatena et al. 2012; Setterfield et al. 2002). Furthermore, anaplastic lymphoma kinase (ALK) positivity

has been observed in rhabdomyosarcoma, particularly in the alveolar subtype, although it is reported to occur in an unusual, dot-like cytoplasmic pattern (Corao et al. 2009). The pattern of ALK staining and CD30 negativity are important in distinguishing RMS from anaplastic large cell lymphoma.

Molecular/Genetics

The translocations t(2;13)(q35;q14) and t(1;13) (p36;q14) are characteristic of conventional alveolar RMS, resulting in the fusion of transcription factors PAX3 or PAX7, respectively, to the transcription factor FOXO1 (also known as FKHR). These fusion gene products have been detected in some cases of primary cutaneous alveolar RMS (Nakagawa et al. 2008; Setterfield et al. 2002). Interestingly, however, these translocations are absent in many cases of neonatal alveolar RMS with metastasis to the skin. Therefore, clinical and histologic features must be considered in adjunct to molecular profiles in neonates when cutaneous metastases of RMS are suspected (Kuroiwa et al. 2009; Marburger et al. 2012).

Fig. 18.34
Rhabdomyosarcoma. Nuclear myogenin immunoreactivity, even when patchy as in this embryonal type, secures the diagnosis (Photograph courtesy of Dr. Jerad Gardner, University of Arkansas for Medical Sciences, Little Rock, AR)

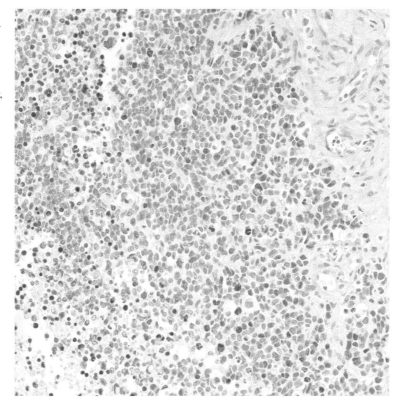

Prognosis/Course

Unlike the more favorable outcomes observed when some other soft tissue tumors present as primary cutaneous neoplasms, the prognosis of cutaneous RMS mirrors that of the soft tissue forms. In fact, it is not uncommon for cutaneous RMS to result in local recurrence, distant metastasis, and even death (Marburger et al. 2012; Nakagawa et al. 2008; Scatena et al. 2012).

Cutaneous Osteosarcoma

Epidemiology

Primary skeletal osteosarcoma (OS), although rare overall, is the most common primary malignant bone tumor, most frequently involving the metaphyses of long bones in children and young adults. While approximately 95 % of skeletal OS metastasize to the lung, metastases to the skin do occur, either exclusively or – more commonly – in addition to pulmonary metastases (Collier et al. 2003; Ragsdale et al. 2011; Setoyama et al. 1996). Extraskeletal osteosarcomas (ESOS) comprise a small fraction of all osteosarcomas (approximately 2–4 %), and only 1–2 % of all soft tissue sarcomas collectively (Riddle et al. 2009; Salamanca et al. 2008). Case reports of ESOS arising as a primary neoplasm from the dermis and subcutis exist (Drut and Barletta 1975; Kobos et al. 1995; Kuo 1992; Llamas-Velasco et al. 2013; Massi et al. 2007; Park et al. 2011; Riddle et al. 2009; Salamanca et al. 2008). Risk factors for primary cutaneous osteosarcoma are similar to those for deep-seated ESOS and include a history of prior irradiation, chemotherapy, and trauma; several cutaneous OS, in fact, have arisen within remote scars (Drut and Barletta 1975; Kuo 1992; Park et al. 2011; Riddle et al. 2009).

Clinical Features

Both primary and metastatic cutaneous OS present as firm, flesh-colored to red or violaceous

Fig. 18.35 Osteosarcoma. Tumor osteoid production is characterized by eosinophilic, fibrillary, immature-appearing deposits between individual tumor cells in a lacelike pattern

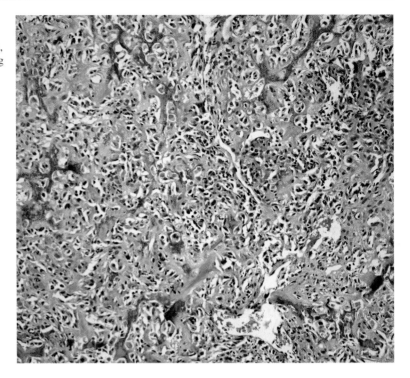

subcutaneous nodules (Collier et al. 2003; Larsen et al. 2010; Llamas-Velasco et al. 2013; Massi et al. 2007; Park et al. 2011). ESOS most commonly occurs within the deep soft tissues of the extremities, and unlike its skeletal counterpart, ESOS primarily affects middle-aged to elderly adults (Park et al. 2011; Riddle et al. 2009). Like deep-seated ESOS, primary cutaneous OS have also been identified in the extremities of older adults (Drut and Barletta 1975; Kobos et al. 1995; Kuo 1992; Park et al. 2011; Riddle et al. 2009; Salamanca et al. 2008). Interestingly, cutaneous OS, whether metastatic or primary in origin, demonstrates a particular proclivity for the scalp (Collier et al. 2003; Massi et al. 2007; Park et al. 2011; Ragsdale et al. 2011).

Histology, Immunohistochemistry, and Differential Diagnosis

Skeletal OS is commonly categorized according to predominant histologic features, and subtypes include osteoblastic OS, osteoclastic/giant cell OS, chondroblastic OS, telangiectatic OS, fibroblastic OS, and small cell OS. The small cell variant is the most likely OS type to resemble other

small round blue cell tumors and lymphoproliferative disorders. No particular subtype appears to be more likely to metastasize to or develop as a primary tumor in the skin (Fernandez-Pineda et al. 2011; Park et al. 2011).

Histologically, cutaneous OS is composed of poorly defined sheets of spindled to pleomorphic tumor cells with hyperchromatic nuclei and little cytoplasm. Neoplastic cells are often admixed with and surrounded by a lacelike, amorphous osteoid matrix and/or immature bony trabeculae (Fig. 18.35). One must be cautioned that osteoid deposition is seen in a variety of other reactive and neoplastic processes, including myositis ossificans, osteoma cutis, ossifying fibromyxoid tumor, and sarcomas or melanomas with osseous metaplasia; the presence of osteoid alone, therefore, must not reflexively give rise to a diagnosis of osteosarcoma (Riddle et al. 2009). Conversely, evidence of bone formation may be absent, particularly in biopsies, and in these cases, immunohistochemistry may be useful (see below) (Salamanca et al. 2008). Mitotic activity is typically brisk and atypical mitotic figures can be seen, but necrosis is usually absent (Massi et al. 2007).

Fig. 18.36 Osteosarcoma. Sheets of pleomorphic cells are admixed with multinucleated giant osteoclasts and anastamosing vascular spaces. Osteoid deposition here is focal

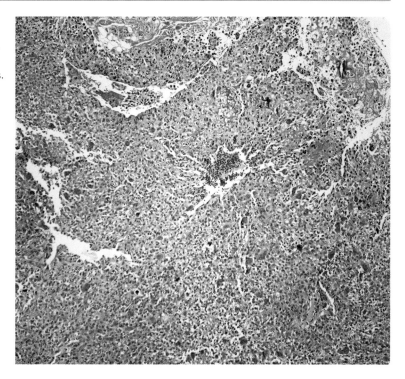

Other features, including multinucleated giant osteoclasts, chondroid differentiation, large anastomosing vascular spaces, and fibroblastic proliferation, may variably be present or predominate the histologic picture (Fig. 18.36).

Tumor cell negativity for CD43, CD45/LCA, and other hematolymphoid markers will exclude the possibility of lymphoma. Tumor cells of osteosarcoma stain positively with vimentin, alkaline phosphatase, anti-osteonectin, and anti-osteocalcin (Covello et al. 2003; Fanburg-Smith et al. 1999; Massi et al. 2007). Osteonectin is sensitive but lacks specificity, as it is also expressed in fibroblasts, pericytes, endothelial cells, chondrocytes, basal epidermal cells, nerves, and osteoclasts. Osteocalcin demonstrates greater specificity. Unfortunately, neither stain is routinely available in all immunohistochemistry laboratories (Fanburg-Smith et al. 1999). If present, chondroid areas may stain with S100.

Molecular/Genetics

Molecular studies are of little utility in the work-up of osteosarcoma, as there are currently no well-established molecular markers of diagnostic or prognostic significance.

Prognosis/Course

ESOS has a 5-year mortality rate approaching 75 % (Covello et al. 2003; Riddle et al. 2009). The clinical behavior of primary OS arising in the skin appears to parallel that of extracutaneous ESOS, in that local recurrence, as well as metastasis and death, may result (Kobos et al. 1995; Park et al. 2011; Riddle et al. 2009; Salamanca et al. 2008). Tumor size appears to most closely correlate with clinical outcome, however, this feature along with other prognostic indicators, including tumor histology, remain controversial (Larsen et al. 2010; Park et al. 2011). Like skeletal OS, extracutaneous ESOS can metastasize to the skin, and often metastasizes to the scalp (Covello et al. 2003; Fernandez-Pineda et al. 2011; Park et al. 2011; Ragsdale et al. 2011).

Cutaneous Angiosarcoma

Epidemiology

Angiosarcoma is a rare but aggressive neoplasm of vascular derivation accounting for approximately 1 % of soft tissue sarcomas. It typically affects older individuals with light skin color,

Fig. 18.37 Angiosarcoma, well differentiated. Vasoformative areas, as demonstrated by the slit-like, irregular vascular spaces lined by hyperchromatic endothelial cells, are fundamental to the diagnosis

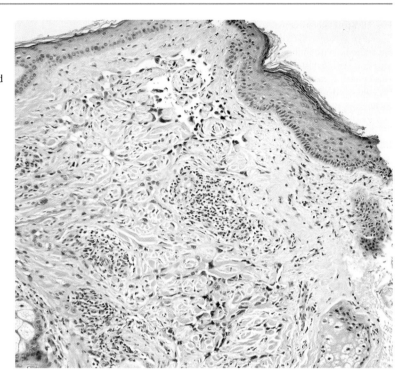

but there is no well-established gender predilection (Albores-Saavedra et al. 2011). These tumors may arise in soft tissues and also in the skin, where they occur most frequently on head and neck sites in elderly individuals. Cutaneous angiosarcoma also has a well-established association with radiation and chronic lymphedema, with tumors presenting after long intervals following irradiation as a treatment modality or after many years of chronic lymphedema; classically, this phenomenon can be seen as the Stewart-Treves syndrome following mastectomy (Requena et al. 2007). Exceptionally, angiosarcoma is reported in children, in which case it appears to more frequently affect the extremities (Bacchi et al. 2010).

Clinical Features

Cutaneous angiosarcoma, given its vascular derivation, usually presents as a violaceous patch or indurated plaque, often resembling a bruise or hematoma. The tumor frequently has ill-defined borders, and an early lesion can be extraordinarily subtle, consisting of only slight erythema and edema (Requena et al. 2007). Idiopathic cutaneous angiosarcomas typically arise on the

scalp or facial region of older individuals, while angiosarcomas related to irradiation or lymphedema arise in patients with relevant history, often on the breast, chest wall, or inner arm. Lesions may be multifocal and/or ulcerated. Angiosarcomas arising from extracutaneous sites may metastasize to the skin (Hart and Mandavilli 2011).

Histology, Immunohistochemistry, and Differential Diagnosis

Angiosarcoma may have a variety of histologic patterns. Well-differentiated variants will show a poorly circumscribed proliferation of irregular, anastamosing vascular channels dissecting through dermal collagen with deep extension. Endothelial cells are hyperchromatic and pleomorphic and will protrude into the lumen of the vascular spaces (hobnailing) (Requena et al. 2007). These vasoformative foci are fundamental to the diagnosis but may be difficult to discern in more poorly differentiated tumors (Fig. 18.37).

Epithelioid angiosarcoma in particular has the capacity to mimic other tumors, including lymphoma, melanoma, and certain carcinomas (Bacchi et al. 2010). Epithelioid angiosarcoma tumor cells tend to aggregate as broad sheets or islands of large, polygonal to round cells (Fig. 18.38). There is typically mild pleomorphism of tumor cells, with enlarged and often eccentrically placed nuclei and prominent nucleoli. The nuclei often have amphophilic to steel grey coloration (Bacchi et al. 2010), and margination of chromatin may lead to a vesicular appearance (Fig. 18.39) (Hart and Mandavilli 2011). Individual cell necrosis or apoptosis is more likely to be identified than frank necrosis (Bacchi et al. 2010). Vasoformative foci may be only focal in this tumor type but should be searched for on microscopic examination. The presence of erythrocytes around tumor cells may be useful. An additional helpful clue is the presence of focal cytoplasmic vacuolization of tumor cells, which is thought to correlate with primitive vascular lumen formation (Hart and Mandavilli 2011; Requena et al. 2007). Rarely, cutaneous angiosarcoma is accompanied by an obscuring inflammatory infiltrate including lymphoid follicles with germinal center formation, thereby mimicking follicle center cell lymphoma or reactive cutaneous lymphoid hyperplasia (Requena et al. 2007).

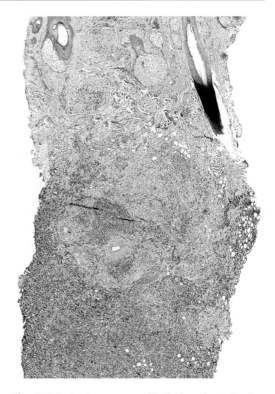

Fig. 18.38 Angiosarcoma, epithelioid variant. On low power, there is a prominent, diffuse infiltrate of blue cells with several interspersed lymphoid aggregates, reminiscent of the sheets of blue cells seen in diffuse large B-cell lymphoma

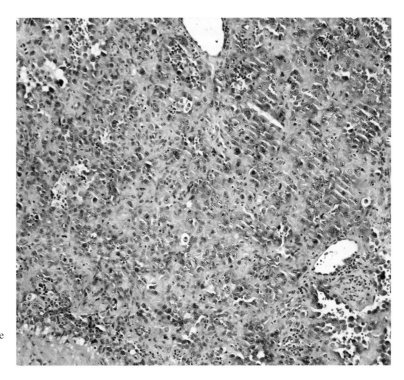

Fig. 18.39 Angiosarcoma, epithelioid variant. High-power examination shows sheets of polygonal epithelioid tumor cells with amphophilic cytoplasm, prominent nucleoli, and mitotic figures. Vasoformative foci are evident in the upper left and lower right

Angiosarcomas express endothelial markers, namely, CD31, CD34, factor VIII-related antigen (von Willebrand factor), FLI-1 protein, and podoplanin (D2-40) (Hart and Mandavilli 2011, Weed and Folpe 2008). CD31 represents a specific marker and demonstrates approximately equivalent sensitivity to some of the other, less specific stains (Bacchi et al. 2010). Recently, the use of the nuclear immunohistochemical stain ERG has been described as having superior sensitivity and specificity in the diagnosis of cutaneous angiosarcoma (McKay et al. 2012). Epithelioid angiosarcoma may express pancytokeratin and, less frequently, epithelial membrane antigen, although the exact frequency of co-expression ranges widely depending on the case series (Bacchi et al. 2010; McCluggage et al. 1995; Meis-Kindblom and Kindblom 1998; Suchak et al. 2011). Aberrant CD30 expression has been reported in an angiosarcoma arising in an irradiated site, thereby mimicking anaplastic large cell lymphoma (Weed and Folpe 2008). In the so-called pseudolymphomatous variant of cutaneous angiosarcoma, the lymphoid infiltrate was composed of a mix of predominantly CD4-positive T cells, with CD20-positive, Bcl-6-co-expressing germinal center cells that demonstrated the expected high proliferative index by MIB-1 (Ki-67) staining for a reactive follicle (Requena et al. 2007). The distinction of this variant from reactive cutaneous lymphoid hyperplasia requires careful evaluation of the tumor for the presence of vasoformative foci which express the previously discussed endothelial markers.

Electron Microscopy

While now uncommonly utilized as a diagnostic modality, ultrastructural examination of angiosarcoma will reveal endothelial cells and associated pericytes. Red blood cells may be identified between and within tumor cells, and Weibel-Pelade bodies may be visualized, assisting with the identification of vascular differentiation (Hart and Mandavilli 2011).

Molecular/Genetics

Cutaneous angiosarcoma associated with prior radiation has been shown to demonstrate MYC amplification as detected by FISH or by strong nuclear immunoreactivity using immunohistochemical staining (Fernandez et al. 2012; Mentzel et al. 2012). Angiosarcomas unassociated with radiation do not seem to exhibit this amplification (Mentzel et al. 2012).

Prognosis/Course

Survival rates for cutaneous angiosarcoma are generally unfavorable and appear to be related to multiple factors, including patient age, site of tumor, and disease stage. Younger patients (less than 50 years old) and those with truncal disease have increased survival rates at 10 years (approximately 75 %) compared to older patients (37 %) or patients with tumors on the head and neck (14 %) (Albores-Saavedra et al. 2011). Predictably, patients with localized cutaneous disease have improved survival compared to those with regional or distant disease (Albores-Saavedra et al. 2011). The presence of a prominent lymphoid infiltrate in angiosarcoma has been proposed as a potential predictor of improved survival; however, additional studies are required (Requena et al. 2007).

Cutaneous Neuroblastoma

Epidemiology

Like some of the previous entities mentioned, cutaneous neuroblastoma (NB) is both exceedingly rare and more likely to occur as a metastatic implant from a primary visceral source than as a primary cutaneous neoplasm. The adrenal gland is the most common primary site for tumor development, but neuroblastoma may develop at any site along the sympathetic nervous system chain (Argenyi and Jokinen 2011; Klapman and Chun 1991; Van Nguyen and Argenyi 1993). Of soft tissue sarcomas, neuroblastoma is one of the most likely to metastasize to the skin; in fact, approximately one-third of patients with congenital neuroblastoma present with cutaneous metastases, and cutaneous metastases are particularly more prevalent in neonates than in any other patient population (Hawthorne et al. 1970; Kao and Yu 1991; Lucky et al. 1982; Wyatt and Hansen 2000).

Fig. 18.40 Neuroblastoma. Sheets of monotonous blue cells are arranged in nests

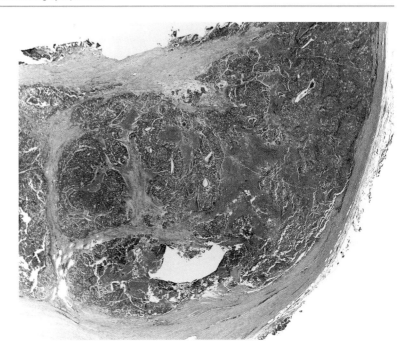

Unlike metastatic NB, cutaneous neuroblastomas of primary origin are recognized almost exclusively in the adult population (Argenyi and Jokinen 2011, Van Nguyen and Argenyi 1993).

Clinical Features

Whether primary or secondary in origin, cutaneous neuroblastoma presents as a rapidly growing blue or purple nodule with characteristic protracted blanching behavior following the application of pressure, a feature of which is likely due to vasoconstriction secondary to the local release of catecholamines (Argenyi and Jokinen 2011; Hawthorne et al. 1970; Lucky et al. 1982). Clinically, mesenchymal neuroblastomas are unique, and, therefore, one may find a review of the patient's history particularly useful when presented with a potential metastatic NB. First, the tumor is associated with increased levels of the serum catecholamines dopamine and norepinephrine and the urine catecholamine metabolites homovanillic acid (HVA) and vanillylmandelic acid (VMA). Visceral neuroblastoma may be confirmed by scintigraphy, a test in which radio-iodinated metaiodobenzylguanidine (^{123}I-MIBG) is administered and then monitored for its uptake by tumor foci (Dabbs 2010). Similar laboratory and imaging studies are not generally performed in cases of primary cutaneous neuroblastoma.

Histology, Immunohistochemistry, and Differential Diagnosis

Whether primary or metastatic in origin, cutaneous neuroblastoma appears microscopically as a poorly demarcated aggregate of tumor cells arranged in infiltrative sheets, nests, or trabeculae (Fig. 18.40) (Argenyi and Jokinen 2011). The neoplastic cells are epithelioid to ovoid in shape with a vesicular chromatin pattern and scant cytoplasm. The tumor cells often assimilate to form Homer Wright rosettes, which are ringlike structures characterized by a rim of palisading neoplastic cells and a central area containing fine, pink fibrillary material (Argenyi and Jokinen 2011). Like in visceral NB, Homer Wright rosettes are pathognomonic for cutaneous NB and, when present, are fundamental clues in differentiating this tumor from the other small round blue cell neoplasms (Fig. 18.41). The presence of ganglion cells, schwannoma-like stroma, and neuropil vary depending on the degree of maturation of the tumor.

Fig. 18.41 Neuroblastoma. On higher examination, rosette formation can be appreciated and karyorrhectic debris is plentiful

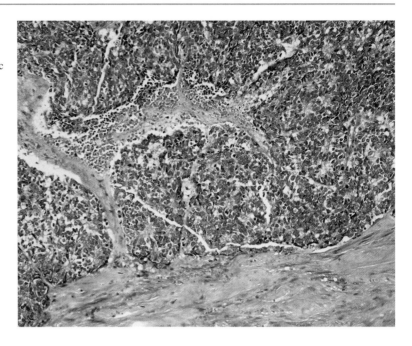

NB tumor cells express neuroblastic markers such as neuron-specific enolase (NSE), CD56, synaptophysin, chromogranin, and neurofilament protein. More recent markers for NB appear to be more specific but less sensitive and include anti-neuroblastoma antibody (NB84), protein gene product 9.5 (PGP 9.5), and anti-GD2, a cell membrane glycolipid identified on neuroblastoma cells (Dabbs 2010; Sariola et al. 1991). A promiscuous stain, ALK 1, is also positive in greater than 90 % of neuroblastomas, and as discussed previously with rhabdomyosarcoma and Merkel cell carcinoma, discretion must be used in its interpretation (Dabbs 2010). Ganglioneuroma-like differentiation has been identified in Merkel cell carcinoma; CK20 stain is helpful in distinguishing this rare variant from cutaneous neuroblastoma (Vanchinathan et al. 2009). Schwannoma-like stroma, when present, stains positively for S100 protein.

Molecular/Genetics

Ancillary studies are primarily of prognostic rather than diagnostic utility: NBs that express TRK-A, a neurotrophic tyrosine kinase receptor important in sympathetic neuronal development, have a more favorable prognosis, while tumors that express TRK-B and/or that demonstrate N-*myc* oncogene amplification are associated with lack of response to therapy and rapid tumor progression, respectively (Brodeur et al. 2009). Currently, molecular tests for the detection of the neurotrophic tyrosine kinase receptors are not widely available. Identification of N-*myc* amplification, however, has been made relatively straightforward through the use of fluorescence in situ hybridization studies (FISH). DNA indexing via flow cytometry is also a useful prognostic indicator in young patients with disseminated neuroblastoma; triploid and hyperdiploid tumors are associated with a more favorable prognosis, while those with near diploid states are associated with more aggressive tumor behavior (Brodeur et al. 2009).

Prognosis/Course

Visceral neuroblastomas display significant prognostic heterogeneity, with survival rates varying from 15 % to 90 % based on the age of the patient and the extent of disease burden. Two staging systems have been proposed for NB. According to the International Neuroblastoma Staging System (INSS), the presence of cutaneous metastases in children upstages the tumor to stage 4 disease, although children less than 1 year of age have substantially greater survival rates than children older than 1 year of age. Importantly, however, if all of the following are true – (1) the primary tumor consists of a single focus that can be completely excised; (2) there are no distant metastases other than dermal metastases; and (3) the patient is less than 1 year of age – then the patient's disease is categorized as stage 4S, and survival rates are comparable to those of stage 1 or 2 disease (75–90 % at 3 years) (ASCO 2012). The more recent International Neuroblastoma Risk Group Staging System (INRGSS) takes into account not only the tumor stage but also the molecular and histologic features of the tumor to classify patients into low-, intermediate-, or high-risk disease categories (ASCO 2012, Cohn et al. 2009). As reports of primary cutaneous neuroblastoma are rare, generalizations about patient outcome are not available, although adult patients appear to have an unfavorable prognosis with rapid disease progression (Klapman and Chun 1991).

Current treatment options range from careful observation to neoadjuvant chemotherapy, surgical excision, and postsurgical chemoradiation therapy, depending on the determined disease risk level (Cohn et al. 2009).

Conclusion

This chapter has sought to describe nonlymphoid malignancies that demonstrate histologic overlap with hematolymphoid infiltrates of the skin. We acknowledge that no such chapter – however broad – can be entirely exhaustive. When presented with a cutaneous infiltrate without clear lineage, one must often go beyond the basic H&E-stained slide evaluation to exploit available supplementary tools and methods of investigation. As is evident in this chapter, diagnostic precision often necessitates the use of immunohistochemistry, molecular testing, and clinical information. However, sometimes simply thinking outside the box and remembering to include a rare entity within one's differential diagnosis will lead down the path to an accurate diagnosis.

References

Albores-Saavedra J, Schwartz AM, Henson DE, Kostun L, Hart A, Angeles-Albores D, et al. Cutaneous angiosarcoma. Analysis of 434 cases from the Surveillance, Epidemiology, and End Results Program, 1973-2007. Ann Diagn Pathol. 2011;15(2):93–7.

Angervall L, Enzinger FM. Extraskeletal neoplasm resembling Ewing's sarcoma. Cancer. 1975;36(1):240–51.

Anne N, Pallapothu R. Lymphoma of the breast: a mimic of inflammatory breast cancer. World J Surg Oncol. 2011;9:125. doi:10.1186/1477-7819-9-125.

Ansai S, Maeda K, Yamakawa M, Matsuda M, Saitoh S, Suwa S, et al. CD56-positive (nasal-type T/NK cell) lymphoma arising on the skin. Report of two cases and review of the literature. J Cutan Pathol. 1997;24(8):468–76.

Aoki R, Mitsui H, Harada K, Kawamura T, Shibagaki N, Tsukamoto K, et al. A case of lymphoepithelioma-like carcinoma of the skin associated with Epstein-Barr virus infection. J Am Acad Dermatol. 2010;62(4):681–4. doi:10.1016/j.jaad.2008.07.024.

Argenyi Z, Jokinen CH. Cutaneous neural neoplasms : a practical guide. New York: Humana Press; 2011. xiv, 135 p.

Arsenovic N. Lymphoepithelioma-like carcinoma of the skin: new case of an exceedingly rare primary skin tumor. Dermatol Online J. 2008;14(8):12.

ASCO. Neuroblastoma-childhood. [Internet]. 2012. [Updated Oct 2012]. Available from: http://www.cancer.net/cancer-types/neuroblastoma-childhood/staging

Azoulay S, Adem C, Pelletier FL, Barete S, Frances C, Capron F. Skin metastases from unknown origin: role of immunohistochemistry in the evaluation of cutaneous metastases of carcinoma of unknown origin. J Cutan Pathol. 2005;32(8):561–6. doi:10.1111/j.0303-6987.2005.00386.x.

Bacchi CE, Silva TR, Zambrano E, Plaza J, Suster S, Luzar B, et al. Epithelioid angiosarcoma of the skin: a study of 18 cases with emphasis on its clinicopathologic spectrum and unusual morphologic features. Am J Surg Pathol. 2010;34(9):1334–43. doi:10.1097/PAS.0b013e3181ee4eaf.

Bagley FH, Cady B, Lee A, Legg MA. Changes in clinical presentation and management of malignant melanoma. Cancer. 1981;47(9):2126–34.

Barnes L, Eveson JW, Reichart R, Sidransky D, World Health Organization, Cancer IAfRo. WHO classification of tumours: Pathology and Genetics of Head and Neck Tumours. 2nd ed. Lyon: IARC Press; 2007. 430 p.

Basler GC, Fader DJ, Yahanda A, Sondak VK, Johnson TM. The utility of fine needle aspiration in the diagnosis of melanoma metastatic to lymph nodes. J Am Acad Dermatol. 1997;36(3 Pt 1):403–8.

Bauer J, Bastian BC. Distinguishing melanocytic nevi from melanoma by DNA copy number changes:

comparative genomic hybridization as a research and diagnostic tool. Dermatol Ther. 2006;19(1):40–9. doi:10.1111/j.1529-8019.2005.00055.x.

Biswas A, Geyvan Pittius D, Stephens M, Smith AG. Recurrent primary cutaneous lymphoma with florid pseudoepitheliomatous hyperplasia masquerading as squamous cell carcinoma. Histopathology. 2008;52(6):755–8. doi:10.1111/j.1365-2559.2008.03013.x.

Blessing K, Grant JJ, Sanders DS, Kennedy MM, Husain A, Coburn P. Small cell malignant melanoma: a variant of naevoid melanoma. Clinicopathological features and histological differential diagnosis. J Clin Pathol. 2000;53(8):591–5.

Boland JM, Folpe AL. Cutaneous neoplasms showing EWSR1 rearrangement. Adv Anat Pathol. 2013;20(2):75–85. doi:10.1097/PAP.0b013e31828625bf.

Brecher AR, Reyes-Mugica M, Kamino H, Chang MW. Congenital primary cutaneous rhabdomyosarcoma in a neonate. Pediatr Dermatol. 2003;20(4):335–8.

Brodeur GM, Minturn JE, Ho R, Simpson AM, Iyer R, Varela CR, et al. Trk receptor expression and inhibition in neuroblastomas. Clin Cancer Res. 2009;15(10):3244–50. doi:10.1158/1078-0432.CCR-08-1815.

Brownstein MH, Helwig EB. Metastatic tumors of the skin. Cancer. 1972;29(5):1298–307.

Buresh CJ, Oliai BR, Miller RT. Reactivity with TdT in Merkel cell carcinoma: a potential diagnostic pitfall. Am J Clin Pathol. 2008;129(6):894–8. doi:10.1309/R494HQ9VRDJWDY30.

Calder KB, Smoller BR. New insights into merkel cell carcinoma. Adv Anat Pathol. 2010;17(3):155–61. doi:10.1097/PAP.0b013e3181d97836.

Cangiarella J, Symmans WF, Shapiro RL, Roses DF, Cohen JM, Chhieng D, et al. Aspiration biopsy and the clinical management of patients with malignant melanoma and palpable regional lymph nodes. Cancer. 2000;90(3):162–6.

Carr KA, Bulengo-Ransby SM, Weiss LM, Nickoloff BJ. Lymphoepitheliomalike carcinoma of the skin. A case report with immunophenotypic analysis and in situ hybridization for Epstein-Barr viral genome. Am J Surg Pathol. 1992;16(9):909–13.

Chapman PB, Hauschild A, Robert C, Haanen JB, Ascierto P, Larkin J, et al. Improved survival with vemurafenib in melanoma with BRAF V600E mutation. N Engl J Med. 2011;364(26):2507–16. doi:10.1056/NEJMoa1103782.

Cheung WL, Patel RR, Leonard A, Firoz B, Meehan SA. Amelanotic melanoma: a detailed morphologic analysis with clinicopathologic correlation of 75 cases. J Cutan Pathol. 2012;39(1):33–9. doi:10.1111/j.1600-0560.2011.01808.x.

Chu P, Wu E, Weiss LM. Cytokeratin 7 and cytokeratin 20 expression in epithelial neoplasms: a survey of 435 cases. Mod Pathol. 2000;13(9):962–72. doi:10.1038/modpathol.3880175.

Cibull TL, Thomas AB, O'Malley DP, Billings SD. Myeloid leukemia cutis: a histologic and immunohistochemical review. J Cutan Pathol. 2008;35(2):180–5. doi:10.1111/j.1600-0560.2007.00784.x.

Cimino-Mathews A, Subhawong AP, Illei PB, Sharma R, Halushka MK, Vang R, et al. GATA3 expression in breast carcinoma: utility in triple-negative, sarcomatoid, and metastatic carcinomas. Hum Pathol. 2013;44(7):1341–9. doi:10.1016/j.humpath.2012.11.003.

Cobanoglu B, Kandi B, Okur I. Primary cutaneous rhabdomyosarcoma in an adult. Dermatol Surg. 2009;35(10):1573–5. doi:10.1111/j.1524-4725.2009.01278.x.

Cohn SL, Pearson AD, London WB, Monclair T, Ambros PF, Brodeur GM, et al. The International Neuroblastoma Risk Group (INRG) classification system: an INRG Task Force report. J Clin Oncol. 2009;27(2):289–97. doi:10.1200/JCO.2008.16.6785.

Collier 3rd AB, Simpson L, Monteleone P. Cutaneous Ewing sarcoma: report of 2 cases and literature review of presentation, treatment, and outcome of 76 other reported cases. J Pediatr Hematol Oncol. 2011;33(8):631–4. doi:10.1097/MPH.0b013e31821b234d.

Collier DA, Busam K, Salob S. Cutaneous metastasis of osteosarcoma. J Am Acad Dermatol. 2003;49(4):757–60.

Corao DA, Biegel JA, Coffin CM, Barr FG, Wainright LM, Ernst LM, et al. ALK expression in rhabdomyosarcomas: correlation with histologic subtype and fusion status. Pediatr Dev Pathol. 2009;12(4):275–83. doi:10.2350/08-03-0434.1.

Covello SP, Humphreys TR, Lee JB. A case of extraskeletal osteosarcoma with metastasis to the skin. J Am Acad Dermatol. 2003;49(1):124–7. doi:10.1067/mjd.2003.297.

D'Agostino M, Cinelli C, Willard R, Hofmann J, Jellinek N, Robinson-Bostom L. Epidermotropic Merkel cell carcinoma: a case series with histopathologic examination. J Am Acad Dermatol. 2010;62(3):463–8. doi:10.1016/j.jaad.2009.06.023.

Dabbs DJ. Diagnostic immunohistochemistry : theranostic and genomic applications. 3rd ed. Philadelphia: Saunders/Elsevier; 2010. xviii, 941 p.

Delaplace M, Lhommet C, de Pinieux G, Vergier B, de Muret A, Machet L. Primary cutaneous Ewing sarcoma: a systematic review focused on treatment and outcome. Br J Dermatol. 2012;166(4):721–6. doi:10.1111/j.1365-2133.2011.10743.x.

Donner LR, Speights VO, Trompler RA. Merkel cell carcinoma with pagetoid spread. Ultrastruct Pathol. 1992;16(1–2):25–8.

Drut R, Barletta L. Osteogenic sarcoma arising in an old burn scar. J Cutan Pathol. 1975;2(6):302–6.

Edge SB, American Joint Committee on Cancer., American Cancer Society. AJCC cancer staging handbook : from the AJCC cancer staging manual. 7th ed. New York: Springer; 2010. xix, 718 p.

Ehrig T, Billings SD, Fanburg-Smith JC. Superficial primitive neuroectodermal tumor/Ewing sarcoma (PN/ES): same tumor as deep PN/ES or new entity? Ann Diagn Pathol. 2007;11(3):153–9. doi:10.1016/j.anndiagpath.2006.12.019.

Essner R. Lymphatic mapping and sentinel lymphadenectomy in primary cutaneous melanoma. Expert Rev

Anticancer Ther. 2010;10(5):723–8. doi:10.1586/era.10.65.

Falini B, Pileri S, Stein H, Dieneman D, Dallenbach F, Delsol G, et al. Variable expression of leucocyte-common (CD45) antigen in CD30 (Ki1)-positive anaplastic large-cell lymphoma: implications for the differential diagnosis between lymphoid and nonlymphoid malignancies. Hum Pathol. 1990;21(6):624–9.

Fanburg-Smith JC, Bratthauer GL, Miettinen M. Osteocalcin and osteonectin immunoreactivity in extraskeletal osteosarcoma: a study of 28 cases. Hum Pathol. 1999;30(1):32–8.

Feng H, Shuda M, Chang Y, Moore PS. Clonal integration of a polyomavirus in human Merkel cell carcinoma. Science. 2008;319(5866):1096–100. doi:10.1126/science.1152586.

Fernandez-Pineda I, Bahrami A, Green JF, McGregor LM, Davidoff AM, Sandoval JA. Isolated subcutaneous metastasis of osteosarcoma 5 years after initial diagnosis. J Pediatr Surg. 2011;46(10):2029–31. doi:10.1016/j.jpedsurg.2011.06.011.

Fernandez AP, Sun Y, Tubbs RR, Goldblum JR, Billings SD. FISH for MYC amplification and anti-MYC immunohistochemistry: useful diagnostic tools in the assessment of secondary angiosarcoma and atypical vascular proliferations. J Cutan Pathol. 2012;39(2):234–42. doi:10.1111/j.1600-0560.2011.01843.x.

Filtenborg-Barnkob BE, Bzorek M. Expression of anaplastic lymphoma kinase in Merkel cell carcinomas. Hum Pathol. 2013. doi:10.1016/j.humpath.2012.11.021.

Folpe AL, Hill CE, Parham DM, O'Shea PA, Weiss SW. Immunohistochemical detection of FLI-1 protein expression: a study of 132 round cell tumors with emphasis on CD99-positive mimics of Ewing's sarcoma/primitive neuroectodermal tumor. Am J Surg Pathol. 2000;24(12):1657–62.

Gast A, Scherer D, Chen B, Bloethner S, Melchert S, Sucker A, et al. Somatic alterations in the melanoma genome: a high-resolution array-based comparative genomic hybridization study. Genes Chromosomes Cancer. 2010;49(8):733–45. doi:10.1002/gcc.20785.

Gerami P, Jewell SS, Morrison LE, Blondin B, Schulz J, Ruffalo T, et al. Fluorescence in situ hybridization (FISH) as an ancillary diagnostic tool in the diagnosis of melanoma. Am J Surg Pathol. 2009;33(8):1146–56. doi:10.1097/PAS.0b013e3181a1ef36.

Gillum PS, Morgan MB, Naylor MF, Everett MA. Absence of Epstein-Barr virus in lymphoepithelioma-like carcinoma of the skin. Polymerase chain reaction evidence and review of five cases. Am J Dermatopathol. 1996;18(5):478–82.

Goessling W, McKee PH, Mayer RJ. Merkel cell carcinoma. J Clin Oncol. 2002;20(2):588–98.

Gul U, Kilic A, Gonul M, Kulcu Cakmak S, Erinckan C. Spectrum of cutaneous metastases in 1287 cases of internal malignancies: a study from Turkey. Acta Derm Venereol. 2007;87(2):160–2. doi:10.2340/00015555-0199.

Hafstrom L, Hugander A, Jonsson PE, Lindberg LG. Fine-needle-aspiration cytodiagnosis of recurrent malignant melanoma. J Surg Oncol. 1980;15(3):229–34.

Hall BJ, Pincus LB, Yu SS, Oh DH, Wilson AR, McCalmont TH. Immunohistochemical prognostication of Merkel cell carcinoma: p63 expression but not polyomavirus status correlates with outcome. J Cutan Pathol. 2012;39(10):911–7. doi:10.1111/j.1600-0560.2012.01964.x.

Hall G, Duncan A, Azurdia R, Leonard N. Lymphoepithelioma-like carcinoma of the skin: a case with lymph node metastases at presentation. Am J Dermatopathol. 2006;28(3):211–5.

Hanson IM, Banerjee SS, Menasce LP, Prescott RJ. A study of eleven cutaneous malignant melanomas in adults with small-cell morphology: emphasis on diagnostic difficulties and unusual features. Histopathology. 2002;40(2):187–95.

Hart J, Mandavilli S. Epithelioid angiosarcoma: a brief diagnostic review and differential diagnosis. Arch Pathol Lab Med. 2011;135(2):268–72. doi:10.1043/1543-2165-135.2.268.

Hasegawa SL, Davison JM, Rutten A, Fletcher JA, Fletcher CD. Primary cutaneous Ewing's sarcoma: immunophenotypic and molecular cytogenetic evaluation of five cases. Am J Surg Pathol. 1998;22(3):310–8.

Hashimoto K, Lee MW, D'Annunzio DR, Balle MR, Narisawa Y. Pagetoid Merkel cell carcinoma: epidermal origin of the tumor. J Cutan Pathol. 1998;25(10):572–9.

Hawthorne Jr HC, Nelson JS, Witzleben CL, Giangiacomo J. Blanching subcutaneous nodules in neonatal neuroblastoma. J Pediatr. 1970;77(2):297–300.

Higaki-Mori H, Kuwamoto S, Iwasaki T, Kato M, Murakami I, Nagata K, et al. Association of Merkel cell polyomavirus infection with clinicopathological differences in Merkel cell carcinoma. Hum Pathol. 2012;43(12):2282–91. doi:10.1016/j.humpath.2012.04.002.

Hsiao CH, Su IJ. Primary cutaneous pre-B lymphoblastic lymphoma immunohistologically mimics Ewing's sarcoma/primitive neuroectodermal tumor. J Formos Med Assoc. 2003;102(3):193–7.

Izquierdo MJ, Pastor MA, Carrasco L, Requena C, Farina MC, Martin L, et al. Cutaneous metastases from Ewing's sarcoma: report of two cases. Clin Exp Dermatol. 2002;27(2):123–8.

Jagirdar J. Application of immunohistochemistry to the diagnosis of primary and metastatic carcinoma to the lung. Arch Pathol Lab Med. 2008;132(3):384–96. doi:10.1043/1543-2165(2008)132[384:AOITTD]2.0.CO;2.

Jimenez F, Clark RE, Buchanan MD, Kamino H. Lymphoepithelioma-like carcinoma of the skin treated with Mohs micrographic surgery in combination with immune staining for cytokeratins. J Am Acad Dermatol. 1995;32(5 Pt 2):878–81.

Kanitakis J, Euvrard S, Chouvet B, Butnaru AC, Claudy A. Merkel cell carcinoma in organ-transplant recipients: report of two cases with unusual histological features and literature review. J Cutan Pathol. 2006;33(10):686–94. doi:10.1111/j.1600-0560.2006.00529.x.

Kao CH, Yu HS. Cutaneous neonatal neuroblastoma: report of a case. J Formos Med Assoc. 1991;90(4):422–5.

Klapman MH, Chun D. Cutaneous and subcutaneous neuroblastoma in children and adults: case reports and population study. J Am Acad Dermatol. 1991;24(6 Pt 1):1025–7.

Kobos JW, Yu GH, Varadarajan S, Brooks JS. Primary cutaneous osteosarcoma. Am J Dermatopathol. 1995;17(1):53–7.

Kolhe R, Reid MD, Lee JR, Cohen C, Ramalingam P. Immunohistochemical expression of PAX5 and TdT by Merkel cell carcinoma and pulmonary small cell carcinoma: a potential diagnostic pitfall but useful discriminatory marker. Int J Clin Exp Pathol. 2013;6(2):142–7.

Kuo TT. Primary osteosarcoma of the skin. J Cutan Pathol. 1992;19(2):151–5.

Kuroiwa M, Sakamoto J, Shimada A, Suzuki N, Hirato J, Park MJ, et al. Manifestation of alveolar rhabdomyosarcoma as primary cutaneous lesions in a neonate with Beckwith-Wiedemann syndrome. J Pediatr Surg. 2009;44(3):e31–5. doi:10.1016/j.jpedsurg.2008.12.010.

Larsen S, Davis DM, Comfere NI, Folpe AL, Sciallis GF. Osteosarcoma of the skin. Int J Dermatol. 2010;49(5):532–40. doi:10.1111/j.1365-4632.2010.04315.x.

Lazova R, Seeley EH, Keenan M, Gueorguieva R, Caprioli RM. Imaging mass spectrometry – a new and promising method to differentiate Spitz nevi from Spitzoid malignant melanomas. Am J Dermatopathol. 2012;34(1):82–90. doi:10.1097/DAD.0b013e31823df1e2.

LeBoit PE, Crutcher WA, Shapiro PE. Pagetoid intraepidermal spread in Merkel cell (primary neuroendocrine) carcinoma of the skin. Am J Surg Pathol. 1992;16(6):584–92.

Lima LL, Rodrigues CA, Pereira PM, Schettini AP, Tupinamba WL. Primary cutaneous alveolar rhabdomyosarcoma in a pediatric patient. An Bras Dermatol. 2011;86(2):363–5.

Llamas-Velasco M, Rutten A, Requena L, Mentzel T. Primary cutaneous osteosarcoma of the skin: a report of 2 cases with emphasis on the differential diagnoses. Am J Dermatopathol. 2013. doi:10.1097/DAD.0b013e31827f0a6f.

Lobo AZ, Tanabe KK, Luo S, Muzikansky A, Sober AJ, Tsao H, et al. The distribution of microscopic melanoma metastases in sentinel lymph nodes: implications for pathology protocols. Am J Surg Pathol. 2012;36(12):1841–8. doi:10.1097/PAS.0b013e31826d25f9.

Lopez V, Martin JM, Santonja N, Molina I, Ramon D, Monteagudo C, et al. Lymphoepithelioma-like carcinoma of the skin: report of three cases. J Cutan Pathol. 2011;38(1):54–8. doi:10.1111/j.1600-0560.2009.01458.x.

Lucky AW, McGuire J, Komp DM. Infantile neuroblastoma presenting with cutaneous blanching nodules. J Am Acad Dermatol. 1982;6(3):389–91.

Marburger TB, Gardner JM, Prieto VG, Billings SD. Primary cutaneous rhabdomyosarcoma: a clinicopathologic review of 11 cases. J Cutan Pathol. 2012;39(11):987–95. doi:10.1111/cup.12007.

Marcoval J, Penin RM, Llatjos R, Martinez-Ballarin I. Cutaneous metastasis from lung cancer: retrospective analysis of 30 patients. Australas J Dermatol. 2012;53(4):288–90. doi:10.1111/j.1440-0960.2011.00828.x.

Marghoob AA, Schoenbach SP, Kopf AW, Orlow SJ, Nossa R, Bart RS. Large congenital melanocytic nevi and the risk for the development of malignant melanoma. A prospective study. Arch Dermatol. 1996;132(2):170–5.

Massi D, Franchi A, Leoncini G, Maio V, Dini M. Primary cutaneous osteosarcoma of the scalp: a case report and review of the literature. J Cutan Pathol. 2007;34(1):61–4. doi:10.1111/j.1600-0560.2006.00562.x.

McCluggage WG, Clarke R, Toner PG. Cutaneous epithelioid angiosarcoma exhibiting cytokeratin positivity. Histopathology. 1995;27(3):291–4.

McGovern VJ. Spontaneous regression of melanoma. Pathology. 1975;7(2):91–9.

McKay KM, Doyle LA, Lazar AJ, Hornick JL. Expression of ERG, an Ets family transcription factor, distinguishes cutaneous angiosarcoma from histological mimics. Histopathology. 2012;61(5):989–91. doi:10.1111/j.1365-2559.2012.04286.x.

McNiff JM, Cowper SE, Lazova R, Subtil A, Glusac EJ. CD56 staining in Merkel cell carcinoma and natural killer-cell lymphoma: magic bullet, diagnostic pitfall, or both? J Cutan Pathol. 2005;32(8):541–5. doi:10.1111/j.0303-6987.2005.00378.x.

Meis-Kindblom JM, Kindblom LG. Angiosarcoma of soft tissue: a study of 80 cases. Am J Surg Pathol. 1998;22(6):683–97.

Menasce LP, Shanks JH, Howarth VS, Banerjee SS. Regressed cutaneous malignant melanoma mimicking lymphoma: a potential diagnostic pitfall. Int J Surg Pathol. 2005;13(3):281–4.

Mentzel T, Schildhaus HU, Palmedo G, Buttner R, Kutzner H. Postradiation cutaneous angiosarcoma after treatment of breast carcinoma is characterized by MYC amplification in contrast to atypical vascular lesions after radiotherapy and control cases: clinicopathological, immunohistochemical and molecular analysis of 66 cases. Mod Pathol. 2012;25(1):75–85. doi:10.1038/modpathol.2011.134.

Mohamed A, Gonzalez RS, Lawson D, Wang J, Cohen C. SOX10 expression in malignant melanoma, carcinoma, and normal tissues. Appl Immunohistochem Mol Morphol. 2012. doi:10.1097/PAI.0b013e318279bc0a.

Mott RT, Smoller BR, Morgan MB. Merkel cell carcinoma: a clinicopathologic study with prognostic implications. J Cutan Pathol. 2004;31(3):217–23.

Murali R, Doubrovsky A, Watson GF, McKenzie PR, Lee CS, McLeod DJ, et al. Diagnosis of metastatic melanoma by fine-needle biopsy: analysis of 2,204 cases. Am J Clin Pathol. 2007;127(3):385–97. doi:10.1309/3QR4FC5PPWXA7N29.

Musette P, Bachelez H, Flageul B, Delarbre C, Kourilsky P, Dubertret L, et al. Immune-mediated destruction of melanocytes in halo nevi is associated with the local expansion of a limited number of T cell clones. J Immunol. 1999;162(3):1789–94.

Nakagawa N, Tsuda T, Yamamoto M, Ito T, Futani H, Yamanishi K. Adult cutaneous alveolar rhabdomyosarcoma on the face diagnosed by the expression of PAX3-FKHR gene fusion transcripts. J Dermatol. 2008;35(7):462–7. doi:10.1111/j.1346-8138.2008.00503.x.

NCCN. Clinical Practice Guidelines in Oncology: merkel cell carcinoma. [Internet]. 2013. [Updated May 14 2013]. Available from: http://www.NCCN.org/professionals/physician_gls/pdf/mcc.pdf

Nelson AA, Tsao H. Melanoma and genetics. Clin Dermatol. 2009;27(1):46–52. doi:10.1016/j.clindermatol.2008.09.005.

Nonaka D, Chiriboga L, Soslow RA. Expression of pax8 as a useful marker in distinguishing ovarian carcinomas from mammary carcinomas. Am J Surg Pathol. 2008;32(10):1566–71. doi:10.1097/PAS.0b013e31816d71ad.

Ormsby AH, Snow JL, Su WP, Goellner JR. Diagnostic immunohistochemistry of cutaneous metastatic breast carcinoma: a statistical analysis of the utility of gross cystic disease fluid protein-15 and estrogen receptor protein. J Am Acad Dermatol. 1995;32(5 Pt 1):711–6.

Park SG, Song JY, Song IG, Kim MS, Shin BS. Cutaneous extraskeletal osteosarcoma on the scar of a previous bone graft. Ann Dermatol. 2011;23 Suppl 2:S160–4. doi:10.5021/ad.2011.23.S2.S160.

Park SY, Kim BH, Kim JH, Lee S, Kang GH. Panels of immunohistochemical markers help determine primary sites of metastatic adenocarcinoma. Arch Pathol Lab Med. 2007;131(10):1561–7. doi:10.1043/1543-2165(2007)131[1561:POIMHD]2.0.CO;2.

Penn I, First MR. Merkel's cell carcinoma in organ recipients: report of 41 cases. Transplantation. 1999;68(11):1717–21.

Perry MD, Gore M, Seigler HF, Johnston WW. Fine needle aspiration biopsy of metastatic melanoma. A morphologic analysis of 174 cases. Acta Cytol. 1986a;30(4):385–96.

Perry MD, Seigler HF, Johnston WW. Diagnosis of metastatic malignant melanoma by fine needle aspiration biopsy: a clinical and pathologic correlation of 298 cases. J Natl Cancer Inst. 1986b;77(5):1013–21.

Poulsen MG, Rischin D, Porter I, Walpole E, Harvey J, Hamilton C, et al. Does chemotherapy improve survival in high-risk stage I and II Merkel cell carcinoma of the skin? Int J Radiat Oncol Biol Phys. 2006;64(1):114–9. doi:10.1016/j.ijrobp.2005.04.042.

Pulitzer M, Brady MS, Blochin E, Amin B, Teruya-Feldstein J. Anaplastic large cell lymphoma: a potential pitfall in the differential diagnosis of melanoma. Arch Pathol Lab Med. 2013;137(2):280–3. doi:10.5858/arpa.2011-0532-CR.

Pulitzer MP, Amin BD, Busam KJ. Merkel cell carcinoma: review. Adv Anat Pathol. 2009;16(3):135–44. doi:10.1097/PAP.0b013e3181a12f5a.

Ragsdale MI, Lehmer LM, Ragsdale BD, Chow WA, Carson RT. Cutaneous metastasis of osteosarcoma in the scalp. Am J Dermatopathol. 2011;33(6):e70–3. doi:10.1097/DAD.0b013e318214a7ea.

Ramos-Herberth FI, Karamchandani J, Kim J, Dadras SS. SOX10 immunostaining distinguishes desmoplastic melanoma from excision scar. J Cutan Pathol. 2010;37(9):944–52. doi:10.1111/j.1600-0560.2010.01568.x.

Requena L, Santonja C, Stutz N, Kaddu S, Weenig RH, Kutzner H, et al. Pseudolymphomatous cutaneous angiosarcoma: a rare variant of cutaneous angiosarcoma readily mistaken for cutaneous lymphoma. Am J Dermatopathol. 2007;29(4):342–50. doi:10.1097/DAD.0b013e31806f1856.

Richardson SK, Tannous ZS, Mihm Jr MC. Congenital and infantile melanoma: review of the literature and report of an uncommon variant, pigment-synthesizing melanoma. J Am Acad Dermatol. 2002;47(1):77–90.

Riddle ND, Bowers JW, Bui MM, Morgan MB. Primary cutaneous osteoblastic osteosarcoma: a case report and review of the current literature. Clin Exp Dermatol. 2009;34(8):e879–80. doi:10.1111/j.1365 2230.2009.03637.x.

Robins P, Perez MI. Lymphoepithelioma-like carcinoma of the skin treated by Mohs micrographic surgery. J Am Acad Dermatol. 1995;32(5 Pt 1):814–6.

Rocamora A, Badia N, Vives R, Carrillo R, Ulloa J, Ledo A. Epidermotropic primary neuroendocrine (Merkel cell) carcinoma of the skin with Pautrier-like microabscesses. Report of three cases and review of the literature. J Am Acad Dermatol. 1987;16(6):1163–8.

Rodrigues LK, Leong SP, Ljung BM, Sagebiel RW, Burnside N, Hu T, et al. Fine needle aspiration in the diagnosis of metastatic melanoma. J Am Acad Dermatol. 2000;42(5 Pt 1):735–40.

Rosen T. Cutaneous metastases. Med Clin North Am. 1980;64(5):885–900.

Rubinstein JC, Sznol M, Pavlick AC, Ariyan S, Cheng E, Bacchiocchi A, et al. Incidence of the V600K mutation among melanoma patients with BRAF mutations, and potential therapeutic response to the specific BRAF inhibitor PLX4032. J Transl Med. 2010;8:67. doi:10.1186/1479-5876-8-67.

Saad RS, Ghorab Z, Khalifa MA, Xu M. CDX2 as a marker for intestinal differentiation: Its utility and limitations. World J Gastrointest Surg. 2011;3(11):159–66. doi:10.4240/wjgs.v3.i11.159.

Saeed S, Keehn CA, Morgan MB. Cutaneous metastasis: a clinical, pathological, and immunohistochemical appraisal. J Cutan Pathol. 2004;31(6):419–30. doi:10.1111/j.0303-6987.2004.00207.x.

Sahi H, Koljonen V, Kavola H, Haglund C, Tukiainen E, Sihto H, et al. Bcl-2 expression indicates better prognosis of Merkel cell carcinoma regardless of the presence of Merkel cell polyomavirus. Virchows Arch. 2012;461(5):553–9. doi:10.1007/s00428-012-1310-3.

Salamanca J, Dhimes P, Pinedo F, Gomez de la Fuente E, Perez Espejo G, Martinez-Tello FJ. Extraskeletal cutaneous chondroblastic osteosarcoma: a case report. J Cutan Pathol. 2008;35(2):231–5. doi:10.1111/j.1600-0560.2007.00785.x.

Samarendra P, Berkowitz L, Kumari S, Alexis R. Primary nodal neuroendocrine (Merkel cell) tumor in a patient with HIV infection. South Med J. 2000;93(9):920–2.

Sariola H, Terava H, Rapola J, Saarinen UM. Cell-surface ganglioside GD2 in the immunohistochemical detection and differential diagnosis of neuroblastoma. Am J Clin Pathol. 1991;96(2):248–52.

Sariya D, Ruth K, Adams-McDonnell R, Cusack C, Xu X, Elenitsas R, et al. Clinicopathologic correlation of cutaneous metastases: experience from a cancer center. Arch Dermatol. 2007;143(5):613–20. doi:10.1001/archderm.143.5.613.

Scatena C, Massi D, Franchi A, De Paoli A, Canzonieri V. Rhabdomyosarcoma of the skin resembling carcinosarcoma: report of a case and literature review. Am J Dermatopathol. 2012;34(1):e1–6. doi:10.1097/DAD.0b013e31822381fas.

SEER. SEER Stat Fact Sheets: melanoma of the skin. [Internet]: National Cancer Institute; 2012. [Updated Nov 2012]. Available from: http://www.seer.cancer.gov/statfacts/html/melan.html

Setoyama M, Kanda A, Kanzaki T. Cutaneous metastasis of an osteosarcoma. A case report. Am J Dermatopathol. 1996;18(6):629–32.

Setterfield J, Sciot R, Debiec-Rychter M, Robson A, Calonje E. Primary cutaneous epidermotropic alveolar rhabdomyosarcoma with t(2;13) in an elderly woman: case report and review of the literature. Am J Surg Pathol. 2002;26(7):938–44.

Sihto H, Kukko H, Koljonen V, Sankila R, Bohling T, Joensuu H. Clinical factors associated with Merkel cell polyomavirus infection in Merkel cell carcinoma. J Natl Cancer Inst. 2009;101(13):938–45. doi:10.1093/jnci/djp139.

Smith PD, Patterson JW. Merkel cell carcinoma (neuroendocrine carcinoma of the skin). Am J Clin Pathol. 2001;115(Suppl):S68–78.

Strum SB, Park JK, Rappaport H. Observation of cells resembling Sternberg-Reed cells in conditions other than Hodgkin's disease. Cancer. 1970;26(1):176–90.

Suchak R, Thway K, Zelger B, Fisher C, Calonje E. Primary cutaneous epithelioid angiosarcoma: a clinicopathologic study of 13 cases of a rare neoplasm occurring outside the setting of conventional angiosarcomas and with predilection for the limbs. Am J Surg Pathol. 2011;35(1):60–9. doi:10.1097/PAS.0b013e3181fee872.

Swanson SA, Cooper PH, Mills SE, Wick MR. Lymphoepithelioma-like carcinoma of the skin. Mod Pathol. 1988;1(5):359–65.

Tai PT, Yu E, Tonita J, Gilchrist J. Merkel cell carcinoma of the skin. J Cutan Med Surg. 2000a;4(4):186–95.

Tai PT, Yu E, Winquist E, Hammond A, Stitt L, Tonita J, et al. Chemotherapy in neuroendocrine/Merkel cell carcinoma of the skin: case series and review of 204 cases. J Clin Oncol. 2000b;18(12):2493–9.

Tarantola TI, Vallow LA, Halyard MY, Weenig RH, Warschaw KE, Grotz TE, et al. Prognostic factors in Merkel cell carcinoma: analysis of 240 cases. J Am Acad Dermatol. 2013;68(3):425–32. doi:10.1016/j.jaad.2012.09.036.

Terashima T, Kanazawa M. Lung cancer with skin metastasis. Chest. 1994;106(5):1448–50.

Terrier-Lacombe MJ, Guillou L, Chibon F, Gallagher G, Benhattar J, Terrier P, et al. Superficial primitive Ewing's sarcoma: a clinicopathologic and molecular cytogenetic analysis of 14 cases. Mod Pathol. 2009;22(1):87–94. doi:10.1038/modpathol.2008.156.

Tilling T, Moll I. Which are the cells of origin in merkel cell carcinoma? J Skin Cancer. 2012;2012:680410. doi:10.1155/2012/680410.

Tokura Y, Yamanaka K, Wakita H, Kurokawa S, Horiguchi D, Usui A, et al. Halo congenital nevus undergoing spontaneous regression. Involvement of T-cell immunity in involution and presence of circulating anti-nevus cell IgM antibodies. Arch Dermatol. 1994;130(8):1036–41.

van Akkooi AC, Voit CA, Verhoef C, Eggermont AM. New developments in sentinel node staging in melanoma: controversies and alternatives. Curr Opin Oncol. 2010;22(3):169–77. doi:10.1097/CCO.0b013e328337aa78.

Van Nguyen A, Argenyi ZB. Cutaneous neuroblastoma. Peripheral neuroblastoma. Am J Dermatopathol. 1993;15(1):7–14.

Vanchinathan V, Marinelli EC, Kartha RV, Uzieblo A, Ranchod M, Sundram UN. A malignant cutaneous neuroendocrine tumor with features of Merkel cell carcinoma and differentiating neuroblastoma. Am J Dermatopathol. 2009;31(2):193–6. doi:10.1097/DAD.0b013e31819114c4.

Voit C, Mayer T, Proebstle TM, Weber L, Kron M, Krupienski M, et al. Ultrasound-guided fine-needle aspiration cytology in the early detection of melanoma metastases. Cancer. 2000;90(3):186–93.

Wallace ML, Longacre TA, Smoller BR. Estrogen and progesterone receptors and anti-gross cystic disease fluid protein 15 (BRST-2) fail to distinguish metastatic breast carcinoma from eccrine neoplasms. Mod Pathol. 1995;8(9):897–901.

Weed BR, Folpe AL. Cutaneous CD30-positive epithelioid angiosarcoma following breast-conserving therapy and irradiation: a potential diagnostic pitfall. Am J Dermatopathol. 2008;30(4):370–2. doi:10.1097/DAD.0b013e31817330ff.

Weedon D. Weedon's skin pathology. 3rd ed. China: Elsevier; 2010. 1041 p.

Weiss LM, Movahed LA, Butler AE, Swanson SA, Frierson Jr HF, Cooper PH, et al. Analysis of lymphoepithelioma and lymphoepithelioma-like carcinomas for Epstein-Barr viral genomes by in situ hybridization. Am J Surg Pathol. 1989;13(8):625–31.

Wick MR, Swanson PE, LeBoit PE, Strickler JG, Cooper PH. Lymphoepithelioma-like carcinoma of the skin with adnexal differentiation. J Cutan Pathol. 1991;18(2):93–102.

Wick MR. Immunohistochemical approaches to the diagnosis of undifferentiated malignant tumors.

Ann Diagn Pathol. 2008;12(1):72–84. doi:10.1016/j.
anndiagpath.2007.10.003.

Wyatt AJ, Hansen RC. Pediatric skin tumors. Pediatr Clin
North Am. 2000;47(4):937–63.

Ziprin P, Smith S, Salerno G, Rosin RD. Two cases of
merkel cell tumour arising in patients with chronic

lymphocytic leukaemia. Br J Dermatol. 2000;
142(3):525–8.

Zur Hausen A, Rennspiess D, Winnepenninckx V, Speel
EJ, Kurz AK. Early B-cell differentiation in Merkel
cell carcinomas: clues to cellular ancestry. Cancer
Res. 2013. doi:10.1158/0008-5472.CAN-13-0616.

Index

A

Acquired immune deficiency syndrome (AIDS)
    bacillary angiomatosis, 423, 424
    CD4+ cells, 423
    differential diagnosis, 423
    EBV infection, 423
    etiology and epidemiology, 422–423
    herpesviruses and human papillomavirus, 423
    histopathology, 423
    HIV-infected individuals, 423
    Kaposi's sarcoma, 423
    North America and Europe, 403
    oral hairy leukoplakia, 423, 424
    pandemic of, 405
Actinic reticuloid (AR)
    chronic actinic dermatitis, 236
    clinical course, 239
    cytomorphology, 237
    diagnosis, 161, 239–240
    differential diagnosis, 137
    epidemiology, 237
    features, 160
    genetics and molecular findings, 161, 239
    histopathology, 160
    Hodgkin's lymphoma, 237
    immunophenotype, 161–162, 238, 239
    infiltration pattern, 237, 238
    lesions, 237
    and MF, 161
    prognosis and clinical course, 161
    reactive erythroderma, 166–168
Addressins, 26, 32
ALCL. *See* Anaplastic large cell lymphoma (ALCL)
ALK. *See* Anaplastic lymphoma kinase gene (ALK)
ALLP. *See* Atypical lymphocytic lobular panniculitis
        (ALLP)
Alopecia
    chronic
        hepatitis C infection, 480
        rubbing, scalp, 160

cutaneous manifestations, 415
    interferon and ribavirin, 478
    syringolymphoid hyperplasia, 114
Amelanotic melanoma, 540–541
Anaplastic large cell lymphoma (ALCL)
    cALCL, 194, 351, 352, 370, 545, 556
    CD30+ tumor cells, 326, 328
    and LyP, 69–73
    myxoid, 351
    NK-/T-cell lymphoma, 530, 531
    primary (*see* Primary cutaneous ALCL)
    Sézary syndrome (SS), 194
    systemic, 109, 254, 356
Anaplastic lymphoma kinase gene (ALK)
    CD246, 35
    CD30 expression, 69, 182
    cytoplasmic activity, 336, 353–354, 356
    and EMA, 69
    gene rearrangement, 224
    lack of, 356
    nonlymphoid tumors, 551, 568, 576
    nucleophosmin, 353–355
    oncoprotein, 202
    single cutaneous, 69
Angioendotheliomatosis, 521, 530, 533
Angioimmunoblastic T cell lymphoma (AITL)
    description, 302
    features, 303
    follicular T helper cells, 34, 303
    histologic patterns, 302–303
    nodular form, erythematous rash, 18
    non-atypical lymphocytes with eosinophils, 303, 304
    systemic, 303
Angiosarcoma
    clinical features, 572
    electron microscopy, 574
    epidemiology, 571, 572
    immunohistochemistry and diagnosis, 572–574
    molecular/genetics, 574
    prognosis/course, 574

H.D. Cualing et al. (eds.), *Cutaneous Hematopathology*,
DOI 10.1007/978-1-4939-0950-6, © Springer Science+Business Media New York 2014

Printed in the United States of America